Prilocaine

Proprietary name	Manufacturer	Percent local anesthetic	Vasoconstrictor	Duration of analgesia	Author's and manufacturer's MRD (mg)
Citanest Plain	Astra Pharmaceutical	4	—	Pulpal: 10 min infiltration; 60 min block Soft tissue: 1½ to 2 hr infiltration; 2 to 4 hr block	6/kg 2.7/lb Absolute max: 400
Citanest Forte	Astra Pharmaceutical	4	Epinephrine 1:200,000	Pulpal: 60 to 90 min Soft tissue: 3 to 8 hr	6/kg 2.7/lb Absolute max: 400

MRD, Maximum recommended dose.

Articaine

Proprietary name	Manufacturer	Percent local anesthetic	Vasoconstrictor	Duration of analgesia	Author's and manufacturer's MRD (mg)
Septanest N Ultracaine D-S	Septodont Hoechst Labs	4	Epinephrine 1:200,000	Pulpal: 45 to 60 min Soft tissue: 2 to 5 hr	Adult: 7/kg, 3.2/lb Absolute max: 500 Children: 5/kg, 2.3/lb
Septanest SP Ultracaine D-S Forte	Septodont Hoechst Labs	4	Epinephrine 1:100,000	Pulpal: 60 to 75 min Soft tissue: 3 to 6 hr	Adult: 7/kg, 3.2/lb Absolute max: 500 Children: 5/kg, 2.3/lb

MRD, Maximum recommended dose.

Bupivacaine

Proprietary name	Manufacturer	Percent local anesthetic	Vasoconstrictor	Duration of analgesia	Author's and manufacturer's MRD (mg)
Marcaine HCl	Cook-Waite Labs	0.5	Epinephrine 1:200,000	Pulpal: 90 to 180 min Soft tissue: 4 to 9 hr, up to 12 hr reported	1.3/kg 0.6/lb Absolute max: 90

MRD, Maximum recommended dose.

Etidocaine

Proprietary name	Manufacturer	Percent local anesthetic	Vasoconstrictor	Duration of analgesia	Author's and manufacturer's MRD (mg)
Duranest	Astra Pharmaceutical	1.5	Epinephrine 1:200,000	Pulpal: 90 to 180 min average Soft tissue: 4 to 9 hr average	8/kg 3.6/lb Absolute max: 400

MRD, Maximum recommended dose.

HANDBOOK OF
LOCAL ANESTHESIA

HANDBOOK OF LOCAL ANESTHESIA

FOURTH EDITION

STANLEY F. MALAMED, D.D.S.

Professor and Chair, Section of Anesthesia and Medicine
University of Southern California School of Dentistry
Los Angeles, California

Original drawings by
Susan B. Clifford, R.D.H., Ed.D.

with 346 illustrations

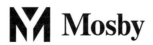

St. Louis Baltimore Boston Carlsbad Chicago Naples New York Philadelphia Portland
London Madrid Mexico City Singapore Sydney Tokyo Toronto Wiesbaden

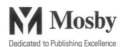

Mosby
Dedicated to Publishing Excellence

A Times Mirror
Company

Vice President and Publisher: Don Ladig
Editor: Linda L. Duncan
Developmental Editor: Melba Steube
Project Manager: Linda Clarke
Associate Production Editor: Kathleen E. Hillock
Composition Specialists: Christine H. Poullain and Pamela Merritt
Designer: Carolyn O'Brien
Cover Design: Nancy McDonald
Manufacturing Manager: William A. Winneberger, Jr.

FOURTH EDITION

Printed in the United States of America
Composition by Mosby Electronic Production, Philadelphia
Lithography by Graphic World, Inc.
Printing/binding by Von Hoffman Press

Mosby-Year Book, Inc.
11830 Westline Industrial Drive
St. Louis, Missouri 63146

Library of Congress Cataloging in Publication Data
Malamed, Stanley F.
    Handbook of local anesthesia / Stanley F. Malamed ; original
drawings by Susan B. Clifford. — 4th ed.
        p.   cm.
    Includes bibliographical references and index.
    ISBN 0-8151-6423-8
    1. Anesthesia in dentistry. 2. Local anesthesia.   I. Title
    [DNLM: 1. Anesthesia, Dental. 2. Anesthesia, Local.
    3. Anesthetics, Local—pharmacology.   WO 460 M236h 1997]
    RK510.M33   1997
    617.9'676—dc20
DNLM/DLC
for Library of Congress   96-22999
                                                            CIP

97 98 99 00 01 / 9 8 7 6 5 4 3 2 1

To Beverly, Heather, Jennifer, and Jeremy

FOREWORD

Stanley Malamed has focused his considerable knowledge and energies here to develop an up-to-date *Handbook of Local Anesthesia.* Local anesthesia, a widely used method of pain control in dentistry, continues to be accepted by most practitioners with matter-of-factness; this is not only a testament to its safety and efficacy but also an indication of our complacency and reluctance to look for even more effective and safer materials and techniques.

This handbook carefully explores and teaches methods that enhance good local anesthesia practices while alerting the reader to specific hazards and errors that may produce both minor and major complications. Advances in all aspects of the science and technology of anesthesia have been notable, and the busy practitioner will benefit from a close reading of this handbook. It will also become more evident that local anesthetics require patient preparation to achieve optimal effects. The atraumatic injection deserves and receives special consideration in Dr. Malamed's book. Appropriate psychological and pharmacological preparations that accompany local anesthesia administration help achieve maximal effectiveness and avoid frustration for both the dentist and the patient.

Modern acceptance of dental treatment can be credited, in large measure, to the freedom from pain that local anesthesia offers. As "Novocain" became a household word, dentistry grew away from its painful image and became an important health and esthetic service. Advances in all phases of local anesthetic practice constitute continuing progress. Materials, methods, and techniques have undergone pronounced changes and warrant our renewed attention.

Norman Trieger D.M.D., M.D.

PREFACE

Publication of this fourth edition of the *Handbook of Local Anesthesia* comes at a time of considerably heightened interest in the field of anesthesiology in dentistry. Interest among students, both those still in dental school and those practicing dentistry, is intense. Attendance at continuing education seminars on this subject has increased sharply over the past 5 years. Why has this occurred?

Local anesthesia is, arguably, *the* technique that has allowed dentistry to become what it is today—enabling dentistry to be transformed from a mere trade to a highly regarded profession. Preventing pain associated with dental care is the goal of all who practice in this profession, as well as the strong desire of all of our patients. Yet despite the usual ease with which pain control can be obtained, the occasional problem does intrude. Problems include the inability to anesthetize certain patients or certain teeth, a patient's inherent fear of receiving "shots" of local anesthetic drugs, and those local and systemic complications that are associated with the administration of intraoral local anesthetics. Many reasons exist for these problems, including biological variation in response to drugs, anatomical differences among patients, and, significant in relation to intraoral local anesthetic administration, fear and anxiety.

The importance of clinically adequate pain control during dental treatment is highlighted by the fact that it is not possible to safely complete treatment in the absence of pain control. Most, if not all, practicing dentists have faced the vexing problem of the inability to provide complete anesthesia to a patient. Though this can occur anywhere in the oral cavity, it is almost a given that this problem occurs most often in mandibular molars. In the absence of complete anesthesia, it is oftentimes not possible to complete the planned dental procedure. Additionally, and of even greater importance, treatment in the absence of adequate pain control is responsible for the development of a significant number of the medical emergencies that occur in dental practice. Matsuura demonstrates that of 22% of emergencies developing during dental treatment, 67% occur either during the extraction of a tooth or during pulpal extir-pation—two procedures where achieving profound pulpal anesthesia is, on occasion, difficult.[1] Additionally, 54.9% of *all* of the emergencies reported in Matsuura's study develop either during the injection or within the first 5 minutes after local anesthetic administration. The vast majority of these emergencies are related to the stress of receiving the injection (psychogenically induced emergencies) or to the uptake of the drug into the cardiovascular system of the patient.

Another reason for the increase in interest in the field of dental pain control is the continual introduction of new techniques, devices, and drugs. It is the expectation of their designers that these innovations represent an improvement on the drugs or devices that preceded them: a drug that when infiltrated on the maxillary buccal surface will diffuse palatally, providing palatal anesthesia without the need for a palatal injection; devices that can help to make the administration of local anesthetics on the palate (or elsewhere) absolutely atraumatic; techniques that will do away with the need for local anesthesia entirely! Try though we might, and as close as we may come in some cases, a panacea for pain control in dentistry has yet to be developed. New drugs, devices, and techniques are discussed in Chapter 19. Yet some new devices seem destined to succeed. One example, in my opinion, is the so-called "safety" syringe. Needle-stick injury with a contaminated needle is a significant fear of health professionals. Syringe/needle devices with which it is virtually impossible to stick oneself or an auxiliary appear to have a place in the pain control armamentarium in dentistry. Several such devices, which have recently been introduced, are discussed in Chapter 5.

Techniques for intraoral anesthesia, especially in the mandible, have evolved to the point where today a dentist has available six techniques for pain control. These include the traditional inferior alveolar nerve block (NB), the mental/incisive NB, the Gow-Gates mandibular NB, the Vazirani-Akinosi mandibular NB, the periodontal ligament (PDL) injection, and intraosseous anesthesia. Many of these techniques did not exist, or were not used, by most dentists as recently as 20 years ago. Today an increasing number of dentists have many or all of these techniques available for clinical use, thereby diminishing the number of patients in whom it is difficult or impossible to achieve profound mandibular pulpal anesthesia.

Despite all of the efforts at improving local anesthesia in dentistry, "the more things change, the more they stay the same." In this fourth edition of the *Handbook of Local Anesthesia,* those basic concepts that are essential to the safe and effective practice of local anesthesia in dentistry, well known and well established for more than 40 years, continue to be emphasized. Without knowledge and understanding of these concepts, the field of local anesthesia and pain control in dentistry is fraught with peril, and the likelihood of therapeutic misadventure is greatly increased.

So this fourth edition contains both the "golden oldies" and the best of the exciting innovations and techniques that promise to make dental pain control both more effective and safer.

As always, there are a number of people whom I must acknowledge, for without their assistance, which took many and varied forms, publication of this fourth edition of the *Handbook of Local Anesthesia* would not have been possible. I must start with the models, Drs. Gabriel Aslanian, Kenneth Leopold, and Greg Trnavsky, who sat and endured many hours of hot lights and needle sticks to provide the new photographs included in this edition. Thanks, too, to several of the manufacturers of local anesthetic drugs and devices in North America: Astra Pharmaceutical Products, Beutlich, Kodak, Hoechst Pharmaceuticals, Novocol, Safety Syringes, and Septodont, for their assistance in preparing the chapters on local anesthetic drugs and armamentarium. I also wish to thank Melba Steube from Mosby–Year Book, who has had the task of dealing with an oftentimes lazy, frequently hard-to-reach, author. Her perseverance has paid off with this fine fourth edition.

Finally, I wish to thank the many, many members of my profession of dentistry, who have provided me with written and verbal input regarding prior editions of this textbook. A good many of their suggestions for additions, deletions, and corrections have been incorporated into this new text. Thank you all!

Stanley F. Malamed

REFERENCE

1. Matsuura H: Analysis of systemic complications and deaths during dental treatment in Japan, *Anesthesia Prog* 36(4-5):223-225, 1989.

The treatment modalities and the indications and doses of all drugs in *Handbook of Local Anesthesia* have been recommended in the medical literature. Unless specifically indicated, drug doses are those recommended for adult patients.

The package insert for each drug should be consulted for use and doses as approved by the FDA. Because standards of usage change, it is advisable to keep abreast of revised recommendations, particularly those concerning new drugs

CONTENTS

HANDBOOK OF
LOCAL ANESTHESIA

in this part

The drugs

In the first section of this book the pharmacological and clinical properties of the classes of drugs known as local anesthetics (Chapter 2) and vasoconstrictors (Chapter 3) are discussed. Knowledge of the pharmacological and clinical properties of these drugs, by all persons permitted to administer them, is absolutely essential for their safe use and for a better understanding of those potentially life-threatening systemic reactions associated with their administration. Emphasis is placed on those local anesthetic drug combinations currently used in anesthesia in dentistry (Chapter 4).

Chapter 1 provides background for an understanding of how local anesthetics work to block nerve conduction and thus prevent pain from being experienced. The anatomy and physiology of normal neurons and nerve conduction are reviewed as a background for the discussion, which, in subsequent chapters, takes up the pharmacology and clinical actions of various specific agents.

one

Neurophysiology

DESIRABLE PROPERTIES OF LOCAL ANESTHETICS

Local anesthesia has been defined as a loss of sensation in a circumscribed area of the body caused by a depression of excitation in nerve endings or an inhibition of the conduction process in peripheral nerves.[1] An important feature of local anesthesia is that it produces this loss of sensation without inducing a loss of consciousness. In this one major area local anesthesia differs dramatically from general anesthesia.

There are many methods of inducing local anesthesia, some of which follow:

1. Mechanical trauma
2. Low temperature
3. Anoxia
4. Chemical irritants
5. Neurolytic agents such as alcohol and phenol
6. Chemical agents such as local anesthetics

However, only those methods or substances that induce a *transient* and *completely reversible* state of anesthesia are used in clinical practice. The following are those properties deemed most desirable for a local anesthetic:

1. It should not be irritating to the tissue to which it is applied.
2. It should not cause any permanent alteration of nerve structure.
3. Its systemic toxicity should be low.
4. It must be effective regardless of whether it is injected into the tissue or applied locally to mucous membranes.
5. The time of onset of anesthesia should be as short as possible.
6. The duration of action must be long enough to permit completion of the procedure yet not so long as to require an extended recovery.

Most local anesthetics discussed in this section meet the first two criteria: they are (relatively) *nonirritating* to tissues and *completely reversible*. Of paramount importance is *systemic toxicity*, since all injectable and most topical local anesthetics are eventually absorbed from their site of administration into the cardiovascular system. Therefore the potential toxicity of a drug is an important factor in its selection for use as a local anesthetic. Toxicity varies greatly among the local anesthetics currently in use. Toxicity is discussed more thoroughly in Chapter 2. Although it is a desirable characteristic, not all local anesthetics in clinical use today meet the criterion of being effective *regardless of whether the drug is injected or applied topically*. Several of the more potent injectable local anesthetics (procaine, mepivacaine) prove to be relatively ineffective when applied topically to mucous membrane. To be effective as topical anesthetics, these drugs must be applied in concentrations that prove to be locally irritating to tissues and increase the risk of systemic toxicity. Dyclonine, a potent topical anesthetic, is not administered by injection because of its tissue-irritating properties. Lidocaine and tetracaine, on the other hand, are both effective anesthetics when administered by injection or topical application in clinically acceptable concentrations. The last factors, *rapid onset of action* and *adequate duration of clinical action*, are met quite satisfactorily by most of the clinically effective local anesthetics in use today. Clinical duration of action does vary considerably among drugs and also among different preparations of the same drug. The duration of anesthesia required to complete a procedure will be a major consideration in the selection of a local anesthetic.

In addition to these qualities, Bennett[2] lists other desirable properties of an ideal local anesthetic:

7. It should have a potency sufficient to give complete anesthesia without the use of harmful concentrated solutions.
8. It should be relatively free from producing allergic reactions.
9. It should be stable in solution and readily undergo biotransformation in the body.
10. It should either be sterile or be capable of being sterilized by heat without deterioration.

The local anesthetics in use today, although they do not satisfy all of these criteria, do meet the majority of them. Research is continuing in an effort to produce newer drugs that possess a maximum of desirable factors and a minimum of negative ones.

FUNDAMENTALS OF IMPULSE GENERATION AND TRANSMISSION

The discovery in the late 1800s of a group of chemicals with the ability to prevent pain without inducing a loss of consciousness was one of the major steps in the advancement of the medical and dental professions. Medical and dental procedures could, for the first time, be carried out easily and in the absence of pain, a fact that is virtually taken for granted by contemporary medical and dental professionals and their patients.

The concept behind the actions of local anesthetics is simple: they prevent both the generation and the conduction of a nerve impulse. In effect, local anesthetics set up a chemical roadblock between the source of the impulse (e.g., the scalpel incision in soft tissues) and the brain. The aborted impulse, prevented from reaching the brain, is not, therefore, interpreted as pain by the patient.

How, in fact, do local anesthetics, the most commonly used drugs in dentistry, function to abolish or prevent pain? The following is a discussion of current theories seeking to explain the mode of action of local anesthetic drugs. To understand the mode of action of local anesthetics better, however, the reader must have an acquaintance with the fundamentals of nerve conduction; thus a review of the relevant characteristics and properties of nerve anatomy and physiology follows.

The Neuron

The neuron or nerve cell is the structural unit of the nervous system. It is able to transmit messages between the central nervous system (CNS) and all parts of the body. There are two basic types of neuron: the sensory (afferent) and the motor (efferent). The basic structure of these two neuronal types differs significantly (Fig. 1-1).

Sensory neurons that are capable of transmitting the sensation of pain consist of three major portions.[3] The *dendritic zone*, which is composed of an arborization of free nerve endings, is the most distal segment of the sensory neuron. These free nerve endings respond to stimulation produced in the tissues in which they lie, provoking an impulse that is transmitted centrally along the *axon*. The axon is a thin cablelike structure that may be quite long (the giant squid axon has been measured at 100 to 200 cm). At its mesial (or central) end there is an arborization similar to that seen in the dendritic zone. However, in this case the arborizations form synapses with various nuclei in the CNS to distribute incoming (sensory) impulses to their appropriate sites within the CNS for interpretation. The *cell body*, or soma, is the third part of the neuron. In the sensory neuron described here, the cell body is located at a distance from the axon, or the main pathway of impulse transmission in this

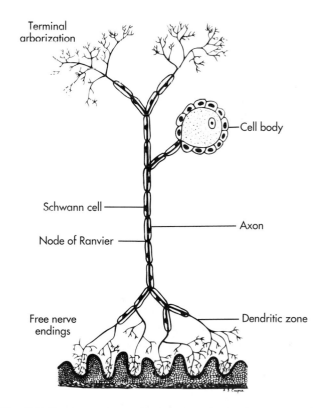

Fig. 1-1 Sensory neuron innervating the oral mucosa. The relative length of the axon in this diagram is foreshortened by a factor of 5000. *(From Jastak JT, Yagiela JA: Regional anesthesia of the oral cavity, St Louis, 1981, Mosby–Year Book.)*

Terminal arborization

Cell body

Schwann cell

Axon

Node of Ranvier

Free nerve endings

Dendritic zone

nerve. The cell body of the sensory nerve is therefore not involved in the process of impulse transmission, its primary function being to provide the vital metabolic support for the entire neuron.

Nerve cells that conduct impulses from the CNS peripherally are termed *motor neurons* and are structurally different from the sensory neurons just described in that their cell body is interposed between the axon and the dendrites. In motor neurons the cell body not only is an integral component of the impulse transmission system but also provides metabolic support for the cell.

The Axon

The single nerve fiber—the axon—is a long cylinder of neural cytoplasm (axoplasm) encased in a thin sheath— the nerve membrane, or axolemma. Nerve cells have a cell body and a nucleus, as do all other cells; however, nerve cells differ from other cells in that nerve cells have an axonal process from which the cell body may be a considerable distance. The axoplasm, a gelatinous substance, is separated from extracellular fluids by a continuous nerve membrane. In some nerves this membrane is itself covered by an insulating lipid-rich layer of myelin.

Current thinking holds that sensory nerve excitability and conduction are both attributable to changes developing within the *nerve membrane*. The cell body and the axoplasm are not essential for nerve conduction. They are important, however: the metabolic support of the membrane is probably derived from the axoplasm.

The nerve (cell) membrane itself is approximately 70 to 80 Å thick. (An angstrom unit is 1/10,000 of a micrometer.) Figure 1-2 represents a currently acceptable configuration. All biologic membranes are organized to (1) block the diffusion of water-soluble molecules; (2) be selectively permeable to certain molecules via specialized pores or channels; and (3) transduce information by protein receptors responsive to chemical or physical stimulation by neurotransmitters or hormones (chemical) or light, vibrations, or pressure (physical).[4] The membrane is described as a flexible nonstretchable structure consisting of two layers of lipid molecules (bilipid layer of phospholipids) and associated proteins, lipids, and carbohydrates. The lipids are oriented with their hydrophilic (polar) ends facing the outer surface and the hydrophobic (nonpolar) ends projecting to the middle of the membrane (Fig. 1-2, *A*). Proteins are visualized as the primary organizational elements of membranes (Fig. 1-2, *B*).[5] Proteins are classified as *transport proteins* (channels, carriers, or pumps) and *receptor sites*. Channel proteins are thought to be continuous pores through the membrane, allowing some ions (Na$^+$, K$^+$, Ca^{++}) to flow passively, whereas other channels are "gated," permitting ion flow only when the gate is "open."[4] The nerve membrane lies at the interface between the extracellular fluid and axoplasm. It separates highly diverse ionic concentrations within the axon from those outside. The *resting nerve membrane* has an electrical resistance about 50 times greater than that of the intracellular and extracellular fluids, thus preventing the passage of sodium, potassium, and chloride ions down their concentration gradients. When a nerve impulse passes, however, electrical conductivity of the nerve membrane increases approximately a hundredfold. This increase in conductivity permits the passage of sodium and potassium ions along their concentration gradients through the nerve membrane. It is the movement of these ions that provides the immediate source of energy for impulse conduction along the nerve.

Some nerve fibers are covered by an insulating lipid layer of myelin. In vertebrates, myelinated nerve fibers include all but the smallest of axons (Table 1-1).[6] Myelinated nerve fibers (Fig. 1-3) are enclosed in spirally wrapped layers of lipoprotein myelin sheaths, which are actually a specialized form of Schwann cell. Although primarily (75%) lipid, the myelin sheath also contains some protein (20%) and carbohydrate (5%).[7] Each myelinated nerve fiber is enclosed in its own myelin sheath. The outermost layer of myelin consists of the Schwann cell cytoplasm and its nucleus. There are constrictions located at regular intervals (approximately every 0.5 to 3 mm)

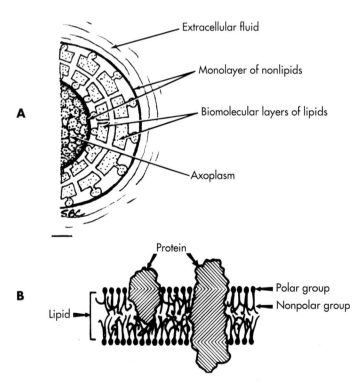

A

B

Fig. 1-2 A, Configuration of a biological membrane. **B,** Heterogeneous lipoprotein membrane as suggested by Singer and Nicolson.[5] *(From Covino BG, Vassalo HG: Local anesthetics: mechanisms of action and clinical use, New York, 1976, Grune & Stratton. Used by permission.)*

TABLE 1-1 Classification and Characteristics of Peripheral Nerve Fibers

Characteristic	Classification					
	A-alpha	A-beta	A-gamma	A-delta	B	C
Myelin	+++	++	++	++	+	−
Diameter (μm)	12 to 20	5 to 12	5 to 12	1 to 4	1 to 3	0.5 to 1
Conduction velocity (m/sec)	70 to 120	30 to 70	30 to 70	12 to 30	14.8	1.2
Onset time	6	5	4	3	1	2
Function	Motor, muscle proprioception	Touch, pressure proprioception	Touch, motor proprioception	Pain, temperature, pressure proprioception	Preganglionic autonomic (sympathetic) activity	Pain, temperature, itch, pressure, postganglionic sympathetic activity

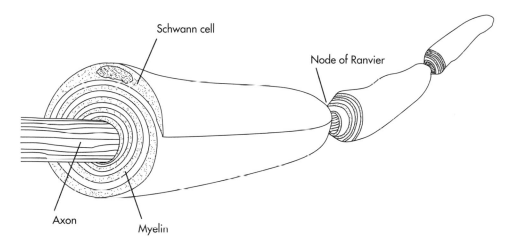

Fig. 1-3 Structure of a myelinated nerve fiber. *(From de Jong RH:* Local anesthetics, *St Louis, 1994, Mosby–Year Book.)*

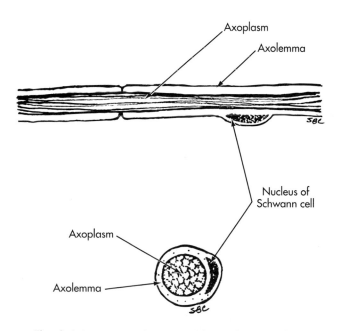

Fig. 1-4 Structure of an unmyelinated nerve fiber.

along the myelinated nerve fiber. These are *nodes of Ranvier*, and they form a gap between two adjoining Schwann cells and their myelin spirals.[8] At these nodes the nerve membrane is exposed directly to the extracellular medium.

Unmyelinated nerve fibers (Fig. 1-4) are also surrounded by a Schwann cell sheath. Groups of unmyelinated nerve fibers share the same sheath. The insulating properties of the myelin sheath enable a myelinated nerve to conduct impulses at a much faster rate than an unmyelinated nerve of equal size can.

Physiology of the Peripheral Nerves

The function of a nerve is to carry messages from one part of the body to another. These messages, in the form of electrical action potentials, are called *impulses*. Action potentials are transient membrane depolarizations that result from a brief increase in the permeability of the membrane to sodium, and usually also from a delayed increase in the permeability to potassium.[9] Impulses are

6   PART ONE   The Drugs

initiated by chemical, thermal, mechanical, or electrical stimuli.

Once an impulse is initiated by a stimulus in any particular nerve fiber, the amplitude and shape of that impulse remain constant, regardless of changes in the quality of the stimulus or its strength. The impulse remains constant without losing strength as it passes along the nerve because the energy used for its propagation is derived from energy that is released by the nerve fiber along its length and not solely from the initial stimulus. de Jong has described impulse conduction as being like the active progress of a spark along a fuse of gunpowder.[10] Once lit, the fuse burns steadily along its length, one burning segment providing the energy required to ignite its neighbor. Such is the situation with impulse propagation along a nerve.

Electrophysiology of Nerve Conduction

The following is a description of electrical events that occur within a nerve during the conduction of an impulse. Subsequent sections describe the precise mechanisms for each of these steps:

Step 1   A nerve possesses a resting potential (Fig. 1-5, *Step 1*). This is a negative electrical potential of −70 mV that exists across the nerve membrane, produced by differing concentrations of ions on either side of the membrane (Table 1-2). The interior of the nerve is negative in relation to the exterior.

Step 2   A stimulus *excites* the nerve, leading to the following sequence of events:

a. An initial phase of *slow depolarization*. The electrical potential within the nerve becomes slightly less negative (Fig. 1-5, *Step 2, A*).
b. When the falling electrical potential reaches a critical level, an extremely rapid phase of depolarization results. This is termed *threshold potential*, or *firing threshold* (Fig. 1-5, *Step 2, B*).
c. This phase of *rapid depolarization* results in a reversal of the electrical potential across the nerve membrane (Fig. 1-5, *Step 2, C*). The interior of the nerve is now electrically positive in relation to the exterior. An electrical potential of +40 mV exists on the interior of the nerve cell.[11]

Step 3   Following these steps of depolarization, *repolarization* occurs (Fig. 1-5, *Step 3*). The electrical potential gradually becomes more negative inside the nerve cell relative to outside until the original resting potential of −70 mV is again achieved.

The entire process (Steps 2 and 3) requires 1 millisecond (msec); depolarization (Step 2) takes 0.3 msec; repolarization (Step 3) takes 0.7 msec.

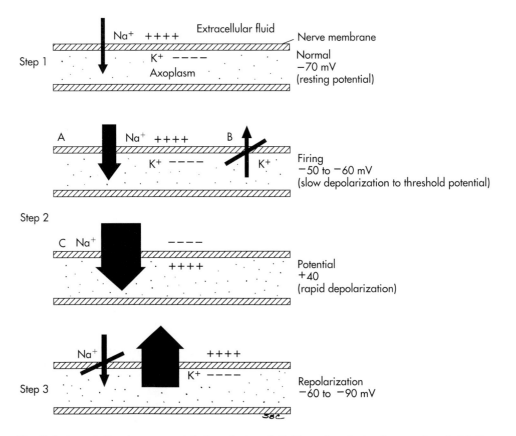

Fig. 1-5 *Step 1,* Resting potential. *Step 2, A* and *B,* Slow depolarization to threshold. *Step 2, C,* Rapid depolarization. *Step 3,* Repolarization.

Electrochemistry of Nerve Conduction

The preceding sequence of events depends on two important factors: (1) the concentrations of electrolytes in the axoplasm (interior of the nerve cell) and extracellular fluids and (2) the permeability of the nerve membrane to sodium and potassium ions.

Table 1-2 shows the differing concentrations of ions found within nerve cells and in the extracellular fluids. Significant differences exist for ions between their intracellular and extracellular concentrations. These ionic gradients differ because the nerve membrane exhibits *selective permeability.*

Resting State

In its resting state the nerve membrane is

- Slightly permeable to sodium ions (Na^+)
- Freely permeable to potassium ions (K^+)
- Freely permeable to chloride ions (Cl^-)

Potassium remains *within* the axoplasm, despite its ability to diffuse freely through the nerve membrane and despite its concentration gradient (passive diffusion usually occurs from a region of greater concentration to one of lesser concentration), because the negative charge of the nerve membrane restrains the positively charged ions by electrostatic attraction.

Chloride remains *outside* the nerve membrane instead of moving along its concentration gradient into the nerve cell because the opposing, nearly equal, electrostatic influence (electrostatic gradient from inside to outside) forces outward migration. The net result is no diffusion of chloride through the membrane.

Sodium migrates *inwardly* because both the concentration (greater outside) and the electrostatic gradient (positive ion attracted by negative intracellular potential) favor such migration. Only the fact that the resting nerve membrane is relatively impermeable to sodium prevents a massive influx of this ion.

Membrane Excitation

Depolarization   Excitation of a nerve segment leads to an increase in permeability of the cell membrane to sodium ions. This is accomplished by a transient widening of transmembrane ion channels sufficient to permit the unhindered passage of hydrated sodium ions (p. 8). The rapid influx of sodium ions to the interior of the nerve cell causes a depolarization of the nerve membrane from its resting level to its firing threshold of approximately −50 to −60 mV (Fig. 1-5, *Step 2, A* and *B*).[12] The firing threshold is actually the *magnitude of the decrease in negative transmembrane potential that is required to initiate an action potential (impulse).*

A decrease in negative transmembrane potential of 15 mV (i.e., from −70 to −55) is required to reach the firing threshold; a voltage difference of less than 15 mV will not initiate an impulse. In a normal nerve the firing threshold remains constant. Exposure of the nerve to a local anesthetic *raises* its firing threshold. Elevating the firing threshold means that more sodium must pass through the membrane to decrease the negative transmembrane potential to a level where depolarization will occur.

When firing threshold is reached, permeability of the membrane to sodium increases dramatically, and sodium ions rapidly enter the axoplasm. At the end of depolarization (the peak of the action potential), the electrical potential of the nerve is actually reversed; an electrical potential of +40 mV exists (Fig. 1-5, *Step 2, C*). The entire depolarization process requires approximately 0.3 msec.

Repolarization   The action potential is terminated when the membrane repolarizes. This is caused by the extinction ("inactivation") of increased permeability to sodium. In many cells permeability to potassium also increases, resulting in the efflux of K^+, leading to a more rapid membrane repolarization and return to its resting potential (Fig. 1-5, *Step 3*).

The movement of sodium ions into the cell during depolarization and the subsequent movement of potassium ions out of the cell during repolarization are passive (not requiring the expenditure of energy), since each ion moves along its concentration gradient. Following the return of the membrane potential to its original level (−70 mV), a slight excess of sodium exists within the nerve cell, and a slight excess of potassium exists extracellularly. A period of metabolic activity then begins.

Active transfer of sodium ions out of the cell occurs via the "sodium pump." An expenditure of energy is needed to move sodium ions *out* of the nerve cell against their concentration gradient, this energy coming from the oxidative metabolism of adenosine triphosphate (ATP). The same pumping mechanism is thought to be responsible for the active transport of potassium ions *into* the cell against their concentration gradient. The entire process of repolarization requires 0.7 msec.

T A B L E 1 - 2 Intracellular and Extracellular Ionic Concentrations			
Ion	Intracellular (mEq/L)	Extracellular (mEq/L)	Ratio (approximate)
Potassium (K^+)	110 to 170	3 to 5	27:1
Sodium (Na^+)	5 to 10	140	1:14
Chloride (Cl^-)	5 to 10	110	1:11

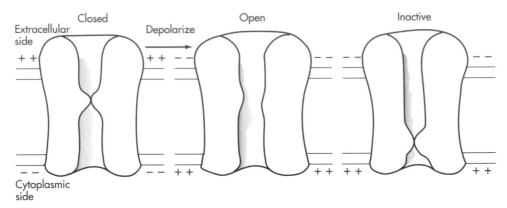

Fig. 1-6 Sodium channel transition stages. Depolarization reverses resting membrane potential from interior negative *(left)* to interior positive *(center)*. The channel proteins undergo corresponding conformational changes from resting state (closed) to ion-conducting state (open). State changes continue from open *(center)* to inactive *(right)*, where channel configuration assumes a different—but still impermeable—state. With repolarization the inactivated refractory channel reverts to the initial resting configuration *(left)*, ready for the next sequence. *(From Siegelbaum SA, Koester F:* Ion channels. *In Kandel ER, editor:* Principles of neural science, *ed 3, Norwalk, Conn, 1991, Appleton-Lange.)*

Immediately after a stimulus has initiated an action potential, a nerve is unable, for a time, to respond to another stimulus, regardless of its strength. This is termed the *absolute refractory period*, and it lasts for about the duration of the main part of the action potential. The absolute refractory period is followed by a *relative refractory period*, during which a new impulse can be initiated but only by a stronger than normal stimulus. The relative refractory period continues to decrease until the normal level of excitability returns, at which point the nerve is said to be repolarized.

During depolarization the major proportion of ionic sodium channels are found in their "open" (O) state (thus permitting the rapid influx of Na$^+$). This is followed by a slower decline into a state of "inactivation" (I) of the channels to a nonconducting state. Inactivation temporarily converts the channels to a state from which they cannot open in response to depolarization (absolute refractory period). This inactivated state is slowly converted back, so the majority of channels are found in their closed (C) resting form when the membrane is repolarized (−70 mV). Upon depolarization the channels change configuration, first to an open ion-conducting (O) state and then to an inactive nonconducting (I) state. Although both C and I states correspond to nonconducting channels, they differ in that depolarization can recruit channels to the conducting O state from C but not from I. Figure 1-6 describes the sodium channel transition stages.[13]

Membrane Channels

Discrete aqueous pores through the excitable nerve membrane, called sodium (or ion) channels, are molecular structures that mediate its sodium permeability. A channel seems to be a lipoglycoprotein firmly situated in the membrane (Fig. 1-2). It consists of an aqueous pore spanning the membrane that is narrow enough at least at one point to discriminate between sodium and other ions (Na$^+$ passes through 12 times more easily than K$^+$). The channel also includes a portion that changes configuration in response to changes in membrane potential, thereby gating the passage of ions through the pore (C, O, I states described above). The presence of these channels helps explain membrane permeability or impermeability to certain ions. Sodium channels have an internal diameter of approximately 0.3×0.5 nm.[14]

A sodium ion is "thinner" than either a potassium or a chloride ion and should therefore diffuse freely down its concentration gradient through membrane channels into the nerve cell. This does not occur, however, because all these ions attract water molecules and thus become hydrated. Hydrated sodium ions have a radius of 3.4 Å, which is approximately 50% greater than the 2.2 Å radius of potassium and chloride ions. Sodium ions are therefore too large to pass through the narrow channels when a nerve is at rest (Fig. 1-7). Potassium and chloride ions can pass through these channels. During *depolarization*, sodium ions readily pass through the nerve membrane because configurational changes that develop within the membrane produce a transient widening of these transmembrane channels to a size adequate to allow the unhindered passage of sodium ions down their concentration gradient into the axoplasm (transformation from the C to the O configuration). This concept can be visualized as the opening of a gate during depolarization that

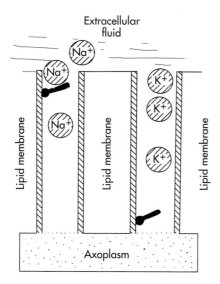

Fig. 1-7 Membrane channels are partially occluded; the nerve is at rest. Hydrated sodium ions *(Na+)* are too large to pass through channels, although potassium ions *(K+)* can pass through unimpeded.

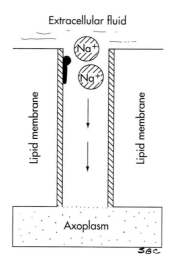

Fig. 1-8 Membrane channels are open; depolarization occurs. Hydrated sodium ions *(Na+)* now pass unimpeded through the sodium channel.

is partially occluding the channel in the resting membrane (C) (Fig. 1-8).

Recent evidence indicates that *channel specificity exists,* in that sodium channels differ from potassium channels.[15] The gates on the sodium channel are located near the external surface of the nerve membrane, whereas those on the potassium channel are located near the internal surface of the nerve membrane.

Impulse Propagation

Following the initiation of an action potential by a stimulus, the impulse must move along the surface of the axon. Energy for impulse propagation is derived from the nerve membrane in the following manner.

The stimulus disrupts the resting equilibrium of the nerve membrane; the transmembrane potential is reversed momentarily—the interior of the cell changing from negative to positive, the exterior changing from positive to negative. This new electrical equilibrium in this segment of nerve produces local currents that begin flowing between the depolarized segment and the adjacent resting area. These local currents flow from positive to negative, extending for several millimeters along the nerve membrane.

As a result of this current flow, the interior of the adjacent area becomes less negative and its exterior less positive. Transmembrane potential decreases, approaching firing threshold for depolarization. When transmembrane potential is decreased by 15 mV from resting potential, firing threshold is reached and complete depolarization occurs. The newly depolarized segment sets up local cur-

rents in adjacent resting membrane, and the entire process starts anew.

Conditions in the segment that has just depolarized return to normal following the absolute and relative refractory periods. Because of this the wave of depolarization can spread in only one direction. Backward (retrograde) movement is prevented by the unexcitable, refractory segment.

Impulse Spread

The propagated impulse travels along the nerve membrane toward the CNS. The spread of this impulse differs depending on whether or not a nerve is myelinated.

Unmyelinated Nerves

An unmyelinated nerve fiber is basically a long cylinder with a high–electrical resistance cell membrane surrounding a low-resistance conducting core of axoplasm, all of which is bathed in low-resistance extracellular fluid.

The high-resistance cell membrane and low-resistance intracellular and extracellular media produce a rapid decrease in the density of current within a short distance of the depolarized segment. In areas immediately adjacent to this depolarized segment, local current flow may be adequate to initiate depolarization in the resting membrane. Farther away it will prove to be inadequate to achieve firing threshold.

The spread of an impulse in an unmyelinated nerve fiber is therefore characterized as a relatively slow forward-creeping process (Fig. 1-9). Conduction rate in unmyelinated C fibers is 1.2 m/sec compared with 14.8 to 120 m/sec in myelinated A-alpha and A-delta fibers.[16]

Impulse

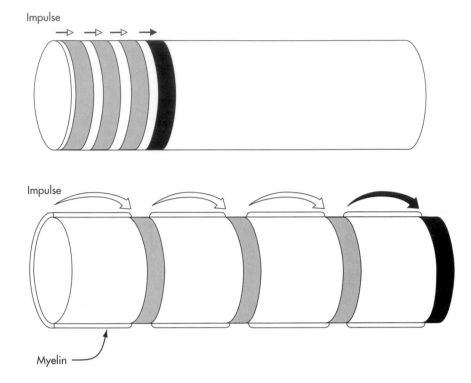

Impulse

Myelin

Fig. 1-9 Saltatory propagation. Comparing impulse propagation in nonmyelinated *(upper)* and myelinated *(lower)* axons. In nonmyelinated axons the impulse moves forward by sequential depolarization of short adjoining membrane segments. Depolarization in myelinated axons, on the other hand, is discontinuous; the impulse leaps forward from node to node. Note how much farther ahead the impulse is in the myelinated axon after four depolarization sequences. *(From de Jong RH:* Local anesthetics, *St Louis, 1994, Mosby–Year Book.)*

Myelinated Nerves

Impulse spread within myelinated nerves differs from that in unmyelinated nerves because of the layer of insulating material separating the intracellular and extracellular charges. The farther apart the charges, the smaller will be the current required to charge the membrane. Local currents can thus travel much farther in a myelinated nerve than in an unmyelinated nerve before becoming incapable of depolarizing the nerve membrane ahead of it.

Impulse conduction in myelinated nerves occurs by means of current leaps from node to node—a process termed *saltatory conduction* (Fig. 1-9) (*saltare* is the Latin verb "to leap"). This form of impulse conduction proves to be much faster and more energy efficient than that which is employed in unmyelinated nerves. The thickness of the myelin sheath increases with increasing diameter of the axon. In addition, the distance between adjacent nodes of Ranvier increases with greater axonal diameter. Because of these two factors, saltatory conduction is more rapid in a thicker axon.

Saltatory conduction usually progresses from one node to the next in a stepwise manner. However, it can be demonstrated that the current flow at the next node still exceeds that necessary to reach the firing threshold of the nodal membrane. If conduction of an impulse is blocked at one node, the local current will skip over that node and prove adequate to raise the membrane poten-

tial at the next node to its firing potential and produce depolarization. A minimum of perhaps 8 to 10 mm of nerve must be covered by anesthetic solution to ensure thorough blockade.[17]

MODE AND SITE OF ACTION OF LOCAL ANESTHETICS

How and where do local anesthetics alter the processes of impulse generation and transmission? It is possible for local anesthetic agents to interfere with the excitation process in a nerve membrane in one or more of the following ways:

1. Altering the basic resting potential of the nerve membrane
2. Altering the threshold potential (firing level)
3. Decreasing the rate of depolarization
4. Prolonging the rate of repolarization

It has been established that the primary effects of local anesthetics occur during the depolarization phase of the action potential.[18] These effects include a decrease in the rate of depolarization, particularly in the phase of slow depolarization. Because of this, cellular depolarization is not sufficient to reduce the membrane potential of a nerve fiber to its firing level, and a propagated action potential does not develop. There is *no* accompanying change in the rate of repolarization.

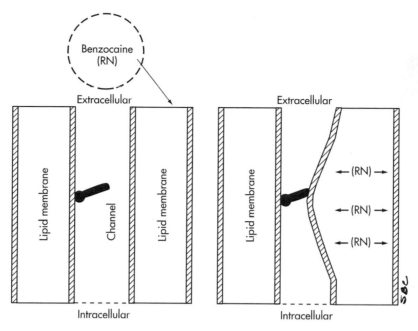

Fig. 1-10 Membrane expansion theory.

Where Do Local Anesthetics Work?

The nerve membrane is the site at which local anesthetic agents exert their pharmacological actions. Many theories have been promulgated over the years to explain the mechanism of action of local anesthetics, including the acetylcholine, calcium displacement, and surface charge theories. The *acetylcholine theory* stated that acetylcholine was involved in nerve conduction in addition to its role as a neurotransmitter at nerve synapses.[19] There is no evidence that acetylcholine is involved in neural transmission along the body of the neuron. The *calcium displacement theory*, once quite popular, maintained that local anesthetic nerve block was produced by the displacement of calcium from some membrane site that controlled permeability to sodium.[20] Evidence that varying the concentration of calcium ions bathing a nerve does not affect local anesthetic potency has diminished the credibility of this theory. The *surface charge (repulsion) theory* proposed that local anesthetics acted by binding to the nerve membrane and changing the electrical potential at the membrane surface.[21] Cationic (RNH^+) (p. 16) drug molecules were aligned at the membrane-water interface, and since some of the local anesthetic molecules carried a net positive charge, they made the electrical potential at the membrane surface more positive, thus decreasing the excitability of the nerve by increasing the threshold potential. Current evidence indicates that the resting potential of the nerve membrane is unaltered by local anesthetics (they do not become hyperpolarized) and that conventional local anesthetics act within the membrane channels rather than at the membrane surface. Also the surface charge theory cannot explain the activity of uncharged anesthetic molecules in blocking nerve impulses (e.g., benzocaine).

Two other theories, membrane expansion and specific receptor, are given some credence today. Of the two, the specific receptor theory is more widely held.

The *membrane expansion theory* states that local anesthetic molecules diffuse to hydrophobic regions of excitable membranes, producing a general disturbance of the bulk membrane structure, expanding some critical region(s) in the membrane, and thus preventing an increase in the permeability to sodium ions.[22,23] Local anesthetics that are highly lipid soluble can easily penetrate the lipid portion of the cell membrane, producing a change in configuration of the lipoprotein matrix of the nerve membrane. This results in a decreased diameter of sodium channels, which leads to an inhibition of both sodium conductance and neural excitation (Fig. 1-10). The membrane expansion theory serves as a possible explanation for the local anesthetic activity of a drug such as benzocaine, which does not exist in cationic form yet still exhibits potent topical anesthetic activity. It has been demonstrated that nerve membranes do, in fact, expand and become more "fluid" when exposed to local anesthetics. However, there is no direct evidence that nerve conduction is entirely blocked by membrane expansion per se.

The *specific receptor theory*, the most favored today, proposes that local anesthetics act by binding to specific receptors on the sodium channel (Fig. 1-11).[24] The

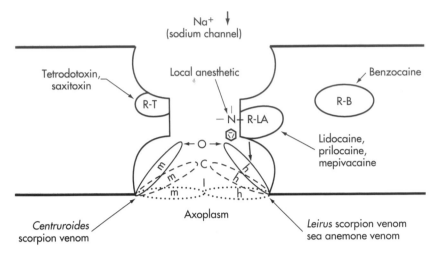

Na⁺ ↓
(sodium channel)

Fig. 1-11 Tertiary amine local anesthetics inhibit the influx of sodium during nerve conduction by binding to a receptor within the sodium channel *(R-LA)*. This blocks the normal activation mechanism (*O* gate configuration, depolarization) and also promotes movement of the activation and inactivation gates (*m* and *h*) to a position resembling that in the inactivated state *(I)*. Biotoxins *(R-T)* block the influx of sodium at an outer surface receptor; various venoms do it by altering the activity of the activation and inactivation gates; and benzocaine *(R-B)* does it by expanding the membrane. *C*, Channel in the closed configuration. *(From Pallasch TJ:* Dent Drug Serv Newslett *4:25, 1983.)*

TABLE 1-3   Classification of Local Anesthetic Substances According to Biological Site and Mode of Action

Classification	Definition	Chemical substance
Class A	Agents acting at receptor site on external surface of nerve membrane	Biotoxins (e.g., tetrodotoxin and saxitoxin)
Class B	Agents acting at receptor sites on internal surface of nerve membrane	Quaternary ammonium analogues of lidocaine Scorpion venom
Class C	Agents acting by a receptor-independent physicochemical mechanism	Benzocaine
Class D	Agents acting by combination of receptor and receptor-independent mechanisms	Most clinically useful local anesthetic agents (e.g., lidocaine, mepivacaine, prilocaine)

Modified from Covino BG, Vassallo HG: *Local anesthetics: mechanisms of action and clinical use,* New York, 1976, Grune & Stratton. Used by permission.

action of the drug is direct, not mediated by some change in the general properties of the cell membrane. Both biochemical and electrophysiological studies have indicated that a specific receptor site for local anesthetic agents exists in the sodium channel either on its external surface or on the internal axoplasmic surface.[25, 26] Once the local anesthetic has gained access to the receptors, permeability to sodium ions is decreased or eliminated and nerve conduction is interrupted.

Local anesthetics are classified by their ability to react with specific receptor sites in the sodium channel. It appears that there are at least four sites within the sodium channel at which drugs can alter nerve conduction (Fig. 1-11):

1. Within the sodium channel (tertiary amine local anesthetics)
2. At the outer surface of the sodium channel (tetrodotoxin, saxitoxin)
3-4. At either the activation or the inactivation gates (scorpion venom)

Table 1-3 is a biological classification of local anesthetics based on their site of action and the active form of the compound. Drugs in Class C exist only in the uncharged form (RN), whereas Class D drugs exist in both charged and uncharged forms. Approximately 90% of the blocking effects of Class D drugs is caused by the cationic form of the drug; only 10% of blocking action is produced by the base (Fig. 1-12).

Myelinated Nerve Fibers

One additional factor needs consideration with regard to the site of action of local anesthetics in myelinated nerves. The myelin sheath insulates the axon both electrically and pharmacologically. The only site at which the molecules of local anesthetic have access to the nerve membrane is at the nodes of Ranvier where sodium channels are found in abundance. The ionic changes that develop during impulse conduction also arise only at the nodes.

Because an impulse may skip over or bypass one or two blocked nodes and continue on its way, it is necessary for at least two or three nodes immediately adjacent

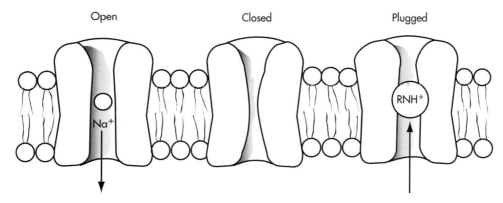

Open   Closed   Plugged

Fig. 1-12 Channel entry. On the left is an open channel, inward permeant to sodium ion. The center channel is in the resting closed configuration; though impermeant to sodium ion here, the channel remains voltage-responsive. The channel on the right, though in open configuration, is impermeant because it has local anesthetic cation bound to the gating receptor site. Note that local anesthetic enters the channel from the axoplasmic (lower) side; the channel filter precludes direct entry via the external mouth. Local anesthetic renders the membrane impermeant to sodium ion; hence inexcitable by local action currents. *(From de Jong RH:* Local anesthetics, *St Louis, 1994, Mosby–Year Book.)*

to the anesthetic solution to be blocked to ensure effective anesthesia, a length of approximately 8 to 10 mm.

Sodium channel densities differ in myelinated and unmyelinated nerves. In small unmyelinated nerves the density of sodium channels is about $35/\mu m^2$, whereas at the nodes of Ranvier in myelinated fibers it may be as high as $20,000/\mu m^2$. On an average nerve-length basis, there are relatively few sodium channels in unmyelinated nerve membranes. For example, in the garfish olfactory nerve the ratio of sodium channels to phospholipid molecules is 1:60,000, corresponding to a mean distance between channels of 0.2 μm, whereas at densely packed nodes of Ranvier the channels are separated by only 70 Å.[27,28]

How Local Anesthetics Work

The primary action of local anesthetics in producing a conduction block is to decrease the permeability of the ion channels to sodium ions (Na^+). Local anesthetics selectively inhibit peak sodium permeability, whose value is normally about 5 to 6 times greater than the minimum required for impulse conduction (i.e., there is a safety factor for conduction of 5× to 6×).[29] Local anesthetics reduce this safety factor, decreasing both the rate of rise of the action potential and its conduction velocity. When the safety factor falls below unity (1.0), conduction fails and nerve block occurs.

Local anesthetics produce a very slight, virtually insignificant decrease in potassium (K^+) conductance through the nerve membrane.

Calcium ions (Ca^{++}), which exist in bound form within the cell membrane, are thought to exert a regulatory role on the movement of sodium ions across the nerve membrane. Release of bound calcium ions from the ion channel receptor site may be the primary factor responsible for the increased sodium permeability of the nerve membrane. This represents the first step in nerve membrane depolarization. Local anesthetic molecules may act by competitive antagonism with calcium for some site on the nerve membrane.

The following sequence is a proposed mechanism of action of local anesthetics:[1]

1. Displacement of calcium ions from the sodium channel receptor site, *which permits ...*
2. Binding of the local anesthetic molecule to this receptor site, *which thus produces ...*
3. Blockade of the sodium channel, *and a ...*
4. Decrease in sodium conductance, *which leads to ...*
5. Depression of the rate of electrical depolarization *and a ...*
6. Failure to achieve the threshold potential level, *along with a ...*
7. Lack of development of propagated action potentials, *which is called ...*
8. Conduction blockade.

The mechanism whereby sodium ions gain entry to the axoplasm of the nerve, thereby initiating an action potential, is altered by local anesthetics. The nerve membrane remains in a polarized state because the ionic movements responsible for the action potential fail to develop. Because the membrane's electrical potential remains unchanged, local currents do not develop and the self-perpetuating mechanism of impulse propagation is stalled. An impulse that arrives at a blocked nerve segment is stopped because it is unable to release the energy needed for its continued propagation. Nerve block produced by local anesthetics is called a *nondepolarizing nerve block*.

ACTIVE FORMS OF LOCAL ANESTHETICS

Local Anesthetic Molecules

The vast majority of injectable local anesthetics are tertiary amines. Only a few (e.g., prilocaine and hexylcaine) are secondary amines. The typical local anesthetic structure is shown in Figs. 1-13 and 1-14. The lipophilic part is the largest portion of the molecule. Aromatic in structure, it is derived from benzoic acid or aniline. All local anesthetics are amphipathic—that is, they possess both lipophilic and hydrophilic characteristics, generally at opposite ends of the molecule. The hydrophilic part is an amino derivative of ethyl alcohol or acetic acid. Local anesthetics without a hydrophilic part are not suited for injection but are good topical anesthetics (e.g., benzocaine). The anesthetic structure is completed by an intermediate hydrocarbon chain containing either an ester or an amide linkage. Other chemicals, especially antihistamines and anticholinergics, share this basic structure with the local anesthetics and commonly exhibit weak local anesthetic properties.

Local anesthetics are classified as either *esters* or *amides* according to their chemical linkages. The nature of the linkage is important in defining several properties of the local anesthetic, including the basic mode of biotransformation. Ester-linked local anesthetics (e.g., procaine) are readily hydrolyzed in aqueous solution. Amide-linked local anesthetics (e.g., lidocaine) are relatively resistant to hydrolysis. A greater percentage of an amide-linked drug is excreted unchanged in the urine than of an ester-linked drug. Procainamide, which is procaine with an amide linkage replacing the ester linkage, is as potent a local anesthetic as procaine; yet, because of its amide linkage, it is hydrolyzed much more slowly. Procaine is hydrolyzed in plasma in only a few minutes, but only approximately 10% of procainamide is hydrolyzed in 1 day.

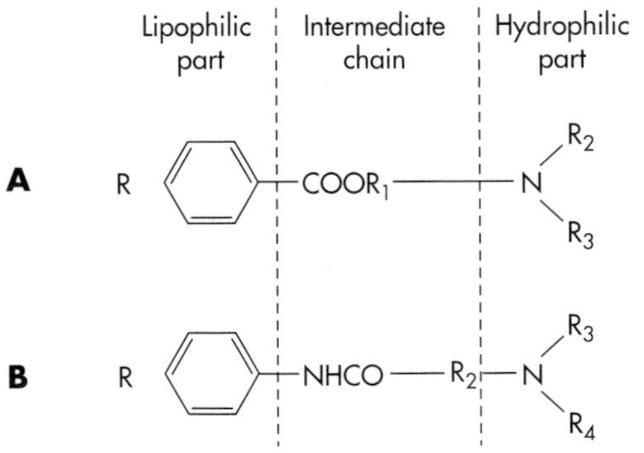

As prepared in the laboratory, local anesthetics are basic compounds, poorly soluble in water, and unstable on exposure to air.[30] Their pK_a values range from 7.5 to 10. In this form they have little or no clinical value. However, being weakly basic, they combine readily with acids to form local anesthetic salts, in which form they are quite soluble in water and comparatively stable. Thus local anesthetics used for injection are dispensed as salts, most commonly the hydrochloride salt, dissolved in either sterile water or saline.

It is well known that the pH of a local anesthetic solution (and the pH of the tissue into which it is injected) greatly influences its nerve-blocking action. *Acidification* of tissue decreases local anesthetic effectiveness. Inadequate anesthesia results when local anesthetics are injected into infected or inflamed areas. The inflammatory process produces acidic products: the pH of normal tissue is 7.4; the pH of an inflamed area is 5 to 6. Local anesthetics containing epinephrine or other vasopressors are acidified by the manufacturer to inhibit the oxidation of the vasopressor (p. 18). The pH of solutions without epinephrine is about 5.5; epinephrine-containing solutions have a pH of about 3.3. Clinically this lower pH is more likely to produce a burning sensation on injection, as well as a slightly slower onset of anesthesia.

Increasing the pH (alkalinization) of a local anesthetic solution speeds the onset of its action, increases its clinical effectiveness, and makes its injection more comfortable. However, the local anesthetic base, because it is quite unstable, precipitates out of alkalinized solutions, and this makes these solutions ill suited for clinical use. Recently, carbonated local anesthetics have received much attention. Sodium bicarbonate or carbon dioxide (CO_2) added to the anesthetic solution immediately prior to injection provides greater comfort and a more rapid onset of anesthesia. (See Chapter 19.)[31,32]

Despite wide pH variation of extracellular fluids, the pH at the interior of a nerve remains quite stable. Normal functioning of a nerve is therefore affected very little by changes in extracellular pH. However, the ability of a local anesthetic to block nerve impulses is profoundly altered by changes in extracellular pH.

Dissociation of Local Anesthetics

As just discussed, local anesthetics are available as salts (usually the hydrochloride) for clinical use. The salt, both water soluble and stable, is dissolved in either sterile water or saline. In this solution it exists simultaneously as (1) uncharged molecules (RN), also called the *base*, and

Fig. 1-13   Typical local anesthetic. **A,** Ester type. **B,** Amide type.

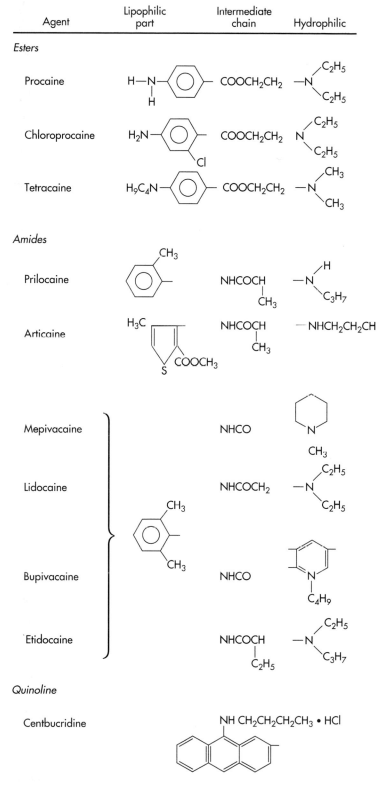

Fig. 1-14 Chemical configuration of local anesthetics.

TABLE 1 - 4 Dissociation Constants (pK_a) of Local Anesthetics

Agent	pK$_a$	Percent base (RN) at pH 7.4	Approximate onset of action (min)
Benzocaine	3.5	100	—
Mepivacaine	7.7	33	2 to 4
Lidocaine	7.8	29	2 to 4
Articaine	7.8	29	2 to 4
Etidocaine	7.9	25	2 to 4
Prilocaine	7.9	25	2 to 4
Ropivacaine	8.1	17	2 to 4
Bupivacaine	8.1	17	5 to 8
Tetracaine	8.4	9	10 to 15
Cocaine	8.6	7	—
Propoxycaine	8.9	4	9 to 14
Procaine	9.1	2	14 to 18
Chloroprocaine	8.7	6	6 to 12
Procainamide	9.3	1	—

(2) positively charged molecules (RNH$^+$), called the *cation*.

$$RNH^+ \rightleftarrows RN + H^+$$

The relative proportion of each ionic form in the solution varies with the pH of the solution or surrounding tissues. In the presence of a high concentration of hydrogen ions (low pH) the equilibrium shifts to the left and most of the anesthetic solution exists in cationic form:

$$RNH^+ > RN + H^+$$

As hydrogen ion concentration decreases (higher pH), the equilibrium shifts toward the free base form:

$$RNH^+ < RN + H^+$$

The relative proportion of ionic forms also depends on the pK$_a$, or dissociation constant, of the specific local anesthetic. The pK$_a$ is a measure of a molecule's affinity for hydrogen ions (H$^+$). When the pH of a solution has the same value as the pK$_a$ of the local anesthetic, exactly half the drug will exist in the RNH$^+$ form and exactly half in the RN form. The percentage of drug existing in either form can be determined from the Henderson-Hasselbalch equation:

$$Log \frac{Base}{Acid} = pH - pK_a$$

Table 1-4 lists the pK$_a$ values for some commonly used local anesthetics.

Actions on Nerve Membranes

The two factors involved in the action of a local anesthetic are *diffusion of the drug through the nerve sheath* and *binding at the receptor site* in the ion chan-nel. The uncharged, lipid-soluble, free base form (RN) of the anesthetic is responsible for diffusion through the nerve sheath. Consider the following example:

1. Assume that 1000 molecules of a local anesthetic with a pK$_a$ of 7.9 are deposited in the tissues outside a nerve. The tissue pH is normal (7.4) (Fig. 1-15).
2. From Table 1-4 and the Henderson-Hasselbalch equation, it can be determined that at this pH 75% of the local anesthetic molecules are present in the cationic form (RNH$^+$) and 25% in the free base form (RN).
3. Theoretically all 250 lipophilic RN molecules diffuse through the nerve sheath to reach the axoplasm of the nerve cell.
4. Extracellularly the equilibrium between RNH$^+$ and RN is disrupted by passage of the free base forms into the nerve cell. The remaining 750 extracellular RNH$^+$ molecules now reequilibrate according to the tissue pH and the drug pK$_a$.

$$RNH^+(570) \rightleftarrows RN(180) + H^+$$

5. The 180 newly created lipophilic RN molecules diffuse into the cell, starting the entire process (Step 4) again. Theoretically this will continue until all local anesthetic molecules have diffused into the axoplasm. In reality, however, not all the anesthetic molecules reach the interior of the nerve cell because of the process of diffusion and because some will be absorbed into local blood vessels and extracellular soft tissues at the injection site.
6. Let us now look inside the nerve. Following penetration of the nerve sheath and entry into the axoplasm by the lipophilic RN form of the anesthetic, a reequilibration takes place since the local anesthetic cannot exist in only the RN form at the intracellular pH of 7.4. Seventy-five percent of the RN molecules present intracellularly revert to the RNH$^+$ form; the remaining molecules stay in the uncharged RN form.
7. From the axoplasmic side of the sodium channel the charged cationic form binds to the channel receptor site and is ultimately responsible for the conduction blockade that results (Figs. 1-11 and 1-12).

Of the two factors—diffusibility and binding—responsible for local anesthetic effectiveness, the former is extremely important in actual practice. An agent's ability to diffuse through the tissues surrounding a nerve is of critical significance, since in clinical situations the local anesthetic cannot be applied directly to the nerve membrane as it can in a laboratory setting. Solutions better able to diffuse through soft tissue are at an advantage in clinical practice.

A local anesthetic with a high pK$_a$ has very few molecules available in the RN form at a tissue pH of 7.4. The anesthetic action of this drug will be poor because too

Neurophysiology CHAPTER 1   17

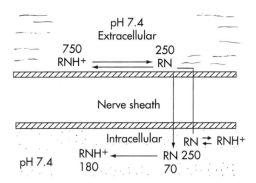

Fig. 1-15 Mechanism of action of the local anesthetic molecule. Anesthetic pK$_a$ of 7.9; tissue pH of 7.4.

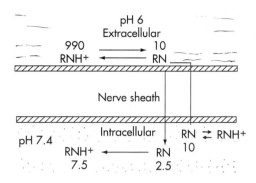

Fig. 1-16 Effect of decreased tissue pH on the actions of a local anesthetic.

few base molecules are available to diffuse through the nerve membrane (e.g., procaine, with a pK$_a$ of 9.1). *The rate of onset of anesthetic action is related to the pKa of the local anesthetic* (Table 1-4).

A local anesthetic with a low pK$_a$ (below 7.5) has a very large number of lipophilic free base molecules, which are able to diffuse through the nerve sheath; however, the anesthetic action of this drug will also prove inadequate because at an intracellular pH of 7.4 only a very small number of base molecules will dissociate back to the cationic form necessary for binding at the receptor site.

In actual clinical situations with the local anesthetics currently available, it is the pH of the *extracellular fluid* that determines the ease with which a local anesthetic moves from the site of its administration into the axoplasm of the nerve cell. The intracellular pH (at the external surface of the nerve membrane) remains quite stable and independent of the extracellular pH. This is because hydrogen ions (H$^+$), like the local anesthetic cations (RNH$^+$), do not readily diffuse through tissues. The pH of extracellular fluid may therefore differ from that at the nerve membrane. The ratio of anesthetic cations to uncharged base molecules (RNH$^+$/RN) may also vary greatly at these sites. Differences in extracellular and intracellular pH are highly significant in pain control where there is inflammation or infection.[33] The effect of a decrease in tissue pH on the actions of a local anesthetic is described in Fig. 1-16. Compare this with the example in Fig. 1-15, involving normal tissue pH.

1. Assume that approximately 1000 molecules of a local anesthetic with a pK$_a$ of 7.9 are deposited outside a nerve. The tissue is inflamed and infected and has a pH of 6.
2. At this tissue pH approximately 99% of the anesthetic molecules are present in the charged cationic (RNH$^+$) form, with fewer than 1% in the lipophilic free base (RN) form.
3. Approximately 10 RN molecules diffuse across the nerve sheath to reach the interior of the cell (con-

trasting with 250 RN molecules in the healthy example). The pH on the interior of the nerve cell remains normal (i.e., 7.4).
4. Extracellularly the equilibrium between RNH$^+$ and RN, which has been disrupted, is reestablished. The relatively few newly created RN molecules diffuse into the cell, starting the entire process again. However, a sum total of fewer RN molecules succeed in eventually crossing the nerve sheath than would succeed at a normal pH because of the greatly increased absorption of anesthetic molecules into the blood vessels in the region (increased vascularity in the area of inflammation and infection).
5. After penetration of the nerve sheath by the base form, reequilibrium occurs. Approximately 75% of the molecules present intracellularly revert to the cationic form (RNH$^+$), 25% remaining in the uncharged free base form (RN).
6. The cationic molecules bind to receptor sites within the sodium channel, resulting in conduction blockade.

Adequate blockade of the nerve is more difficult to achieve in infected or inflamed tissues because of the scarcity of molecules able to cross the nerve sheath (RN) and the increased absorption of the remaining anesthetic molecules into dilated blood vessels in this region. Although a potential problem in all aspects of dental practice, this situation develops most frequently in endodontics. Possible remedies are described in Chapter 16.

Clinical Implications of pH and Local Anesthetic Activity

Most commercially prepared solutions of local anesthetics without a vasoconstrictor have a pH between 5.5 and 7. When these solutions are deposited into tissue, the vast buffering capacity of the tissue fluids rapidly returns the pH at the injection site to a normal 7.4. Local anesthetic solutions that contain a vasopressor (e.g., epinephrine) are acidified by the manufacturer to retard oxidation of the vasoconstrictor, thereby prolonging the period of the drug's effectiveness. (See Chapter 3 for a discussion of the appropriate use of vasoconstrictors in local anesthetics.)

Epinephrine may be added to a local anesthetic solution immediately prior to its administration without the addition of antioxidants; however, if the solution is not used in a short time it will oxidize, becoming reddish brown.

Rapid oxidation of the vasoactive substance may be delayed, thereby increasing the shelf life of the product, through the addition of antioxidants. Sodium bisulfite is commonly used, in a concentration between 0.05% and 0.1%. A 2% solution of lidocaine, with a pH of 6.8, is acidified to 4.2 by the addition of sodium bisulfite.

Even in this situation the large buffering capacity of the tissues tends to maintain a normal tissue pH; however, it does require a longer time to do so following injection of a pH 4.2 solution than with a pH 6.8 solution. During this time the local anesthetic is not able to function at its full effectiveness, resulting in a slower onset of clinical action for local anesthetics with vasoconstrictors when compared with their "plain" counterparts.

Local anesthetics are clinically effective on both axons and free nerve endings. Free nerve endings lying below intact skin may be reached only by the injection of anesthetic beneath the skin. Intact skin forms an impenetrable barrier to the diffusion of local anesthetic agents. The recently formulated EMLA (eutectic mixture of local anesthetics) enables local anesthetics to penetrate intact skin, albeit quite slowly.[34]

Mucous membranes and injured skin (e.g., burns and abrasions) lack the protection afforded by intact skin, permitting topically applied local anesthetics to diffuse through to reach free nerve endings. Topical anesthetics can be employed effectively wherever skin is no longer intact because of injury and on mucous membranes (e.g., cornea, gingiva, pharynx, trachea, larynx, esophagus, and bladder).[35]

The buffering capacity of mucous membrane is quite poor; thus the topical application of a local anesthetic with a pH between 5.5 and 6.5 lowers the regional pH to below normal, and less local anesthetic base is formed. Diffusion of the drug across the mucous membrane to free nerve endings is limited, and nerve block is ineffective. Increasing the pH of the drug provides more RN form, thereby increasing potency of the topical anesthetic; however, the drug in this form is more rapidly oxidized. The effective shelf life of the anesthetic is decreased as the drug's pH increases.[30]

To make topical anesthetics clinically more effective, a more concentrated form of the drug is commonly used (5% or 10% lidocaine) than for injection (2% lidocaine). Although only a small percentage of the drug will be available in base form, raising the concentration provides more RN molecules for diffusion and dissociation to the active cation form at free nerve endings.

Some topical anesthetics, such as benzocaine, are not ionized in solution; thus their anesthetic effectiveness is unaffected by pH. Because of benzocaine's poor water solubility, its absorption from the site of application is minimal, and systemic reactions (e.g., overdose) are rarely encountered.

KINETICS OF LOCAL ANESTHETIC ONSET AND DURATION OF ACTION
Barriers to Diffusion of the Solution

A peripheral nerve is composed of hundreds to thousands of tightly packed axons. These axons are protected, supported, and nourished by several layers of fibrous and elastic tissues. Nutrient blood vessels and lymphatics course throughout the layers.

Individual nerve fibers (axons) are covered with, and also separated from each other by, the *endoneurium*. The *perineurium* then binds these nerve fibers together into bundles called *fasciculi*. The radial nerve, located in the wrist, contains between 5 and 10 fasciculi. Each fasciculus contains between 500 and 1000 individual nerve fibers. Five thousand nerve fibers occupy approximately 1 mm^2 of space.

The thickness of the perineurium varies with the diameter of the fasciculus it surrounds. The thicker the perineurium, the slower the rate of local anesthetic diffusion across it.[36] The innermost layer of perineurium is the perilemma. It is covered with a smooth mesothelial membrane. The perilemma represents the main barrier to diffusion into a nerve.

Fasciculi are contained within a loose network of areolar connective tissue called the *epineurium*. The epineurium constitutes between 30% and 75% of the total cross-section of a nerve. Local anesthetics are readily able to diffuse through the epineurium because of its loose consistency. Nutrient blood vessels and lym-

T A B L E   1 - 5   Organization of a Peripheral Nerve

Structure	Description
Nerve fiber	Single nerve cell
Endoneurium	Covers each nerve fiber
Fasciculi	Bundles of 500 to 1000 nerve fibers
Perineurium*	Covers fasciculi
Perilemma*	Innermost layer of perineurium
Epineurium	Alveolar connective tissue supporting fasciculi and carrying nutrient vessels
Epineural sheath	Outer layer of epineurium

*The perineurium and perilemma constitute the greatest anatomical barriers to diffusion in a peripheral nerve.

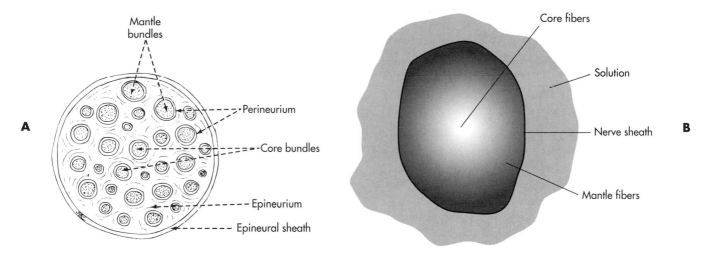

Fig. 1-17 A, Composition of nerve fibers and bundles within a peripheral nerve. **B,** In a large peripheral nerve (containing hundreds or thousands of axons), local anesthetic solution must diffuse inward toward the nerve core from the extraneural site of injection. Local anesthetic molecules are removed by tissue uptake, while tissue fluid mixes with the carrier solvent. This results in a gradual dilution of the local anesthetic solution as it penetrates the nerve toward the core. A concentration gradient occurs during induction so that the outer mantle fibers are solidly blocked, whereas the inner core fibers are not yet blocked. Core fibers are not only exposed to a lower local anesthetic concentration, but the drug also arrives later. Delay depends on the tissue mass to be penetrated and the diffusivity of the local anesthetic. *(**B**, From de Jong RH: Local anesthetics, St Louis, 1994, Mosby–Year Book.)*

phatics traverse the epineurium. These vessels absorb local anesthetic molecules, thus removing them from the nerve.

The outer layer of the epineurium surrounding the nerve is denser and thickened, forming what is termed the *epineural sheath,* or *nerve sheath.* The epineural sheath does not constitute a barrier to diffusion of local anesthetic into a nerve.

Table 1-5 summarizes the layers of a typical peripheral nerve.

Induction of Local Anesthesia

Following the administration of a local anesthetic into the soft tissues near a nerve, molecules of the local anesthetic traverse the distance from one site to another according to their concentration gradient. During the induction phase of anesthesia, the local anesthetic moves from its extraneural site of deposition toward the nerve (as well as in all other directions). This process is termed *diffusion.* It is the unhindered migration of molecules or ions through a fluid medium under the influence of the concentration gradient. *Penetration* of an anatomical barrier to diffusion occurs when a drug passes through a tissue that tends to restrict free molecular movement. The perineurium is the greatest barrier to penetration of local anesthetics.

Diffusion

The rate of diffusion is governed by several factors, the most significant of which is the *concentration gradient.* The greater the initial concentration of the local anesthetic, the faster will be the diffusion of its molecules and the more rapid its onset of action.

Fasciculi that are located near the surface of the nerve are termed *mantle bundles* (Fig. 1-17, *A*). Mantle bundles are the first ones reached by the local anesthetic and are exposed to a higher concentration of it. Mantle bundles are usually blocked completely shortly after the injection of a local anesthetic (Fig. 1-17, *B*).

Fasciculi found closer to the center of the nerve are called *core bundles.* Core bundles are contacted by a local anesthetic only after much delay and by a lower anesthetic concentration because of the greater distance that the solution must traverse and the greater number of barriers it must cross.

As the local anesthetic diffuses into the nerve, it becomes increasingly diluted by tissue fluids and is absorbed by capillaries and lymphatics; ester anesthetics undergo almost immediate enzymatic hydrolysis. Thus the core fibers are exposed to a decreased concentration of local anesthetic, a fact that may explain the clinical situation of inadequate pulpal anesthesia developing in the presence of subjective symptoms of adequate soft tissue anesthesia. Complete conduction block of all nerve fibers in a peripheral nerve requires that an adequate *volume* as well as an adequate *concentration* of the local anesthetic be deposited. In no clinical situation are 100% of the fibers within a peripheral nerve blocked, even in cases of clinically excellent pain control.[37] Fibers near the surface of the nerve (mantle fibers) tend to innervate more proximal regions (e.g., the molar area with an inferior alveolar nerve block), whereas fibers in the core bundles innervate the more distal points of nerve distribution (e.g., the central and lateral incisors with an inferior alveolar block).

Blocking Process

Following deposition as close to the nerve as possible, the local anesthetic solution diffuses in many directions according to prevailing concentration gradients. A portion of the injected anesthetic diffuses toward the nerve and into the nerve. However, a significant portion of the injected drug also diffuses away from the nerve. The following reactions then occur:

1. Some of the drug is absorbed by nonneural tissues (e.g., muscle and fat).
2. Some is diluted by interstitial fluid.
3. Some is removed by capillaries and lymphatics from the injection site.
4. Ester-type anesthetics are hydrolyzed.

The sum total of these factors is to decrease the local anesthetic concentration outside the nerve; however, the concentration of local anesthetic within the nerve continues to rise as diffusion progresses. These processes continue until an equilibrium results between the intraneural and extraneural concentrations of anesthetic solution.

Induction Time

Induction time is defined as the period from deposition of the anesthetic solution to complete conduction blockade. Several factors control the induction time of a given drug. Those under the operator's control are the concentration of the drug and the pH of the local anesthetic solution. Factors not under the clinician's control are the diffusion constant of the anesthetic drug and the anatomical diffusion barriers of the nerve.

Physical Properties and Clinical Actions

There are other physicochemical factors of a local anesthetic that influence its clinical characteristics.

The effect of the *dissociation constant* (pK_a) on the rate of onset of anesthesia has been described. Although both molecular forms of the anesthetic are important in neural blockade, drugs with a lower pK_a possess a more rapid onset of action than do those with a higher pK_a.[38]

Lipid solubility of a local anesthetic appears to be related to its intrinsic potency. The approximate lipid solubilities of various local anesthetics are presented in Table 1-6. Increased lipid solubility permits the anesthetic to penetrate the nerve membrane (which itself is 90% lipid) more easily. This is reflected biologically in an increased potency of the anesthetic. Local anesthetics with greater lipid solubility produce more effective conduction blockade at lower concentrations (lower percentage solutions or smaller volumes deposited) than do the less lipid-soluble solutions.

The degree of *protein binding* of the anesthetic molecule is responsible for the duration of local anesthetic activity. After penetration of the nerve sheath, a reequilibrium occurs between the base and cationic forms of the anesthetic. Now, in the sodium channel itself, the RNH^+ ions bind at the receptor site. Proteins constitute approximately 10% of the nerve membrane, and local anesthetics (e.g., etidocaine and bupivacaine) possessing a greater degree of protein binding (Table 1-6) than others (e.g., procaine) appear to attach more securely to the protein receptor sites and to possess a longer duration of clinical activity.[39]

Vasoactivity affects both the anesthetic potency and the duration of anesthesia provided by a drug. Injection of local anesthetics, such as procaine, with greater vasodilating properties increases perfusion of the local site with blood. The injected local anesthetic is therefore absorbed into the cardiovascular compartment more rapidly and carried away from the injection site and from the nerve, thus providing for a shortened duration of anesthesia as well as decreased potency of the drug. Table 1-7 summarizes the influence of various factors on local anesthetic action.

Recovery from Local Anesthetic Block

Emergence from a local anesthetic nerve block follows the same diffusion patterns as does induction; however, it does so in the *reverse order.*

The extraneural concentration of local anesthetic is continually depleted by diffusion, dispersion, and uptake of the drug, whereas the intraneural concentration of the local anesthetic remains relatively stable. The concentration gradient is thus reversed, the intraneural concentration exceeding the extraneural concentration, and the anesthetic molecules begin to diffuse out of the nerve.

Fasciculi in the mantle begin to lose the local anesthetic much earlier than the core bundles do. Recovery from block anesthesia appears first in the proximally innervated regions (e.g., third molars before the central incisors). Core fibers gradually lose their local anesthetic concentration. Recovery is usually a slower process than induction because the local anesthetic is bound to the drug receptor site in the sodium channel and is therefore released more slowly than it is absorbed.

TABLE 1-6 Chemical Structure, Physicochemical Properties, and Pharmacological Properties of Local Anesthetic Agents

Agent	Chemical Configuration			Physicochemical Properties			Approx. lipid solubility	Pharmacological Properties		
	Aromatic lipophilic	Intermediate chain	Amine hydrophilic	Molecular weight (base)	pKa (36°C)	Onset		Usual effective concentration %	Protein binding	Duration
Esters										
Procaine	*(structure)*			236	8.9	Slow	1.0	2 to 4	5	Short
Chloroprocaine	*(structure)*			271	9.1	Fast	NA	NA	NA	Short
Tetracaine	*(structure)*			264	8.4	Slow	80	0.15	85	Long
Amides										
Mepivacaine	*(structure)*			246	7.7	Fast	1.0	2 to 3	75	Moderate
Prilocaine	*(structure)*			220	7.8	Fast	1.5	4	55	Moderate
Lidocaine	*(structure)*			234	7.3	Fast	4.0	2	65	Moderate
Ropivacaine	*(structure)*			274	8.1	Moderate	NA	NA	NA	Long
Bupivacaine	*(structure)*			283	8.1	Moderate	30	0.5 to 0.75	95	Long
Etidocaine	*(structure)*			276	7.9	Fast	140	0.5 to 1.5	94	Long

Modified from Rogers MC, et al, editors: *Principles and practice of anesthesiology*, St Louis, 1993, Mosby–Year Book.
NA, Not available.

TABLE 1-7 Factors Affecting Local Anesthetic Action

Factor	Action affected	Description
pK_a	Onset	Lower pK_a = More rapid onset of action, more RN molecules present to diffuse through nerve sheath; thus onset time is decreased
Lipid solubility	Anesthetic potency	Increased lipid solubility = Increased potency (example: procaine = 1; etidocaine = 140)
		Etidocaine produces conduction blockade at very low concentrations, whereas procaine poorly suppresses nerve conduction, even at higher concentrations
Protein binding	Duration	Increased protein binding allows anesthetic cations (RNH+) to be more firmly attached to proteins located at receptor sites; thus duration of action is increased
Nonnervous tissue diffusibility	Onset	Increased diffusibility = Decreased time of onset
Vasodilator activity	Anesthetic potency and duration	Greater vasodilator activity = Increased blood flow to region = Rapid removal of anesthetic molecules from injection site; thus decreased anesthetic potency and decreased duration

From Cohen S, Burns RC: *Pathways of the pulp*, ed 6, St Louis, 1994, Mosby–Year Book.

Reinjection of Local Anesthetic

Not infrequently a dental procedure will outlast the duration of clinically effective pain control and a repeat injection of local anesthetic will be required. Usually this repeat injection immediately results in a return of profound anesthesia; on other occasions, however, the clinician may encounter greater difficulty in reestablishing adequate pain control.

Recurrence of Immediate Profound Anesthesia

At the time of reinjection, the concentration of local anesthetic in the mantle fibers is below that in the more centrally located core fibers. The partially recovered mantle fibers still contain some local anesthetic, although not enough to provide complete anesthesia. After deposition of a new high concentration of anesthetic near the nerve, the mantle fibers are once again exposed to a concentration gradient directed inward toward the nerve. This combination of residual local anesthetic (in the nerve) and the newly deposited supply results in a rapid onset of profound anesthesia with a smaller volume of local anesthetic drug being administered.

Difficulty Reachieving Profound Anesthesia

In this second situation, as in the first, the dental procedure has outlasted the clinical effectiveness of the anesthetic drug and the patient is experiencing pain. The doctor readministers a volume of local anesthetic but, unlike the first scenario, effective control of pain does not occur.

Tachyphylaxis In this second clinical situation a process known as tachyphylaxis occurs. *Tachyphylaxis* is defined as an increasing tolerance to a drug that is administered repeatedly. It is much more likely to develop if nerve function is allowed to return prior to reinjection (i.e., if the patient complains of pain). The duration, intensity, and spread of anesthesia with reinjection are greatly reduced.[40]

Although difficult to explain, tachyphylaxis is probably brought about through some or all of the following factors: edema, localized hemorrhage, clot formation, transudation, hypernatremia, and decreased pH of tissues. The first four factors isolate the nerve from contact with the local anesthetic solution. The fifth, hypernatremia, raises the sodium ion gradient, thus counteracting the decrease in sodium ion conduction brought about by the local anesthetic. The last factor, a decrease in pH of the tissues, is brought about by the first injection of the acidic local anesthetic. The ambient pH in the area of injection may be somewhat lower, so that fewer local anesthetic molecules are transformed into the free base (RN) on reinjection.

Duration of Anesthesia

As the local anesthetic is removed from the nerve, the function of the nerve returns, rapidly at first but then gradually slowing. Compared with the onset of the nerve block, which is rapid, recovery from nerve block is much slower because the local anesthetic is bound to the nerve membrane. Longer-acting local anesthetics, such as bupivacaine and tetracaine, are more firmly bound to the nerve membrane (increased protein binding) than are shorter-acting drugs, such as procaine and lidocaine, and are therefore released from the receptor sites in the sodium channels more slowly. The rate at which an anesthetic is removed from a nerve has an effect on the duration of neural blockade; in addition to increased *protein binding* other factors that influence the rate of a drug's removal from the injection site are the *vascularity of the injection site* and the *presence or absence of a vasoactive substance*. Anesthetic duration is increased in areas of decreased vascularity; and the addition of a vasopressor decreases tissue perfusion to a local area, thus increasing the duration of the block.

REFERENCES

1. Covino BG, Vassallo HG: *Local anesthetics: mechanisms of action and clinical use,* New York, 1976, Grune & Stratton.
2. Bennett CR: *Monheim's local anesthesia and pain control in dental practice,* ed 5, St Louis, 1974, Mosby–Year Book.
3. Fitzgerald MJT: *Neuroanatomy: basic and clinical,* London, 1992, Bailliere Tindall.
4. Noback CR, Strominger NL, Demarest RJ: *The human nervous system: introduction and review,* ed 4, Philadelphia, 1991, Lea & Febiger.
5. Singer SJ, Nicholson GL: The fluid mosaic model of the structure of cell membranes, *Science* 175:720-731, 1972.
6. Guyton AC: *Basic neuroscience: anatomy and physiology,* Philadelphia, 1987, WB Saunders.
7. Guidotti G: The composition of biological membranes, *Arch Intern Med* 129:194-201, 1972.
8. Denson DD, Maziot JX: *Physiology, pharmacology, and toxicity of local anesthetics: adult and pediatric considerations.* In Raj PP, editor: *Clinical practice of regional anesthesia,* New York, 1991, Churchill Livingstone.
9. Heavner JE: *Molecular action of local anesthetics.* In Raj PP, editor: *Clinical practice of regional anesthesia,* New York, 1991, Churchill Livingstone.
10. de Jong: *Local anesthetics,* ed 2, Springfield, Ill, 1977, Charles C Thomas.
11. Hodgkin AL, Huxley AF: A quantitative description of membrane current and its application to conduction and excitation in nerve, *J Physiol (London)* 117:500-544, 1954.
12. Noback CR, Demarest RJ: *The human nervous system: basic principles of neurobiology,* ed 3, New York, 1981, McGraw-Hill, pp 44-45.
13. Keynes RD: Ion channels in the nerve-cell membrane, *Sci Am* 240(3):126-135, 1979.
14. Cattarall WA: Structure and function of voltage-sensitive ion channels, *Science* 242:50-61, 1988.
15. Hille B: Ionic selectivity, saturation, and block in sodium channels: a four-barrier model, *J Gen Physiol* 66:535-560, 1975.
16. Ritchie JM: *Physiological basis for conduction in myelinated nerve fibers.* In Morell P, editor: *Myelin,* ed 2, New York, 1984, Plenum Press, pp 117-145.
17. Franz DN, Perry RS: Mechanisms for differential block among single myelinated and non-myelinated axons by procaine, *J Physiol* 235:193-210, 1974.
18. de Jong RH, Wagman IH: Physiological mechanisms of peripheral nerve block by local anesthetics, *Anesthesiology* 24:684-727, 1963.
19. Dettbarn WD: The acetylcholine system in peripheral nerve, *Ann NY Acad Sci* 144:483-503, 1967.
20. Goldman DE, Blaustein MP: Ions, drugs and the axon membrane, *Ann NY Acad Sci* 137:967-981, 1966.
21. Wei LY: Role of surface dipoles on axon membrane, *Science* 163:280-282, 1969.
22. Lee AG: Model for action of local anesthetics, *Nature* 262:545-548, 1976.
23. Seeman P: The membrane actions of anesthetics and tranquilizers, *Pharmacol Rev* 24:583-655, 1972.
24. Strichartz GR, Ritchie JM: *The action of local anesthetics on ion channels of excitable tissues.* In Strichartz GR, editor: *Local anesthetics,* New York, 1987, Springer-Verlag.
25. Butterworth JF IV, Strichartz GR: Molecular mechanisms of local anesthesia: a review, *Anesthesiology* 72:711-734, 1990.
26. Ritchie JM: Mechanisms of action of local anesthetic agents and biotoxins, *Br J Anaesth* 47:191-198, 1975.
27. Rasminsky M: *Conduction in normal and pathological nerve fibers.* In Swash M, Kennard C, editors: *Scientific basis of clinical neurology,* Edinburgh, 1985, Churchill Livingstone.
28. Ritchie JM: *The distribution of sodium and potassium channels in mammalian myelinated nerve.* In Ritchie JM, Keyes RD, Bolis L, editors: *Ion channels in neural membranes,* New York, 1986, Alan R Liss.
29. Hille B, Courtney K, Dum R: *Rate and site of action of local anesthetics in myelinated nerve fibers.* In Fink BR, editor: *Molecular mechanisms of anesthesia,* New York, 1975, Raven Press, pp 13-20.
30. Setnikar I: Ionization of bases with limited solubility: investigation of substances with local anesthetic activity, *J Pharm Sci* 55:1190-1195, 1990.
31. Stewart JH, Chinn SE, Cole GW, Klein JA: Neutralized lidocaine with epinephrine for local anesthesia—II, *J Dermatol Surg Oncol* 16(9):842-845, 1990.
32. Bokesch PM, Raymond SA, Strichartz GR: Dependence of lidocaine potency on pH and pCO2, *Anesth Analg* 66.9-17, 1987.
33. Bieter RN: Applied pharmacology of local anesthetics, *Am J Surg* 34:500-510, 1936.
34. Buckley MM, Benfield P: Eutectic lidocaine/prilocaine cream: a review of the topical anaesthetic/analgesic efficacy of a eutectic mixture of local anaesthetics (EMLA), *Drugs* 46(1):126-151, 1993.
35. Campbell AH, Stasse JA, Lord GH, Willson JE: In vivo evaluation of local anesthetics applied topically, *J Pharm Sci* 57:2045-2048, 1968.
36. Noback CR, Demarest RJ: *The human nervous system: basic principles of neurobiology,* ed 3, New York, 1981, McGraw-Hill.
37. de Jong RH: *Local anesthetics,* ed 2, Springfield, Ill, 1977, Charles C Thomas, pp 66-68.
38. Ritchie JM, Ritchie B, Greengard P: The active structure of local anesthetics, *J Pharmacol Exp Ther* 150:152, 1965.
39. Tucker GT: Plasma binding and disposition of local anaesthetics, *Int Anesthesiol Clin* 13:33, 1975.
40. Cohen EN, Levine DA, Colliss JE, Gunther RE: The role of pH in the development of tachyphylaxis to local anesthetic agents, *Anesthesiology* 29:994-1001, 1968.

two

Pharmacology of Local Anesthetics

Local anesthetics, when used for the management of pain, differ from most other drugs commonly used in medicine and dentistry in one very important manner. Virtually all other drugs, regardless of the route through which they are administered, must ultimately enter into the circulatory system in sufficiently high concentrations (i.e., attain therapeutic blood levels) *before* they can begin to exert a clinical action. Local anesthetics, however, when used for pain control, *cease* to provide a clinical effect when they are absorbed from the site of administration into the circulation. One prime factor involved in the termination of action of local anesthetics used for pain control is their absorption into the cardiovascular system.

The presence of a local anesthetic in the circulatory system means that the drug will be carried to every cell in the body. Local anesthetics have the potential to produce an alteration in the functioning of many of these cells. In this chapter the actions of local anesthetics, other than their ability to block conduction in nerve axons of the peripheral nervous system, are reviewed. The following is a classification of local anesthetics:

Esters

Esters of benzoic acid:

    Butacaine

    Cocaine

    Ethyl aminobenzoate (benzocaine)

    Hexylcaine

    Piperocaine

    Tetracaine

Esters of para-aminobenzoic acid:

    Chloroprocaine

    Procaine

    Propoxycaine

Amides

Articaine

Bupivacaine

Dibucaine

Etidocaine

Lidocaine

Mepivacaine

Prilocaine

Quinoline

Centbucridine

PHARMACOKINETICS OF LOCAL ANESTHETICS

Uptake

When injected into soft tissues, local anesthetics exert a pharmacological action on the blood vessels in the area. All local anesthetics possess a degree of vasoactivity, most producing dilation of the vascular bed into which they are deposited, although the degree of vasodilation may vary, and some may produce vasoconstriction. To a slight degree these effects may be concentration dependent.[1] Relative vasodilating values of amide local anesthetics are shown in Table 2-1.

Ester local anesthetics are also potent vasodilating drugs. *Procaine* is probably the most potent vasodilator and is often used clinically for vasodilation when peripheral blood flow has been compromised due to (accidental) intraarterial (IA) injection of a drug (e.g., thiopental).[2] IA administration of an irritating drug such as thiopental may produce arteriospasm with an attendant decrease in tissue perfusion, which could lead, if prolonged, to tissue death, gangrene, and loss of the limb. In this situation procaine is administered IA in an attempt to break the arteriospasm and reestablish blood flow to the affected limb. *Tetracaine, chloroprocaine,* and *propoxycaine* also possess vasodilating properties to varying degrees but not to the degree of procaine.

Cocaine is the only local anesthetic that consistently produces vasoconstriction.[3] The initial action of cocaine is vasodilation, which is followed by an intense and prolonged vasoconstriction. It is produced by an inhibition of the uptake of catecholamines (especially norepinephrine) into tissue binding sites. This results in an excess of free norepinephrine, which leads to a prolonged and intense state of vasoconstriction. The property of inhibiting the reuptake of norepinephrine has not been demonstrated to occur with other local anesthetics, such as lidocaine and bupivacaine.

A significant clinical effect of vasodilation is an increase in the rate of absorption of the local anesthetic into the blood, thus decreasing the duration of pain control while increasing the anesthetic blood level and the potential for overdose. The rates at which local anesthetics are absorbed into the bloodstream and reach their peak blood level vary according to the route of administration:

Route	Time to peak level (min)
Intravenous	1
Topical	5 (approx)
Intramuscular	5-10
Subcutaneous	30-90

Oral Route

With the exception of cocaine, local anesthetic drugs are absorbed poorly, if at all, from the gastrointestinal tract following oral administration. Additionally, most local anesthetics (especially lidocaine) undergo a significant *hepatic first-pass effect* following oral administration. Following absorption of lidocaine from the gastrointestinal tract into the enterohepatic circulation, a fraction of the drug dose is carried to the liver, where approximately 72% of the dose is biotransformed into inactive metabolites.[4] This has seriously hampered the use of lidocaine as an oral antidysrhythmic drug. In November 1984, Astra Pharmaceuticals and Merck Sharp & Dohme introduced an analogue of lidocaine, tocainide hydrochloride, which is effective orally.[5] The chemical structures of tocainide and lidocaine are presented in Fig. 2-1.

Topical Route

Local anesthetics are absorbed at differing rates after application to mucous membranes: in the *tracheal mucosa,* uptake is almost as rapid as with intravenous (IV) administration (indeed, intratracheal drug administration [epinephrine, lidocaine, atropine, naloxone, and flumazenil] is used in certain emergency situations); in *the pharyngeal mucosa,* uptake is slower; and in the *esophageal* or *bladder mucosa,* uptake is even slower than occurs through the pharynx. Wherever there is no layer of intact skin present, local anesthetics exert their action following topical application. Sunburn remedies usually contain lidocaine, benzocaine, or other anesthetics in an ointment formulation. Applied to intact skin, they do not provide an anesthetic action, but with skin damaged by sunburn they bring rapid relief of pain. A

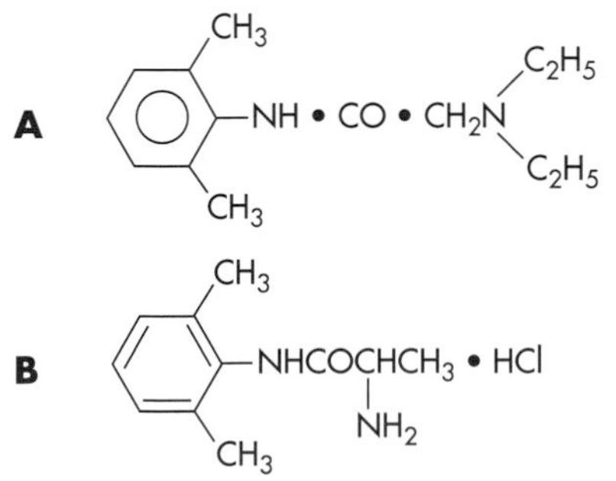

		Mean % increase in femoral artery blood flow in dogs after intraarterial injection*	
	Vasodilating activity	1 min	5 min
Articaine	1 (approx)	NA	NA
Bupivacaine	2.5	45.4	30
Etidocaine	2.5	44.3	26.6
Lidocaine	1	25.8	7.5
Mepivacaine	0.8	35.7	9.5
Prilocaine	0.5	42.1	6.3
Tetracaine	NA	37.6	14

TABLE 2-1 Relative Vasodilating Values of Amide-Type Local Anesthetics

Modified from Blair MR: Cardiovascular pharmacology of local anaesthetics, *Br J Anaesth* 47(suppl):247-252, 1975.
*Each agent injected rapidly in a dose of 1 mg/0.1 ml saline.
NA, Not available.

Fig. 2-1 Tocainide. **A,** Represents a modification of a lidocaine, **B,** that is able to pass through the liver after oral administration with minimal hepatic first-pass effect.

eutectic mixture of local anesthetics (EMLA) has been developed to provide surface anesthesia for intact skin.[6] (EMLA is discussed in Chapter 19.)

Injection

The rate of uptake (absorption) of local anesthetics after injection (subcutaneous, intramuscular, or IV) is related to both the vascularity of the injection site and the vasoactivity of the drug.

IV administration of local anesthetics provides the most rapid elevation of blood levels and is used in the primary treatment of ventricular dysrhythmias.[7] Rapid IV administration can lead to overly high local anesthetic blood levels, which can produce serious toxic reactions. The benefits to be gained from IV drug administration must always be weighed against the risks associated with IV administration. Only if the benefits clearly outweigh the risks should the drug be administered, as is the case with ventricular dysrhythmias such as premature ventricular contractions (PVCs).[8]

Distribution

Once absorbed into the blood, local anesthetics are distributed throughout the body to all tissues. Highly perfused organs (and areas) such as the brain, head, liver, kidneys, lungs, and spleen initially have higher blood levels of the anesthetic than do less highly perfused organs. Skeletal muscle, although not as highly perfused as these organs, contains the greatest percentage of local anesthetic of any tissue or organ in the body, since it makes up the largest mass of tissue in the body.

The level of a local anesthetic drug in the blood (in certain "target" organs) has a significant bearing on the potential toxicity of the drug. The blood level of the local anesthetic is influenced by the following factors:

1. Rate at which the drug is absorbed into the cardiovascular system
2. Rate of distribution of the drug from the vascular compartment to the tissues (more rapid in healthy patients than in those who are medically compromised [e.g., congestive heart failure], thus leading to lower blood levels in healthier patients)
3. Elimination of the drug through metabolic and/or excretory pathways

The latter two factors act to decrease the blood level of the local anesthetic.

The rate at which a local anesthetic is removed from the blood is described as the elimination half-life of the drug. Simply stated, the half-life is the time required for a 50% reduction in the blood level (one half-life = 50% reduction; two half-lives = 75% reduction; three half-lives = 87.5% reduction; four half-lives = 94% reduction; five half-lives = 97% reduction; six half-lives = 98.5% reduction).

Drug	Half-life (hr)
2-Chloroprocaine*	0.1
Procaine*	0.1
Tetracaine*	0.3
Cocaine*	0.7
Prilocaine†	1.6
Lidocaine†	1.6
Mepivacaine†	1.9
Articaine†	2.0
Etidocaine†	2.6
Bupivacaine†	3.5
Propoxycaine*	NA

*Ester.
†Amide.
NA, Not available.

All local anesthetics readily cross the blood-brain barrier. They also readily cross the placenta and enter the circulatory system of the developing fetus.

Metabolism (Biotransformation)

A significant difference between the two major classes of local anesthetics, the esters and the amides, is the means by which they undergo metabolic breakdown. Metabolism (or biotransformation) of local anesthetics is important, because the overall toxicity of a drug depends on a balance between its rate of absorption into the bloodstream at the site of injection and its rate of removal from the blood through the processes of tissue uptake and metabolism.

Ester Local Anesthetics

Ester local anesthetics are hydrolyzed in the plasma by the enzyme *pseudocholinesterase*.[9] The rate at which hydrolysis of different esters occurs varies considerably:

Drug	Rate of hydrolysis (µmol/ml/hr)
Chloroprocaine	4.7
Procaine	1.1
Tetracaine	0.3

The rate of hydrolysis has an impact on the potential toxicity of a local anesthetic. *Chloroprocaine,* the most rapidly hydrolyzed, is the least toxic, whereas *tetracaine,* hydrolyzed 16 times more slowly than chloroprocaine, has the greatest potential toxicity. Procaine undergoes hydrolysis to para-aminobenzoic acid (PABA), which is excreted unchanged in the urine, and to diethylamino alcohol, which undergoes further biotransformation prior to excretion (Fig. 2-2). *Allergic reactions* that occur in response to ester drugs are usually *not* related to the parent compound (e.g., procaine) but rather to PABA, which is a major metabolic product of ester local anesthetics.

Approximately 1 out of every 2800 persons has an *atypical form of pseudocholinesterase,* which causes an inability to hydrolyze ester local anesthetics and other

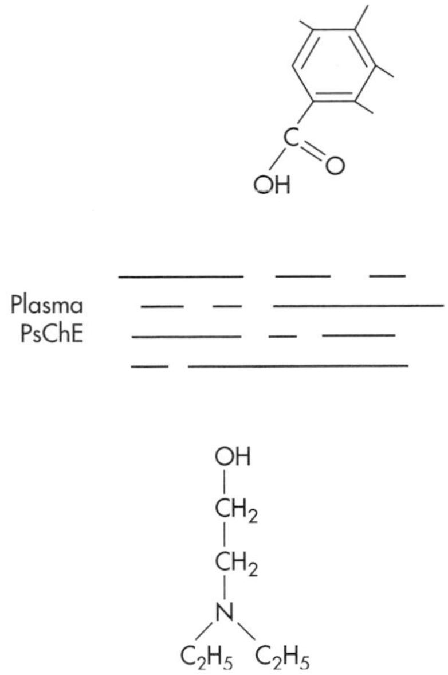

Fig. 2-2 Metabolic hydrolysis of procaine. *PsChE,* Pseudocholinesterase. *(From Tucker GT: Biotransformation and toxicity of local anesthetics,* Acta Anaesthesiol Belg *26(suppl):123, 1975.)*

chemically related drugs (e.g., succinylcholine).[10] Its presence leads to a prolongation of higher blood levels of the local anesthetic and an increased potential for toxicity.

Succinylcholine is a short-acting muscle relaxant employed frequently during the induction phase of general anesthesia. It produces respiratory arrest (apnea) for a period of approximately 2 to 3 minutes. Then plasma pseudocholinesterase hydrolyzes succinylcholine, blood levels fall, and spontaneous respiration resumes. Persons with atypical pseudocholinesterase are unable to hydrolyze succinylcholine at a normal rate; therefore the duration of apnea is prolonged. Atypical pseudocholinesterase is a *hereditary* trait. Any familial history of "difficulty" during general anesthesia should be carefully evaluated by the doctor prior to any dental care. A confirmed or strongly suspected history, in the patient or biological family, of atypical pseudocholinesterase represents a relative contraindication to the use of ester local anesthetics.

There are absolute and relative contraindications to drug administration. An *absolute contraindication* infers that under no circumstance should this drug be administered to this patient because the possibility of potentially toxic or lethal reactions is increased. A *relative contraindication* means that the drug in question may be administered to the patient after carefully weighing the risk of using the drug to its potential benefit, and if an acceptable alternative drug is not available. However, the smallest clinically effective dose should always be used. There is a *somewhat increased* possibility of adverse reaction to this drug in this patient.

TABLE 2-2 Lidocaine Disposition in Various Groups of Patients

Group	Half-life (hr)	Mean total body clearance (ml/kg/min)
Normal	1.8	10
Heart failure	1.9	6.3
Hepatic disease	4.9	6
Renal disease	1.3	13.7

Data from Thomson PD, et al: Lidocaine pharmacokinetics in advanced heart failure, liver disease, and renal failure in humans, *Ann Intern Med* 78:499-513, 1973.

Amide Local Anesthetics

The metabolism of the amide local anesthetics is more complex than that of the esters. The primary site of biotransformation of amide drugs is the *liver.* Virtually the entire metabolic process occurs in the liver for lidocaine, mepivacaine, articaine, etidocaine, and bupivacaine. *Prilocaine* undergoes primary metabolism in the liver, with some also possibly occurring in the lung.[11,12]

The rates of biotransformation of lidocaine, mepivacaine, articaine, etidocaine, and bupivacaine are quite similar. Prilocaine undergoes more rapid biotransformation than the other amides. Liver function and hepatic perfusion therefore significantly influence the rate of biotransformation of an amide local anesthetic. Approximately 70% of a dose of injected lidocaine undergoes biotransformation in patients with normal liver function.[4] Patients with lower than usual hepatic blood flow (hypotension, congestive heart failure) or poor liver function (cirrhosis) are unable to biotransform amide local anesthetics at a normal rate.[13,14] This slower than normal biotransformation rate leads to increased anesthetic blood levels and potentially increased toxicity. Significant liver dysfunction (ASA IV to VI) or heart failure (ASA IV to VI) represent a *relative contraindication* to the administration of amide local anesthetic drugs (Table 2-2).

The biotransformation products of certain local anesthetics are capable of producing significant clinical activity if permitted to accumulate in the blood. This is seen in renal or cardiac failure and during periods of prolonged drug administration. A clinical example is the production of *methemoglobinemia* in patients receiving large doses of prilocaine or articaine.[15,16] Prilocaine, the parent compound, cannot produce methemoglobinemia; but orthotoluidine, a primary metabolite of prilocaine, does induce the formation of methemoglobin, which is responsible for methemoglobinemia. If methemoglobin blood levels become elevated, clinical signs and symptoms will be observed. This is discussed more fully in Chapter 10. Another example of pharmacologically active metabolites is the sedative effect occasionally

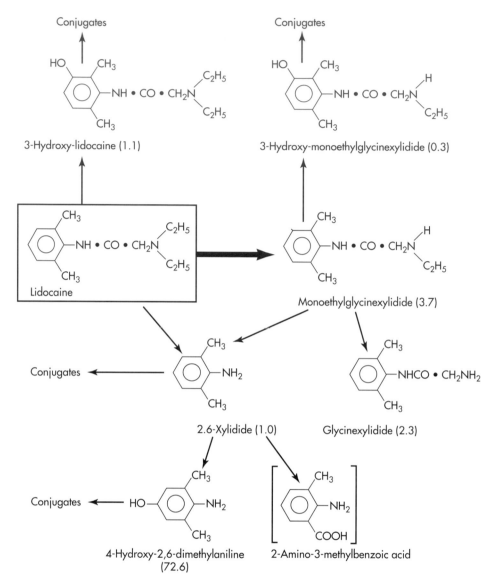

Fig. 2-3 Metabolic pathways of lidocaine. Percentages of dose found in urine are indicated in parentheses. *(From Cousins JM, Bridenbaugh PO, editors:* Neural blockade, *Philadelphia, 1980, JB Lippincott.)*

observed following lidocaine administration. Lidocaine does not produce sedation; however, two metabolites—monoethylglycinexylidide and glycinexylidide—are currently thought to be responsible for this clinical action.[17]

The metabolic pathways of lidocaine and prilocaine are shown in Figs. 2-3 and 2-4.

Excretion

The kidneys are the primary excretory organ for both the local anesthetic and its metabolites. A percentage of a given dose of local anesthetic drug will be excreted unchanged in the urine. This percentage varies according to the drug. *Esters* appear in only very small concentrations as the parent compound in the urine. This is

because they are hydrolyzed almost completely in the plasma. Procaine appears in the urine as PABA (90%) and 2% unchanged. Ten percent of a cocaine dose is found in the urine unchanged. *Amides* are usually present in the urine as the parent compound in a greater percentage than are esters, primarily because of their more complex process of biotransformation. Though the percentages of parent drug found in urine vary from study to study, less than 3% lidocaine, 1% mepivacaine, and 1% etidocaine are found unchanged in the urine.

Patients with *significant renal impairment* may be unable to eliminate the parent local anesthetic compound or its major metabolites from the blood, resulting in slightly elevated blood levels and an increased poten-

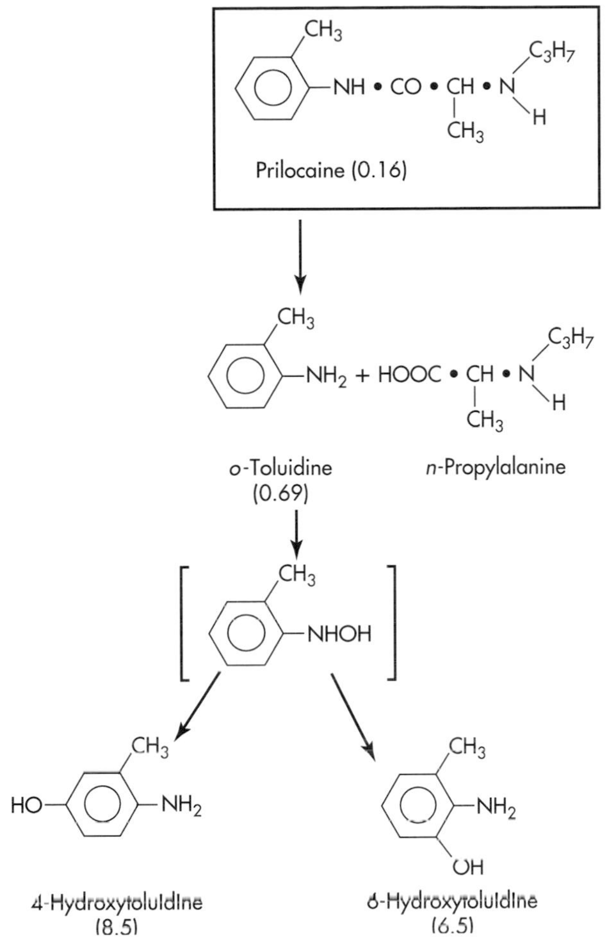

Fig. 2-4 Metabolic pathways of prilocaine. Percentages of dose found in urine are indicated in parentheses. *(From Ackerman B, Astrom A, Ross S, et al: Studies on the absorption, distribution, and metabolism of labelled prilocaine and lidocaine in some animal species,* Acta Pharmacol [Kobenhavn] *24:389-403, 1966.)*

tial for toxicity. This may occur with either the esters or the amides and is especially likely with cocaine. Thus significant renal disease (ASA IV to VI) represents a *relative contraindication* to the administration of local anesthetics. This includes patients undergoing renal dialysis and those with chronic glomerulonephritis and/or pyelonephritis.

SYSTEMIC ACTIONS OF LOCAL ANESTHETICS

Local anesthetics are chemicals that reversibly block action potentials in all excitable membranes. The central nervous system (CNS) and the cardiovascular system (CVS) are therefore especially susceptible to their actions. Most of the systemic actions of local anesthetics are related to their *blood* or *plasma* level. The higher the level, the greater will be the clinical action.

Centbucridine (a quinoline derivative), has proved to be 5 to 8 times as potent a local anesthetic as lidocaine, with an equally rapid onset of action as well as an equivalent duration.[18,19] Of potentially great importance is the finding that it does not affect the CNS or CVS adversely except in very high doses. (Centbucridine is discussed more fully in Chapter 19.)

Local anesthetics are absorbed from their site of administration into the circulatory system, which effectively dilutes them and carries them to all cells of the body. The blood level of the anesthetic depends on its rate of uptake from its site of administration *into* the circulatory system (increasing the blood level) and on the rates of distribution in tissue and biotransformation (in the liver), which remove the drug *from* the blood (decreasing the blood level).

Central Nervous System

Local anesthetics readily cross the blood-brain barrier. Their pharmacological action on the CNS is depression. At low (therapeutic, nontoxic) blood levels, there are no CNS effects of any significance. At higher (toxic, overdose) levels, the primary clinical manifestation is a generalized tonic-clonic convulsive episode. Between these two extremes there exists a spectrum of other clinical signs and symptoms. (See "Preconvulsive signs and symptoms," on the next page.)

Anticonvulsant Properties

Some local anesthetics (procaine, lidocaine, mepivacaine, prilocaine, and even cocaine) have demonstrated *anticonvulsant* properties.[20,21] These occur at a blood level considerably *below* that at which the same drugs produce seizure activity. Values for anticonvulsive blood levels of lidocaine follow[22]:

Clinical situation	Blood level
Anticonvulsive level	0.5 to 4 µg/ml
Preseizure signs and symptoms	4.5 to 7 µg/ml
Tonic-clonic seizure	>7.5 µg/ml

Procaine, mepivacaine, and lidocaine have been used intravenously to terminate or decrease the duration of both grand mal and petit mal seizures.[20,23] The anticonvulsant blood level of lidocaine (about 1 to 4.5 µg/ml) is very close to its cardiotherapeutic range (see the following material). It has been demonstrated to be effective in temporarily arresting seizure activity in a majority of human epileptics.[24] It was especially effective in interrupting status epilepticus at therapeutic doses of 2 to 3 mg/kg given at a rate of 40 to 50 mg/min.

Mechanism of anticonvulsant properties Epileptic patients possess hyperexcitable cortical neurons at a site within the brain where the convulsive episode originates (epileptic focus). Local anesthetics, by their depressant actions on the CNS, raise the seizure threshold by decreasing the excitability of these neurons, thereby preventing or terminating seizures.

Preconvulsive Signs and Symptoms

With a further increase in the blood level of a local anesthetic above its "therapeutic" value, adverse actions may be observed. Because the CNS is much more susceptible to the actions of local anesthetics than other systems, it is not surprising that the initial clinical signs and symptoms of overdose (toxicity) are CNS in origin. With lidocaine this second phase is observed at a level between 4.5 and 7 μg/ml in the average normal healthy patient.* Initial clinical signs and symptoms of CNS toxicity are usually *excitatory* in nature:

Signs (objectively observable)	Symptoms (subjectively felt)
Slurred speech	Numbness of tongue and circumoral region
Shivering	Warm, flushed feeling of skin
Muscular twitching	Pleasant dreamlike state
Tremor in muscles of face and distal extremities	Generalized light-headedness
	Dizziness
	Visual disturbances (inability to focus)
	Auditory disturbance (tinnitus)
	Drowsiness
	Disorientation

These clinical signs and symptoms are all related to the direct depressant action of the local anesthetic on the CNS, except for the sensation of circumoral and lingual numbness. Numbness of the tongue and circumoral regions is *not* caused by the CNS effects of the local anesthetic drug.[25] Rather it is the result of a direct anesthetic action of the drug, which is present in high concentrations in these highly vascularized tissues, on free nerve endings. The anesthetic has been transported to these tissues by the CVS. A dentist might have difficulty conceptualizing why anesthesia of the tongue is considered to be a sign of a toxic reaction when lingual anesthesia is commonly produced following mandibular nerve blocks. Consider for a moment a physician administering a local anesthetic into the patient's foot. Overly high blood levels would produce a *bilateral* numbness of the tongue, as contrasted to the usual *unilateral* anesthesia seen following dental nerve blocks.

Lidocaine and procaine differ somewhat from other local anesthetic drugs in that the usual progression of signs and symptoms just noted may *not* be seen. Lidocaine

and procaine frequently produce an initial *mild sedation* or *drowsiness* (more common with lidocaine).[26]

Sedation may develop *in place of* the excitatory signs. If either excitation or sedation is observed in the initial 5 to 10 minutes following the intraoral administration of a local anesthetic, it should serve as a warning to the clinician of a rising local anesthetic blood level and the possibility (if the blood level continues to rise) of a more serious reaction, possibly leading to a generalized convulsive episode.

Convulsive Phase

Further elevation of the local anesthetic blood level produces clinical signs and symptoms consistent with a generalized tonic-clonic convulsive episode. The duration of seizure activity is related to the local anesthetic level in the blood and inversely related to the arterial P_{CO_2} level.[27] At a normal P_{CO_2} a lidocaine blood level between 7.5 and 10 μg/ml will usually result in a convulsive episode. Where CO_2 levels are increased, the amount of local anesthetic necessary for seizures will be decreased while the duration of the seizure will be increased.[27] Seizure activity is generally self-limiting, since cardiovascular activity usually is not significantly impaired and biotransformation and redistribution of the local anesthetic continue throughout the episode. This results in a decrease of the anesthetic blood level and termination of seizure activity.

However, several other mechanisms are also at work that unfortunately act to prolong the convulsive episode. Both cerebral blood flow and cerebral metabolism increase during local anesthetic-induced convulsions. *Increased blood flow* to the brain leads to an increase in the volume of local anesthetic delivered to the brain, tending to prolong the seizure. *Increased cerebral metabolism* leads to a progressive metabolic acidosis as the seizure continues, and this tends to *prolong* the seizure activity (by *lowering* the blood level of anesthetic required to provoke a seizure), even in the presence of a declining local anesthetic level in the blood. As noted in Tables 2-3 and 2-4, the dose of local anesthetic required to induce seizures is markedly diminished in the presence of hypercarbia (Table 2-3) and/or acidosis (Table 2-4).[27,28]

Further increases in local anesthetic blood level result in a cessation of seizure activity. Electroencephalographic (EEG) tracings become flattened, indicating a generalized CNS depression. Respiratory depression occurs at this time, leading eventually to respiratory arrest if the anesthetic blood levels continue to rise. Respiratory effects are a result of the depressant action of the local anesthetic drug on the CNS.

Mechanism of preconvulsant and convulsant actions   It is known that local anesthetics exert a *depressant* action on excitable membranes, yet the pri-

---

*Individual variation in response to drugs, as depicted in the normal distribution curve, may produce clinical symptoms at levels lower than these (in hyperresponders) or may fail to produce them at higher levels (in hyporesponders).

TABLE 2-3 Effects of P_{CO_2} on the Convulsive Threshold (CD_{100}) of Various Local Anesthetics in Cats

Agent	CD_{100} (mg/kg)		Percent change in CD_{100}
	P_{CO_2} (25-40 torr)	P_{CO_2} (65-81 torr)	
Procaine	35	17	51
Mepivacaine	18	10	44
Prilocaine	22	12	45
Lidocaine	15	7	53
Bupivacaine	5	2.5	50

Data from Englesson S, Grevsten S, Olin A: Some numerical methods of estimating acid-base variables in normal human blood with a haemoglobin concentration of 5 g-100 cm³, *Scand J Lab Clin Invest* 32:289-295, 1973.

TABLE 2-4 Convulsant Dose (CD_{100}) and Acid-Base Status*

	pH 7.10	pH 7.20	pH 7.30	pH 7.40
P_{CO_2} 30	—	—	27.5	26.6
P_{CO_2} 40	—	20.6	21.4	22.0
P_{CO_2} 60	13.1	15.4	17.5	—
P_{CO_2} 80	11.3	14.3	—	—

From Englesson S: The influence of acid-base changes on central nervous toxicity of local anaesthetic agents, *Acta Anaesth Scand* 18:88-103, 1974.
*Intravenous lidocaine 5 mg/kg/min, cats; doses in mg/kg.

mary clinical manifestation associated with high local anesthetic blood levels is related to varying degrees of CNS *stimulation.* How can a drug that is primarily a CNS depressant be responsible for the production of varying degrees of CNS stimulation, including tonic-clonic seizure activity? It is thought that local anesthetics produce clinical signs and symptoms of CNS excitation (including convulsions) through a selective blockade of inhibitory pathways in the cerebral cortex.[29-31] de Jong states that "inhibition of inhibition thus is a presynaptic event that follows local anesthetic blockade of impulses traveling along inhibitory pathways."[32]

The cerebral cortex has pathways of neurons that are essentially inhibitory and others that are facilitory (excitatory). A state of balance is normally maintained between the degrees of effect exerted by these neuronal paths (Fig. 2-5). At *preconvulsant* anesthetic blood levels, the observed clinical signs and symptoms are produced because the local anesthetic selectively *depresses* the action of inhibitory neurons (Fig. 2-6). The state of balance is then tipped slightly in favor of excessive facilitory (excitatory) input, leading to the feeling of tremor and slight agitation.

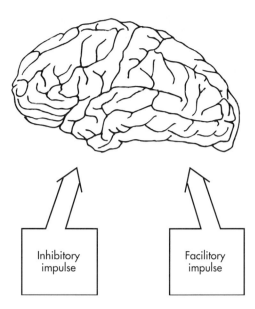

Fig. 2-5 Balance between inhibitory and facilitory impulses in a normal cerebral cortex.

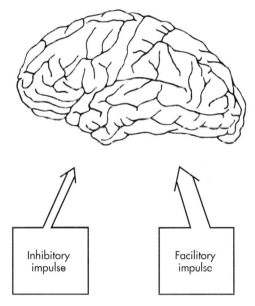

Fig. 2-6 In the preconvulsive stage of local anesthetic action, the inhibitory impulse is more profoundly depressed than the facilitory impulse.

At higher *(convulsive)* blood levels the inhibitory neuron function is entirely depressed, allowing facilitory neurons to function unopposed (Fig. 2-7). Pure facilitory input without inhibition produces the tonic-clonic activity observed at these levels.

Further increases in anesthetic blood level lead to depression of the facilitory as well as the inhibitory pathways, producing generalized CNS depression (Fig. 2-8).

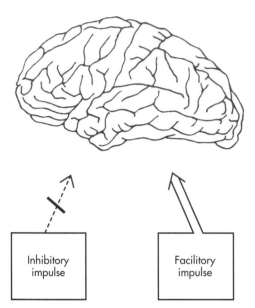

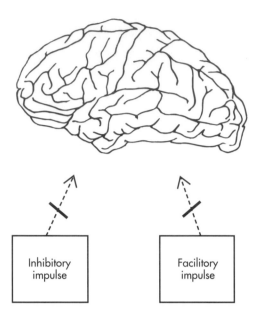

Fig. 2-7 In the convulsive stage of local anesthetic action, the inhibitory impulse is totally depressed, permitting unopposed facilitory impulse activity.

Fig. 2-8 In the final stage of local anesthetic action, both inhibitory and facilitory impulses are totally depressed, producing generalized CNS depression.

The precise site of action of the local anesthetic within the CNS is not known but is thought to be either at the inhibitory cortical synapses or directly on the inhibitory cortical neurons.

Analgesia

There is a second action that local anesthetics possess in relation to the CNS. Administered intravenously, they increase the pain reaction threshold and also produce a degree of analgesia.

In the 1940s and 1950s procaine was administered intravenously for the management of chronic pain and arthritis.[33] The *procaine unit* was commonly used for this purpose; it consisted of 4 mg/kg of body weight administered over 20 minutes. The technique was ineffective for acute pain. Because of the relatively narrow safety margin between procaine's analgesic actions and the occurrence of signs and symptoms of overdose, this technique is rarely used today.

Mood Elevation

The use of local anesthetic drugs for mood elevation and for rejuvenation has persisted for centuries, despite documenation of both catastrophic events (mood elevation) and a lack of effect (rejuvenation).

Cocaine has long been used for both its euphoria-inducing and fatigue-lessening actions, dating back to the chewing of coca leaves by Incans and other South American natives.[34,35] Unfortunately, as is well known today, the prolonged use of cocaine leads to habituation. William Halsted, the father of American surgery, cocaine researcher, and the first person to administer a local anes-

thetic nerve block, suffered greatly because of an addiction to cocaine.[36] In more modern times the sudden, unexpected deaths of several prominent athletes due to cocaine, and the addiction of many others, clearly demonstrate the dangers involved in the casual use of potent drugs.

More benign, but totally unsubstantiated, is the use of procaine (Novocain) as a rejuvenating drug. Clinics professing to "restore youthful vigor" claim that procaine is a literal Fountain of Youth. These clinics operate primarily in central Europe and Mexico, where procaine is used under the proprietary name "Gerovital." de Jong states that "whatever the retarding effect on aging, it probably is relegated most charitably to mood elevation."[37]

Cardiovascular System

Local anesthetic drugs have a *direct* action on the myocardium and peripheral vasculature. In general, however, the cardiovascular system appears to be more resistant to the effects of local anesthetic drugs than is the CNS[38] (Table 2-5).

Direct Actions on the Myocardium

Local anesthetics modify electrophysiological events in the myocardium in a manner similar to their actions on peripheral nerves. As the anesthetic blood level increases, the rate of rise of various phases of myocardial depolarization is reduced. There is no significant change in resting membrane potential, and no significant prolongation of the phases of repolarization.[39]

Local anesthetics produce a *depression* of the myocardium related to the anesthetic level in the blood.

Local anesthetic drug action decreases electrical excitability of the myocardium, decreases the conduction rate, and decreases the force of contraction.[40-42]

Therapeutic advantage is taken of this depressant action in managing the hyperexcitable myocardium, which manifests itself as various cardiac dysrhythmias. Although many local anesthetics have demonstrated antidysrhythmic actions in animals, only *procaine* and *lidocaine* have gained significant clinical reliability in humans. Lidocaine is the most widely used and intensively studied local anesthetic in this regard.[8,26,43,44] *Procainamide* is the procaine molecule with an amide linkage replacing the ester linkage. Because of this it is hydrolyzed much more slowly than procaine.[45] Tocainide, a chemical analogue of lidocaine, was introduced in 1984 as an oral antidysrhythmic drug since lidocaine is ineffective following oral administration.[46] Tocainide is also effective in ventricular dysrhythmias but is associated with a 40% incidence of adverse effects including nausea, vomiting, tremor, paresthesias, agranulocytosis, and pulmonary fibrosis.[47,48] Tocainide worsens symptoms of congestive heart failure in about 5% of patients and may provoke dysrhythmias (is prodysrhythmic) in from 1% to 8%.[49]

Levels of lidocaine in the blood that normally occur following intraoral injection of one or two dental cartridges (0.5 to 2 μg/ml) are not associated with cardiodepressant activity. Increasing lidocaine blood levels slightly is still nontoxic and is associated with antidysrhythmic actions. Therapeutic blood levels of lidocaine for antidysrhythmic activity range from 1.8 to 6 μg/ml.[50,51]

Lidocaine is usually administered intravenously in a bolus of 50 to 100 mg at a rate of 25 to 50 mg/min. This dose is based on 1 mg/kg of body weight and frequently is followed by a continuous IV infusion of 2 to 4 mg/min. Signs and symptoms of local anesthetic overdose will be noted if the blood level rises beyond 6 μg/ml of blood.[50]

Lidocaine is used clinically primarily in the management of PVCs and ventricular tachycardia. It is also used as a fundamental drug in advanced cardiac life support and in managing cardiac arrest caused by ventricular fibrillation.[52]

Direct cardiac actions of local anesthetics at blood levels greater than the therapeutic (antidysrhythmic) level include a decrease in myocardial contractility and decreased cardiac output, both of which lead to circulatory collapse (Table 2-5).

Table 2-6 summarizes the CNS and cardiovascular effects of increasing local anesthetic blood levels.

T A B L E   2 - 5   Intravenous Dose of Local Anesthetic Agents Required for Convulsive Activity (CD_{100}) and Irreversible Cardiovascular Collapse (LD_{100}) in Dogs

Agent	CD_{100} (mg/kg)	LD_{100} (mg/kg)	LD_{100}/CD_{100} ratio
Lidocaine	22	76	3.5
Etidocaine	8	40	5.0
Bupivacaine	4	20	5.0
Tetracaine	5	27	5.4

Data from Liu P, et al: Acute cardiovascular toxicity of intravenous amide local anesthetics in anesthetized ventilated dogs, *Anesth Analg* 61:317-322, 1982.

T A B L E   2 - 6   Clinical Manifestations of Local Anesthetic Overdose

Signs	Symptoms
Low to moderate overdose levels	
Confusion	Headache
Talkativeness	Lightheadedness
Apprehension	Dizziness
Excitedness	Blurred vision, unable to focus
Slurred speech	Ringing in ears
Generalized stutter	Numbness of tongue and perioral tissues
Muscular twitching and tremor of the face and extremities	Flushed or chilled feeling
Nystagmus	Drowsiness
Elevated blood pressure	Disorientation
Elevated heart rate	Loss of consciousness
Elevated respiratory rate	
Moderate to high blood levels	
Generalized tonic-clonic seizure, followed by:	
Generalized CNS depression	
Depressed blood pressure, heart rate, and respiratory rate	

From Malamed SF: *Medical emergencies in the dental office*, ed 4, St Louis, 1993, Mosby–Year Book.

Direct Action on the Peripheral Vasculature

Cocaine is the only local anesthetic drug that consistently produces *vasoconstriction* at commonly employed dosages.[3] Ropivacaine causes cutaneous vasoconstriction, whereas its congener bupivacaine produces vasodilation.[53] All other local anesthetics produce a peripheral *vasodilation,* through relaxation of the smooth muscle in the walls of blood vessels. This results in an increased blood flow to and from the site of local anesthetic deposition (Table 2-1). The increase in local blood flow increases the rate of drug absorption, which in turn leads to a decreased duration of local anesthetic action, increased bleeding in the treatment area, and increased local anesthetic blood levels (with a greater possibility of toxicity).

Table 2-7 provides examples of peak blood levels achieved following local anesthetic injection with and without the presence of a vasopressor.[53-55]

The primary effect of local anesthetics on blood pressure is *hypotension.* Procaine produces hypotension more frequently and to a more profound degree than does lidocaine; 50% of patients in one study receiving procaine became hypotensive, compared with 6% of those receiving lidocaine.[57] This action is produced by direct depression of the myocardium and smooth muscle relaxation in the vessel walls by the local anesthetic.

In summary, negative effects on the cardiovascular system are not noted until significantly elevated local anesthetic blood levels are reached. The usual sequence of local anesthetic–induced actions on the cardiovascular system is as follows:

At *nonoverdose levels* there is a slight increase or no change in blood pressure because of increased cardiac output and heart rate, as a result of enhanced sympathetic activity; and there is direct vasoconstriction of certain peripheral vascular beds.

At *levels approaching, yet still below, overdose level* a mild degree of hypotension is noted; this is produced by a direct relaxant action on the vascular smooth muscle.

At *overdose levels* there is profound hypotension caused by decreased myocardial contractility, decreased cardiac output, and decreased peripheral resistance.

At *lethal levels* cardiovascular collapse is noted. This is caused by massive peripheral vasodilation, decreased myocardial contractility, and decreased heart rate (sinus bradycardia).

Certain local anesthetics such as bupivacaine (and to a lesser degree ropivacaine and etidocaine) may precipitate potentially fatal ventricular fibrillation.[58,59]

Local Tissue Toxicity

Skeletal muscle appears to be more sensitive to the local irritant properties of local anesthetics than other tissues. Intramuscular and intraoral injection of lidocaine, mepivacaine, prilocaine, bupivacaine, and etidocaine can produce skeletal muscle alterations.[60-63] It appears that the longer-acting local anesthetics cause more localized skeletal muscle damage than shorter-acting drugs. The changes occurring in skeletal muscle are reversible, with muscle regeneration being complete within 2 weeks following local anesthetic administration. These muscle changes have not been associated with any overt clinical signs of local irritation.

Respiratory System

Local anesthetic drugs exert a dual effect on respiration. At nonoverdose levels they have a direct relaxant action on bronchial smooth muscle; at overdose levels they may produce respiratory arrest as a result of generalized CNS depression. In general, respiratory function is unaffected

TABLE 2-7 Peak Plasma Levels following Local Anesthetic Administration with and without Vasopressor

Injection site	Anesthetic	Dose (mg)	Epinephrine dilution	Peak level (µg/ml)
Infiltration	Lidocaine	400	None	2.0
Infiltration	Lidocaine	400	1:200,000	1.0
Intercostal	Lidocaine	400	None	6.5
Intercostal	Lidocaine	400	1:200,000	5.3
Intercostal	Lidocaine	400	1:80,000	4.9
Infiltration	Mepivacaine	5 mg/kg	None	1.2
Infiltration	Mepivacaine	5 mg/kg	1:200,000	0.7

Data from Kopacz DJ, Carpenter RL, MacKay DL: Effect of ropivacaine on cutaneous capillary flow in pigs, *Anesthesiology* 71:69, 1989; Scott DB, et al: Factors affecting plasma levels of lignocaine and prilocaine, *Br J Anaesth* 44:1040-1049, 1972; Duhner KG, et al: Blood levels of mepivacaine after regional anaesthesia, *Br J Anaesth* 37:746-752, 1965.

by local anesthetic drugs until near overdose levels are achieved.

Miscellaneous Actions

Neuromuscular Blockade

Many local anesthetics have been demonstrated to block neuromuscular transmission in humans. This is a result of the inhibition of sodium diffusion through a blockade of sodium channels in the cell membrane. This action is normally slight and usually clinically insignificant. On occasion, however, it can be additive to that produced by both depolarizing (e.g., succinylcholine) and nondepolarizing (e.g., curare) muscle relaxants, and this may lead to abnormally prolonged periods of muscle paralysis. Such actions are unlikely to occur in the dental outpatient.

Drug Interactions

In general, CNS depressants (e.g., opioids, antianxiety drugs, phenothiazines, and barbiturates), when administered in conjunction with local anesthetics, lead to potentiation of the CNS-depressant actions of the local anesthetic. The conjoint use of local anesthetics and drugs that share a common metabolic pathway can produce adverse reactions. Both ester local anesthetics and the depolarizing muscle relaxant succinylcholine require plasma pseudocholinesterase for hydrolysis. Prolonged apnea may result from the concomitant use of these drugs.

Drugs that induce the production of hepatic microsomal enzymes (e.g., barbiturates) may alter the rate at which amide local anesthetics are metabolized. Increased hepatic microsomal enzyme induction will *increase* the rate of metabolism of the local anesthetic.

Malignant Hyperthermia

Malignant hyperthermia (MH; hyperpyrexia) is a pharmacogenic disorder in which a genetic variant in the individual alters that person's response to certain drugs. Acute clinical manifestations of MH include tachycardia, tachypnea, unstable blood pressure, cyanosis, respiratory and metabolic acidosis, fever (as high as 108° F [42° C] or more), muscle rigidity, and death. Mortality ranges from 63% to 73%. Many commonly used anesthetic drugs can trigger MH in certain individuals.

Until recently the amide local anesthetics were thought to be capable of provoking MH and were considered to be absolutely contraindicated in MH-susceptible patients.[64] Information from the Malignant Hyperthermia Association of the United States, however, has raised considerable doubt about this.[65,66] The presence of MH is considered today a *relative contraindication* to local anesthetic administration. Ester local anesthetics may be administered with no increase in risk when a familial history of MH is known. These include

procaine/propoxycaine, tetracaine, and chloroprocaine. MH is discussed in some detail in Chapter 10.

REFERENCES

1. Aps C, Reynolds F: The effect of concentration in vasoactivity of bupivacaine and lignocaine, *Br J Anaesth* 48:1171-1174, 1976.
2. Kao FF, Jalar UH: The central action of lignocaine and its effects on cardiac output, *Br J Pharmacol* 14:522-526, 1959.
3. MacMillan WH: A hypothesis concerning the effect of cocaine on the action of sympathomimetic amines, *Br J Pharmacol* 14:385, 1959.
4. Arthur GR: *Pharmacokinetics of local anesthetics.* In Strichartz GR, editor: *Local anesthetics: handbook of experimental pharmacology,* vol 81, Berlin, 1987, Springer-Verlag.
5. Hohnloser SH, Lange HW, Raeder E, et al: Short- and long-term therapy with tocainide for malignant ventricular tachyarrhythmias, *Circulation* 73:143, 1986.
6. Soliman IE, Broadman LM, Hannallah RS, et al: Comparison of the analgesic effects of EMLA (eutectic mixture of local anesthetics) to intradermal lidocaine infiltration prior to venous cannulation in unpremedicated children, *Anesthesiology* 68:804, 1988.
7. Standards and guidelines for cardiopulmonary resuscitation (CPR) and emergency cardiac care (ECC), *JAMA* 255:2905-2989, 1986.
8. Collingsworth KA, Kalman SM, Harrison DC: The clinical pharmacology of lidocaine as an anti-arrhythmic drug, *Circulation* 50:1217-1230, 1974.
9. Kalow W: Hydrolysis of local anesthetics by human serum cholinesterase, *J Pharmacol Exp Ther* 104:122-134, 1952.
10. Foldes FF, Foldes VM, Smith JC, et al: The relation between plasma cholinesterase and prolonged apnea caused by succinylcholine, *Anesthesiology* 24:208-216, 1963.
11. Harris WH, Cole DW, Mital M, Laver MB: Methemoglobin formation and oxygen transport following intravenous regional anesthesia using prilocaine, *Anesthesiology* 29:65, 1968.
12. Arthur GR: *Distribution and elimination of local anesthetic agents: the role of the lung, liver, and kidneys,* PhD thesis, Edinburgh, 1981, University of Edinburgh.
13. Nation RL, Triggs EJ: Lidocaine kinetics in cardiac patients and aged subjects, *Br J Clin Pharmacol* 4:439-448, 1977.
14. Thompson P, Melmon K, Richardson J, et al: Lidocaine pharmacokinetics in advanced heart failure, liver disease, and renal failure in humans, *Ann Intern Med* 78:499, 1973.
15. Prilocaine-induced methemoglobinemia—Wisconsin, 1993, *MMWR Morb Mortal Wkly Rep* 43(35):655-657, 1994.
16. Daly DJ, Davenport J, Newland MC: Methemoglobinemia following the use of prilocaine, *Br J Anaesth* 36:737-739, 1964.
17. Strong JM, Parker M, Atkinson AJ Jr: Identification of glycinexylidide in patients treated with intravenous lidocaine, *Clin Pharmacol Ther* 14:67-72, 1973.
18. Gupta PP, Tangri AN, Saxena RC, Dhawan BN: Clinical pharmacology studies on 4-N-butylamino-1,2,3,4,-tetrahydroacridine hydrochloride (centbucridine), a new local anaesthetic agent, *Indian J Exp Biol* 20:344-346, 1982.
19. Vacharajani GN, Parikh N, Paul T, Satoskar RS: A comparative study of centbucridine and lidocaine in dental extraction, *Int J Clin Pharmacol Res* 3:251-255, 1983.
20. Bernhard CG, Bohm E: *Local anaesthetics as anticonvulsants: a study on experimental and clinical epilepsy,* Stockholm, 1965, Almqvist & Wiksell.
21. Bernhard CG, Bohm E, Wiesel T: On the evaluation of the anticonvulsive effect of different local anesthetics, *Arch Int Pharmacodyn Ther* 108:392-407, 1956.
22. Julien RM: Lidocaine in experiental epilepsy: correlation of anticonvulsant effect with blood concentrations, *Electroencephalogr Clin Neurophysiol* 34:639-645, 1973.

23. Berry CA, Sanner JH, Keasling HH: A comparison of the anticonvulsant activity of mepivacaine and lidocaine, *J Pharmacol Exp Ther* 133:357-363, 1961.

24. Bohm E, Flodmark S, Petersen I: Effect of lidocaine (Xylocaine) on seizure and interseizure electroencephalograms in epileptics, *Arch Neurol Psychiat* 81:550-556, 1959.

25. Adriani J: The clinical pharmacology of local anesthetics, *Clin Pharmacol Ther* 1:645-673, 1960.

26. Lie KI, Wellens HJ, van Capelle FJ, Durrer D: Lidocaine in the prevention of primary ventricular fibrillation: a double-blind, randomized study of 212 consecutive patients, *N Engl J Med* 291:1324-1326, 1974.

27. Englesson S: The influence of acid-base changes on central nervous system toxicity of local anesthetic agents. I. An experimental study in cats, *Acta Anaesthesiol Scand* 18:79, 1974.

28. Englesson S, Grevsten S, Olin A: Some numerical methods of estimating acid-base variables in normal human blood with a haemoglobin concentration of 5g-100cm^3, *Scand J Lab Clin Invest* 32:289-295, 1973.

29. de Jong RH, Robles R, Corbin RW: Central actions of lidocaine—synaptic transmission, *Anesthesiology* 30:19, 1969.

30. Huffman RD, Yim GKW: Effects of diphenylaminoethanol and lidocaine on central inhibition, *Int J Neuropharmacol* 8:217, 1969.

31. Tanaka K, Yamasaki M: Blocking of cortical inhibitory synapses by intravenous lidocaine, *Nature* 209:207, 1966.

32. de Jong RH: *Local anesthetics,* ed 2, Springfield, Ill, 1977, Charles C Thomas, p 102.

33. Graubard DJ, Peterson MC: *Clinical uses of intravenous procaine,* Springfield, Ill, 1950, Charles C Thomas.

34. Garcilasso de la Vega: *Commentarios reales de los Incas.* 1609-1617. In Freud S: *Uber Coca,* Wien, 1884, Verlag von Moritz Perles.

35. *Disertacion sobre el aspecto, cultivo, comercio y virtudes de la famosa planta del Peru nombrado Coca. Lima, 1794.* In Freud S: *Uber Coca,* Wien, 1884, Verlag von Moritz Perles.

36. Olch PD, William S: Halsted and local anesthesia: contributions and complications, *Anesthesiology* 42:479-486, 1975.

37. de Jong RH: *Local anesthetics,* ed 2, Springfield, Ill, 1977, Charles C Thomas, p 89.

38. Scott DB: Toxicity caused by local anaesthetic drugs, *Br J Anaesth* 53:553-554, 1981.

39. Gettes LS: Physiology and pharmacology of antiarrhythmic drugs, *Hosp Pract* 16:89, 1981.

40. Block A, Covino BG: Effect of local anesthetic agents on cardiac conduction and contractility, *Reg Anesth* 6:55, 1982.

41. Feldman HS, Covino BM, Sage DJ: Direct chronotropic and inotropic effects of local anesthetic agents in isolated guinea pig atria, *Reg Anesth* 7:149, 1982.

42. Harrison DC, Sprouse JH, Morrow AG: The antiarrhythmic properties of lidocaine and procaine amide: clinical and physiologic studies of their cardiovascular effects in man, *Circulation* 28:486, 1963.

43. Kupersmith J, Antman EM, Hoffman BF: In vivo electrophysiologic effects of lidocaine in canine acute myocardial ischemia, *Am Heart J* 97:360-366, 1979.

44. DeSilva RA, Hennekens CH, Lown B, Casseells W: Lignocaine prophylaxis in acute myocardial infarction: an evaluation of randomized trials, *Lancet* 2:855-858, 1981.

45. Fenster PE, Comess KA, Marsh R, et al: Conversion of atrial fibrillation to sinus rhythm by acute intravenous procainamide infusion, *Am Heart J* 106:501-506, 1983.

46. Lalka D, Meyer MB, Duce BR, et al: Kinetics of the oral antiarrhythmic lidocaine congener, tocainide, *Clin Pharmacol Ther* 19:757, 1976.

47. Perlow GM, Jain BP, Pauker SC, et al: Tocainide-associated interstitial pneumonitis, *Ann Intern Med* 94:489, 1981.

48. Volosin K, Greenberg RM, Greenspon AJ: Tocainide associated agranulocytosis, *Am Heart J* 109:1392, 1985.

49. Bronheim D, Thys DM: *Cardiovascular drugs.* In Rogers MC, Tinker JH, Covino BG, Longnecker DE, editors: *Principles and practice of anesthesiology,* St Louis, 1993, Mosby–Year Book.

50. Benowitz N, Forsyth RP, Melmon KL, Rowland M: Lidocaine disposition kinetics in monkey and man. I. Prediction of a perfusion model, *Clin Pharmacol Ther* 16:87-98, 1974.

51. Stargel WW, Shand DG, Routledge PA, et al: Clinical comparison of rapid infusion and multiple injection methods for lidocaine loading, *Am Heart J* 102:972-976, 1981.

52. American Heart Association: *Textbook of Advanced Cardiac Life Support,* Dallas, 1987, The Association.

53. Kopacz DJ, Carpenter RL, MacKay DL: Effect of ropivacaine on cutaneous capillary flow in pigs, *Anesthesiology* 71:69, 1989.

54. Scott DB, Jebson PJR, Braid DP, et al: Factors affecting plasma levels of lignocaine and prilocaine, *Br J Anaesth* 44:1040-1049, 1972.

55. Duhner KG, Harthon JGL, Hebring BG, Lie T: Blood levels of mepivacaine after regional anaesthesia, *Br J Anaesth* 37:746-752, 1965.

56. de Jong RH: *Local anesthetics,* ed 2, Springfield, Ill, 1977, Charles C Thomas, p 199.

57. Kimmey JR, Steinhaus JE: Cardiovascular effects of procaine and lidocaine (Xylocaine) during general anesthesia, *Acta Anaesthesiol Scand* 3:9-15, 1959.

58. de Jong RH, Ronfeld R, DeRosa R: Cardiovascular effects of convulsant and supraconvulsant doses of amide local anesthetics, *Anesth Analg* 61:3, 1982.

59. Feldman HS, Arthur GR, Covino BG: Comparative systemic toxicity of convulsant and supraconvulsant doses of intravenous ropivacaine, bupivacaine and lidocaine in the conscious dog, *Anesth Analg* 69:794, 1989.

60. Benoit PW, Belt WD: Destruction and regeneration of skeletal muscle after treatment with a local anesthetic, bupivacaine (Marcaine), *J Anat* 107:547, 1970.

61. Libelius R, Sonesson B, Stamenovic BA, et al: Denervation-like changes in skeletal muscle after treatment with a local anesthetic (Marcaine), *J Anat* 106:297, 1970.

62. Benoit PW, Yagiela JA, Fort NF: Pharmacologic correlation between local anesthetic–induced myotoxicity and disturbances of intracellular calcium distribution, *Toxicol Appl Pharmacol* 52:187-198, 1980.

63. Hinton RJ, Dechow PC, Carlson DS: Recovery of jaw muscle function following injection of a myotoxic agent (lidocaine-epinephrine), *Oral Surg Oral Med Oral Pathol* 59:247-251, 1986.

64. Denborough MA, Forster JF, Lovell RR, et al: Anaesthetic deaths in a family, *Br J Anaesth* 34:395-396, 1962.

65. Ording H: Incidence of malignant hyperthermia in Denmark, *Anesth Analg* 64:700-704, 1985.

66. Paasuke RT, Brownell AKW: Amine local anaesthetics and malignant hyperthermia, *Can Anaesth Soc J* 33:126-129, 1986 (editorial).

CHAPTER
three

Pharmacology of Vasoconstrictors

All clinically effective injectable local anesthetics possess some degree of vasodilating activity. The degree of vasodilation varies from significant (procaine) to minimal (prilocaine, mepivacaine) and may vary with injection site and individual patient response. After local anesthetic injection into tissues, blood vessels in the area dilate, resulting in an increased blood flow to the site. This increase in perfusion leads to the following reactions:

1. Increased rate of absorption of the local anesthetic into the cardiovascular system, which in turn removes it from the injection site
2. Higher plasma levels of the local anesthetic, with an attendant increased risk of local anesthetic toxicity
3. Decreased duration of action and decreased depth of anesthesia because it diffuses away from the injection site more rapidly
4. Increased bleeding at the site of local anesthetic administration due to increased perfusion

Vasoconstrictors are drugs that constrict blood vessels and thereby control tissue perfusion. They are added to local anesthetic solutions to oppose the vasodilating actions of the local anesthetics. Vasoconstrictors are highly important additions to a local anesthetic solution for the following reasons:

1. By constricting blood vessels, vasoconstrictors decrease blood flow (perfusion) to the site of injection.
2. Absorption of the local anesthetic into the cardiovascular system is slowed, resulting in lower anesthetic blood levels.[1,2] Table 3-1 illustrates levels of local anesthetic in the blood with and without a vasoconstrictor.
3. Lower local anesthetic blood levels decrease the risk of local anesthetic toxicity.
4. Higher volumes of the local anesthetic agent remain in and around the nerve for longer periods, thereby increasing (in some cases significantly,[3] in others minimally[4]) the duration of action of most local anesthetics.
5. Vasoconstrictors decrease bleeding at the site of their administration and are useful, therefore, when increased bleeding is anticipated (i.e., during a surgical procedure).[5,6]

The vasoconstrictors used in conjunction with injected local anesthetics are chemically identical or quite similar to the sympathetic nervous system mediators epinephrine and norepinephrine. The actions of the vasoconstrictors so resemble the response of adrenergic nerves to stimulation that they are classified as *sympathomimetic,* or *adrenergic,* drugs. These drugs have many clinical actions besides vasoconstriction.

• • •

Sympathomimetic drugs may also be classified according to their chemical structure and mode of action.

CHEMICAL STRUCTURE

Classification of sympathomimetic drugs by chemical structure is related to the presence or absence of a catechol nucleus. Catechol is orthodihydroxybenzene.

Sympathomimetic drugs that have hydroxyl (OH) substitutions in the third and fourth positions of the aromatic ring are termed *catechols.*

$$HO-\text{\Large⟨ring⟩}-C-C$$
$$HO-$$

If they also contain an amine group (NH_2) attached to the aliphatic side chain, they are then called *catecholamines.* Epinephrine, norepinephrine, and dopamine are the naturally occurring catecholamines of the sympathetic nervous system. Isoproterenol and levonordefrin are synthetic catecholamines.

Vasoconstrictors not possessing OH groups in the third and fourth positions of the aromatic molecule are not catechols, but all are amines because they have an NH_2 group attached to the aliphatic side chain.

Catecholamines	Noncatecholamines
Epinephrine	Amphetamine
Norepinephrine	Methamphetamine
Levonordefrin	Ephedrine
Isoproterenol	Mephentermine
Dopamine	Hydroxyamphetamine
	Metaraminol
	Methoxamine
	Phenylephrine

Felypressin, a synthetic analogue of the polypeptide vasopressin (antidiuretic hormone), is available in many countries as a vasoconstrictor. At present (September 1995), however, it is not available in the United States.

MODES OF ACTION

There are three categories of sympathomimetic amines: (1) *direct-acting drugs,* which exert their action directly on adrenergic receptors; (2) *indirect-acting drugs,* which act by releasing norepinephrine from adrenergic nerve terminals; and (3) *mixed-acting drugs,* with both direct and indirect actions.

Direct-acting	Indirect-acting	Mixed-acting
Epinephrine	Tyramine	Metaraminol
Norepinephrine	Amphetamine	Ephedrine
Levonordefrin	Methamphetamine	
Isoproterenol	Hydroxyamphetamine	
Dopamine		
Methoxamine		
Phenylephrine		

Adrenergic Receptors

Adrenergic receptors are found in most tissues of the body. The concept of adrenergic receptors was proposed by Ahlquist in 1948 and is well accepted today.[7] Ahlquist recognized two types of adrenergic receptors, termed *alpha* (α) and *beta* (β) based on the inhibitory or excitatory actions of the catecholamines on smooth muscle.

Activation of α receptors by a sympathomimetic drug usually produces a response that includes the contraction of smooth muscle in blood vessels (vasoconstriction). Based on differences in their function and location, α receptors have since been subcategorized. Whereas α_1 receptors are excitatory-postsynaptic, α_2 receptors are inhibitory-postsynaptic.[8]

Activation of β receptors produces smooth muscle relaxation (vasodilation and bronchodilation) and cardiac stimulation (increased heart rate and strength of contractions).

Beta receptors are further divided into β_1 and β_2—the former is found in the heart and small intestines and responsible for cardiac stimulation and lipolysis; the latter is found in the bronchi, vascular beds, and uterus and produces bronchodilation and vasodilation.[9]

Table 3-2 illustrates the differences in the varying degrees of α and β receptor activity of three commonly used vasoconstrictors.

Table 3-3 lists the systemic effects, based on α and β receptor activity, of the sympathomimetic drugs.

Release of Catecholamines

Other sympathomimetic drugs, such as tyramine and amphetamine, act *indirectly* by causing release of the catecholamine norepinephrine from stores in the adren-

TABLE 3-1   Effect of Vasoconstrictor (Epinephrine 1:200,000) on Peak Local Anesthetic Level in Blood

Local anesthetic	Dose (mg)	Peak level (µg/ml) Without vasoconstrictor	Peak level (µg/ml) With vasoconstrictor
Mepivacaine	500	4.7	3
Lidocaine	400	4.3	3
Prilocaine	400	2.8	2.6
Etidocaine	300	1.4	1.3

TABLE 3-2   Adrenergic Receptor Activity of Vasoconstrictors

Drug	α_1	α_2	β_1	β_2
Epinephrine	+++	+++	+++	+++
Norepinephrine	++	++	++	+
Levonordefrin	+	++	++	+

From Jastak JT, Yagiela JA, Donaldson D: *Local anesthesia of the oral cavity,* Philadelphia, 1995, WB Saunders.
Relative potency of drugs is indicated as follows: +++ = high, ++ = intermediate, and + = low.

TABLE 3-3   Systemic Effects of Sympathomimetic Amines

Effector organ or function	Epinephrine	Norepinephrine
Cardiovascular system		
Heart rate	+	−
Stroke volume	++	++
Cardiac output	+++	0, −
Arrhythmias	++++	++++
Coronary blood flow	++	++
Blood pressure		
Systolic arterial	+++	+++
Mean arterial	+	++
Diastolic arterial	+, 0, −	++
Peripheral circulation		
Total peripheral resistance	−	++
Cerebral blood flow	+	0, −
Cutaneous blood flow	−	−
Splanchnic blood flow	+++	0, +
Respiratory system		
Bronchodilation	+++	0
Genitourinary system		
Renal blood flow	−	−
Skeletal muscle		
Muscle blood flow	+++	0, −
Metabolic effects		
Oxygen consumption	++	0, +
Blood glucose	+++	0, +
Blood lactic acid	+++	0, +

After Goldenberg M, Aranow H Jr, Smith AA, Faber M: Pheochromocytoma and essential hypertensive vascular disease, *Arch Intern Med* 86:823-836, 1950.

ergic nerve terminals. In addition, these drugs may also exert a direct action on α and β receptors.

The clinical actions of this group of drugs are therefore quite similar to the actions of norepinephrine. Successively repeated doses of these drugs will prove to be less effective than those given previously because of the depletion of norepinephrine stores. This phenomenon is termed *tachyphylaxis* and is *not* seen with drugs that act directly on adrenergic receptors.

DILUTIONS OF VASOCONSTRICTORS

The dilution of vasoconstrictors is commonly referred to as a ratio (e.g., 1 to 1000 [written 1:1000]). Because max-

imum doses of vasoconstrictors are presented in milligrams, the following interpretations should enable the reader to convert these terms readily:

- 1:1000 means that there is 1 gram (or 1000 mg) of solute (drug) contained in 1000 ml of solution.
- Therefore a 1:1000 dilution contains 1000 mg in 1000 ml or 1.0 mg/ml of solution.

Vasoconstrictors used in dental local anesthetic solutions are much less concentrated than the 1:1000 described above. To produce these more dilute, clinically safer, yet quite effective dilutions, the 1:1000 dilution must be diluted further. This process is described below.

- To produce a 1:10,000 dilution, 1 ml of a 1:1000 solution is added to 9 ml of solvent (e.g., sterile water); therefore 1:10,000 = 0.1 mg/ml.
- To produce a 1:100,000 dilution, 1 ml of a 1:10,000 dilution is added to 9 ml of solvent; therefore 1:100,000 = 0.01 mg/ml.

The milligram per milliliter values of the various vasoconstrictor dilutions used in medicine and dentistry follow:

Dilution	Milligrams per milliliter	Therapeutic use
1:1,000	1.0	Emergency medicine (*IM/SC anaphylaxis*)
1:2,500	0.4	Phenylephrine
1:10,000	0.1	Emergency medicine (*IV cardiac arrest*)
1:20,000	0.05	Levonordefrin
1:30,000	0.033	Norepinephrine
1:50,000	0.02	Local anesthesia
1:80,000	0.0125	Local anesthesia (United Kingdom)
1:100,000	0.01	Local anesthesia
1:200,000	0.005	Local anesthesia

The genesis of vasoconstrictor dilutions in local anesthetics began with the discovery of adrenalin in 1897 by Abel. In 1903 Braun suggested using adrenalin as a "chemical tourniquet" to prolong the duration of local anesthetics.[10] Braun recommended the use of a 1:10,000 dilution of epinephrine, ranging to as great as 1:100,000, for use with cocaine when used for nasal surgery. It appears, currently, that a dilution of 1:200,000 provides comparable results, with fewer systemic side effects of epinephrine. The 1:200,000 dilution, which contains 5 μg/ml (or 0.005 mg/ml), has become widely used in both medicine and dentistry and is currently found in articaine, prilocaine, lidocaine (not in the United States, September 1995), etidocaine, and bupivacaine.

Though the most used vasoconstrictor in both medicine and dentistry, epinephrine is not an ideal drug. The benefits to be gained from adding a vasoconstrictor to a local anesthetic solution must be weighed against any risks that might be present. Epinephrine is absorbed from the site of injection, just as is the local anesthetic. Measurable epinephrine blood levels are obtained, which influence the heart and blood vessels. Resting plasma epinephrine levels (39 pg/ml) are doubled following the administration of one cartridge of lidocaine with 1:100,000 epinephrine.[11] The elevation of epinephrine plasma levels is linearly dose-dependent and persists from several minutes to half an hour.[12] Contrary to a previously held position that the intraoral administration of "usual" volumes of epinephrine produced no cardiovascular response and that patients were more at risk from endogenously released epinephrine than they were from exogenously administered epinephrine,[13,14] recent evidence demonstrates that epinephrine plasma levels equivalent to those achieved during moderate to heavy exercise may occur following intraoral injection.[15,16] These are associated with moderate increases in cardiac output and stroke volume (see the following section). Blood pressure and heart rate are minimally affected at these dosages.[17]

In patients with preexisting cardiovascular or thyroid disease, the side effects of absorbed epinephrine must be weighed against those of elevated local anesthetic blood levels. It is currently thought that the cardiovascular effects of conventional epinephrine doses are of little practical concern, even in patients with heart disease.[12] However, even following usual precautions (aspiration, slow injection), sufficient epinephrine can be absorbed to cause sympathomimetic reactions such as apprehension, tachycardia, sweating, and pounding in the chest (palpitation), the so-called "epinephrine reaction."[18]

Intravascular administration of vasoconstrictors as well as their administration to "sensitive" individuals (hyperresponders), or the occurrence of unanticipated drug-drug interactions can, however, produce significant clinical manifestations. Intravenous administration of 0.015 mg of epinephrine with lidocaine results in increases in the heart rate ranging from 25 to 70 beats per minute, with elevations in the systolic blood from 20 to 70 mm Hg.[12,19,20] Occasional rhythm disturbances may also be observed, premature ventricular contractions (PVCs) being the most often noted.

Other vasoconstrictors used in medicine and dentistry include norepinephrine, phenylephrine, levonordefrin, and octapressin. *Norepinephrine,* lacking significant β_2 actions, produces intense peripheral vasoconstriction with possible dramatic elevation of blood pressure, and is associated with a side effect ratio nine times higher than that of epinephrine.[21] Although currently available in many countries in local anesthetic solutions, norepinephrine's use as a vasopressor in dentistry is not recommended. The use of a mixture of epinephrine and norepinephrine is to be

absolutely avoided.[22] *Phenylephrine,* a pure α-adrenergic agonist, theoretically possesses advantages over other vasoconstrictors. However, in clinical trials peak blood levels of lidocaine were actually higher with phenylephrine 1:20,000 (2.4 µg/ml) than with epinephrine 1:200,000 (1.4 µg/ml).[23] The cardiovascular effects of *levonordefrin* most closely resemble those of norepinephrine.[24] *Octapressin* was shown to be about as effective as epinephrine in reducing cutaneous blood flow.[5]

Epinephrine remains the most effective and most used vasoconstrictor in medicine and dentistry.

PHARMACOLOGY OF SPECIFIC AGENTS

The pharmacological actions of the sympathomimetic amines commonly used as vasoconstrictors in local anesthetics are reviewed. *Epinephrine* is the most useful and best example of a drug that mimics the activity of sympathetic discharge. Its clinical actions are therefore worthy of an in-depth review. The actions of other drugs are compared with those of epinephrine.

Epinephrine

Proprietary name Adrenalin.

Chemical structure Epinephrine as the acid salt is highly soluble in water. Slightly acid solutions are relatively stable if they are protected from air. Deterioration (through oxidation) is hastened by heat and the presence of heavy metal ions. *Sodium bisulfite* is usually added to epinephrine solutions to delay this deterioration. The shelf life of a local anesthetic cartridge containing a vasoconstrictor is somewhat shorter than that of a cartridge containing no vasoconstrictor.

Source Epinephrine is available as a synthetic and is also obtained from the adrenal medulla of animals (approximately 80% of adrenal medullary secretions being epinephrine). It exists in both levorotatory and dextrorotatory forms; the levorotatory form is approximately 15 times as potent as the dextrorotatory.

Mode of action Epinephrine acts directly on both α- and β-adrenergic receptors; β effects predominate.

Systemic Actions

Myocardium Epinephrine stimulates the β_1 receptors of the myocardium. There is a positive inotropic (force of contraction) and positive chronotropic (rate of contraction) effect. Both cardiac output and heart rate are increased.

Pacemaker cells Epinephrine stimulates β_1 receptors and increases the irritability of pacemaker cells, leading to a greater incidence of dysrhythmias. Ventricular tachycardia and premature ventricular contractions are not uncommon.

Coronary arteries Epinephrine produces dilation of the coronary arteries, leading to an increased coronary artery blood flow.

Blood pressure Systolic blood pressure is *increased.* The diastolic pressure is *decreased* when small doses are administered, because of the greater sensitivity to epinephrine of β_2 receptors than of α receptors in vessels supplying the skeletal muscles. Diastolic pressure is *increased* when larger doses are administered, because of the constriction of vessels supplying the skeletal muscles produced by α-receptor stimulation.

Cardiovascular dynamics The overall action of epinephrine on the heart and cardiovascular system is direct stimulation:

Increased systolic and diastolic pressures
Increased cardiac output
Increased stroke volume
Increased heart rate
Increased strength of contraction
Increased myocardial oxygen consumption

These actions lead to an overall *decrease* in cardiac efficiency.

The cardiovascular responses of increased systolic blood pressure and increased heart rate will develop with the administration of one to two dental cartridges of a 1:100,000 epinephrine dilution.[25] Administration of four cartridges of 1:100,000 epinephrine will bring about a slight decrease in diastolic blood pressure.

Vasculature The primary action of epinephrine is on smaller arterioles and precapillary sphincters. Vessels supplying the skin, mucous membranes, and kidneys contain primarily α receptors. Epinephrine produces constriction in these vessels. Vessels supplying the skeletal muscles contain both α and β_2 receptors, with β_2 predominating. Small epinephrine doses produce dilation of these vessels as a result of β_2 actions. Beta-2 receptors are more sensitive to epinephrine than are α receptors. Larger doses produce vasoconstriction because the α receptors are stimulated.

Clinically epinephrine is frequently used as a vasoconstrictor for hemostasis during surgical procedures. The injection of epinephrine directly into surgical sites leads to high tissue concentrations, a predominant α-receptor stimulation, and hemostasis. As epinephrine tissue levels decrease with time the primary action on blood vessels will revert to vasodilation, as β_2 actions predominate. It is

not uncommon, therefore, for some bleeding to be noted at about 6 hours following the surgery. In a clinical trial involving extraction of third molars, postsurgical bleeding occurred in 13 of 16 patients receiving epinephrine with their local anesthetic for hemostasis, whereas 0 of 16 patients receiving local anesthetic without vasoconstrictor (mepivacaine plain) had bleeding at 6 hours postsurgery.[26] Additional findings of increased postsurgical pain and delayed wound healing were also noted.[26]

Respiratory system Epinephrine is a potent dilator (β_2 effect) of the smooth muscle of the bronchioles. It is the drug of choice for management of acute asthma (bronchospasm).

Central nervous system In usual therapeutic dosages epinephrine is *not* a potent CNS stimulant. Its CNS-stimulating actions become prominent when an excessive dose is administered.

Metabolism Epinephrine increases oxygen consumption in all tissues. Through a β action it stimulates glycogenolysis in the liver and skeletal muscle, producing an elevation of the blood sugar level at plasma epinephrine concentrations of 150 to 200 pg/ml.[25] The equivalent of four dental local anesthetic cartridges of 1:100,000 epinephrine must be administered to elicit this response.[27]

Termination of action and elimination The action of epinephrine is terminated primarily by its reuptake by adrenergic nerves. Epinephrine that escapes reuptake is rapidly inactivated in the blood by the enzymes catechol-O-methyltransferase (COMT) and monoamine oxidase (MAO), both of which are present in the liver.[28] Only small amounts (approximately 1%) of epinephrine are excreted unchanged in the urine.

Side effects and overdose The clinical manifestations of epinephrine overdose relate to CNS stimulation and include increasing fear and anxiety, tension, restlessness, throbbing headache, tremor, weakness, dizziness, pallor, respiratory difficulty, and palpitation.

With increasing levels of epinephrine in the blood, cardiac dysrhythmias become more common; ventricular fibrillation is a rare but possible consequence. Dramatic increases in both systolic (>300 mm Hg) and diastolic (>200 mm Hg) pressures may be noted, which have led to cerebral hemorrhage.[29] Anginal episodes may be precipitated in patients with coronary insufficiency. Because of the rapid inactivation of epinephrine, the stimulatory phase of the overdose reaction is usually very brief. Vasoconstrictor overdose is discussed in greater depth in Chapter 18.

Clinical Applications—Epinephrine

- Management of acute allergic reactions
- Management of bronchospasm
- Treatment of cardiac arrest
- As a vasoconstrictor, for hemostasis

- As a vasoconstrictor in local anesthetics, to decrease absorption into the cardiovascular system
- As a vasoconstrictor in local anesthetics, to increase duration of action
- To produce mydriasis

Availability in dentistry   Epinephrine is the most potent and widely used vasoconstrictor in dentistry. It is available in the following dilutions and drugs:

Dilution with epinephrine	Local anesthetic (generic)
1:50,000	Lidocaine
1:80,000	Lidocaine (United Kingdom)
1:100,000	Articaine*
	Lidocaine
1:200,000	Articaine*
	Bupivacaine
	Etidocaine
	Lidocaine*
	Mepivacaine*
	Prilocaine

*Not available in the United States as of September 1995.

Maximum Doses

For pain control   *The least concentrated solution that produces effective pain control should be used.* Lidocaine is available with two dilutions of epinephrine—1:50,000 and 1:100,000 in the United States and Canada—and with 1:80,000 and 1:200,000 in other countries. The duration of effective pulpal and soft tissue anesthesia is equivalent with all forms. Therefore it is recommended that the 1:100,000 epinephrine dilution be used with lidocaine when extended pain control is required. Where 1:200,000 epinephrine is available in lidocaine, this is the preferred form for pain control.[30]

The following dosages represent recommended maximums as suggested by me and others.[31] They are, in fact, rather conservative figures but still provide the dental practitioner with adequate volumes to produce clinically acceptable anesthesia. The American Heart Association (1964) has stated that "the typical concentrations of vasoconstrictors contained in local anesthetics are not contraindicated in patients with cardiovascular disease so long as preliminary aspiration is practiced, the agent is injected slowly, and the smallest effective dose is administered."[32] In 1954 the New York Heart Association recommended that maximal epinephrine doses be limited to 0.2 mg per appointment.[33] More recently the American Heart Association has recommended the restriction of epinephrine in local anesthetics when administered to patients with ischemic heart disease.[34]

In cardiovascularly compromised patients it seems prudent to limit or avoid exposure to vasoconstrictors, if possible. These include poorly controlled ASA III, and all ASA IV and greater, cardiovascular risk patients.

AMERICAN SOCIETY OF ANESTHESIOLOGISTS PHYSICAL STATUS CLASSIFICATION

I   Normal healthy individual

II   Patient with mild to moderate systemic disease

III   Patient with severe systemic disease that limits activity but is not incapacitating

IV   Patient with severe systemic disease that limits activity and is a constant threat to life

V   Moribund patient not expected to survive 24 hours with or without an operation

VI   Clinically dead patient being maintained for harvesting of organs

However, as was previously stated, the risk of epinephrine administration must be weighed against the benefits to be gained from its inclusion in the local anesthetic solution. Can clinically adequate pain control be provided for this patient without epinephrine in the solution? What is the potential deleterious effect of poor anesthesia on the endogenous release of catecholamines in response to sudden, unexpected pain?

Normal healthy patient: 0.2 mg per appointment
   10 ml of a 1:50,000 dilution (5 cartridges)
   20 ml of a 1:100,000 dilution (11 cartridges)*
   40 ml of a 1:200,000 dilution (22 cartridges)*

Patient with clinically significant cardiovascular disease (ASA III or IV): 0.04 mg per appointment
   2 ml of a 1:50,000 dilution (1 cartridge)
   4 ml of a 1:100,000 dilution (2 cartridges)
   8 ml of a 1:200,000 dilution (4 cartridges)

The use of vasoconstrictors for cardiovascularly compromised patients is reviewed in greater depth in Chapter 20.

Hemostasis   Epinephrine-containing local anesthetic solutions are used, via infiltration into the site of operation, to prevent or minimize bleeding during surgical and other procedures. The 1:50,000 dilution of epinephrine is more effective in this regard than less concentrated, 1:100,000 or 1:200,000, solutions.[35] Epinephrine dilutions of 1:50,000 and 1:100,000 are considerably more effective in restricting surgical blood loss than local anesthetics without vasoconstrictor additives.[26]

Clinical experience has shown that effective hemostasis can be obtained with dilutions of 1:100,000 epi-

*Maximum volume for administration limited by local anesthetic.

nephrine. Although the small volumes of 1:50,000 epinephrine required for hemostasis do not increase a patient's risk, consideration should always be given to use of the 1:100,000 dilution, especially in patients known to be more sensitive to catecholamines. These include the ASA III or IV risk cardiovascularly compromised individual and the geriatric patient.

Norepinephrine (Levarterenol)

Proprietary names Levophed, Noradrenalin; levarterenol is the official name of norepinephrine.

Chemical structure Norepinephrine (as the bitartrate) in dental cartridges is relatively stable in acid solutions, deteriorating on exposure to light and air. The shelf life of a cartridge containing norepinephrine bitartrate is 18 months. Acetone–sodium bisulfite is added to the cartridge to retard deterioration.

Source Norepinephrine is available in both synthetic and natural forms. The natural form constitutes approximately 20% of the catecholamine production of the adrenal medulla. In patients with pheochromocytoma, a tumor of the adrenal medulla, norepinephrine may comprise up to 80% of adrenal medullary secretions. It exists in both levorotatory and dextrorotatory forms; the levorotatory form is 40 times as potent. Norepinephrine is synthesized and stored at postganglionic adrenergic nerve terminals.

Mode of action The actions of norepinephrine are almost exclusively on α receptors (90%). It also stimulates β actions in the heart (10%). Norepinephrine is one fourth as potent as epinephrine.

Systemic Actions

Myocardium Norepinephrine has a positive inotropic action on the myocardium through β_1 stimulation.

Pacemaker cells Norepinephrine stimulates pacemaker cells and increases their irritability, which leads to a greater incidence of cardiac dysrhythmias (β_1 action).

Coronary arteries Norepinephrine produces an increase in coronary artery blood flow through a vasodilatory effect.

Heart rate It produces a *decrease* in heart rate caused by reflex action of the carotid and aortic baroreceptors and the vagus nerve following a marked increase in both systolic and diastolic pressures.

Blood pressure Both the systolic and the diastolic pressure are increased, the systolic to a greater extent. This is produced through the α-stimulating actions of norepi-

nephrine, which lead to peripheral vasoconstriction and a concomitant increase in peripheral vascular resistance.

Cardiovascular dynamics The overall action of norepinephrine on the heart and cardiovascular system is as follows:

Increased systolic pressure
Increased diastolic pressure
Decreased heart rate
Unchanged or slightly decreased cardiac output
Increased stroke volume
Increased total peripheral resistance

Vasculature Norepinephrine, through α stimulation, produces constriction of cutaneous blood vessels. This leads to increased total peripheral resistance and increased systolic and diastolic blood pressures.

The degree and duration of ischemia noted following norepinephrine infiltration into the palate have led to soft tissue necrosis (Fig. 3-1).

Respiratory system Norepinephrine does not relax bronchial smooth muscle as does epinephrine. It does, however, produce α-induced constriction of lung arterioles, which reduces airway resistance to a small degree. Norepinephrine is *not* clinically effective in the management of bronchospasm.

Central nervous system As with epinephrine, norepinephrine does *not* exhibit CNS-stimulating actions at usual therapeutic doses; its CNS-stimulating properties are most prominent following overdose. Clinical manifestations are similar to those of epinephrine overdose (p. 41) but are less frequent and usually not as severe.

Metabolism Norepinephrine increases basal metabolic rate. Tissue oxygen consumption is also increased in the area of injection. Norepinephrine produces an elevation in the blood sugar level in the same manner as does epinephrine, but to a lesser degree.

Termination of action and elimination The action of norepinephrine is terminated through its reup-

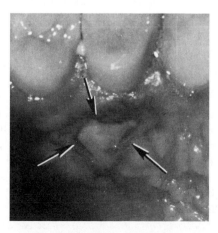

Fig. 3-1 Sterile abscess on the palate produced by excessive use of a vasoconstrictor (norepinephrine).

take at adrenergic nerve terminals and its oxidation by MAO. Exogenous norepinephrine is inactivated by COMT.

Side effects and overdose The clinical manifestations of norepinephrine overdose are similar to, but less frequent and less severe than, those of epinephrine. They normally involve CNS stimulation. Excessive levels of norepinephrine in the blood produce markedly elevated systolic and diastolic pressures with an increased risk of hemorrhagic "stroke," headache, anginal episodes in susceptible patients, and cardiac dysrhythmias.

The extravascular injection of norepinephrine into tissues may produce necrosis and sloughing because of intense α stimulation. In the oral cavity the most likely site to encounter this phenomenon is the hard palate (Fig. 3-1). Norepinephrine should be avoided for vasoconstricting purposes (e.g., hemostasis). Several authorities have stated that norepinephrine should not be used at all with local anesthetics.[30,36]

Clinical applications It is used as a vasoconstrictor in local anesthetics and for the management of hypotension.

Availability in dentistry In the United States norepinephrine was included with the local anesthetics propoxycaine and procaine in a 1:30,000 dilution. In other countries norepinephrine is included with lidocaine (Germany) and mepivacaine (Germany) or as the combination of norepinephrine and epinephrine with lidocaine (Germany) or with tolycaine (Japan).[21]

Maximum doses When used, norepinephrine should be used for *pain control only,* there being little or no justification for its use in obtaining hemostasis. It is approximately 25% as potent a vasopressor as epinephrine and is therefore used clinically as a 1:30,000 dilution.

Recent recommendations of the International Federation of Dental Anesthesiology Societies suggest that norepinephrine be eliminated as a vasoconstrictor in dental local anesthetics.[30]

Normal healthy patient: 0.34 mg per appointment
  10 ml of a 1:30,000 solution

Patient with clinically significant cardiovascular disease (ASA III or IV): 0.14 mg per appointment
  approximately 4 ml of a 1:30,000 solution

Levonordefrin

Proprietary name Neo-Cobefrin.
Chemical structure Levonordefrin is freely soluble in dilute acidic solutions. Sodium bisulfite is added to the solution to delay its deterioration. The shelf life of a cartridge containing levonordefrin–sodium bisulfite is 18 months.

Source Levonordefrin, a synthetic vasoconstrictor, is prepared by the resolution of nordefrin into its optically active isomers. The dextrorotatory form of nordefrin is virtually inert.

Mode of action It appears to act through direct α receptor stimulation (75%) with some β activity (25%), but to a lesser degree than epinephrine. Levonordefrin is 15% as potent a vasopressor as epinephrine.

Systemic Actions

Levonordefrin produces less cardiac and CNS stimulation than epinephrine does.

Myocardium Same action as epinephrine, but to a lesser degree.

Pacemaker cells Same action as epinephrine, but to a lesser degree.

Coronary arteries Same action as epinephrine, but to a lesser degree.

Heart rate Same effect as epinephrine, but to a lesser degree.

Vasculature Same as epinephrine, but to a lesser degree.

Respiratory system Some bronchodilation, but to a much smaller degree than with epinephrine.

Central nervous system Same actions as epinephrine, but to a lesser extent.

Metabolism Same action as epinephrine, but to a lesser extent.

Termination of action and elimination Levonordefrin is eliminated through the actions of COMT and MAO.

Side effects and overdose Same as with epinephrine, but to a lesser extent. In higher doses additional side effects include hypertension, ventricular tachycardia, and anginal episodes in patients with coronary insufficiency.

Clinical applications Levonordefrin is used as a vasoconstrictor in local anesthetics.

Availability in dentistry It can be obtained with mepivacaine or with propoxycaine/procaine in a 1:20,000 dilution.

Maximum doses Levonordefrin is considered one sixth (15%) as effective a vasopressor as epinephrine; therefore it is used in a lesser dilution (1:20,000).

For all patients the maximum dose should be 1 mg per appointment
  20 ml of a 1:20,000 dilution (11 cartridges)*

In the dilution at which it is available, levonordefrin has the same effect on clinical activity of local anesthetics does as 1:50,000 or 1:100,000 epinephrine.

Phenylephrine Hydrochloride

Proprietary name Neo-Synephrine

---

*Maximum volume for administration limited by local anesthetic.

Chemical structure Phenylephrine is quite soluble in water. It is the most stable and the weakest vasoconstrictor employed in dentistry.

$$HO-\text{benzene ring}-CH(OH)-CH_2-N(H)-CH_3$$

Source Phenylephrine is a synthetic sympathomimetic amine.

Mode of action There is direct α receptor stimulation (95%). Although the effect is less than with epinephrine, the duration is longer. Phenylephrine exerts little or no β action on the heart. Only a small portion of its activity is due to its ability to release norepinephrine. Phenylephrine is only 5% as potent as epinephrine.

Systemic Actions

Myocardium Little chronotropic or inotropic effect on the heart.

Pacemaker cells Little effect.

Coronary arteries Increased blood flow, caused by dilation.

Blood pressure Alpha action produces increases in both systolic and diastolic pressures.

Heart rate Bradycardia is produced by reflex actions of the carotid-aortic baroreceptors and the vagus nerve. Cardiac dysrhythmias are rarely noted, even following large doses of phenylephrine.

Cardiovascular dynamics Overall, the cardiovascular actions of phenylephrine are as follows:

Increased systolic and diastolic pressures
Reflex bradycardia
Slightly decreased cardiac output (resulting from increased blood pressure and bradycardia)
Powerful vasoconstriction (most vascular beds constricted, peripheral resistance increased significantly) but without marked venous congestion
Rarely associated with provoking cardiac dysrhythmias

Respiratory system The bronchi are dilated but to a lesser degree than with epinephrine. Phenylephrine is *not* effective in treating bronchospasm.

Central nervous system Minimum effect on activity.

Metabolism Some increase in the metabolic rate is noted. Other actions (e.g., glycogenolysis) are similar to those produced by epinephrine.

Termination of action and elimination Phenylephrine undergoes hydroxylation to epinephrine, then oxidation to metanephrine, following which it is eliminated in the same manner as epinephrine.

Side effects and overdose CNS effects are minimal with phenylephrine. Headache and ventricular dys-

rhythmias have been noted following overdose. Tachyphylaxis is observed with chronic use.

Clinical applications It is used as a vasoconstrictor in local anesthetics, for the management of hypotension, as a nasal decongestant, and in ophthalmic solutions to produce mydriasis.

Availability in dentistry It is used with 4% procaine in a 1:2500 dilution (no longer available in dental cartridges).

Maximum doses Phenylephrine is considered only one twentieth as potent as epinephrine, hence its use in a 1:2500 dilution. It is an excellent vasoconstrictor, with few significant side effects.

Normal healthy patient: 4 mg per appointment
10 ml of a 1:2500 solution

Patient with clinically significant cardiovascular impairment (ASA III or IV): 1.6 mg per appointment
equivalent to 4 ml of a 1:2500 solution

Felypressin

Proprietary name Octapressin.
Chemical structure

Cys-Phe-Phe-Gly-Asn-Cys-Pro-Lys-GlyNH$_2$

Source Felypressin is a synthetic analogue of the antidiuretic hormone vasopressin. It is a nonsympathomimetic amine, categorized as a vasoconstrictor.

Mode of action It acts as a direct stimulant of vascular smooth muscle. Its actions appear to be more pronounced on the venous than on the arteriolar microcirculation.[37]

Systemic Actions

Myocardium No direct effects.

Pacemaker cells Felypressin is nondysrhythmogenic, in contradistinction to the sympathomimetic amines (e.g., epinephrine and norepinephrine).

Coronary arteries When administered in high doses (greater than therapeutic), it may impair blood flow through the coronary arteries.

Vasculature In high doses (greater than therapeutic), felypressin-induced constriction of cutaneous blood vessels may produce facial pallor.

Central nervous system Felypressin has no effect on adrenergic nerve transmission; thus it may be safely administered to hyperthyroid patients and to anyone receiving MAO inhibitors or tricyclic antidepressants.

Uterus It has both antidiuretic and oxytocic actions, the latter contraindicating its use in pregnant patients.

Side effects and overdose Laboratory and clinical studies with felypressin in animals and humans have demonstrated a wide margin of safety.[38] The drug is well tolerated by tissues into which it is deposited, with little irritation developing. The incidence of systemic reactions to felypressin is minimal.

Clinical applications   It is used as a vasoconstrictor in local anesthetics to decrease their absorption as well as increase their duration of action.

Availability in dentistry   Felypressin is employed in a dilution of 0.03 IU/ml (International Units) with 3% prilocaine in Japan, Germany, and other countries. It is not available as a vasoconstrictor in the United States.

Maximum doses   Felypressin-containing solutions are *not recommended for use when hemostasis is required* because of their predominant effect on the venous rather than the arterial circulation.[39]

Patients with clinically significant cardiovascular impairment (ASA III or IV): maximum recommended dose 0.27 IU

   9 ml of 0.03 IU/ml

SELECTION OF A VASOCONSTRICTOR

Two vasoconstrictors are currently available in local anesthetic solutions in the United States. In order of their effectiveness, they are epinephrine and levonordefrin.

In the selection of an appropriate vasoconstrictor, if any, for use with a local anesthetic, several factors must be considered: (1) the length of the dental procedure, (2) the need for hemostasis during and following the procedure, (3) the requirement for postoperative pain control, and (4) the medical status of the patient.

Length of the Dental Procedure

The addition of a vasoactive drug will prolong the duration of clinically effective pulpal and soft tissue anesthesia of most local anesthetics. For example, pulpal and hard tissue anesthesia with 2% lidocaine lasts approximately 10 minutes; the addition of 1:50,000, 1:100,000, or 1:200,000 epinephrine prolongs this to approximately 60 minutes. The addition of a vasoconstrictor to prilocaine, on the other hand, does not significantly increase the duration of clinically effective pain control. Prilocaine 4% provides pulpal anesthesia of about 40 to 60 minutes duration, the addition of a 1:200,000 epinephrine dilution increasing this but slightly (to about 60 to 90 minutes).[4,40]

Average durations of pulpal and hard tissue anesthesia expected from commonly used local anesthetics without vasoconstrictors are as follows:

2% Lidocaine	5 to 10 minutes
3% Mepivacaine	20 to 40 minutes
4% Prilocaine	5 to 15 minutes (infiltration)
	Up to 60 minutes (block anesthesia)

The typical dental appointment today lasts approximately 1 hour. For routine restorative procedures it might

be estimated that pulpal anesthesia will be required for approximately 40 to 50 minutes. As can be seen from this list, it is difficult to achieve consistently reliable pulpal anesthesia without the inclusion of a vasoconstrictor.

Requirement for Hemostasis

Epinephrine is effective in preventing or minimizing blood loss during surgical procedures. However, most vasoconstrictors also possess the disturbing action of producing a rebound vasodilatory effect as the tissue level of epinephrine declines. This leads to possible bleeding postoperatively, which may also interfere with wound healing.[26]

Epinephrine, possessing both α and β actions, produces vasoconstriction through its α effects. Used in a 1:50,000 dilution, and even at 1:100,000 (but to a lesser extent), it will produce a definite rebound β effect once the α-induced vasoconstriction has ceased. This leads to increased postoperative blood loss, which, if significant (usually in dentistry it is not), may compromise a patient's cardiovascular status.

Phenylephrine, a longer-acting, almost pure α-stimulating vasoconstrictor, does not produce a rebound β effect because its β actions are minimal. Therefore, since it is not as potent a vasoconstrictor as epinephrine, hemostasis *during* the procedure is not as effective; however, because of the long duration of action of phenylephrine compared with that of epinephrine, the postoperative period passes with less bleeding. Total blood loss is usually lower when phenylephrine is used.

Norepinephrine is a potent α stimulator and vasoconstrictor that has produced documented cases of tissue necrosis and slough. It cannot be recommended as a vasoconstrictor in dentistry, since its disadvantages outweigh its advantages. Other, more or equally effective, agents are available that do not possess norepinephrine's disadvantages.[41,42]

Felypressin stimulates the venous circulation more than the arteriolar circulation and therefore is of minimum value for hemostasis.

Vasoconstrictors used to achieve hemostasis must be deposited locally into the area of bleeding to be effective. They act directly on α receptors in the vascular smooth muscle. Only small volumes of local anesthetic solutions with vasoconstrictor are required to achieve hemostasis.

Medical Status of the Patient

There are few contraindications to vasoconstrictor administration in the dilutions in which they are found in dental local anesthetic solutions. For all patients, but for some in particular, the benefits and risks of including the vasopressor in the anesthetic solution must be weighed against the benefits and risks of using a "plain" anesthetic solution.[43-45] In general, these groups are:

Patients with more significant cardiovascular disease
Patients with certain noncardiovascular diseases (such as thyroid dysfunction, diabetes, sulfite sensitivity)
Patients receiving MAO inhibitors, tricyclic antidepressants, and phenothiazines

In each of these situations it is necessary to determine the degree of severity of the underlying disorder to determine whether a vasoconstrictor may safely be included or should be excluded from the local anesthetic solution. It is not uncommon for a medical consultation to be obtained to aid in determining this information.

Management of these patients is discussed in depth in Chapters 10 and 20. Briefly, however, it may be stated that local anesthetics with vasoconstrictors are not absolutely contraindicated for a patient whose medical condition has been diagnosed and is under control through medical or surgical means (ASA II or III risk) and if the vasoconstrictor is administered slowly, in minimal doses, and after negative aspiration has been ensured.

Patients with a resting blood pressure (minimum 5-minute rest) of either greater than 200 mm Hg systolic or greater than 115 mm Hg diastolic should not receive elective dental care until their more significant medical problem of high blood pressure is corrected. Patients with severe cardiovascular disease (ASA IV+ risk) may be at too great a risk for elective dental therapy—for example, a patient who has had an acute myocardial infarction within the past 6 months, a patient who has been experiencing acute anginal episodes on a daily basis or whose signs and symptoms are increasing in severity (preinfarction or unstable angina), or a patient whose cardiac dysrhythmias continue despite antiarrhythmic drug therapy.[43] Epinephrine and other vasoconstrictors can be administered in moderation to patients with mild to moderate cardiovascular disease (ASA II or III). Felypressin has minimum cardiovascular stimulatory actions and is nondysrhythmogenic; it is the recommended drug for ASA III and IV cardiovascular risk patients.

Epinephrine is also contraindicated in patients exhibiting clinical evidence of the hyperthyroid state.[44] Signs and symptoms include exophthalmos, hyperhydrosis, tremor, irritability and nervousness, increased body temperature, inability to tolerate heat, increased heart rate, and increased blood pressure. Epinephrine should not be used as a vasoconstrictor during general anesthesia when a patient (in any ASA category) is receiving a halogenated anesthetic (halothane, methoxyflurane, or ethrane). These inhalation general anesthetics sensitize the myocardium such that epinephrine administration is usually associated with the occurrence of cardiac dysrhythmias (PVCs or ventricular fibrillation). Felypressin is recommended in these situations; however, because of its potential oxytocic actions, felypressin is not recommended for pregnant patients. Once the impaired medical status of the patient is improved, routine dental care involving the administration of local anesthetics with vasoconstrictors is again indicated.

Patients being treated with MAO inhibitors may receive vasoconstrictors within the usual dental dosage parameters without increased risk.[45,46] Patients receiving tricyclic antidepressants are at a greater risk of developing dysrhythmias with epinephrine administration. It is recommended that when epinephrine is administered, its dose be minimal. The administration of either levonordefrin or norepinephrine is absolutely contraindicated in patients receiving tricyclic antidepressants. Large doses of vasoconstrictor may induce severe (exaggerated) responses.

Local anesthetic solutions containing a vasoconstrictor also contain an antioxidant (to retard oxidation of the vasoconstrictor). *Sodium bisulfite* is the most commonly used antioxidant in dental cartridges. It prolongs the shelf life of the anesthetic solution with vasoconstrictor to approximately 18 months. However, sodium bisulfite renders the local anesthetic considerably more *acidic* than the same solution without a vasoconstrictor. Acidic solutions of local anesthetics contain a greater proportion of charged cation molecules (RNH^+) than of uncharged base molecules (RN). Because of this, the diffusion of local anesthetic solution into the axoplasm is slower, resulting in a delayed onset of anesthesia when local anesthetics containing sodium bisulfite (and vasoconstrictors) are injected.

Vasoconstrictors are important additions to local anesthetic solutions. Numerous studies have demonstrated conclusively that epinephrine, added to short- or medium-duration local anesthetic solutions, slows the rate of absorption, lowers the systemic blood level, delays cresting of the peak blood level, prolongs duration of anesthesia, intensifies "depth" of anesthesia, and reduces the incidence of systemic reactions.[18] In modern dentistry, adequate pain control of sufficient clinical duration is difficult to achieve without the inclusion of vasoconstrictors in the local anesthetic solution. Unless specifically contraindicated by a patient's medical status or by the required duration of treatment (short), the inclusion of a vasoconstrictor should be considered. Whenever these drugs are used, however, care must always be taken to avoid the inadvertent intravascular administration of the vasoconstrictor (and the local anesthetic) through careful aspiration and the slow administration of minimum dilutions.

REFERENCES

1. Cannall H, Walters H, Beckett AH, Saunders A: Circulating blood levels of lignocaine after peri-oral injections, *Br Dent J* 138:87-93, 1975.
2. Wildsmith JAW, Tucker GT, Cooper S, et al: Plasma concentrations of local anaesthetics after interscalene brachial plexus block, *Br J Anaesth* 49:461, 1977.

3. Brown G: The influence of adrenaline, noradrenaline vasoconstrictors on the efficacy of lidocaine, *J Oral Ther Pharmacol* 4:398-405, 1968.

4. Cowan A: Further clinical evaluation of prilocaine (Citanest), with and without epinephrine, *Oral Surg Oral Med Oral Pathol* 26:304-311, 1968.

5. Carpenter RL, Kopacz DJ, Mackey DC: Accuracy of Doppler capillary flow measurements for predicting blood loss from skin incisions in pigs, *Anesth Analg* 68:308-311, 1989.

6. Myers RR, Heckman HM: Effects of local anesthesia on nerve blood flow: studies using lidocaine with and without epinephrine, *Anesthesiology* 71:757-762, 1989.

7. Ahlquist RP: A study of adrenotropic receptors, *Am J Physiol* 153:586-600, 1948.

8. Langer SZ: Presynaptic regulation of catecholamine release, *Biochem Pharmacol* 23:1793-1800, 1974.

9. Lands AM, Arnold A, McAuliff JP, et al: Differentiation of receptor systems activated by sympathomimetic amines, *Nature* 214:597-598, 1967.

10. Braun H: Uber den Einfluss der Vitalitat der Gewebe auf die ortlichen und allgemeinen Giftwirkungen localabaesthesierender Mittel, und uber die Bedeutung des Adrerenalins fur die Lokalanasthesie, *Arch Klin Chir* 69:541-591, 1903.

11. Tolas AG, Pflug AE, Halter JB: Arterial plasma epinephrine concentrations and hemodynamic responses after dental injection of local anesthetic with epinephrine, *J Am Dent Assoc* 104:41-43, 1982.

12. Jastak JT, Yagiela JAY, Donaldson D, editors: *Local anesthesia of the oral cavity,* Philadelphia, 1995, WB Saunders.

13. Holroyd SV, Requa-Clark B: *Local anesthetics.* In Holroyd SV, Wynn RL, editors: *Clinical pharmacology in dental practice,* ed 3, St Louis, 1983, Mosby–Year Book.

14. Malamed SF: *Handbook of local anesthesia,* ed 3, St Louis, 1990, Mosby–Year Book.

15. Cryer PE: Physiology and pathophysiology of the human sympathoadrenal neuroendocrine system, *N Engl J Med* 303:436-444, 1980.

16. Yagiela JA: Epinephrine and the compromised heart, *Orofac Pain Manage* 1(5):1-8, 1991.

17. Kaneko Y, Ichinohe T, Sakurai M, et al: Relationship between changes in circulation due to epinephrine oral injection and its plasma concentration, *Anesth Prog* 36:188-190, 1989.

18. de Jong RH: *Uptake, distribution, and elimination.* In de Jong RH: *Local anesthetics,* St Louis, 1994, Mosby–Year Book.

19. Huang KC: Effect of intravenous epinephrine on heart rate as monitored with a computerized tachometer, *Anesthesiology* 73:A762, 1990.

20. Narchi P, Mazoit J-X, Cohen S, Samii K: Heart rate response to an IV test dose of adrenaline and lignocaine with and without atropine pretreatment, *Br J Anaesth* 66:583-586, 1991.

21. Malamed SF, Sykes P, Kubota Y, et al: Local anesthesia: a review, *Anesth Pain Control Dent* 1:11-24, 1992.

22. Lipp M, Dick W, Daublander M: Examination of the central venous epinephrine level during local dental infiltration and block anesthesia using tritium marked epinephrine as vasoconstrictor, *Anesthesiology* 69:371, 1988.

23. Stanton-Hicks Md'A, Berges PU, Bonica JJ: Circulatory effects of peridural block: IV. Comparison of the effects of epinephrine and phenylephrine, *Anesthesiology* 39:308-314, 1973.

24. Robertson VJ, Taylor SE, Gage TW: Quantitative and qualitative analysis of the pressor effects of levonordefrin, *J Cardiovasc Pharmacol* 6(5):929-935, 1984.

25. Clutter WE, Bier DM, Shah SD, Cryer PE: Epinephrine plasma metabolic clearance rates and physiologic thresholds for metabolic and hemodynamic actions in man, *J Clin Invest* 66:94-101, 1980.

26. Sveen K: Effect of the addition of a vasoconstrictor to local anesthetic solution on operative and postoperative bleeding, analgesia, and wound healing, *Int J Oral Surg* 8:301-306, 1979.

27. Meechan JG: The effects of dental local anaesthetics on blood glucose concentration in healthy volunteers and in patients having third molar surgery, *Br Dent J* 170:373-376, 1991.

28. Lefkowitz RJ, Hoffman BB, Taylor P: *Neurohumoral transmission: the autonomic and somatic motor nervous system.* In Gilman AG, et al, editors: *Goodman and Gilman's the pharmacological basis of therapeutics,* ed 8, New York, 1990, Pergamon Press.

29. Campbell RL: Cardiovascular effects of epinephrine overdose: case report, *Anesth Prog* 24:190-193, 1977.

30. Jakob W: Local anaesthesia and vasoconstrictive additional components, *Newslett Int Fed Dent Anesthesiol Soc* 2(1):3, 1989.

31. Bennett CR: *Monheim's local anesthesia and pain control in dental practice,* ed 7, St Louis, 1983, Mosby–Year Book.

32. Management of dental problems in patients with cardiovascular disease: report of a working conference jointly sponsored by the American Dental Association and American Heart Association, *J Am Dent Assoc* 68:333-342, 1964.

33. Use of epinephrine in connection with procaine in dental procedures: report of the Special Committee of the New York Heart Association, Inc., on the use of epinephrine in connection with procaine in dental procedures, *J Am Dent Assoc* 50.108, 1955.

34. Kaplan EL, editor: *Cardiovascular Disease in Dental Practice,* Dallas, 1986, American Heart Association.

35. Buckley JA, Ciancio SG, McMullen JA: Efficacy of epinephrine concentration in local anesthesia during periodontal surgery, *J Periodontol* 55:653-657, 1984.

36. Holroyd SV: *Clinical pharmacology in dental practice,* ed 2, St Louis, 1978, Mosby–Year Book.

37. Altura BM, Hershey SG, Zweifach BW: Effects of a synthetic analogue of vasopressin on vascular smooth muscle, *Proc Soc Exp Biol Med* 119:258-261, 1965.

38. Klingenstrom P, Nylen B, Westermark L: A clinical comparison between adrenalin and octapressin as vasoconstrictors in local anaesthesia, *Acta Anaesthesiol Scand* 11:35, 1967.

39. Newcomb GM, Waite IM: The effectiveness of local analgesic preparations in reducing haemorrhage during periodontal surgery, *J Dent* 1:37-42, 1972.

40. Epstein S: Clinical study of prilocaine with varying concentrations of epinephrine, *J Am Dent Assoc* 78:85-90, 1969.

41. van der Bijl P, Victor AM: Adverse reactions associated with norepinephrine in dental local anesthesia, *Anesth Prog* 39(3):87-89, 1992.

42. Hirota Y, Hori T, Kay K, Matsuura H: Effects of epinephrine and norepinephrine contained in 2% lidocaine on hemodynamics of the carotid and cerebral circulation in older and younger adults, *Anesth Pain Control Dent* 1(3):143-151, 1992.

43. Goulet JP, Perusse R, Turcotte JY: Contraindications to vasoconstrictors in dentistry: Part I. Cardiovascular diseases, *Oral Surg Oral Med Oral Pathol* 74(5):679-686, 1992.

44. Goulet JP, Perusse R, Turcotte JY: Contraindications to vasoconstrictors in dentistry: Part II. Hyperthyroidism, diabetes, sulfite sensitivity, cortico-dependent asthma, and pheochromocytoma, *Oral Surg Oral Med Oral Pathol* 74(5):687-691, 1992.

45. Goulet JP, Perusse R, Turcotte JY: Contraindications to vasoconstrictors in dentistry: Part III. Pharmacologic interactions, *Oral Surg Oral Med Oral Pathol* 74(5):692-697, 1992.

46. Verrill PJ: Adverse reactions to local anaesthetics and vasoconstrictor drugs, *Practitioner* 214:380-387, 1975.

CHAPTER
four

Clinical Action
of Specific Agents

Although many drugs are classified as local anesthetics and find use within the health professions, only a handful are currently used in dentistry. When the first edition of this text was published in 1980, five local anesthetics were available in dental cartridge form in the United States: *lidocaine, mepivacaine, prilocaine,* and the combination of *procaine* and *propoxycaine*.[1] In the 15 years since that first edition, increased demand for longer-acting local anesthetics has led to the introduction, in dental cartridges, of *bupivacaine* (1982 Canada, 1983 United States) and *etidocaine* (1985). In 1983 the thiophene ring-containing amide *articaine* became available in many areas (Europe, United Kingdom, Canada), but not yet in the United States (April 1996). Articaine is classified as an intermediate-duration local anesthetic. Procaine/propoxycaine was withdrawn from the U.S. market in January 1996.

With the availability of this increasing number of local anesthetics, there has been a renewal of interest in the all-important area of dental pain control. It is now possible for a doctor to select from a broad spectrum of local anesthetics a drug possessing the specific properties required by the patient for a given dental procedure. Table 4-1 lists local anesthetics and the various combinations in which they are currently available in the United States and Canada, and Table 4-2 lists these combinations by their expected duration of clinical action.

In this chapter each of the local anesthetics in its various combinations is described. In addition, the rationale for the selection of an appropriate local anesthetic for a given patient at a given appointment is presented. It is strongly suggested that the reader, the potential adminis-

trator of these drugs, become familiar with this material, including the contraindications to the administration of certain local anesthetic agents (Table 4-6).

In the following discussion of the clinical properties of specific local anesthetic combinations, several concepts are presented that require some prior discussion. These are the *duration of action* of the drug and the determination of the *maximum recommended dose.*

DURATION

The duration of pulpal (hard tissue) and soft tissue (total) anesthesia cited for each drug is an approximation. Factors exist that will affect both the depth and the duration of a drug's anesthetic action, either prolonging or (much more commonly) decreasing it. These factors include:

1. Individual variation in response to the drug administered
2. Accuracy in administration of the drug
3. Status of the tissues at the site of drug deposition (vascularity, pH)
4. Anatomical variation
5. Type of injection administered (supraperiosteal ["infiltration"] or nerve block)

The durations of anesthesia (pulpal and soft tissue) will be presented as a range (e.g., 40 to 60 minutes). This is an attempt to take into account the above-mentioned factors that can influence drug action.

Variation in individual response to a drug is quite common and is depicted in the so-called "bell" or normal

TABLE 4-1   Local Anesthetics Available in the United States and Canada (April 1996)

Agent	Duration of action*	Category
Articaine hydrochloride†		Amide
4% + epinephrine 1:100,000	Intermediate	
4% + epinephrine 1:200,000	Intermediate	
Bupivacaine hydrochloride		Amide
0.5% + epinephrine 1:200,000	Long	
Chloroprocaine hydrochloride		Ester
2%‡	Short	
Etidocaine hydrochloride		Amide
1.5% + epinephrine 1:200,000	Long	
Lidocaine hydrochloride		Amide
2%	Short	
2% + epinephrine 1:50,000	Intermediate	
2% + epinephrine 1:100,000	Intermediate	
Mepivacaine hydrochloride		Amide
3%	Short/intermediate	
2% + levonordefrin 1:20,000	Intermediate	
2% + epinephrine 1:200,000†	Intermediate	
Prilocaine hydrochloride		Amide
4%	Short	
4% + epinephrine 1:200,000	Long	
Procaine hydrochloride 2%/		Ester
propoxycaine hydrochloride†		Ester
0.4% + levonordefrin 1:20,000	Intermediate	

*The classification of duration of action is approximate, for extreme variations may be noted among patients. Short-duration drugs provide pulpal or deep anesthesia for less than 30 minutes; intermediate-duration drugs for about 60 minutes; and long-duration drugs for longer than 90 minutes.
†Not available in the United States (April 1996).
‡Not available in a glass cartridge for use in a dental aspirating syringe (April 1996).

TABLE 4-2   Approximate Duration of Action of Local Anesthetics

Short duration (pulpal about 30 min)
Chloroprocaine 2%†
Lidocaine 2%
Prilocaine 4% (infiltration)
Mepivacaine 3%

Intermediate (pulpal 60 min)
Articaine 4% + epinephrine 1:100,000*
Articaine 4% + epinephrine 1:200,000*
Lidocaine 2% + epinephrine 1:50,000
Lidocaine 2% + epinephrine 1:100,000
Mepivacaine 2% + levonordefrin 1:20,000
Mepivacaine 2% + epinephrine 1:200,000*
Prilocaine 4% (nerve block)
Prilocaine 4% + epinephrine 1:200,000
Procaine 2%/propoxycaine 0.4% + levonordefrin
   1:20,000*

Long (pulpal 90+ min)
Bupivacaine 0.5% + epinephrine 1:200,000
Etidocaine 1.5% + epinephrine 1:200,000 (nerve block)

*Not available in the United States (April 1996).
†Not available in glass cartridges for use in a dental aspirating
   syringe (April 1996).

distribution curve. A majority of patients will respond in a predictable manner to a drug's actions (i.e., 40 to 60 minutes). However, some patients will (with none of the other factors that influence drug action obviously present) have either a shorter or a longer duration of anesthesia. *This is to be expected and is entirely normal.*

Accuracy in the administration of an injected local anesthetic is the second factor influencing drug action. Though not as significant in certain techniques (i.e., supraperiosteal), accuracy in deposition is a major factor in many nerve blocks in which a considerable thickness of soft tissue must be penetrated to access the nerve to be blocked. The inferior alveolar nerve block is a prime example of a technique in which the duration of anesthesia is greatly influenced by the accuracy of injection. Deposition of the anesthetic close to a nerve will provide greater depth and duration of anesthesia compared with an anesthetic deposited at a greater distance from the nerve to be blocked.

The *status of the tissues* into which a local anesthetic is deposited will influence the observed duration of anesthetic action. The presence of normal healthy tissue at the site of drug deposition is assumed. Inflammation, infection, or pain (acute or chronic) usually decrease the anticipated duration of action. Increased vascularity at an injection site results in a more rapid absorption of the local anesthetic and a decreased duration of anesthesia. This is most notable in areas of infection and inflammation but is also a consideration in "normal" anatomy. The neck of the mandibular condyle, the target for local anesthetic deposition in the Gow-Gates mandibular nerve block, is considerably less vascular than the target area for the inferior alveolar nerve block. The expected duration of anesthesia for any local anesthetic will be greater in the less vascular region.

Anatomical variation will also influence clinical anesthesia. In Chapter 12 the normal anatomy of the maxilla and mandible is described. If anything, the most notable aspect of "normal" anatomy is the presence of extreme variation (in size and shape of the head, for example) from person to person. The techniques presented in later chapters are based on the middle of the bell curve, the so-called "normal responders." Anatomical variations away from this "norm" will adversely influence the duration of clinical drug action. Though most obvious in the mandible (height of the mandibular foramen, width of the ramus), such variation may also be noted in the maxilla. Supraperiosteal infiltration, usually quite effective in providing pulpal anesthesia for maxillary teeth, will provide shorter than expected or inadequate anesthesia where the alveolar bone is more dense than usual. Where the zygomatic arch is lower (primarily in children, but occasionally in adults), infiltration anesthesia of the maxillary first and second molars may provide a shorter duration or even fail to provide adequate pulpal anesthesia. In other cases the palatal root of maxillary molars may not be adequately anesthetized, even in the presence of a normal alveolar bony thickness, when that root flares greatly toward the midline of the palate.

Finally, the duration of clinical anesthesia will be influenced by the *type of injection administered.* For all the drugs presented, administration of a nerve block will provide a longer duration of both pulpal and soft tissue anesthesia than will supraperiosteal injection. This assumes that the recommended minimum volume of anesthetic is injected. Smaller than recommended volumes will decrease the duration of action. Larger than recommended doses will *not* provide increased duration. For example, a duration of 40 minutes may be expected to follow a supraperiosteal injection, whereas a 60-minute duration is to be expected with a nerve block.

MAXIMUM DOSES OF LOCAL ANESTHETICS

The doses of local anesthetic drugs are presented in terms of milligrams of drug per unit of body weight, either milligrams per kilogram (mg/kg) or milligrams per pound (mg/lb). These numbers, like the ones presented for duration, reflect approximate values, for there is a wide range in patient responses to blood levels of local anesthetics (or of any drug).

In patients whose responses to anesthetic blood levels lie in the middle of the normal distribution curve, the administration of a maximum dose based on body weight will produce a local anesthetic blood level just below the threshold for an overdose (toxic) reaction. The response observed if an overdose reaction develops will be mild (e.g., tremor of the arms and legs, drowsiness). Patients who are "hyporesponders" to elevated local anesthetic blood levels will not experience adverse reactions until their local anesthetic blood level is above this "normal" threshold. These patients represent little or no increased risk when local anesthetics are administered in "usual" dental doses. However, "hyperresponders" may demonstrate clinical signs and symptoms of local anesthetic overdose at blood levels that are somewhat lower than those normally required to produce such reactions. To increase safety during the administration of local anesthetics for all patients, but especially in this latter group, *one should always minimize drug doses, using the smallest clinically effective dose.* Recommended volumes of anesthetics are presented for each injection technique in Chapters 13, 14, and 15.

Maximum doses for many of the local anesthetics have been modified since the first edition of this book. The Council on Dental Therapeutics of the American Dental Association and the United States Pharmacopeial (USP) Convention reviewed (independently) maximum recommended doses for local anesthetics and no longer adjust them for inclusion of a vasoconstrictor.[2,3] The doses recommended in this chapter represent the more conservative of those recommended by either the Council, the USP, or the drug's manufacturer.[4,5]

Before this change the maximum recommended adult dose of lidocaine, for example, without a vasoconstrictor was 300 mg, whereas if epinephrine was included in the solution the maximum dose was 500 mg.[4] Such distinctions will no longer be made.

Maximum doses are unlikely to be reached in most dental patients, especially adults of normal body weight for most dental procedures. Two groups of patients, however, constitute a potentially increased risk from overly high local anesthetic blood levels: the smaller (well-behaved) child and the debilitated elderly individual. Considerable attention should be given drug administration in these two groups.

The maximum calculated drug dose should always be decreased in medically compromised, debilitated, or elderly persons.

Changes in liver function, plasma protein binding, blood volume, and other important physiological functions influence the manner in which local anesthetics are distributed and biotransformed in the body.[6] The net result of these changes is to increase plasma blood levels of the drug, thereby increasing the relative risk of overdose reactions. The half-lives of amide local anesthetics are significantly increased in the presence of decreased liver function or perfusion.[7] Maximum plasma blood levels tend to be higher and to remain so longer in these situations. The calculated drug dose (based on body weight) should be decreased in all "at risk" individuals. Unfortunately, there is no sure-fire formula to aid in determining the degree of dose reduction for a given patient. It is suggested that the doctor evaluate each patient's dental care needs and then devise a treatment plan that takes into account that person's requirement for smaller doses of local anesthetic at every treatment appointment.

A commonly asked question is, *"How do I determine the dose of each local anesthetic administered in situations where I need to administer more than one drug?"* The answer, again, is that no guaranteed formula exists for determining this number. However the method I use is simply that *the total dose of both local anesthetics should not exceed the lower of the two maximum doses for the individual agents.*

For example, a 100 lb (45 kg) patient receiving 4% prilocaine with epinephrine may be given 2.7 mg/lb (or 270 mg) during a 90-minute procedure (the approximate half-life of prilocaine). She receives two cartridges (144 mg), but anesthesia is inadequate for the treatment to proceed. As is commonly the case, the doctor believes that the lack of anesthesia is due to the anesthetic drug (I've got a "bad batch of local") (but not due to technique or to patient anatomy, as is more likely to be the case) and elects to change to lidocaine 2% with epinephrine 1:100,000 to provide anesthesia. How does one determine the maximum dose of lidocaine that may be used?

If lidocaine were being administered alone to this patient, its maximum dose would be 100 (lb) × 2 (mg/lb), or 200 mg. However, she has already received 144 mg of prilocaine in the past few minutes. The amount of lidocaine permitted will thus be the smaller total maximum dose (which in this case is 200 mg [lidocaine] versus 270 mg [prilocaine]) minus the dose of prilocaine already administered (144 mg), which permits a dose of 56 mg of lidocaine, or 1.5 cartridges, to be administered to this patient.

As is discussed later, it is highly unlikely that a "bad batch" of local anesthetic has been distributed to the doctor. The most common causes for failure to achieve adequate anesthesia are anatomical variation and faulty technique. (However, blaming the failure on the anesthetic drug serves to soothe the doctor's ego.)

The concept of maximum dose is discussed more fully in Chapter 18.

• • •

Clinically available local anesthetics—the amides: lidocaine, mepivacaine, prilocaine, articaine, bupivacaine, and etidocaine; and the esters: propoxycaine and procaine—are discussed. Agents available for topical application (topical anesthetics) are also discussed.

TABLE 4-3 Local Anesthetic Use by Dentists in Ontario, Canada (n = 2426)

Specific drug combinations

Drug combination	Percent of cartridges used
Lidocaine with epinephrine 1:100,000	23.38
Articaine with epinephrine 1:200,000	19.91
Articaine with epinephrine 1:100,000	17.93
Prilocaine with epinephrine 1:200,000	16.36
Mepivacaine with levonordefrin 1:20,000	6.35
Mepivacaine plain	6.29
Prilocaine plain	3.87
Lidocaine with epinephrine 1:50,000	2.97
Bupivacaine 0.5% with epinephrine 1:200,000	2.08
Mepivacaine with epinephrine 1:100,000	0.85

Anesthetic drug utilization

Local anesthetic	Percent of cartridges used
Articaine	37.84
Lidocaine	26.35
Prilocaine	20.23
Mepivacaine	13.49
Bupivacaine	2.08

Data modified from Haas DA, Lennon D: Local anesthetic use by dentists in Ontario, *J Can Dent Assoc* 61:297-304, 1995.

Which local anesthetic combinations are most commonly used in dental practice? In a survey of dentists in Ontario (Canada), three drugs—lidocaine, articaine, and prilocaine—are the most commonly used.[8] Table 4-3 presents the results of this survey.

PROCAINE

Pertinent Information

Classification Ester.

Chemical formula 2-Diethylaminoethyl 4-aminobenzoate hydrochloride.

$$H_2N-\bigcirc-COOCH_2CH_2N\begin{array}{c}C_2H_5\\C_2H_5\end{array}$$

Prepared by Alfred Einhorn, 1904 to 1905.

Potency 1 (procaine = 1).

Toxicity 1 (procaine = 1).

Metabolism Hydrolyzed rapidly in plasma by plasma pseudocholinesterase.

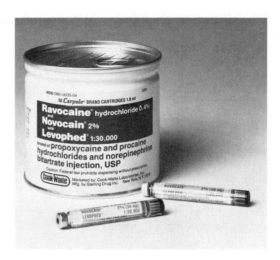

Fig. 4-1 Procaine 2% and propoxycaine 0.4% with levophed 1:30,000. *(Courtesy Cooke-Waite Laboratories, New York.)*

Excretion More than 2% unchanged in the urine (90% as para-aminobenzoic acid [PABA], 8% as diethylaminoethanol).

Vasodilating properties Produces the greatest vasodilation of all currently used local anesthetics.

pK_a 9.1.

pH of plain solution 5.0 to 6.5.

pH of vasoconstrictor-containing solution 3.5 to 5.5.

Onset of action 6 to 10 minutes.

Effective dental concentration 2% to 4%.

Anesthetic half-life 0.1 hour.

Topical anesthetic action Not in clinically acceptable concentration.

Comments

Procaine, the first injectable local anesthetic synthesized, is no longer available as a sole agent in dental cartridges. Its proprietary name, Novocain, however, is synonymous throughout the world with local anesthesia. Procaine was found until recently (January 1996) in dental cartridges in combination with a second ester anesthetic, propoxycaine (Fig. 4-1).

Used as the sole local anesthetic agent for pain control in dentistry, as it was for many years following its introduction in 1904, 2% procaine (plain) provides essentially *no* pulpal anesthesia and from 15 to 30 minutes of soft tissue anesthesia. This is due to its profound vasodilating properties. Procaine produces the most vasodilation of all clinically used local anesthetics.[9] Thus a clean operating field will be more difficult to maintain with procaine because of increased bleeding.

Procaine is an important drug in the immediate management of accidental intraarterial (IA) injection of a drug; its vasodilating properties are used to aid in breaking arteriospasm.[10]

Though not extremely common, the incidence of allergy to both procaine and other ester local anesthetics is significantly greater than that to amide local anesthetics.[11]

Metabolized in the blood by plasma cholinesterase, procaine does not exhibit increased toxicity in patients with hepatic dysfunction.

The maximum recommended dose of procaine, used for peripheral nerve blocks, is 1000 mg.[12]

With a pK_a of 9.1, procaine has a slow clinical onset of anesthesia (6 to 10 minutes), a reason for the inclusion of propoxycaine in the anesthetic cartridge.

PROPOXYCAINE

Pertinent Information

Classification Ester.

Chemical formula 2-Diethylaminoethyl-4-amino-2-propoxybenzoate hydrochloride.

Prepared by Clinton and Laskowski, 1952.

Potency 7 to 8 (procaine = 1).

Toxicity 7 to 8 (procaine = 1).

Metabolism Hydrolyzed in both plasma and the liver.

Excretion Via the kidneys; almost entirely hydrolyzed.

Vasodilating properties Yes, but not as profound as those of procaine.

pK_a Not available.

pH of plain solution Not available.

Onset of action Rapid (2 to 3 minutes).

Effective dental concentration 0.4%.

Anesthetic half-life Not available.

Topical anesthetic action Not in clinically acceptable concentrations.

Comments

Propoxycaine is combined with procaine (Fig. 4-1) in solution to provide a more rapid onset and a more profound and longer-lasting anesthesia than can be obtained with procaine alone. Propoxycaine is not available alone because its high toxicity (7 to 8 times that of procaine) limits its usefulness as a sole agent.

PROCAINE + PROPOXYCAINE

Although seldom used as the drug of choice in contemporary dental practice, the combination of two ester anesthetics, propoxycaine+procaine, is worthy of consideration for inclusion in a dentist's armamentarium of local anesthetics. It is useful when amide agents are absolutely contraindicated (i.e., because of documented allergy [though this is an extremely unlikely occurrence]) or when several amide anesthetics fail to provide clinically adequate anesthesia. Until its removal from the U.S. market in January 1996, the combination of procaine/propoxycaine was the only ester local anesthetic available in dental cartridge form.

0.4% Propoxycaine/2% procaine with 1:20,000 levonordefrin (United States) or *with 1:30,000 norepinephrine* (Canada) provides approximately 40 minutes of pulpal anesthesia and 2 to 3 hours of soft tissue anesthesia. The use of norepinephrine in local anesthetic solutions is not recommended, especially in areas where prolonged ischemia can lead to tissue necrosis. In the oral cavity this is most likely to develop in the palate.

Maximum recommended dose   Manufacturer's recommended maximum dose is 3.0 mg/lb or 6.6 mg/kg of body weight for the adult patient.[13] For children a dose of 3.0 mg/lb is recommended up to a maximum of five cartridges.

Procaine/Propoxycaine*

Proprietary name	Manufacturer	Percent local anesthetic	Vasoconstrictor	Duration of analgesia	Maximum dose (mg)
Novocain/ Ravocaine	Cook-Waite Labs	0.4 Propoxycaine 2 Procaine	Neo-Cobefrin 1:20,000	Pulpal: 30 to 60 min Soft tissue: 2 to 3 hr	6.6/kg 3/lb
	Cook-Waite Labs	0.4 Propoxycaine 2 Procaine	Levophed 1:30,000		Absolute max: 400 of *total* amine (procaine and propoxycaine)

*Procaine/propoxycaine was withdrawn from the U.S. market in January 1996.

DRUG: Procaine/Propoxycaine—with Vasoconstrictor

Concentration: 0.4% (2% procaine)

Cartridge contains:
propoxycaine 7.2 mg
procaine 36 mg
total anesthetic 43.2 mg

Max dose: 6.6 mg/kg			Max dose: 3.0 mg/lb*		
Weight (kg)	mg	Cartridges†	Weight (lb)	mg	Cartridges†
10	66	1.5	20	60	1.5
20	132	3	40	120	3
30	198	4.5	60	180	4
40	264	6	80	240	5.5
50	330	7.5	100	300	7
60	396	9	120	360	8.5
70	400	9	140	400	9
80	400	9	160	400	9
90	400	9	180	400	9
100	400	9	200	400	9

1. As with all local anesthetics, the dose varies and depends on the area to be anesthetized, the vascularity of the tissues, individual tolerance, and the technique of anesthesia. The lowest dose needed to provide effective anesthesia should be administered.
2. Doses indicated are the maximum suggested for normal healthy individuals: they should be decreased for debilitated or elderly patients.
3. Children: Based on a dose of 3.0 mg/lb body weight, 5 cartridges maximum.

*From *Drug information sheet: Ravocaine and Novocain with Levophed,* New York, 1993, Cook-Waite, Sterling Winthrop.
†Rounded to the nearest half-cartridge.

LIDOCAINE

Pertinent Information

Classification   Amide.

Chemical formula   2-Diethylamino 2´,6-acetoxylidide hydrochloride.

Prepared by   Nils Löfgren, 1943.

Introduced   1948.

Potency   2 (compared with procaine) (procaine = 1; today lidocaine is used as the standard of comparison [lidocaine = 1] for all local anesthetics).

Toxicity   2 (compared with procaine).

Metabolism   In the liver, by the microsomal fixed-function oxidases, to monoethylglyceine and xylidide; xylidide is a local anesthetic and potentially toxic.[14] (See Fig. 2-3.)

Excretion   Via the kidneys; less than 10% unchanged, more than 80% various metabolites.

Vasodilating properties   Considerably less than those of procaine; however, more than those of prilocaine or mepivacaine.

pK$_a$ 7.9.

pH of plain solution   6.5.

pH of vasoconstrictor-containing solution 5.0 to 5.5.

Onset of action   Rapid (2 to 3 minutes).
Effective dental concentration   2%.
Anesthetic half-life   1.6 hours.
Topical anesthetic action   Yes (in clinically acceptable concentrations [5%]).

Maximum recommended dose *Manufacturer's* recommended maximum dose of lidocaine with epinephrine is 3.2 mg/lb or 7.0 mg/kg of body weight for the adult patient, not to exceed a dose of 500 mg. For children, the same dose for lidocaine with epinephrine of 3.2 mg/lb is recommended by the manufacturer.[15] The manufacturer also recommends a dose of 2.0 mg/lb (4.4 mg/kg), not to exceed 300 mg for lidocaine without a vasoconstrictor. I recommend the more conservative dosage regimen for lidocaine suggested by the Council on Dental Therapeutics of the American Dental Association and the USP Convention.[2,3] This dose is 2.0 mg/lb (4.4 mg/kg) for lidocaine with or without a vasoconstrictor additive. This dose still allows for a significant volume of drug to be used to achieve profound clinical anesthesia with a somewhat diminished risk of development of toxic (overdose) reactions.

Comments

Lidocaine was synthesized in 1943 and, in 1948, became the first amide local anesthetic to be marketed. Its entry into clinical practice transformed dentistry, replacing procaine (Novocain) as the drug of choice for pain control. Compared with procaine, lidocaine possesses a more rapid onset of action (2 minutes versus 6 to 10 minutes), produces more profound anesthesia, has a longer duration of action, and has a greater potency.

Allergy to amide local anesthetics is virtually nonexistent; true, documented, and reproducible allergic reactions are extremely rare, though possible.[16-20] This is a major clinical advantage of lidocaine (and all amides) over ester local anesthetics.[11]

Within a few years of its introduction, lidocaine replaced procaine as the most widely used local anesthetic in both medicine and dentistry, a position it maintains today in most countries. It is, today, the "gold standard" against which all new local anesthetics are compared.

Lidocaine is available in three formulations—2% without a vasoconstrictor, 2% with epinephrine 1:50,000, and 2% with epinephrine 1:100,000 (Fig. 4-2). Recently, 2% lidocaine with epinephrine 1:200,000 has become available in several countries (though not in North America as of April 1996).

Two percent lidocaine without a vasoconstrictor (lidocaine plain) has a vasodilating effect that limits pulpal anesthesia to only 5 to 10 minutes. The vasodilatory effect produces higher blood levels of the drug, with a consequent increase in the risk of adverse reaction along with an increase in bleeding in the region of drug deposition. There are today few clinical indications for the use of 2% lidocaine without a vasoconstrictor in a typical dental practice. Indeed several major manufacturers of local anesthetics in North America have ceased marketing lidocaine plain in dental cartridges.[21,22]

Two percent lidocaine with epinephrine 1:50,000 causes a decrease in blood flow (perfusion) to the area of injection. The anesthetic blood level will be

Lidocaine						

Proprietary name	Manufacturer	Percent local anesthetic	Vasoconstrictor	Duration of analgesia	Manufacturer's MRD (mg)	Author's MRD (mg)
Lidocaine HCl Alphacaine HCl Xylocaine HCl	Many generics Carlisle Labs Astra Pharmaceutical	2	—	Pulpal: 5 to 10 min Soft tissue: 60 to 120 min	4.4/kg 2.0/lb Absolute max: 300	4.4/kg 2.0/lb Absolute max: 300
Lidocaine HCl Alphacaine HCl Lignospan Octocaine HCl Xylocaine HCl	Many generics Carlisle Labs Septodont Novocol Chemical Astra Pharmaceutical	2	Epinephrine 1:50,000	Pulpal: 60 min Soft tissue: 3 to 5 hr	6.6/kg 3.0/lb Absolute max: 500	4.4/kg 2.0/lb Absolute max: 300
Lidocaine HCl Alphacaine HCl Lignospan Octocaine HCl Xylocaine HCl	Many generics Carlisle Labs Septodont Novocol Chemical Astra Pharmaceutical	2	Epinephrine 1:100,000	Pulpal: 60 min Soft tissue: 3 to 5 hr	6.6/kg 3.0/lb Absolute max: 500	4.4/kg 2.0/lb Absolute max: 300

MRD, Maximum recommended dose.

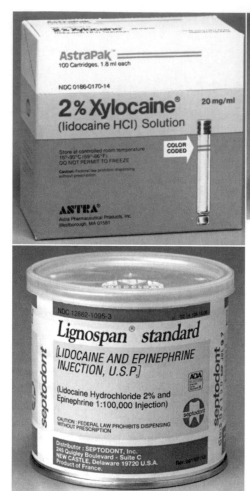

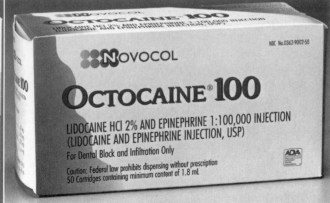

Fig. 4-2 **A,** Lidocaine 2%. **B** and **C,** Lidocaine 2% with epinephrine 1:100,000. (*A, Courtesy Astra Pharmaceutical Products, Westborough, Mass. B, Courtesy Novocol Pharmaceutical of Canada, Cambridge, Ontario. C, Courtesy Septodont, New Castle, Del.*)

decreased, leading to decreased bleeding in the area of injection due to the α-stimulating actions of the epinephrine. Because the local anesthetic is absorbed more slowly (thereby remaining at the site of administration longer), an increased duration of action is noted: approximately 60 minutes of pulpal anesthesia and 3 to 5 hours of soft tissue anesthesia. The epinephrine dilution is 0.02 mg/ml of solution, or 0.036 mg per cartridge. For patients weighing more than 100 lb (approximately 45 kg), the limiting factor in determination of the dose of this drug combination is the maximum epinephrine dose of 0.2 mg for healthy patients. The maximum recommended dose for epinephrine-sensitive individuals—such as certain cardiac patients and clinically hyperthyroid patients—is 0.04 mg per appointment. This is the equivalent of *one* cartridge of 1:50,000 epinephrine. (See Chapter 20.)

My only recommended use of 2% lidocaine with 1:50,000 epinephrine is for hemostasis.

Two percent lidocaine with epinephrine 1:100,000 decreases blood flow into the area of injection. There is also an increased duration of action: approximately 60 minutes of pulpal anesthesia and 3 to 5 hours of soft tissue anesthesia. In addition to the lower blood level of lidocaine, less bleeding occurs in the area of injection. The epinephrine dilution is 0.01 mg/ml of solution, or 0.018 mg per cartridge. Epinephrine-sensitive patients should be limited to *two* cartridges of 1:100,000 epinephrine per appointment.

The duration and depth of pulpal anesthesia obtained with both lidocaine-epinephrine solutions (1:50,000 and 1:100,000) are equivalent. Each may provide 60 minutes of pulpal anesthesia in ideal circumstances and soft tissue anesthesia of 3 to 5 hours' duration. Indeed, 2% lidocaine with 1:200,000 or 1:250,000 epinephrine will provide the same duration of pulpal and soft tissue anesthesia, though not the same level of hemostasis.[23]

For *duration* and *depth* of pain control for most dental procedures in a typical dental patient, 2% lidocaine with 1:100,000 epinephrine is recommended over 2% lidocaine with 1:50,000 epinephrine. Both provide equal duration and depth, but the 1:100,000 solution contains half as much epinephrine as the 1:50,000. Although the dose of epinephrine in the 1:50,000 is not dangerous to most patients, ASA III and IV risks with histories of cardiovascular disease might prove overly sensitive to these dilutions. Additionally, an elderly patient is likely to be more sensitive to vasoconstrictors. In these individuals the greater dilution (1:100,000 or 1:200,000) should be used.

For *hemostasis* in procedures in which bleeding is definitely or potentially a problem, 2% lidocaine with 1:50,000 epinephrine is recommended as it decreases bleeding (during periodontal surgery) by 50% compared with a 1:100,000 epinephrine dilution.[24] Vasoconstrictors act directly in the area of injection to decrease tissue perfusion, and the 1:50,000 provides excellent hemostatic action. A 1:100,000 dilution can also be used for hemostasis, but is not as effective. Rebound vasodilation will occur with both 1:50,000 and 1:100,000 epinephrine dilutions. Minimum volumes need be administered to provide excellent hemostasis.

Signs and symptoms of lidocaine toxicity (overdose) may be the same (CNS stimulation followed by CNS depression) as described in Chapter 2. However, the stimulatory phase may be quite brief or may not develop at all.[25] The first signs and symptoms of lidocaine overdose may be drowsiness, leading to a loss of consciousness and respiratory arrest.

DRUG: Lidocaine—without Vasoconstrictor

Concentration: 2%   Cartridge contains: 36 mg

Max dose: 4.4 mg/kg			Max dose: 2 mg/lb		
Weight (kg)	mg	Cartridges*	Weight (lb)	mg	Cartridges*
10	44	1	20	40	1
20	88	2	40	80	2
30	132	3.5	60	120	3
40	176	4.5	80	160	4
50	220	6	100	200	5.5
60	264	7	120	240	6.5
70	300	8	140	280	7.5
80	300	8	160	300	8
90	300	8	180	300	8
100	300	8	200	300	8

1. As with all local anesthetics, the dose varies and depends on the area to be anesthetized, the vascularity of the tissues, individual tolerance, and the technique of anesthesia. The lowest dose needed to provide effective anesthesia should be administered.
2. Doses indicated are the maximum suggested for normal healthy individuals: they should be decreased for debilitated or elderly patients.
*Rounded to the nearest half-cartridge.

DRUG: Lidocaine—with Epinephrine 1:50,000 Author's Maximum Recommended Dose

Concentration: 2%   Cartridge contains: 36 mg

Max dose: 4.4 mg/kg			Max dose: 2.0 mg/lb		
Weight (kg)	mg	Cartridges*	Weight (lb)	mg	Cartridges*
10	44	1	20	40	1
20	88	2	40	80	2
30	132	3.5	60	120	3
40	176	4.5	80	160	4
50	220	6	100	200	5.5
60	220	6†	120	200	5.5†
70	220	6†	140	200	5.5†
80	220	6†	160	200	5.5†
90	220	6†	180	200	5.5†
100	220	6†	200	200	5.5†

1. As with all local anesthetics, the dose varies and depends on the area to be anesthetized, the vascularity of the tissues, individual tolerance, and the technique of anesthesia. The lowest dose needed to provide effective anesthesia should be administered.
2. Doses indicated are the maximum suggested for normal healthy individuals: they should be decreased for debilitated or elderly patients.
*Rounded to the nearest half-cartridge.
†Two tenths milligram of epinephrine the dose-limiting factor.

DRUG: Lidocaine—with Epinephrine 1:50,000 Manufacturer's Maximum Recommended Dose

Concentration: 2%   Cartridge contains: 36 mg

Max dose: 6.6 mg/kg			Max dose: 3.0 mg/lb		
Weight (kg)	mg	Cartridges*	Weight (lb)	mg	Cartridges*
10	66	2	20	60	1.5
20	132	3.5	40	120	3
30	198	5.5	60	180	5
40	264	7	80	240	6.5
50	330	9	100	300	8
60	396	11	120	360	10
70	462	13	140	420	11.5
80	500	13.5	160	480	13
90	500	13.5	180	500	13.5
100	500	13.5	200	500	13.5

1. As with all local anesthetics, the dose varies and depends on the area to be anesthetized, the vascularity of the tissues, individual tolerance, and the technique of anesthesia. The lowest dose needed to provide effective anesthesia should be administered.
2. Doses indicated are the maximum suggested for normal healthy individuals: they should be decreased for debilitated or elderly patients.
*Rounded to the nearest half-cartridge.

DRUG: Lidocaine—with Epinephrine 1:100,000 Author's Maximum Recommended Dose

Concentration: 2%   Cartridge contains: 36 mg

Max dose: 4.4 mg/kg			Max dose: 2.0 mg/lb		
Weight (kg)	mg	Cartridges*	Weight (lb)	mg	Cartridges*
10	44	1	20	40	1
20	88	2	40	80	2
30	132	3.5	60	120	3
40	176	4.5	80	160	4
50	220	6	100	200	5.5
60	264	7	120	240	6.5
70	300	8	140	280	7.5
80	300	8	160	300	8
90	300	8	180	300	8
100	300	8	200	300	8

1. As with all local anesthetics, the dose varies and depends on the area to be anesthetized, the vascularity of the tissues, individual tolerance, and the technique of anesthesia. The lowest dose needed to provide effective anesthesia should be administered.
2. Doses indicated are the maximum suggested for normal healthy individuals: they should be decreased for debilitated or elderly patients.
*Rounded to the nearest half-cartridge.

DRUG: Lidocaine—with Epinephrine 1:100,000 Manufacturer's Maximum Recommended Dose

Concentration: 2%   Cartridge contains: 36 mg

Max dose: 6.6 mg/kg			Max dose: 3.0 mg/lb		
Weight (kg)	mg	Cartridges*	Weight (lb)	mg	Cartridges*
10	66	2	20	60	1.5
20	132	3.5	40	120	3
30	198	5.5	60	180	5
40	264	7	80	240	6.5
50	330	9	100	300	8
60	396	11	120	360	10
70	462	13	140	420	11.5
80	500	13.5	160	480	13
90	500	13.5	180	500	13.5
100	500	13.5	200	500	13.5

1. As with all local anesthetics, the dose varies and depends on the area to be anesthetized, the vascularity of the tissues, individual tolerance, and the technique of anesthesia. The lowest dose needed to provide effective anesthesia should be administered.
2. Doses indicated are the maximum suggested for normal healthy individuals: they should be decreased for debilitated or elderly patients.
*Rounded to the nearest half-cartridge.

MEPIVACAINE

Pertinent Information

Classification   Amide.

Chemical formula   1-methyl 2',6'-pipecoloxylidide hydrochloride.

Prepared by   A. F. Ekenstam, 1957, and introduced into dentistry in 1960 as a 2% solution containing the synthetic vasopressor levonordefrin, and in 1961 as a 3% solution without a vasoconstrictor.

Potency   2 (procaine = 1; lidocaine = 2).

Toxicity   1.5 to 2 (procaine = 1; lidocaine = 2).

Metabolism   In the liver, by microsomal fixed-function oxidases. Hydroxylation and N-demethylation play important roles in the metabolism of mepivacaine.

Excretion   Via the kidneys; approximately 1% to 16% of anesthetic dose is excreted unchanged.

Vasodilating properties   Mepivacaine produces only slight vasodilation. The duration of pulpal anesthesia with mepivacaine without a vasoconstrictor is 20 to 40 minutes (that with lidocaine without a vasoconstrictor is 5 minutes; that with procaine without a vasoconstrictor, up to 2 minutes).

pKa   7.6.

pH of plain solution   4.5.

pH of vasoconstrictor-containing solution   3.0 to 3.5.

Onset of action   Rapid (1½ to 2 minutes).

Effective dental concentration   3% without a vasoconstrictor; 2% with a vasoconstrictor.

Anesthetic half-life   1.9 hours.

Topical anesthetic action   Not in clinically acceptable concentrations.

Maximum recommended dose   Manufacturer's recommended maximum dose is 3.0 mg/lb or 6.6 mg/kg of body weight, not to exceed 400 mg for the adult patient.[22] For children a dose of 3.0 mg/lb is recommended up to a maximum of five cartridges of either the 2% or 3% form of the drug. My maximum recommended dose for mepivacaine is 2.0 mg/lb (4.4 mg/kg), not to exceed 300 mg for either adult or child.

Comments

The mild vasodilating properties of mepivacaine provide a longer duration of anesthesia than most other local anesthetics when the drug is administered without a vasoconstrictor. Mepivacaine plain provides 20 to 40 minutes of pulpal anesthesia and 2 to 3 hours of soft tissue anesthesia. *Three percent mepivacaine without a vasoconstrictor* (Fig. 4-3) is recommended for patients in whom a vasoconstrictor is not indicated and for dental procedures not requiring lengthy pulpal anesthesia. Mepivacaine plain is among the most used

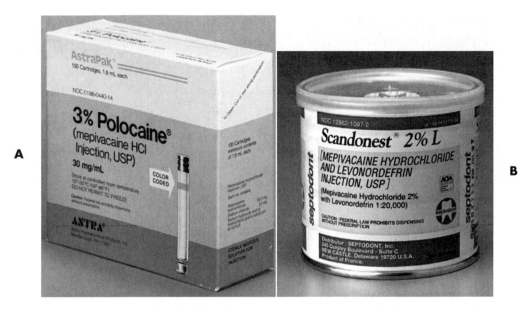

Fig. 4-3 **A,** Mepivacaine 3%. **B,** Mepivacaine 2% with levonordefrin 1:20,000. *(A, Courtesy Astra Pharmaceutical Products, Westborough, Mass. B, Courtesy Septodont, New Castle, Del.)*

Mepivacaine

Proprietary name	Manufacturer	Percent local anesthetic	Vasoconstrictor	Duration of analgesia	Manufacturer's MRD (mg)	Author's MRD (mg)
Mepivacaine HCl Arestocaine HCl Carbocaine HCl Isocaine HCl Polocaine HCl Scandonest HCl	Many generics Carlisle Labs Cook-Waite Labs Novocol Chemical Astra Pharmaceutical Septodont	3		Pulpal: 20 to 40 min Average (20 min infiltration; 40 min block) Soft tissue: 2 to 3 hr average	6.6/kg 3.0/lb Absolute max: 400	4.4/kg 2.0/lb Absolute max: 300
Mepivacaine HCl Arestocaine HCl Isocaine HCl Polocaine HCl Carbocaine HCl	Many generics Carlisle Labs Novocol Chemical Astra Pharmaceutical Cook-Waite Labs	2	Levonordefrin 1:20,000 Neo-Cobefrin 1:20,000	Pulpal: 60 to 90 min average Soft tissue: 3 to 5 hr average	6.6/kg 3.0/lb Absolute max: 400	4.4/kg 2.0/lb Absolute max: 300
Carbocaine HCl	Cooke-Waite Labs	2	Epinephrine 1:200,000	Pulpal: 45 to 60 min Soft tissue: 2 to 4 hr	6.6/kg 3.0/lb Absolute max: 400	4.4/kg 2.0/lb Absolute max: 300
Scandonest 2% Special	Septodont	2	Epinephrine 1:100,000	Pulpal: 60 min Soft tissue: 2 to 5 hr	6.6/kg 3.0/lb Absolute max: 400	4.4/kg 2.0/lb Absolute max: 300

MRD, Maximum recommended dose.

local anesthetics in pediatric dentistry and is often very appropriate in the management of geriatric patients. *Two percent mepivacaine with a vasoconstrictor* provides a depth and duration of both pulpal (hard tissue) and soft tissue (total) anesthesia similar to those observed with the lidocaine-epinephrine solutions. Pulpal anesthesia of approximately 60 minutes' duration and soft tissue anesthesia of 3 to 5 hours are to be expected. Two vasoconstrictors, levonordefrin (1:20,000) and epinephrine (1:100,000), are available

DRUG: Mepivacaine
Author's Maximum Recommended Dose

Concentration: 3%   Cartridge contains: 54 mg

Max dose: 4.4 mg/kg			Max dose: 2.0 mg/lb		
Weight (kg)	mg	Cartridges*	Weight (lb)	mg	Cartridges*
10	44	1	20	40	1
20	88	1.5	40	80	1.5
30	132	2.5	60	120	2
40	176	3	80	160	3
50	220	4	100	200	3.5
60	264	4.5	120	240	4
70	300	5.5	140	280	5
80	300	5.5	160	300	5.5
90	300	5.5	180	300	5.5
100	300	5.5	200	300	5.5

1. As with all local anesthetics, the dose varies and depends on the area to be anesthetized, the vascularity of the tissues, individual tolerance, and the technique of anesthesia. The lowest dose needed to provide effective anesthesia should be administered.
2. Doses indicated are the maximum suggested for normal healthy individuals: they should be decreased for debilitated or elderly patients.
*Rounded to the nearest half-cartridge.

DRUG: Mepivacaine
Manufacturer's Maximum Recommended Dose

Concentration: 3%   Cartridge contains: 54 mg

Max dose: 6.6 mg/kg			Max dose: 3.0 mg/lb		
Weight (kg)	mg	Cartridges*	Weight (lb)	mg	Cartridges*
10	66	1	20	60	1
20	132	1.5	40	120	2
30	198	3.5	60	180	3
40	264	5	80	240	4.5
50	330	6.5	100	300	5.5
60	396	8	120	360	6.5
70	400	8	140	400	7.5
80	400	8	160	400	7.5
90	400	8	180	400	7.5
100	400	8	200	400	7.5

1. As with all local anesthetics, the dose varies and depends on the area to be anesthetized, the vascularity of the tissues, individual tolerance, and the technique of anesthesia. The lowest dose needed to provide effective anesthesia should be administered.
2. Doses indicated are the maximum suggested for normal healthy individuals: they should be decreased for debilitated or elderly patients.
*Rounded to the nearest half-cartridge.

DRUG: Mepivacaine—with Vasoconstrictor
Author's Maximum Recommended Dose

Concentration: 2%   Cartridge contains: 36 mg

Max dose: 4.4 mg/kg			Max dose: 2.0 mg/lb		
Weight (kg)	mg	Cartridges*	Weight (lb)	mg	Cartridges*
10	44	1	20	40	1
20	88	2	40	80	2
30	132	3.5	60	120	3
40	176	4.5	80	160	4
50	220	6	100	200	5.5
60	264	7	120	240	6.5
70	300	8	140	280	7.5
80	300	8	160	300	8
90	300	8	180	300	8
100	300	8	200	300	8

1. As with all local anesthetics, the dose varies and depends on the area to be anesthetized, the vascularity of the tissues, individual tolerance, and the technique of anesthesia. The lowest dose needed to provide effective anesthesia should be administered.
2. Doses indicated are the maximum suggested for normal healthy individuals: they should be decreased for debilitated or elderly patients.
*Rounded to the nearest half-cartridge.

DRUG: Mepivacaine—with Vasoconstrictor
Manufacturer's Maximum Recommended Dose

Concentration: 2%   Cartridge contains: 36 mg

Max dose: 6.6 mg/kg			Max dose: 3.0 mg/lb		
Weight (kg)	mg	Cartridges*	Weight (lb)	mg	Cartridges*
10	66	2	20	60	1.5
20	132	3.5	40	120	3
30	198	5.5	60	180	5
40	264	7	80	240	6.5
50	330	9	100	300	8
60	396	11	120	360	10
70	400	11	140	400	11
80	400	11	160	400	11
90	400	11	180	400	11
100	400	11	200	400	11

1. As with all local anesthetics, the dose varies and depends on the area to be anesthetized, the vascularity of the tissues, individual tolerance, and the technique of anesthesia. The lowest dose needed to provide effective anesthesia should be administered.
2. Doses indicated are the maximum suggested for normal healthy individuals: they should be decreased for debilitated or elderly patients.
*Rounded to the nearest half-cartridge.

with mepivacaine. Though hemostasis is present, levo-nordefrin does not provide the intensity of hemostasis noted with epinephrine 1:100,000.

The incidence of true, documented, and reproducible allergy to mepivacaine, an amide local anesthetic, is virtually nonexistent.

Signs and symptoms of mepivacaine overdose usually follow the more typical pattern of CNS stimulation followed by depression. Although possible, the absence of stimulation with immediate CNS depression (i.e., drowsiness and unconsciousness, as is seen with lidocaine) is quite rare with mepivacaine.

PRILOCAINE

Pertinent Information

Classification   Amide.

Other chemical name   Propitocaine.

Chemical formula   2-Propylamino-*o*-propionotoluidide hydrochloride.

$$\text{CH}_3 - \text{C}_6\text{H}_4 - \text{NH} \cdot \text{CO} \cdot \text{CH}(\text{CH}_3) \cdot \text{N}(\text{C}_3\text{H}_7)(\text{H})$$

Prepared by   Löfgren and Tegnér, 1953; reported in 1960.

Potency   2 (procaine = 1; lidocaine = 2).

Toxicity   1 (procaine = 1; lidocaine = 2); 40% less toxic than lidocaine.

Metabolism   Differs significantly from that of lidocaine and mepivacaine. Being a secondary amine, prilocaine is hydrolyzed straightforwardly by hepatic amidases into orthotoluidine and *N*-propylalanine. Carbon dioxide is a major end-product of prilocaine transformation. The efficiency of the body's degradation of prilocaine is demonstrated by the extremely small fraction of intact prilocaine recoverable in the urine.[26] Orthotoluidine can induce the formation of methemoglobin, producing methemoglobinemia, if large doses are administered. Minor degrees of methemoglobinemia have been observed with both benzocaine and lidocaine administration,[27,28] but prilocaine consistently reduces the blood's oxygen-carrying capacity, at times sufficiently to cause observable cyanosis.[29] Limiting the total prilocaine dose to 600 mg (as recommended by the manufacturer) avoids symptomatic cyanosis. Methemoglobin levels of less than 20% usually do not produce clinical signs or symptoms (which are grayish or slate blue cyanosis of the lips, mucous membranes, and nail beds and [infrequently] respiratory and circulatory distress).

Methemoglobinemia may be reversed within 15 minutes with administration of 1 to 2 mg/kg body weight of 1% methylene blue solution intravenously over a 5-minute period.[28] The mechanism of methemoglobin production is discussed in Chapter 10. Prilocaine undergoes biotransformation more rapidly and completely than lidocaine, taking place not only in the liver, but also to a smaller degree in the kidney and lung.[29] Plasma levels of prilocaine decrease more rapidly than lidocaine.[30] Prilocaine is thus considered to be less toxic systemically than comparably potent local anesthetic amides.[31] Signs of CNS toxicity following prilocaine administration in humans are briefer and less severe than following the same intravenous dose of lidocaine.[32]

Excretion   Prilocaine and its metabolites are excreted primarily via the kidneys. Renal clearance of prilocaine is faster than that for other amides, resulting in its faster removal from the circulation.[33]

Vasodilating properties   Prilocaine is a vasodilating agent. It produces greater vasodilation than does mepivacaine but less than lidocaine and significantly less than procaine.

pK$_a$ 7.9.

pH of plain solution   4.5.

pH of vasoconstrictor-containing solution   3.0 to 4.0.

Onset of action   Slightly slower than that of lidocaine (2 to 4 minutes).

Effective dental concentration   4%.

Anesthetic half-life   1.6 hours.

Topical anesthetic action   Not in clinically acceptable concentrations.

Prilocaine, in its uncharged base form, has recently been released as an integral part of EMLA (eutectic mixture of local anesthetics) cream, which permits the anesthetics (lidocaine/prilocaine) to penetrate the imposing anatomic barrier of intact skin. EMLA cream is used to provide topical anesthesia of skin prior to venipuncture.[34]

Prilocaine

Proprietary name	Manufacturer	Percent local anesthetic	Vasoconstrictor	Duration of analgesia	Author's and manufacturer's MRD (mg)
Citanest Plain	Astra Pharmaceutical	4	—	Pulpal: 10 min infiltration; 60 min block Soft tissue: 1½ to 2 hr infiltration; 2 to 4 hr block	6/kg 2.7/lb Absolute max: 400
Citanest Forte	Astra Pharmaceutical	4	Epinephrine 1:200,000	Pulpal: 60 to 90 min Soft tissue: 3 to 8 hr	6/kg 2.7/lb Absolute max: 400

MRD, Maximum recommended dose.

Maximum recommended dose   Both the manufacturer's and my maximum recommended dose for prilocaine is 2.7 mg/lb or 6.0 mg/kg of body weight for the adult patient, to a maximum recommended dose of 400 mg.[35]

Comments

Clinical actions of *prilocaine plain*   (Fig. 4-4) vary greatly with the type of anesthetic technique used. Though true for all anesthetics, the variation between supraperiosteal and nerve block is more pronounced with prilocaine plain. Infiltration (supraperiosteal) provides short durations of pulpal (5 to 10 minutes) and soft tissue (1½ to 2 hours) anesthesia, whereas regional block (e.g., inferior alveolar nerve block) provides pulpal anesthesia for up to 60 minutes (most often between 40 and 60 minutes) and soft tissue anesthesia for 2 to 4 hours. Thus prilocaine plain is frequently able to provide anesthesia that is equal in duration to that obtained from lidocaine or mepivacaine with a vasoconstrictor.

Clinical actions of *prilocaine with 1:200,000 epinephrine* are not as dependent on anesthetic technique. Prilocaine with epinephrine provides lengthy anesthesia while offering the least concentrated epinephrine dilution currently available: 1:200,000. Pulpal anesthesia of 60 to 90 minutes' duration and soft tissue anesthesia of 3 to 8 hours may be obtained. The cartridge contains 0.009 ml of epinephrine; therefore epinephrine-sensitive individuals—such as the ASA III cardiovascular disease patient—may receive up to four cartridges (0.036 mg) of prilocaine with epinephrine.

In epinephrine-sensitive patients requiring prolonged pulpal anesthesia (≥60 minutes), prilocaine plain or with 1:200,000 epinephrine is strongly recommended. It is rapidly biotransformed and, for this reason, is considered by some the safest of all amide local anesthetics (i.e., lower toxicity).[31]

Prilocaine is *relatively contraindicated* in patients with idiopathic or congenital methemoglobinemia, hemoglobinopathies (sickle cell anemia), anemia, or cardiac or respiratory failure evidenced by hypoxia, as methemoglobin levels are increased, decreasing oxygen-carrying capacity. Prilocaine administration is also *relatively contraindicated* in patients receiving *acetaminophen* or *phenacetin*, both of which produce elevations in methemoglobin levels.

DRUG: Prilocaine—with and without Vasoconstrictor

Concentration: 4%   Cartridge contains: 72 mg

Max dose: 6 mg/kg			Max dose: 2.7 mg/lb		
Weight (kg)	mg	Cartridges*	Weight (lb)	mg	Cartridges*
10	60	1	20	54	1
20	120	1.5	40	108	1.5
30	180	2.5	60	162	2
40	240	3	80	216	3
50	300	4	100	270	3.5
60	360	5	120	324	4.5
70	400	5.5	140	378	5
80	400	5.5	160	400	5.5
90	400	5.5	180	400	5.5
100	400	5.5	200	400	5.5

1. As with all local anesthetics, the dose varies and depends on the area to be anesthetized, the vascularity of the tissues, individual tolerance, and the technique of anesthesia. The lowest dose needed to provide effective anesthesia should be administered.
2. Doses indicated are the maximum suggested for normal healthy individuals: they should be decreased for debilitated or elderly patients.

*Rounded to the nearest half-cartridge.

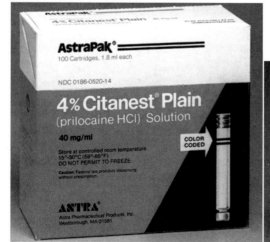
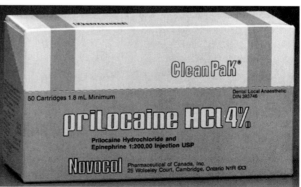

Fig. 4-4   Prilocaine 4%. **A,** Without epinephrine. **B,** With epinephrine 1:200,000. *(A, Courtesy Astra Pharmaceutical Products, Westborough, Mass. B, Courtesy Novocol Pharmaceutical of Canada, Cambridge, Ontario.)*

ARTICAINE

Pertinent Information

Classification   Amide.

Chemical formula   3-*N*-Propylamino-proprionyl-amino-2-carbomethoxy-4-methylthiophene hydrochloride.

$$S$$

COOCH$_3$

• HCl

H$_3$C   NHCOCHNHCH$_2$CH$_2$CH$_3$

CH$_3$

Prepared by   H. Rusching et al, 1969.

Introduced   1976 in Germany and Switzerland, 1978 in the Netherlands, 1980 in Austria and Spain, 1983 in Canada. Not available in the United States (April 1996).

Potency   1.5 times that of lidocaine and 1.9 times that of procaine.

Toxicity   Similar to lidocaine and procaine.

Metabolism   In both the plasma and liver, degradation of articaine is initiated by hydrolysis of the carboxylic and ester groups to give free carboxylic acid.[36] From that point the reaction can follow several pathways: cleavage of the carboxylic acid, formation of an acid amide group by internal cyclization, and oxidation.

Excretion   Via the kidneys; approximately 5% to 10% unchanged, approximately 90% metabolites (M$_1$ at 87%, M$_2$ at 2%).

Vasodilating properties   Articaine has a vasodilating effect equal to that of lidocaine. Procaine is slightly more vasoactive.

pK$_a$ 7.8.

pH of plain solution   Not available.

pH of vasoconstrictor-containing solution   4.4 to 5.2 for 1:100,000; 4.6 to 5.4 for 1:200,000.

Onset of action   Articaine 1:200,000, infiltration 1 to 2 minutes, mandibular block 2 to 3 minutes; articaine 1:100,000, infiltration 1 to 2 minutes, mandibular block 2 to 2½ minutes.

Effective dental concentration   4% with 1:100,000 or 1:200,000 epinephrine.

Anesthetic half-life   1.25 hours.

Topical anesthetic action   Not in clinically acceptable concentration.

Maximum recommended dose   Manufacturer's recommended maximum dose is 3.2 mg/lb or 7.0 mg/kg of body weight for the adult patient.[5,37] For children between the ages of 4 and 12 years, the manufacturer recommends a dose of 2.27 mg/lb or 5.0 mg/kg.[37]

Comments

Originally known as carticaine, the generic nomenclature of this local anesthetic was changed in 1984 to articaine. Literature appearing before 1984 should be reviewed under the original name.

Articaine is the first and only anesthetic of the amide type to possess a thiophene ring as its lipophilic moiety. It has many of the physicochemical properties of other local anesthetics, with the exception of the aromatic moiety and the degree of protein binding.

Articaine has been available in Europe and Canada since 1984 in two formulations: 4% *with 1:100,000 epinephrine* and 4% *with 1:200,000 epinephrine* (Fig. 4-5). The formulation with 1:100:000 epinephrine provides approximately 75 minutes of pulpal anesthesia; the 1:200,000 formulation, approximately 45 minutes.[38,39]

It has been claimed that articaine is able to diffuse through soft and hard tissues more reliably than other anesthetics.[40] However, controlled comparisons between articaine and standard local anesthetics have failed to corroborate this claim.[41,42]

Methemoglobinemia is a potential side effect of the administration of large doses of articaine. Such a reaction

Articaine					
Proprietary name	Manufacturer	Percent local anesthetic	Vasoconstrictor	Duration of analgesia	Author's and manufacturer's MRD (mg)
Septanest N Ultracaine D-S	Septodont Hoechst Labs	4	Epinephrine 1:200,000	Pulpal: 45 to 60 min Soft tissue: 2 to 5 hr	Adult: 7/kg, 3.2/lb Absolute max: 500 Children: 5/kg, 2.3/lb
Septanest SP Ultracaine D-S Forte	Septodont Hoechst Labs	4	Epinephrine 1:100,000	Pulpal: 60 to 75 min Soft tissue: 3 to 6 hr	Adult: 7/kg, 3.2/lb Absolute max: 500 Children: 5/kg, 2.3/lb

MRD, Maximum recommended dose.

DRUG: Articaine—with Vasoconstrictor, for Adults. Author's and Manufacturer's Maximum Recommended Dose

Concentration: 4%   Cartridge contains: 72 mg

Max dose: 7 mg/kg			Max dose: 3.2 mg/lb		
Weight (kg)	mg	Cartridges*	Weight (lb)	mg	Cartridges*
30	210	3	60	192	2.5
40	280	4	80	256	3.5
50	350	5	100	320	4.5
60	420	6	120	384	5.5
70	490	7	140	448	6
80	500	7	160	500	7
90	500	7	180	500	7
100	500	7	200	500	7

1. As with all local anesthetics, the dose varies and depends on the area to be anesthetized, the vascularity of the tissues, individual tolerance, and the technique of anesthesia. The lowest dose needed to provide effective anesthesia should be administered.
2. Doses indicated are the maximum suggested for normal healthy individuals: they should be decreased for debilitated or elderly patients.
*Rounded to the nearest half-cartridge.

DRUG: Articaine—with Vasoconstrictor, for Children. Author's and Manufacturer's Maximum Recommended Dose

Concentration: 4%   Cartridge contains: 72 mg

Max dose: 5 mg/kg			Max dose: 2.3 mg/lb		
Weight (kg)	mg	Cartridges*	Weight (lb)	mg	Cartridges*
10	50	0.5	20	46	0.5
13	65	1	26	60	1
16	80	1	32	74	1
19	95	1.5	38	87	1
22	110	1.5	44	101	1.5
25	125	1.5	50	115	1.5
28	140	2	56	129	2
31	155	2	62	143	2

1. As with all local anesthetics, the dose varies and depends on the area to be anesthetized, the vascularity of the tissues, individual tolerance, and the technique of anesthesia. The lowest dose needed to provide effective anesthesia should be administered.
2. Doses indicated are the maximum suggested for normal healthy individuals: they should be decreased for debilitated or elderly patients.
*Rounded to the nearest half-cartridge.

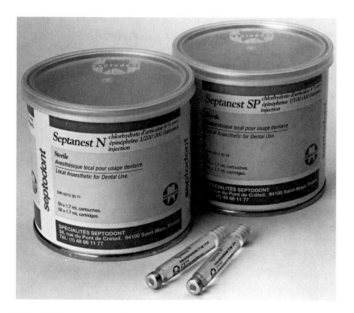

Fig. 4-5 Articaine 4% with epinephrine 1:100,000 and epinephrine 1:200,000. (*Courtesy Spécialités Septodont, France.*)

has been noted following intravenous administration for regional anesthetic purposes; no cases have yet been reported when articaine was administered in the usual manner and volume for dental procedures. The mechanism for methemoglobin production is discussed in Chapter 10.

Articaine is contraindicated in patients with idiopathic or congenital methemoglobinemia, anemia, or cardiac or respiratory failure evidenced by hypoxia (ASA III and IV). Another contraindication is the presence of a documented allergy to sulfur-containing drugs. Articaine is the only local anesthetic possessing the latter contraindication. A case of an allergic reaction to articaine in a dental situation was recently reported.[43]

As originally marketed, cartridges of articaine contained the preservative methylparaben. Although the incidence of allergy to paraben-type preservatives is quite low, methylparaben has been removed from all other available local anesthetic cartridges in the United States and Canada. Formulations of articaine without methylparaben are now available.

BUPIVACAINE

Pertinent Information

Classification   Amide.

Chemical formula   1-Butyl-2′,6′-pipecoloxylidide hydrochloride; structurally related to mepivacaine except for a butyl group replacing a methyl group.

Prepared by   A. F. Ekenstam, 1957.

Potency Some 4 times that of lidocaine, mepivacaine, and prilocaine.

Toxicity Less than 4 times that of lidocaine and mepivacaine.

Metabolism Metabolized in the liver by amidases.

Excretion Via the kidney; 16% unchanged bupivacaine has been recovered from human urine.

Vasodilating properties Relatively significant: greater than those of lidocaine, prilocaine, and mepivacaine, yet considerably less than those of procaine.

pK_a 8.1.

pH of plain solution 4.5 to 6.0.

pH of vasoconstrictor-containing solution 3.0 to 4.5.

Onset of action Occasionally similar to that of lidocaine, mepivacaine, and prilocaine, but usually requires longer onset time (i.e., 6 to 10 minutes).

Effective dental concentration 0.5%.

Anesthetic half-life 2.7 hours.

Topical anesthetic action Not in clinically acceptable concentrations.

Maximum recommended dose Manufacturer's maximum recommended dose is 0.6 mg/lb or 1.3 mg/kg of body weight for the adult patient, with a maximum dose not to exceed 90 mg.[44]

Comments

Bupivacaine has been available in cartridge form since February 1982 in Canada and July 1983 in the United States. Available as a 0.5% solution with 1:200,000 epinephrine (Fig. 4-6), there are two primary indications for its utilization in dentistry:

1. Lengthy dental procedures for which pulpal (deep) anesthesia in excess of 90 minutes is required (e.g., full mouth reconstruction, implant surgery, and extensive periodontal procedures)
2. Management of postoperative pain (e.g., endodontic, periodontal, and surgical)

The patient's requirement for postoperative opioid analgesics is considerably lessened when bupivacaine is administered for pain control.[45] For postoperative pain

control following a short procedure, the bupivacaine may be administered at the start of the procedure; for postoperative pain control in a lengthy procedure, it might be reasonable to administer the bupivacaine at the conclusion of the procedure, immediately before the patient's discharge from the office.

In recent years a regimen for management of postsurgical pain has been developed that is clinically quite effective.[46] It suggests the pretreatment administration of one or two oral doses of a nonsteroidal antiinflammatory drug (NSAID), followed by the administration of a suitable (i.e., intermediate-duration) local anesthetic to manage the periprocedural pain. A long-duration anesthetic (bupivacaine, etidocaine) is administered immediately before patient discharge (if deemed necessary), with the patient continuing the NSAID every "x" hours as indicated (not "prn pain") for "x" number of days. The requirement for opioid agonist analgesics is significantly diminished with this protocol.

For many patients receiving bupivacaine the onset of anesthesia will be similar to that observed with other amide anesthetics (2 to 4 minutes); however, in many patients the onset of anesthesia will be delayed for from

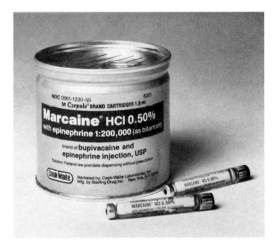

Fig. 4-6 Bupivacaine 0.5% with epinephrine 1:200,000. *(Courtesy Cooke-Waite Laboratories, New York.)*

Bupivacaine					
Proprietary name	Manufacturer	Percent local anesthetic	Vasoconstrictor	Duration of analgesia	Author's and manufacturer's MRD (mg)
Marcaine HCl	Cook-Waite Labs	0.5	Epinephrine 1:200,000	Pulpal: 90 to 180 min Soft tissue: 4 to 9 hr, up to 12 hr reported	1.3/kg 0.6/lb Absolute max: 90

MRD, Maximum recommended dose.

DRUG: Bupivacaine—with Epinephrine 1:200,000

Concentration: 0.5%   Cartridge contains: 9 mg

Weight (kg)	mg	Cartridges*	Weight (lb)	mg	Cartridges*
	Max dose: 1.3 mg/kg			Max dose: 0.6 mg/lb	
10	13	1.5	20	12	1
20	26	3	40	24	2.5
30	39	4	60	36	4
40	52	5.5	80	48	5
50	65	7	100	60	6.5
60	78	8.5	120	72	8
70	90	10	140	84	9
80	90	10	160	90	10
90	90	10	180	90	10
100	90	10	200	90	10

1. As with all local anesthetics, the dose varies and depends on the area to be anesthetized, the vascularity of the tissues, individual tolerance, and the technique of anesthesia. The lowest dose needed to provide effective anesthesia should be administered.
2. Doses indicated are the maximum suggested for normal healthy individuals: they should be decreased for debilitated or elderly patients.
*Rounded to the nearest half-cartridge.

6 to 10 minutes, a finding understandable in view of bupivacaine's pK_a of 8.1. If this occurs it may be advisable, at subsequent appointments, to initiate procedural pain control with a more rapid-acting amide (e.g., mepivacaine, lidocaine, or prilocaine), which provides clinically acceptable pain control within a few moments and permits the procedure to commence more promptly. Follow this with an injection of bupivacaine for long-duration anesthesia.

Bupivacaine is not recommended in younger patients or in those for whom the risk of postoperative soft tissue injury produced by self-mutilation is increased, such as physically and mentally disabled persons. Bupivacaine is rarely indicated in children because pediatric dental procedures are usually of short duration.

ETIDOCAINE

Pertinent Information

Classification   Amide.

Chemical formula   2-(N-Ethylpropylamino) butyro-2,6-xylidide hydrochloride; structurally similar to lidocaine.

Prepared by   Takman, 1971.

Potency   4 times that of lidocaine.

Toxicity   2 times as toxic as lidocaine following subcutaneous administration; 4 times as toxic as lidocaine following rapid intravenous administration.

Metabolism   Undergoes N-dealkylation; can also be hydroxylated on the aromatic ring. Hydrolytic metabolism appears less important than for lidocaine and prilocaine, with less than 10% of the dose appearing in the urine as both 2,6-xylidine and its hydroxylated product, as opposed to over 70% for lidocaine.[47]

Excretion   Etidocaine and its metabolites are excreted primarily via the kidneys.

Vasodilating properties   Relatively significant: greater than those of lidocaine, prilocaine, and mepivacaine yet considerably less than those of procaine.

pK_a   7.7.

pH of plain solution   4.5.

pH of vasoconstrictor-containing solution   3.0 to 3.5.

Onset of action   Equivalent to that of lidocaine, mepivacaine, and prilocaine ($1\frac{1}{2}$ to 3 minutes).

Effective dental concentration   1.5%.

Anesthetic half-life   2.6 hours.

Topical anesthetic action   Not in clinically acceptable concentrations.

Maximum recommended dose   Manufacturer's maximum recommended dose is 3.6 mg/lb or 8.0 mg/kg of body weight for the adult patient, with an absolute maximum dose of 400 mg.[48]

Comments

Etidocaine is a long-acting local anesthetic, chemically related to lidocaine. Its clinical indications are identical to those of bupivacaine. The primary differences in clinical activity between the two are their onset of anesthetic action and duration for infiltration anesthesia. Etidocaine (with a pK_a of 7.7) has an onset of action of about 3 minutes, whereas bupivacaine (with a pK_a of

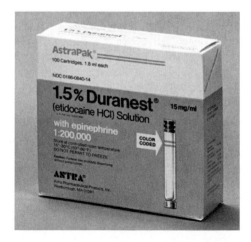

Fig. 4-7   Etidocaine 1.5% with epinephrine 1:200,000. *(Courtesy Astra Pharmaceutical Products, Westborough, Mass.)*

Etidocaine

Proprietary name	Manufacturer	Percent local anesthetic	Vasoconstrictor	Duration of analgesia	Author's and manufacturer's MRD (mg)
Duranest	Astra Pharmaceutical	1.5	Epinephrine 1:200,000	Pulpal: 90 to 180 min average Soft tissue: 4 to 9 hr average	8/kg 3.6/lb Absolute max: 400

MRD, Maximum recommended dose.

DRUG: Etidocaine—with Epinephrine 1:200,000

Concentration: 1.5%   Cartridge contains: 27 mg

Weight (kg)	mg	Cartridges*	Weight (lb)	mg	Cartridges*
	Max dose: 8.0 mg/kg			Max dose: 3.6 mg/lb	
10	80	3	20	72	2.5
20	160	6	40	144	5
30	240	9	60	216	8
40	320	12	80	288	10.5
50	400	15	100	360	13
60	400	15	120	400	15
70	400	15	140	400	15
80	400	15	160	400	15
90	400	15	180	400	15
100	400	15	200	400	15

1. As with all local anesthetics, the dose varies and depends on the area to be anesthetized, the vascularity of the tissues, individual tolerance, and the technique of anesthesia. The lowest dose needed to provide effective anesthesia should be administered.
2. Doses indicated are the maximum suggested for normal healthy individuals: they should be decreased for debilitated or elderly patients.
*Rounded to the nearest half-cartridge.

TABLE 4-4 Effective Concentrations for Injection and Topical Application of Local Anesthetics

Agent	Effective concentration		Useful as topical
	Injection (%)	Topical (%)	
Lidocaine	2	2 to 5	Yes
Mepivacaine	2 to 3	12 to 15	No
Procaine	2 to 4	10 to 20	No
Tetracaine	0.25 to 1	0.2 to 1	Yes

8.1) has an onset of 6 to 10 minutes. In addition, the duration of clinical action of etidocaine is extremely dependent on the type of injection administered. Following infiltration (supraperiosteal) administration, pulpal anesthesia is extremely variable in duration and depth, whereas following nerve block the duration of pulpal anesthesia is considerably longer, ranging from 90 to 180 minutes.[49]

Dental cartridges of etidocaine are a 1.5% solution containing 1:200,000 epinephrine (Fig. 4-7).

ANESTHETICS FOR TOPICAL APPLICATION

The use of topically applied local anesthetics is an important component of the atraumatic administration of regional block anesthesia. (See Chapter 11.) Topical anesthetics are unable to penetrate intact skin but do penetrate abraded skin or any mucous membranes.*

The concentration of an anesthetic used topically is typically greater than that same agent administered by injection. The higher concentration facilitates diffusion of the drug through the mucous membrane. Higher concentration also leads to a greater potential toxicity, both locally to the tissues and systemically.[50] Because topical anesthetics do not contain vasoconstrictors and anesthetics are inherently vasodilators, vascular absorption of some topical formulations is rapid, and levels in the blood may soon reach those achieved by direct intravenous administration.[50]

Many local anesthetics used effectively via injection are ineffective as topical anesthetics (e.g., mepivacaine, prilocaine, and procaine) because the concentrations required to produce anesthesia via topical application are high, with significant overdose and local tissue toxicity potential (Table 4-4).

As a rule, topical anesthesia is effective only on surface tissues (2 to 3 mm). Tissues deep to the area of application are poorly anesthetized. However, surface anesthesia does allow for atraumatic needle penetration of the mucous membrane.[51]

The topical anesthetics benzocaine and lidocaine base are insoluble in water. They are, however, soluble in

*EMLA: Eutectic mixture of local anesthetics, containing lidocaine and prilocaine in a nonionized base form, is able to penetrate intact skin. Its primary use is in preparation for venipuncture. EMLA is discussed more fully in Chapter 19.

alcohol, propylene glycol, polyethylene glycol, and other vehicles suitable for surface application. Benzocaine and lidocaine base are slowly absorbed into the cardiovascular system and therefore less likely to produce overdose reaction.

Some topical anesthetics are marketed in pressurized spray containers. Although they are no more effective than other forms, it is difficult to control the amount of solution expelled and to confine it to the desired site. Spray devices that do not deliver *measured doses* should not be used intraorally.

Benzocaine

Benzocaine (ethyl *p*-aminobenzoate) is an ester local anesthetic.

$$H_2N - \bigcirc - CO \cdot OC_2H_5$$

1. Poor solubility in water.
2. Poor absorption into cardiovascular system.
3. Systemic toxic (overdose) reactions virtually unknown.
4. Remains at the site of application longer, providing a prolonged duration of action.
5. Not suitable for injection.
6. Localized allergic reactions may occur following prolonged or repeated use. Though allergic reaction to ester anesthetics is rare, ester local anesthetics are more allergenic than amide local anesthetics.[52]
7. Reported to inhibit the antibacterial action of sulfonamides.[53]
8. Availability (Fig. 4-8)
    a. *Cetacaine,* liquid and gel topical anesthetic (Cetylite Industries): *tetracaine* 2%, *benzocaine* 14%, butylaminobenzoate 2%, benzalkonium chloride 0.5%, and cetyl dimethyl ethyl ammonium bromide 0.005% in a bland water-soluble base.
    b. *Gingicaine* liquid and gel (Belport Co., Inc.): each 100 g of gel contains 20 g of *benzocaine* with flavoring and coloring agents in a water-soluble polyethylene glycol base.
    c. *Healthco* topical anesthetic gel (Healthco, Inc.): 20% *benzocaine* with flavoring and coloring agents in a water-soluble polyethylene glycol base.
    d. *Hurricaine* liquid, gel, and spray, topical anesthetic (Beutlich, Inc.): 20% *benzocaine* with flavoring and coloring agents in a polyethylene glycol base.
    e. *Nephron* benzocaine ointment (Nephron Corp.): 18% *benzocaine* with flavoring agents in a polyethylene glycol base.
    f. *Novol-benzocaine solution* (Novocol Chemical Mfg. Co., Inc.): 10% *benzocaine* and essential oils 0.3 g/100 ml in a water-soluble base.
    g. *Oradent* Topical Anesthetic (Oradent Chemical Co.): *benzocaine* 16%, chlorobutanol 5 g/100 g, dioctyl sodium sulfosuccinate 1 g, peppermint oil and clove oil 0.155 g, polyoxyethylene sorbitan monolaurate 23.4 g, certified color, and propylene glycol.
    h. *Pennwhite* liquid and ointment topical anesthetic (S.S.White Retail): each 100 g contains 20 g of *benzocaine* with coloring and flavoring agents in a polyethylene glycol base.
    i. *PreJect* topical anesthetic gel (Hoyt Laboratories): each 100 g contains 20 g of *benzocaine* in a water-soluble polyethylene glycol base; available in orange, fruit, and cherry flavors.
    j. *Topex* metered spray (Sultan Chemists, Inc.): *benzocaine* 20%, ethyl alcohol 70.36%, and polyethylene glycol 7.5% with flavoring agents 2.14% in propellant A46; Topex anesthetic liquid and gel do not contain propellant A46.
    k. *Topicale* gel, liquid, and ointment (Premier Dental Products): *benzocaine* 18% and benzalkonium chloride 0.1% with flavoring agents in a water-soluble polyethylene glycol base.

Butacaine Sulfate

Butacaine sulfate (3-dibutylaminopropyl-4aminobenzoate sulfate) is a local anesthetic used as a substitute for cocaine in topical anesthesia of the eyes, ears, nose, and throat.

1. Has twice the anesthetic potency of cocaine, but is two or three times more toxic than cocaine.
2. Not suitable for injection.
3. Recommended dose is a total of 5 ml of a 4% solution (200 mg), which should not be exceeded.
4. Available as *Butyn* dental ointment (Abbott Laboratories): *butacaine* base 4% and benzyl alcohol (preservative) approximately 1%.

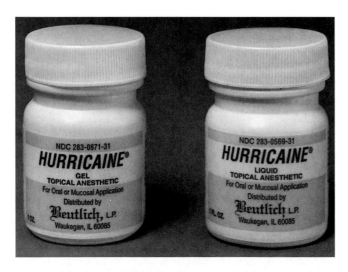

Fig. 4-8 Topical anesthetics containing benzocaine.

Cocaine Hydrochloride

Cocaine hydrochloride (benzoylmethylecgonine hydrochloride) occurs naturally as a white crystalline solid that is *highly soluble in water.*

1. Used exclusively via topical application. Injection contraindicated because of the ready availability of more effective and less toxic local anesthetics. Cocaine is an ester local anesthetic.
2. Onset of topical anesthetic action is quite rapid, usually developing within 1 minute.
3. Duration of anesthetic action may be as long as 2 hours.
4. Absorbed rapidly but eliminated slowly.
5. Undergoes metabolism in the liver. The liver is able to detoxify one minimal lethal dose of cocaine per hour.
6. Unchanged cocaine may be found in the urine.
7. Only local anesthetic consistently demonstrated to produce vasoconstriction, which develops as a result of its ability to potentiate the actions of endogenous epinephrine and norepinephrine.[29] Addition of vasoconstrictors to cocaine is therefore unnecessary, and also potentially dangerous, increasing the likelihood of dysrhythmias, including ventricular fibrillation.
8. Classified as a Schedule II drug under the Controlled Substances Act. Repeated use results in psychic dependence and tolerance.
9. Overdose of cocaine is not uncommon, primarily because the drug is readily absorbed and its dosage is not carefully monitored.
10. Clinical manifestations of mild overdose: euphoria, excitement, restlessness, tremor, hypertension, tachycardia, and tachypnea.
11. Clinical manifestations of acute cocaine overdose: excitement, restlessness, confusion, tremor, hypertension, tachycardia, tachypnea, nausea and vomiting, abdominal pain, exophthalmos, and mydriasis; followed by depression (CNS, cardiovascular, respiratory) and death from respiratory arrest.
12. Available in concentrations ranging from 2% to 10%.
13. It is recommended that the concentration of cocaine not exceed 4% for topical application to oral mucous membranes.
14. Solutions of cocaine are unstable and deteriorate on standing.
15. *Because of the extreme abuse potential of cocaine, its use as a topical anesthetic in dentistry is not recommended.*

Dyclonine Hydrochloride

Dyclonine hydrochloride (4'-butoxy-3-piperidinopropiophenone hydrochloride) is chemically unique from all other local anesthetics in that it is a ketone.

1. Cross-sensitization with other local anesthetics does not occur; therefore dyclonine may be used in patients with known sensitivities to local anesthetics of other chemical groups.
2. Slightly soluble in water.
3. Potency equal to that of cocaine.
4. Onset of anesthesia slow, requiring up to 10 minutes.
5. Duration of anesthesia may be as long as 1 hour.
6. Systemic toxicity extremely low, primarily because of the agent's poor water solubility.
7. Not indicated for use by injection or infiltration; irritating to tissues at the site of application.
8. A 0.5% solution is used in dentistry. Maximum recommended dose is 200 mg (40 ml of a 0.5% solution).
9. Available as *Dyclone* solution 0.5% (Astra Pharmaceutical Products, Inc.): each 100 ml of solution contains 500 mg of dyclonine HCl, 300 mg of chlorobutanol as a preservative, sodium chloride for isotonicity, and hydrochloric acid, as needed, to adjust pH.

Lidocaine

Lidocaine is available in two forms for topical application: (1) *lidocaine base,* which is poorly soluble in water, used as a 5% concentration, and is indicated for use on ulcerated, abraded, or lacerated tissue; and (2) *lidocaine hydrochloride,* which is available as a water-soluble preparation used in a 2% concentration. This water-soluble form of lidocaine penetrates tissue more efficiently than base form. However, systemic absorption is also greater, providing a greater risk of toxicity than base form.

1. Lidocaine is an amide local anesthetic with an *exceptionally low* incidence of allergic reactions.
2. Maximum recommended dose is 200 mg.
3. Availability (Fig. 4-9)

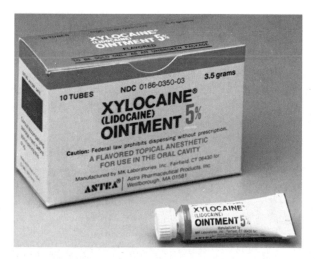

Fig. 4-9 Topical lidocaine ointment. *(Courtesy Astra Pharmaceutical Products, Westborough, Mass.)*

a. *Alphacaine* ointment 5% (Carlisle Laboratories, Inc.): 5.2 g of *lidocaine base* in an ointment consisting of polyethylene glycol–4000, polyethylene glycol–200, propylene glycol, saccharin, and flavor in every 100 g.

b. *Lidocaine* gel 5% topical anesthetic (Premier Dental Products): each 100 g contains 5 g *lidocaine* in a nonirritating, flavored, water-soluble glycol vehicle.

c. *Lidocaine* liquid 5% flavored (Graham Chemical Corp.): 5 g of *lidocaine base* in a solution containing a mixture of propylene glycol, glycerine, and flavoring agents in every 100 ml.

d. *Lidocaine* ointment 5% flavored (Graham Chemical Corp.): 5 g of *lidocaine base* in an ointment consisting of polyethylene glycol–1500, polyethylene glycol–4000, propylene glycol, and flavor in every 100 g.

e. *Xylocaine* liquid 5% flavored (Astra Pharmaceutical Products, Inc.): 5 g of *lidocaine base* in a solution containing a mixture of propylene glycol, glycerine, and flavoring agents in every 100 ml.

f. *Xylocaine* ointment 5% flavored (Astra Pharmaceutical Products, Inc.): 5 g of *lidocaine base* in an ointment consisting of polyethylene glycol–1500, polyethylene glycol–4000, propylene glycol, and flavor in every 100 g.

g. *Xylocaine* 10% aerosol (Astra Pharmaceutical Products, Inc.): 10% *lidocaine,* 7.13% ethyl alcohol, 20.79% polyethylene glycol–400, 0.001% cetylpyridinium chloride, 60.6% propellant mixture, and flavoring agents. (*Note:* is equipped with a metered-dose valve, 10 mg per spray.)

Tetracaine Hydrochloride

Tetracaine hydrochloride (2-dimethylaminoethyl-4-butyl-aminobenzoate hydrochloride) is a long-duration ester local anesthetic agent that can be injected or applied topically.

1. Highly soluble in water.
2. Applied topically, 5 to 8 times more potent than cocaine.
3. Onset of action following topical application is slow.
4. Duration of action is approximately 45 minutes following topical application.
5. Metabolized in plasma and the liver by plasma pseudocholinesterase at a slower rate than procaine.
6. Used for injection, available as a 0.15% concentration.
7. For topical application a 2% concentration is used.
8. Rapidly absorbed through mucous membranes. Use should be limited to small areas to avoid rapid absorption. Other, more slowly or poorly absorbed, agents should be used in lieu of tetracaine when larger areas of topical anesthesia are required.
9. Recommended maximum dose of 20 mg when used for topical application. This is 1 ml of a 2% solution.
10. Extreme caution urged because of the great potential for systemic toxicity.
11. Available as Cetacaine liquid topical anesthetic (Cetylite Industries): 2% tetracaine, 14% benzocaine, 2% butylaminobenzoate, 0.5% benzalkonium chloride, and 0.005% cetyldimethylethyl ammonium bromide in a water-soluble base.

SELECTION OF A LOCAL ANESTHETIC

With so many local anesthetic combinations available for injection, it becomes difficult to select an ideal drug for a given patient. Many dentists deal with this by simply using one local anesthetic for all procedures, regardless of their duration. For example, the dentist may elect to use 2% lidocaine with 1:100,000 epinephrine for procedures lasting 5 to 10 minutes as well as for procedures involving 90 minutes of treatment time. Although the duration of pulpal anesthesia achievable with this drug in ideal circumstances *may* permit pain-free treatment in both these instances, the patient requiring only 10 minutes of pulpal anesthesia will remain anesthetized unnecessarily for an additional 3 to 5 hours (soft tissues), whereas the patient requiring 90 minutes of pulpal anesthesia may experience discomfort toward the end of the procedure.

A rational approach to the selection of a local anesthetic for a patient includes a consideration of the *length of time for which pain control is required.* Table 4-5 lists the commonly used anesthetics according to their usual duration of anesthesia. The average, expected duration of pulpal and soft tissue anesthesia is listed. Again, take note, these numbers are approximations, and the actual duration of clinical anesthesia may be somewhat longer or shorter than indicated.

A second consideration in the selection of a local anesthetic must be the *requirement for pain control following treatment.* Long-duration anesthetics can be administered when postoperative pain is thought to be a factor. Drugs providing a shorter duration of soft tissue anesthesia can be used for nontraumatic procedures.

When postoperative pain is considered likely, 0.5% bupivacaine or 1.5% etidocaine (both with 1:200,000 epinephrine [for 8 to 12 hours of soft tissue anesthesia]) or 4% prilocaine with 1:200,000 epinephrine (for 5 to 8 hours of soft tissue anesthesia) are suggested.

For patients in whom postoperative anesthesia is a potential hazard, shorter-duration anesthetics should be used. These patients include younger children and the physically or mentally disabled, who might accidentally

T A B L E 4 - 5 Duration of Pulpal and Soft Tissue Anesthesia for Available Local Anesthetics

Agent	Duration (approx min)	
	Pulpal	Soft tissue
Chloroprocaine 2%	<10	30 to 45
Lidocaine 2%	5 to 10	60 to 120
Prilocaine 4% (infiltration)	5 to 10	90 to 120
Mepivacaine 3%	20 to 40	120 to 180
Articaine 4%, epinephrine 1:200,000	45	180 to 240
Mepivacaine 2%, epinephrine 1:200,000	45	120 to 240
Procaine 2%, propoxycaine 0.4%, levonordefrin 1:20,000	30 to 60	120 to 180
Lidocaine 2%, epinephrine 1:50,000	60	180 to 240
Lidocaine 2%, epinephrine 1:100,000	60	180 to 240
Mepivacaine 2%, levonordefrin 1:20,000	60	180 to 240
Prilocaine 4% (block)	60	120 to 240
Articaine 4%, epinephrine 1:100,000	75	180 to 300
Prilocaine 4%, epinephrine 1:200,000	60 to 90	120 to 240
Bupivacaine 0.5%, epinephrine 1:200,000	>90	240 to 540
Etidocaine 0.5%, epinephrine 1:200,000	>90	240 to 540

T A B L E 4 - 6 Contraindications for Local Anesthetics

Medical problem	Drugs to avoid	Type of contraindication	Alternative drug
Local anesthetic allergy, documented	All local anesthetics in same chemical class (e.g., esters)	Absolute	Local anesthetics in different chemical class (e.g., amides)
Sulfa allergy	Articaine	Absolute	Non–sulfur containing local anesthetic
Bisulfite allergy	Vasoconstrictor-containing local anesthetics	Absolute	Any local anesthetic without vasoconstrictor
Atypical plasma cholinesterase	Esters	Relative	Amides
Methemoglobinemia, idiopathic or congenital	Articaine, prilocaine	Relative	Other amides or esters
Significant liver dysfunction (ASA III-IV)	Amides	Relative	Amides or esters, but judiciously
Significant renal dysfunction (ASA III-IV)	Amides or esters	Relative	Amides or esters, but judiciously
Significant cardiovascular disease (ASA III-IV)	High concentrations of vasoconstrictors (as in racemic epinephrine gingival retraction cords)	Relative	Local anesthetics with epinephrine concentrations of 1:200,000 or 1:100,000 or mepivacaine 3% or prilocaine 4% (nerve blocks)
Clinical hyperthyroidism (ASA III-IV)	High concentrations of vasoconstrictors (as in racemic epinephrine gingival retraction cords)	Relative	Local anesthetics with epinephrine concentrations of 1:200,000 or 1:100,000 or mepivacaine 3% or prilocaine 4% (nerve blocks)

bite or chew their lips or tongue. For these patients 3% mepivacaine or 4% prilocaine (for infiltration) is recommended for use in short procedures.

A third factor is the need for *hemostasis* during the procedure. Anesthetic solutions containing epinephrine in a 1:50,000 or 1:100,000 dilution are recommended, via local infiltration, when hemostasis is considered necessary.

A fourth factor in the selection of a local anesthetic involves the *physical status of the patient.* Table 4-6 lists contraindications for local anesthetics based on this criterion.

Absolute contraindications require that the offending drug(s) not be administered to the patient under any condition. The risk that a life-threatening situation will arise is

---

**FACTORS IN SELECTION OF
LOCAL ANESTHETIC**

1. Length of time that pain control is required
2. Potential for discomfort in the posttreatment period
3. Possibility of self-mutilation in the postoperative period
4. Requirement for hemostasis during treatment
5. Medical status of the patient

---

increased. One absolute contraindication to local anesthetic administration exists: *documented reproducible allergy.* Fortunately this is an extremely rare occurrence, although the incidence of alleged local anesthetic allergy is quite high. Management of *alleged* and documented allergy to local anesthetics is discussed in Chapter 18.

In cases of a *relative contraindication* it is preferable to avoid administration of the drug in question because of an increased risk that an adverse response will develop. An alternative drug that is not contraindicated is recommended. However, if an acceptable alternative is not available, the drug in question may be used, but judiciously, with use of the minimum dose that will provide adequate pain control. One example of a relative contraindication is the presence of atypical plasma (pseudo)cholinesterase, which decreases the rate of biotransformation of ester local anesthetics. The amides may be used with no increase in risk in these patients. Relative contraindications are reviewed in Chapter 10.

The box above summarizes the criteria used in the selection of a local anesthetic for administration to a given patient at a given dental appointment.

The local anesthetic armamentarium for a practicing dentist or dental hygienist ought therefore to include drugs of varying durations of action such as the selection that follows. A minimum of two agents is recommended for most offices. Amides are preferred to esters whenever possible.

1. Short-duration pulpal anesthesia (30 minutes)
2. Intermediate-duration pulpal anesthesia (approximately 60 minutes)
3. Long-duration pupal anesthesia (90 or more minutes)
4. Availability of an ester local anesthetic, for use when amide agents prove ineffective or are contraindicated
5. Topical anesthetic for tissue preparation prior to injection of local anesthetic

REFERENCES

1. Malamed SF: *Handbook of local anesthesia,* St Louis, 1980, Mosby-Year Book.
2. Council on Dental Therapeutics of the American Dental Association: *Accepted dental therapeutics,* ed 40, Chicago, 1984, American Dental Association.
3. *USP dispensing information,* ed 13, Rockville, Md, 1993, United States Pharmacopeial Convention.
4. *Prescribing information: dental,* Westboro, Mass, 1990, Astra Pharmaceutical Products.
5. *Prescribing information,* Montreal, 1993, Hoechst AG.
6. Nation RL, Triggs EJ: Lidocaine kinetics in cardiac patients and aged subjects, *Br J Clin Pharmacol* 4:439-448, 1977.
7. Thompson P, Melmon K, Richardson J, et al: Lidocaine pharmacokinetics in advanced heart failure, liver disease, and renal failure in humans, *Ann Intern Med* 78:499, 1973.
8. Haas DA, Lennon D: Local anesthetic use by dentists in Ontario, *J Can Dent Assoc* 61(4):297-304, 1995.
9. Kao FF, Jalar UH: The central action of lignocaine and its effects on cardiac output, *Br J Pharmacol* 14:522-526, 1959.
10. Malamed SF: *Sedation: a guide to patient management,* ed 3, St Louis, 1995, Mosby-Year Book, pp 439-440.
11. Aldrete JA, Johnson DA: Evaluation of intracutaneous testing for investigation of allergy to local anesthetic agents, *Anesth Analg* 49:173-181, 1970.
12. Covino BG: *Clinical pharmacology of local anesthetic agents.* In Cousins MJ, Bridenbaugh PO, editors: *Neural blockade in clinical anesthesia and management of pain,* ed 2, Philadelphia, 1988, JB Lippincott.
13. *Prescribing information: Ravocaine and Novocain with Levophed,* New York, 1993, Cook-Waite, Sterling Winthrop.
14. *Astra standard times,* Westborough, Mass, 1988, Astra Pharmaceutical Products.
15. *Prescribing information: Xylocaine hydrochloride,* Westborough, Mass, 1992, Astra Pharmaceutical Products.
16. Assem ESK, Punnia-Moorthy A: Allergy to local anaesthetics: an approach to definitive diagnosis, *Br Dent J* 164:44-47, 1988.
17. Jackson D, Chen AH, Bennett CR: Identifying true lidocaine allergy, *J Am Dent Assoc* 125(10):1362-1366, 1994.
18. Sindel LJ, deShazo RD: Accidents resulting from local anesthetics. True or false allergy? *Clin Rev Allergy* 9:379-395, 1991.
19. Seng GF, Kraus K, Cartwright G, et al: Confirmed allergic reactions to amide local anesthetics, *Gen Dent* 44(1):52-54, 1996.
20. Scheitler LA: Unusual allergic reaction follows allergy testing, *J Am Dent Assoc* 122:88-90, 1991.
21. *Astra dental anesthetics: times to count on,* Mississauga, Ontario, 1995, Astra Pharmaceutical Products.
22. *Kodak Dental Products: prescribing information,* Rochester, NY, 1993, Eastman Kodak Company Dental Products.
23. Young ER, Mason DR, Saso MA, Albert BS: Some clinical properties of Octocaine 200 (2 percent lidocaine with epinephrine 1:200,000), *J Can Dent Assoc* 55(12):987-991, 1989.
24. Buckley JA, Ciancio SG, McMullen JA: Efficacy of epinephrine concentration in local anesthesia during periodontal surgery, *J Periodontol* 55:653-657, 1984.
25. Scott DB: Evaluation of clinical tolerance of local anaesthetic agents, *Br J Anaesth* 47:328-331, 1975.
26. Geddes IC: Metabolism of local anesthetic agents, *Int Anesthesiol Clin* 5:525-549, 1967.
27. Severinghaus JW, Xu F-D, Spellman MJ: Benzocaine and methemoglobin: recommended actions, *Anesthesiology* 74:385-386, 1991.
28. Hjelm M, Holmdahl MH: Methaemoglobinaemia following lignocaine, *Lancet* 1:53-54, 1965.
29. de Jong RH: *Local anesthetics,* St Louis, 1994, Mosby-Year Book.
30. Akerman B, Astrom A, Ross S, et al: Studies on the absorption, distribution, and metabolism of labelled prilocaine and lidocaine in some animal species, *Acta Pharmacol Toxicol* 24:389-403, 1966.
31. Foldes FF, Molloy R, McNall PG, et al: Comparison of toxicity of intravenously given local anesthetic agents in man, *JAMA* 172:1493-1498, 1960.

32. Englesson S, Eriksson E, Wahlqvist S, et al: Differences in tolerance to intravenous Xylocaine and Citanest (L67), a new local anesthetic: a double blind study in man, *Proc 1st Eur Congr Anesthesiol* 2:206-209, 1962.

33. Deriksson E, Granberg PO: Studies on the renal excretion of Citanest and Xylocaine, *Acta Anaesth Scand Suppl* 16:79-85, 1985.

34. Lahteenmaki T, Lillieborg S, Ohlsen L, et al: Topical analgesia for the cutting of split-skin grafts: a multicenter comparison of two doses of a lidocaine/prilocaine cream, *Plast Reconstr Surg* 82:458-462, 1988.

35. *Citanest and Citanest Forte: drug prescribing information,* Westborough, Mass, 1994, Astra Pharmaceutical Products.

36. van Oss GECJM, Vree TB, Baars AM, Termond EFS, Booji LHDJ: Pharmacokinetics, metabolism, and renal excretion of articaine and its metabolite articainic acid in patients after epidural administration, *Eur J Anaesthesiol* 6:49-56, 1989.

37. *Ultracaine D-S and Ultracaine D-S forte: drug prescribing information,* Montreal, Quebec, 1994, Hoechst-Roussel Canada.

38. Donaldson D, James-Perdok L, Craig BJ, Derkson GD, Richardson AS: A comparison of Ultracaine DS (articaine Hcl) and Citanest Forte (prilocaine HCl) in maxillary infiltration and mandibular nerve block, *J Can Dent Assoc* 53:38-42, 1987.

39. Knoll-Kohler E, Rupprecht S: Articaine for local anaesthesia in dentistry: a lidocaine controlled double blind cross-over study, *Eur J Pain* 13:59-63, 1992.

40. Schulze-Husmann M: *Experimental evaluation of the new local anesthetic Ultracaine in dental practice,* doctoral dissertation, Bonn, 1974, University of Bonn.

41. Haas DA, Harper DG, Saso MA, Young ER: Comparison of articaine and prilocaine anesthesia by infiltration in maxillary and mandibular arches, *Anesth Prog* 37:230-237, 1990.

42. Haas DA, Harper DG, Saso MA, Young ER: Lack of differential effect by Ultracaine (articaine HCl) and Citanest (prilocaine HCl) in infiltration anesthesia, *J Can Dent Assoc* 57:217-223, 1991.

43. MacColl S, Young ER: An allergic reaction following injection of local anesthetic: a case report, *J Can Dent Assoc* 55(12): 981-984, 1989.

44. *Marcaine HCl: drug prescribing information,* New York, 1990, Winthrop Pharmaceuticals.

45. Moore PA: Bupivacaine: a long-lasting local anesthetic for dentistry, *Oral Surg* 58:369, 1984.

46. Acute Pain Management Guideline Panel: *Acute pain management: operative or medical procedures and trauma. Clinical practice guideline,* AHCPR Pub. No. 92-0032, Rockville, Md, 1992, Agency for Health Care Policy and Research, Public Health Service, US Department of Health and Human Services.

47. Vine J, Morgan D, Thomas D: The identification of eight hydroxylated metabolites of etidocaine by chemical ionization mass spectrometry, *Xenobiotica* 8:509-513, 1978.

48. *Duranest HCl: drug prescribing information,* Westborough, Mass, 1989, Astra Pharmaceutical Products.

49. Moore PA: Long-acting local anesthetics: a review of clinical efficacy in dentistry, *Compendium* 11(1):22, 24-26, 28-30, 1990.

50. Adriani J, Campbell D: Fatalities following topical aplication of local anesthetics to mucous membranes, *JAMA* 162:1527, 1956.

51. Rosivack RG, Koenigsberg SR, Maxwell KC: An analysis of the effectiveness of two topical anesthetics, *Anesth Prog* 37:290-292, 1990.

52. Patterson RP, Anderson J: Allergic reactions to drugs and biologic agents, *JAMA* 248:2637-2645, 1982.

53. Alston TA: Antagonism of sulfonamides by benzocaine and chloroprocaine, *Anesthesiology* 76(3):475-476, 1992.

in this part

The armamentarium

The equipment necessary for the administration of local anesthetics is introduced and discussed in this section. This includes the syringe, the needle, the local anesthetic cartridge, and additional items of equipment. In addition to a discussion of the armamentarium, each chapter reviews the proper care and handling of the equipment and problems that may be encountered with its use. The section closes with a discussion of the proper technique for preparing the equipment.

Increased concern over the risk of needle-stick injury among health professionals has led to the development of needles and syringes designed to minimize this occurrence. These "safety" needles and "safety" syringes are introduced.

CHAPTER
five

The Syringe

The syringe is one of the three essential components of the local anesthetic armamentarium (others being the needle and the cartridge). It is the vehicle whereby the contents of the anesthetic cartridge are delivered through the needle to the patient.

TYPES

There are seven types of syringe for local anesthetic administration in use in dentistry today. They represent a considerable improvement over the local anesthetic syringes formerly used. The various types of syringes are listed below:

1. Nondisposable
   a. Breech-loading, metallic, cartridge-type, aspirating
   b. Breech-loading, plastic, cartridge-type, aspirating
   c. Breech-loading, metallic, cartridge-type, self-aspirating
   d. Pressure
   e. Jet injector
2. Disposable
3. "Safety" syringes

Syringes not designed to permit easy aspiration (e.g., nonaspirating syringes) are not reviewed because their use unacceptably increases the risk of inadvertent intravascular drug administration. Use of syringes capable of aspiration represents the standard of care.

American Dental Association criteria for acceptance of local anesthetic syringes include the following[1,2]:

1. They must be durable and able to withstand repeat-ed sterilization without damage. (If the unit is disposable, it should be packaged in a sterile container.)
2. They should be capable of accepting a wide variety of cartridges and needles of different manufacture, and they should permit repeated use.
3. They should be inexpensive, self-contained, lightweight, and simple to use with one hand.
4. They should provide for effective aspiration and be constructed so that blood may be easily observed in the cartridge.

Nondisposable Syringes

Breech-loading, Metallic, Cartridge-type, Aspirating

The breech-loading, metallic, cartridge-type syringe (Fig. 5-1) is the most commonly used in dental practice today. The term *breech-loading* implies that the cartridge is inserted into the syringe from the side. A needle is attached to the barrel of the syringe at the needle adaptor. The needle penetrates the barrel and punctures the rubber diaphragm of the anesthetic cartridge. The needle adaptor (screw hub or convertible tip) is removable and is sometimes discarded inadvertently with the disposable needle.

The *aspirating* syringe has a device, such as a tip or harpoon, that is attached to the piston and is used to penetrate the thick rubber or silicone stopper at the opposite end of the cartridge (from the needle). Provided the needle gauge is adequate, when negative pressure is exerted on the thumb ring by the administrator, blood will enter the needle lumen and become visible in the cartridge if

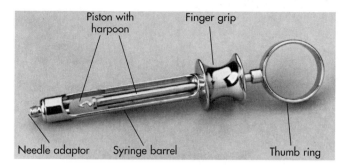

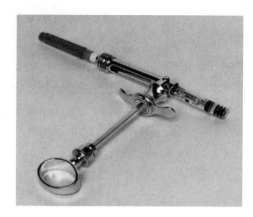

Fig. 5-1 Breech-loading, metallic, cartridge-type syringe.

Fig. 5-3 Articaine syringe, which is loaded from the top rather than from the side.

A nondisposable, metallic, *top-loading*, aspirating syringe is manufactured for use with cartridges of Ultracaine (articaine) in Canada and Europe (articaine is not available in the United States as of April 1996). The piston contains three metal claws that engage the recessed rubber plunger on the cartridge (Fig. 5-3). Although it is useful, the fact that this syringe can be used with only one manufacturer's anesthetic cartridges severely limits its applicability.

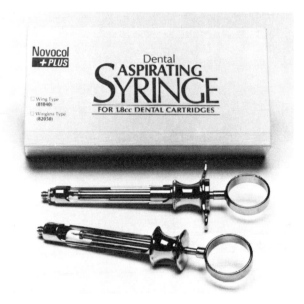

Fig. 5-2 Harpoon aspirating syringes. *(Courtesy Novocol Chemical Manufacturing, Hicksville, NY.)*

Breech-loading, Plastic, Cartridge-type, Aspirating

A *plastic*, reusable, dental aspirating syringe (Fig. 5-4) is also available. With recent advances in the plastics industry, this syringe is both autoclavable and chemically sterilizable. With proper care and handling, multiple uses may be obtained from this syringe before it is discarded. Advantages and disadvantages of the plastic, reusable, aspirating syringe include the following:

Advantages	Disadvantages
Plastic eliminates metallic, clinical look	Size (may be too big for small operators)
Lightweight: provides better "feel" during injection	Possibility of infection with improper care
Cartridge is visible	Deterioration of plastic with repeated auto-
Aspiration with one hand	claving
Rust resistant	
Long lasting with proper maintenance	
Lower cost	

the needle tip rests within a blood vessel. Positive pressure applied to the thumb ring forces local anesthetic into the needle lumen and into the patient's tissues where the needle tip lies. Thumb rings and finger grips give the administrator added control over the syringe.

Most metallic, breech-loading, aspirating syringes are constructed of chrome-plated brass and stainless steel. Examples are the Astra aspirating syringe (2 ml size), the Novocol aspirating syringe, and the Cook-Waite Carpule aspirator (Fig. 5-2).

Advantages and disadvantages of the metallic, breech-loading, aspirating syringe follow:

Breech-loading, Metallic, Cartridge-type, Self-aspirating

The hazards of intravascular administration of local anesthetics are great and are discussed more fully in Chapter 18. The incidence of positive aspiration may be as high as 10% to 15% in some injection techniques.[3] It is fully accepted by the dental profession that an aspiration test prior to administration of a local anesthetic drug is of great importance. Unfortunately, it is abundantly clear

Advantages	Disadvantages
Visible cartridge	Weight (heavier than plastic syringe)
Aspiration with one hand	Size (may be too big for small operators)
Autoclavable	
Rust resistant	Possibility of infection with improper care
Long lasting with proper maintenance	

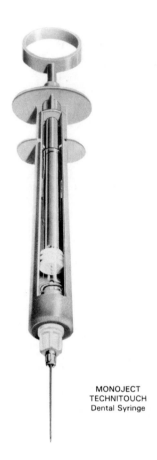

Fig. 5-4 Plastic, reusable, aspirating syringe. *(Courtesy Sherwood Medical Industries, St Louis.)*

MONOJECT
TECHNITOUCH
Dental Syringe

T A B L E 5 - 1 Percentages of Dentists Who Aspirate prior to Injection		
	Inferior alveolar nerve block	Maxillary infiltration
Always	63.2	40.2
Sometimes	14.2	24.1
Rarely	9.2	18.4
Never	13.2	17.3

From Malamed SF: Results of a survey of 209 dentists, Unpublished data, 1975.

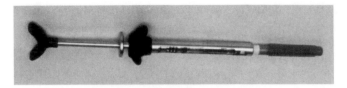

Fig. 5-5 Self-aspirating syringe.

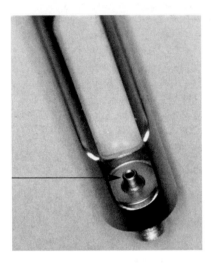

Fig. 5-6 A metal projection within the barrel (*arrow*) depresses the diaphragm and directs the needle into the cartridge.

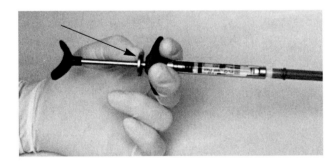

Fig. 5-7 Pressure on the thumb disk (*arrow*) increases the pressure within the cartridge. Release of this is all that is required for an aspiration test.

that in actual clinical practice too little attention is paid to this procedure (Table 5-1).

With the more commonly used breech-loading, metallic, cartridge-type syringes, an aspiration test must knowingly be carried out by the administrator either prior to or during drug deposition. The key word here is *knowingly*. However, as demonstrated in Table 5-1, many dentists knowingly do not perform an aspiration test prior to injection of the anesthetic drug.

To increase the ease of aspiration, several self-aspirating syringe systems have been developed (Fig. 5-5).

These syringes use the elasticity of the rubber diaphragm in the anesthetic cartridge to obtain the required negative pressure for aspiration. The diaphragm rests on a metal projection inside the syringe that directs the needle into the cartridge (Fig. 5-6). Pressure acting directly on the cartridge through the thumb disk (Fig. 5-7) or indirectly through the plunger shaft distorts (stretches) the rubber diaphragm, producing a positive pressure within the anesthetic cartridge. When that pressure is released, sufficient negative pressure develops within the cartridge to permit aspiration. The thumb ring produces twice as much negative pressure as the plunger shaft (Fig. 5-7). The use of a self-aspirating dental syringe permits multiple aspirations to be performed easily throughout the period of local anesthetic deposition.

The Astra self-aspirating syringe was introduced into the United States in 1981. After an initial period of enthusiasm, the popularity of this syringe has decreased. I have been contacted by a number of doctors who did not feel that the self-aspirating syringe provided the same reliable degree of aspiration as that possible with the harpoon-aspirating syringe. It has been demonstrated, however, that this syringe does in fact aspirate as reliably as the harpoon-aspirating syringe.[4,5] Because the administrator does not need to pull back on the thumb ring to aspirate, but rather has only to depress and release the thumb ring, this feeling that aspiration may not be as reliable can occur. Moving the thumb off the thumb ring and onto the thumb disk for aspiration has also been mentioned by many doctors as being uncomfortable for them. Although this is the preferred means of obtaining a satisfactory aspiration test with these syringes, pressure adequate for aspiration may also be obtained by simply releasing pressure of the thumb on the thumb ring. The second generation of the Astra self-aspirating syringe (Fig. 5-5) has eliminated the thumb disk.

The major factor influencing ability to aspirate is the *gauge of the needle* being used. Additionally, most doctors using the harpoon-aspirating syringe tend to overaspirate—that is, they retract the thumb ring back too far and with excessive force (frequently pulling the harpoon out of the stopper). These doctors especially feel insecure with the self-aspirating syringe. Aspiration techniques are discussed in Chapter 11.

Advantages	Disadvantages
Cartridge visible	Weight
Easier to aspirate with small hands	Feeling of "insecurity" for doctors accustomed to harpoon-type syringe
Autoclavable	
Rust resistant	
Long lasting with proper maintenance	Finger must be moved from thumb ring to thumb disk to aspirate
Piston is scored (indicates volume of drug administered)	Possibility of infection with improper care

Pressure Syringes

Introduced in the late 1970s, pressure syringes brought about a renewed interest in the periodontal ligament (PDL) injection (also known as the intraligamentary injection [ILI]) technique. Discussed in Chapter 16, the PDL injection, though usable for any tooth, has made it possible to achieve consistently reliable pulpal anesthesia of one isolated tooth in the mandibular arch, whereas in the past, nerve block anesthesia, with its attendant potential problem for prolonged soft tissue (e.g., lingual) anesthesia, was necessary.

The original pressure devices, Peripress (Universal Dental Implements) and Ligmaject (IMA Associates) (Fig. 5-8), appear to be modeled after a device that was available in dentistry in 1905—the Wilcox-Jewett Obtunder (Fig. 5-9). These first-generation devices, using a pistol-grip, are somewhat larger than the newer, pen-grip, devices (Fig. 5-10). Although special syringes such as these are not required for the PDL injection to be administered successfully, there are several advantages attendant to their use, not the least of which is the mechanical advantage they give the administrator, making the anesthetic somewhat easier to deliver. This same mechanical advantage, however, makes the injection somewhat "too easy" to administer, leading to the too

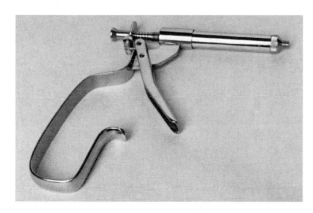

Fig. 5-8 Original pressure syringe designed for a periodontal ligament injection or intraligamentary injection.

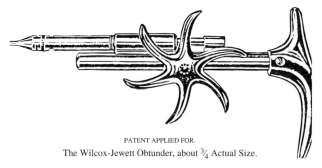

THE WILCOX-JEWETT OBTUNDER.

Lee S. Smith & Son, Pittsburg.

PATENT APPLIED FOR.
The Wilcox-Jewett Obtunder, about ¾ Actual Size.

Fig. 5-9 Pressure syringe (1905) designed for a peridental injection.

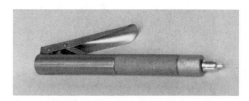

Fig. 5-10 Second-generation syringe for a PDL injection.

rapid injection of the anesthetic solution and to patient discomfort both during the injection and later, when the anesthesia has worn off. However, when used as recommended (slowly) by the manufacturers, these pressure syringes are of some benefit in the administration of this valuable technique of anesthesia.

Pressure syringes offer advantages over the conventional syringe when used for PDL injections because the trigger permits measured dose administration and enables the relatively weak administrator to overcome the significant tissue resistance that is encountered when this technique is administered properly. This mechanical advantage may also prove to be detrimental if the administrator deposits the anesthetic solution too quickly (<20 sec/0.2 ml dose). All of the pressure syringes completely enclose the glass dental cartridge, thereby protecting the patient in the unlikely event that the cartridge cracks or shatters during injection. The original devices looked somewhat threatening, having the appearance of a gun. Newer ones are smaller and are considerably less threatening.

Probably the greatest disadvantage to the use of these devices is their cost, most priced at considerably more than $100 U.S. (1995). For this reason, among others, my recommendation is that pressure devices be considered for use only after the PDL injection has been found to be ineffective following several attempts with a conventional syringe and needle.

Advantages	Disadvantages
Measured dose	Cost
Overcomes tissue resistance	Easy to inject too rapidly
Cartridge protected	Threatening (original devices)
Nonthreatening (newer devices)	

Jet Injector

In 1947 Figge and Scherer introduced a new approach to parenteral injection—the jet or needleless injection.[6] This represented the first fundamental change in the basic principles of injection since 1853, when Alexander Wood introduced the hypodermic syringe. The first report of the use of jet injections in dentistry was in 1958 by Margetis et al.[7] Jet injection is based on the principle that liquids forced through very small openings, called jets, at very high pressure can penetrate skin or mucous membrane (visualize water flowing through a garden hose that is being crimped). The most used jet injectors in dentistry are the Syrijet Mark II (Mizzy, Inc.) and the Madajet (Mada Medical Products, Inc.) (Fig. 5-11). The Syrijet holds any 1.8 ml dental cartridge of local anesthetic. It is calibrated to deliver 0.05 to 0.2 ml of solution at 2000 psi.

The primary use of the jet injector is to obtain topical anesthesia prior to the insertion of a needle. In addition, it may be used to obtain mucosal anesthesia of the palate. Regional nerve blocks or supraperiosteal injections are still required for complete anesthesia. In my experience the jet injector has not proved to be an adequate substitute for the more traditional needle and syringe in obtaining pulpal or regional block anesthesia. Additionally, many patients dislike the feeling that accompanies use of the jet injector, as well as the postinjection soreness of soft tissue areas that may develop even with proper use of the device. Topical anesthetics, applied properly, serve the same purpose as jet injectors at a fraction of the cost and with minimum risk. Following are the advantages and disadvantages of this method:

Advantages	Disadvantages
Does not require use of a needle (recommended for needle-phobics)	Inadequate for pulpal or regional block
Delivers very small volumes of local anesthetic solution	Some patients are disturbed by the "jolt" of jet injection
Used in lieu of topical anesthesia	Cost
	May damage periodontal tissues

Disposable Syringes

Plastic disposable syringes (Fig. 5-12) are available in a variety of sizes and with an assortment of needle gauges. They are most often used for intramuscular or intravenous drug administration but may also be used for intraoral injections.

These syringes contain a Luer-Lok screw-on needle attachment but no aspirating tip. One can, however, perform aspiration by pulling back on the plunger of the syringe prior to or during injection. Because of the lack of a thumb ring, aspiration with the plastic disposable syringe requires the use of both hands. These syringes do not accept dental cartridges. The needle, attached to the syringe, must be inserted into a vial or cartridge of local anesthetic drug and an appropriate volume of solution removed. Care must be taken to avoid contaminating the vial during this procedure. Two- and three-milliliter syringes with 23- or 25-gauge needles are recommended

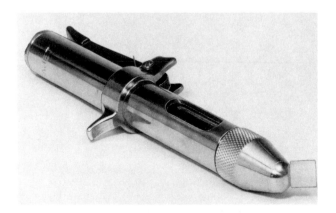

Fig. 5-11 Jet injector.

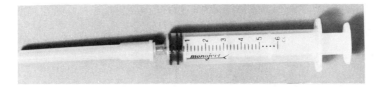

Fig. 5-12 Plastic disposable syringe.

when the system is used for intraoral local anesthetic administration.

I do not recommend the plastic, disposable, non–cartridge-containing syringe for routine use. It should be used only when a traditional syringe is not available. This system may be practical when diphenhydramine is used as a local anesthetic in cases of presumed local anesthetic allergy. (See Chapter 18.)

Following are the advantages and disadvantages of the disposable syringe:

Advantages	Disadvantages
Disposable, single use	Does not accept prefilled dental cartridges
Sterile until opened	Difficult aspiration, requiring two hands
Lightweight (better tactile sensation)	May feel awkward to a first-time user

Safety Syringes

In recent years there has been a move toward the development and introduction of "safety" syringes in both medicine and dentistry. Use of a safety syringe would minimize the risk of accidental needle-stick injury occurring to a dental health provider with a contaminated needle after the administration of a local anesthetic. These syringes possess a sheath that "locks" over the needle when it is removed from the patient's tissues, preventing accidental needle stick.

Two such devices, the UltraSafe aspirating syringe* and Safety Plus,[†] were available as of April 1996.

The UltraSafe aspirating syringe system contains a syringe body assembly and plunger assembly (Fig. 5-13). Once the syringe is properly assembled and the injection administered, the syringe may be made "safe" with one hand by gently moving the index and middle fingers against the front collar of the guard and then pulling the thumb ring back until the needle is retracted into the guard and the guard legs lock into the body notches (Fig. 5-14, *A*). The two-handed guarding technique is recommended for administrators with small hands or when the entire cartridge has not been administered. The two-handed guarding technique is accomplished by grasping

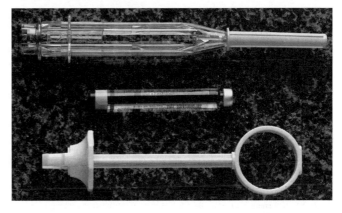

Fig. 5-13 Components of the safety syringe.

the guard near its collar with the free hand (Fig. 5-14, *B*) and pulling the body back until the needle is retracted into the guard and the guard locks into the body notches. Once "guarded," the now-contaminated needle is "safe," so that it is virtually impossible to be injured with the needle. The entire syringe is discarded into the proper receptacle (e.g., sharps container).

Safety Plus is similar though somewhat different in design. It consists of an autoclavable syringe handle and a disposable self-contained injection unit. The dental anesthetic cartridge is clearly visible because the clear plastic design of the injection unit makes the result of aspiration easy to discern. The cartridge also incorporates a self-aspiration system similar to those described above. Upon completion of the injection the autoprotective system is used, markedly diminishing the risk of accidental needle-stick injury. The system provides two options after the injection. The protective sheath can either be slid forward to an intermediate locking position, if multiple injections are required, or to the final locking position for safe disposal.

Both safety syringes are designed to be single-use items (changed after each injection), though they both permit reinjection. Reloading the syringe with a second anesthetic cartridge and reinjecting with the same syringe is discouraged, as this obviates the important safety aspect of the device.

Almost a year's clinical experience with safety syringe systems has demonstrated to me the ease with which these systems may be learned, their simplicity, and the

---

*Safety Syringes, Inc., 250 W. Colorado Boulevard, Suite 101, Arcadia, CA 91007; 818-821-1121.
†Septodont, 245 Quigley Boulevard, Suite C, New Castle, DE 19720; PO Box 11926, Wilmington, DE 19850-1926; 800-872-8305.

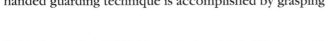

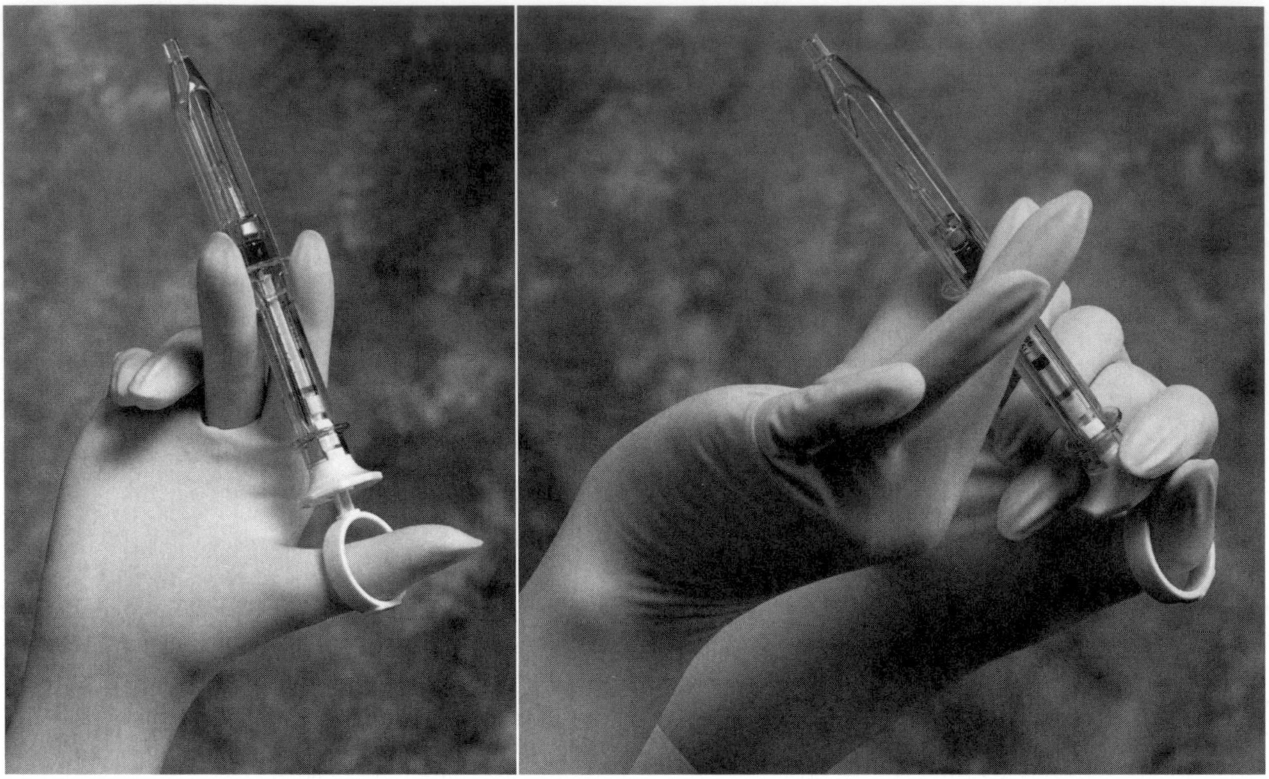

Fig. 5-14 One-handed (A) and two-handed (B) guarding techniques for the safety syringe.

importance of the safety syringe. Use of a safety syringe system is strongly recommended.

Following are the advantages and disadvantages of the safety syringe:

Advantages	Disadvantages
Disposable, single use	Cost: more expensive than reusable syringe
Sterile until opened	May feel awkward to a first-time user
Lightweight (better tactile sensation)	

CARE AND HANDLING

Metal and plastic reusable syringes are designed to provide long-term service if properly maintained. Following is a summary of manufacturers' recommendations concerning care of these syringes:

1. After each use, thoroughly wash and rinse the syringe free of any local anesthetic solution, saliva, or other foreign matter. Autoclave the syringe in the same manner as other surgical instruments.
2. After every five autoclavings, dismantle the syringe and lightly lubricate all threaded joints and where the piston contacts the thumb ring and guide bearing.

3. Clean the harpoon with a brush after each use.
4. Although the harpoon is designed for long-term wear, prolonged use will result in decreased sharpness and failure to remain embedded within the stopper of the cartridge. Replacement pistons and harpoons are readily available at low cost.

PROBLEMS
Leakage During Injection
When reloading a syringe with a second local anesthetic cartridge and a needle already in place, one should be sure that the needle penetrates the center of the rubber diaphragm. An off-center perforation will produce an ovoid puncture of the diaphragm that permits leakage of the anesthetic solution around the outside of the metal needle and into the patient's mouth (Fig. 5-15). (For further information, see Chapter 7.)

Broken Cartridge
A badly worn syringe may damage the cartridge, leading to breakage. This can also result from a bent harpoon. A needle that is bent at its proximal end (Fig. 5-16) may not perforate the diaphragm on the cartridge. Positive pressure on the thumb ring increases intracartridge pressure, which can cause the cartridge to break.

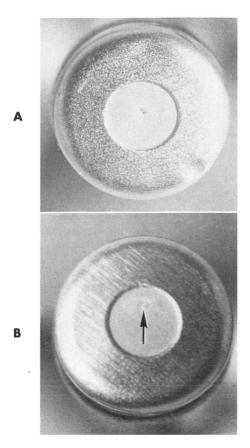

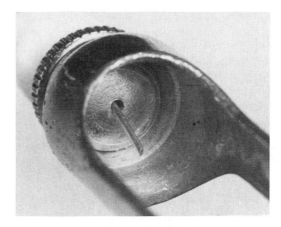

Fig. 5-16 A needle bent at the proximal end may not perforate the cartridge diaphragm. Pressure on the thumb ring can lead to cartridge breakage.

Fig. 5-15 **A**, Centric perforation of the diaphragm by a needle prevents leakage during injection. **B**, Off-center perforation (*arrow*) permits leakage of anesthetic solution into the patient's mouth.

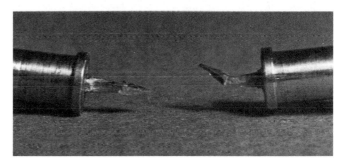

Fig. 5-17 Notice the bent harpoon of the syringe on the left.

Bent Harpoon

The harpoon must be sharp and straight (Fig. 5-17). A bent harpoon produces an off-center puncture of the rubber plunger, causing the plunger to rotate as it moves down the glass cartridge. This may occasionally result in cartridge breakage.

Disengagement of the Harpoon from the Plunger during Aspiration

Disengagement occurs if the harpoon is dull or if the administrator applies too much pressure to the thumb ring during aspiration. If this occurs the harpoon should be cleaned and sharpened or replaced with a new sharp harpoon. A very gentle backward motion of the plunger is all that is required for successful aspiration. Forceful action is not necessary. (See the discussion in Chapter 11.)

Surface Deposits

An accumulation of debris, saliva, and disinfectant solution interferes with syringe function and appearance. Deposits, which can resemble rust, may be removed with

a thorough scrubbing. Ultrasonic cleaning will not harm syringes.

RECOMMENDATIONS

I have not found any one manufacturer's syringe to be superior. Therefore the ultimate decision in selection of a syringe must be left to the discretion of the buyer. It is recommended, however, that before purchasing any syringe, the buyer should place a full dental cartridge in it. Pick up the syringe as if to use it. Note whether the fingers (thumb to other fingers) are stretched maximally. Remember, to aspirate with a harpoon-type syringe one must be able to pull the thumb ring back several millimeters. If not able to do so, reliable aspiration is not possible. Although all syringes available today are of approximately the same dimensions, some variation does exist. Some manufacturers market syringes with smaller thumb rings or shorter pistons. These changes will make aspiration easier to accomplish for persons with smaller hands.

Following are additional recommendations:

1. A safety syringe, minimizing the risk of accidental needle-stick injury, is strongly recommended for use during all local anesthetic injections.
2. A self-aspirating syringe is recommended for practitioners with small hands.
3. Any syringe system used must be capable of aspiration. Nonaspirating syringes should never be used for local anesthetic injections.
4. All reusable syringes must be capable of being sterilized.
5. Nonreusable syringes must be disposed of properly.

REFERENCES

1. Council on Dental Materials and Devices: New American National Standards Institute/American Dental Association specification no. 34 for dental aspirating syringes, *J Am Dent Assoc* 97:236-238, 1978.
2. Council on Dental Materials, Instruments, and Equipment: Addendum to American National Standards Institute/American Dental Association specification no. 34 for dental aspirating syringes, *J Am Dent Assoc* 104:69-70, 1982.
3. Bartlett SZ: Clinical observations on the effects of injections of local anesthetic preceded by aspiration, *Oral Surg* 33:520, 1972.
4. Meechan JG, Blair GS, McCabe JF: Local anaesthesia in dental practice: II. A laboratory investigation of a self-aspirating system, *Br Dent J* 159:109-113, 1985.
5. Meechan JG: A comparison of three different automatic aspirating dental cartridge syringes, *J Dent* 16:40-43, 1988.
6. Figge FHJ, Scherer RP: Anatomical studies on jet penetration of human skin for subcutaneous medication without the use of needles, *Anat Rec* 97:335, 1947 (abstract).
7. Margetis PM, Quarantillo EP, Lindberg RB: Jet injection local anesthesia in dentistry: a report of 66 cases, *US Armed Forces Med J* 9:625-634, 1958.

CHAPTER
six

The Needle

TYPES

The needle permits the local anesthetic solution to travel from the dental cartridge into the tissues surrounding the needle tip. Most needles used in dentistry are stainless steel and are disposable. Other needles are constructed of platinum or an iridium-platinum or ruthenium-platinum alloy. The stainless steel needle is highly recommended. Needles currently available for dental practices are presterilized and disposable.

Reusable needles should not be used for injections.

PARTS

All needles have several components in common (Fig. 6-1). These include the bevel, the shank, the hub, and the syringe-penetrating end.

The *bevel* defines the point or tip of the needle. Bevels are described by manufacturers as long, medium, and short. Several authors have confirmed that the greater the angle of the bevel with the long axis of the needle, the greater will be the degree of deflection as the needle passes through hydrocolloid (and soft tissues of the mouth) (Fig. 6-2).[1-3] A needle whose point is centered on the long axis (e.g., the Huber point and the Truject needle) (Fig. 6-3) will deflect considerably less than a beveled-point needle whose point is eccentric (Fig. 6-4 and Table 6-1).

The *shank* or shaft of the needle consists of the diameter of the needle lumen (needle gauge) and the length of the shank from point to hub.

The *hub* is the plastic or metal piece through which the needle attaches to the syringe. The interior surface of the *plastic syringe adaptor* of the needle is not prethreaded. Therefore to attach a plastic-hubbed needle to a syringe, the needle must be pushed onto the syringe while being screwed on. Metallic-hubbed needles are usually prethreaded.

The *syringe-penetrating end* of the dental needle is placed into the needle adaptor and perforates the rubber diaphragm of the local anesthetic cartridge. Its tip rests within the cartridge.

• • •

When needles are selected for use in various injection techniques, there are two factors of importance that must be considered: the *gauge* and the *length*.

GAUGE

Gauge refers to the diameter of the lumen of the needle: the smaller the number, the greater the diameter of the lumen. A 30-gauge needle has a smaller internal diameter than a 25-gauge needle.

There is a growing trend toward the use of smaller-diameter (higher-gauge) needles on the supposition that they are less traumatic to the patient than needles with larger diameters (Table 6-2). This assumption is unwarranted. Hamburg[4] demonstrated in 1972 that patients cannot differentiate among 23-, 25-, 27-, and 30-gauge needles, a test that I have also used on many occasions. A clinical experiment will prove this point:

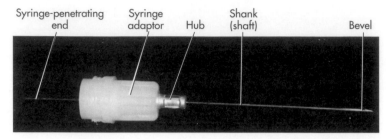

Fig. 6-1 Components of the needle.

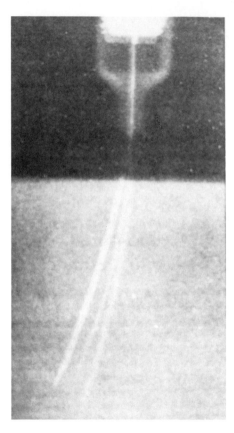

Fig. 6-2 Radiograph demonstrating varying degrees of needle deflection with different gauges (*left to right*, 30, 27, and 25). *(From Robison SE, et al: Comparative study of deflection characteristics and fragility of 25-, 27- and 30-gauge short dental needles,* J Am Dent Assoc *109:920-924, 1984.)*

1. Use 25-, 27-, and 30-gauge needles.
2. Dry the buccal mucosa over the maxillary anterior teeth.
3. Do *not* use topical anesthetic.
4. Be sure that the mucosa is taut.
5. Gently penetrate the mucosa (about 2 to 3 mm) with each needle without revealing to the patient which needle is being used. Select a different site for each penetration.

T A B L E   6 - 1   Deflection of Needles Inserted in Hydrocolloid Tubes to Their Hubs

Needle type	Length (mm, tip to hub)	Maximum tip deflection (mm, ± SD)
25-Gauge long (conventional)	35	7.1 ± 0.81*
27-Gauge long (conventional)	36	8.4 ± 1.2*
27-Gauge short (conventional)	26	4.6 ± 0.97†
28-Gauge long (nondeflecting)	31	1.1 ± 0.82
28-Gauge short (nondeflecting)	22	0.8 ± 0.91

Data modified from Jeske AH, Boshart BF: Deflection of conventional versus non-deflecting dental needles in vitro, *Anesth Prog* 32:62-64, 1985.
*A statistically significant difference from the nondeflecting long needle ($p < 0.01$); n = 10 needles in each group.
†A statistically significant difference from the nondeflecting short needle ($p < 0.01$); n = 10 needles in each group.

6. Question the patient about the needles: Which did you feel the most? Which the least?

In hundreds of clinical demonstrations I have not found a single patient who could correctly determine the gauge of each needle. The usual response has been that he or she could not discern any difference.

Larger-gauge needles (i.e., 25-gauge) have distinct advantages over smaller ones: *Less deflection* occurs as the needle passes through tissues (Table 6-1 and Fig. 6-2). This leads to *greater accuracy* and hopefully to increased success rates, especially for techniques in which the depth of soft tissue being penetrated is significant (e.g., the inferior alveolar, Gow-Gates mandibular, Akinosi mandibular, and infraorbital nerve blocks). Needle breakage, although not common with disposable needles, is much less likely to occur with a larger needle. Numerous authors[5-8] have stated that aspiration of blood is easier and more reliable through a larger lumen. Foldes

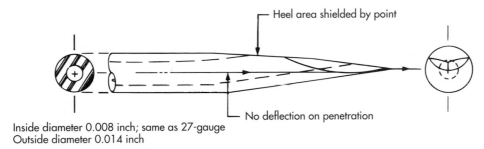

Fig. 6-3 The tip of a nondeflecting needle is located in the center of the shaft, thereby minimizing deflection as the needle penetrates soft tissues.

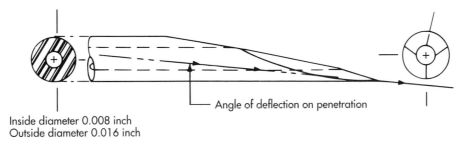

Fig. 6-4 Conventional dental needle. The needle tip lies at the lower edge of the needle shaft, thereby producing deflection as the needle passes through soft tissue.

TABLE 6-2 Needle Gauges Used in Practice		
Gauge	Inferior alveolar nerve block (%)	Maxillary infiltration (%)
23	1.1	0.0
25	66.9	19.1
27	32.0	60.1
30	0.0	20.8

From Malamed SF: Results of a survey of 209 dentists, Unpublished data, 1975.

and McNall,[5] reporting on an unpublished study by Monheim, stated the following:

1. 100% positive aspirations were achieved from blood vessels with 25-gauge needles.
2. 87% positive aspirations were achieved from blood vessels with 27-gauge needles.
3. 2% positive aspirations were achieved from blood vessels with 30-gauge needles.

Trapp and Davies,[9] however, reported that in vivo human blood may be aspirated through 23-, 25-, 27-, and 30-gauge needles without a clinically significant difference in resistance to flow.

Despite this ambiguity concerning ability to aspirate blood through various-gauge needles, I highly recommend using larger needles (i.e., 25-gauge) for any injection technique into a highly vascular area or when needle deflection through soft tissue is a factor. Although blood may presumably be aspirated through all 23- through 30-gauge needles, more pressure is required to aspirate when smaller needles are being used, increasing the likelihood that the harpoon will become dislodged from the rubber plunger during aspiration.

Industry standards for needle gauge have been in place for years, yet Wittrock and Fischer[10] showed in 1968 that variations in internal diameter do exist (Table 6-3), and 27 years later such differences are still encountered. Larger-gauge needles (i.e., 25) should be used when there is a greater risk of positive aspiration, as during an inferior alveolar, posterior superior alveolar, or mental/incisive nerve block.

The most commonly used needles in dentistry are the 25-, 27-, and 30-gauge. The 25-gauge needle is preferred for all injections posing a high risk of positive aspiration. The 27-gauge can be used for all other injection techniques, provided the aspiration percentage is exceedingly low and tissue penetration depth is not great (increased deflection). I cannot recommend the 30-gauge needle for any injection, although it can be used in instances of local infiltration, as when obtaining hemostasis during periodontal therapy.

Deflection becomes important when the needle must penetrate greater thicknesses of soft tissue. On the stan-

T A B L E   6 - 3   Seven Manufacturers' Specifications for Three Needle Gauges and the Industrial Tubing Standards

	Interior diameter (inches) of needle lumens		
Manufacturers	25-gauge (standard, 0.0095)	27-gauge (standard, 0.0075)	30-gauge (standard, 0.006)
1	0.010	0.008	0.006
2	0.0095	0.0075	0.006
3	0.010	0.008	0.005
4	0.0095	0.0075	0.003
5	0.018	0.014	0.010
6	0.010	0.008	0.006
7	0.009	0.0075	0.006

From Wittrock JW, Fischer WE: The aspiration of blood through small-gauge needles, *J Am Dent Assoc* 76:79-81, 1968.

dard dental needle (Fig. 6-4), the tip of the point is located eccentrically. As the needle penetrates soft tissue, the point is deflected by the tissue through which it passes. The greater the angle of the bevel, the greater the degree of needle deflection. Every decade or so a needle is introduced (Truject) (Fig. 6-3) on which the tip of the point is located in the center of the lumen, thereby minimizing deflection as the needle passes through soft tissue. Jeske and Boshart[2] demonstrated (Table 6-1) the effectiveness of this new "nondeflecting" needle. However, it needs to be shown clinically that a lesser degree of needle deflection occurring as the needle passes through soft tissues actually results in an increased rate of successful anesthesia compared to that observed with standard needles. Dentists have become accustomed to the deflecting needles and have modified their injection technique to accommodate this deflection. Changing to a nondeflecting needle might initially lead to lower success rates.

LENGTH

Dental needles are available in two lengths—long (approximately 1⅝ inches or 40 mm) and short (approximately 1 inch or 25 mm). Despite the claim for uniformity of length by manufacturers, Aldous[1] reported that the range of needle lengths is quite wide: 19.4, 19.9, 21.5, 25.5, 28.9, 30.8, 34.9, 35.0, 36.0, and 41.5 mm. The average length of a short needle is 20 mm (measured hub to tip) and 32 mm for the long dental needle.

Needles should not be inserted into tissues to their hubs unless it is absolutely necessary for the success of the injection. There are several reasons for this rule: needle breakage, although rare, does occur. The weakest portion of the needle is at its hub. This is where needle break-

> *Needles should not be inserted into tissues to their hubs unless it is absolutely necessary for the success of the injection.*

age occurs. When a needle inserted in soft tissues to its hub breaks, the elastic properties of the tissues permit them to rebound and cover the needle entirely. Retrieval usually proves to be quite difficult (as discussed in Chapter 17). If even a small portion (5 mm or more) of the needle shaft remains visible in the oral cavity, it can be easily retrieved with a hemostat or pickup forceps.

Long needles are preferred for all injection techniques requiring penetration of significant thicknesses of soft tissue (e.g., the inferior alveolar, Gow-Gates mandibular, Akinosi mandibular, infraorbital, and maxillary nerve blocks). Short needles may be used for injections that do not require the penetration of significant depths of soft tissue.

CARE AND HANDLING

Needles available to the dental profession today are presterilized and disposable. With proper care and handling, they should not be the cause of significant difficulties.

1. Needles must *never* be used on more than one patient.
2. Needles should be changed after several (three or four) tissue penetrations in the same patient.
   a. After three or four insertions, stainless steel disposable needles become dull. Tissue penetration is more traumatic with each insertion, producing pain on insertion and soreness when sensation returns after the procedure.
3. Needles should be covered with a protective sheath when not being used, to prevent accidental needle stick with a contaminated needle. (See the discussion in Chapter 9.)
4. Always be aware of the position of the uncovered needle tip, whether inside or outside the patient's mouth. This will minimize the risk of potential injury to the patient and the administrator.
5. Needles must be properly disposed of after use, to prevent possible injury or reuse by unauthorized individuals. Needles can be destroyed in any of the following ways:
   a. Dispose of contaminated needles (as well as all other items contaminated with blood or saliva) in special "contaminated" containers (Fig. 6-5).
   b. Proper use of a self-sheathing ("safe" needle) needle/syringe unit (as discussed in Chapter 5) minimizes risk of accidental needle stick.

which can be used for all the anesthetic techniques discussed in this book. It provides a rigidity not available with higher-gauge (smaller-diameter) needles, which is required in the periodontal ligament (PDL) and intraseptal injections; it deflects to a lesser degree than smaller needles, and in my opinion provides easier and more reliable aspiration. Because there is no increase in patient discomfort with the 25-gauge long needle, its value is increased still further. In reality, however, it is practical to have a second needle available: the 25- or 27-gauge short needle will be used for injection techniques in which the thickness of soft tissue to be penetrated is less than 20 mm and when the risk of positive aspiration is minimal, as well as in areas of the oral cavity where stabilization of a long needle might prove difficult (e.g., maxillary anteriors and the palate).

PROBLEMS

Pain on Insertion

The use of a dull needle can lead to pain on initial penetration of the mucosa. This may be avoided by using sharp, new, disposable needles and the application of topical anesthetic at the penetration site. Change the needle after three or four penetrations of mucosa, if reinsertion is necessary.

Breakage

Bending weakens needles, making them more likely to break on subsequent contact with hard tissues, such as bone. Needles should not be bent if they are to be inserted into soft tissue to a depth of more than 5 mm. *There is no injection technique used in dentistry that mandates a needle be bent for the injection to be successful.* Most often needles are bent by doctors administering the inferior alveolar nerve block (IANB), the posterior superior alveolar (PSA) nerve block, the intrapulpal injection, and the PDL injection. The two nerve blocks mentioned can readily be administered successfully with a straight (unbent) needle. (See Chapters 13 and 14.) The PDL and intrapulpal injections can usually be administered without bending the needle; however, occasions will arise, such as at the distal root of a mandibular second molar (PDL) or root canals in posterior teeth (intrapulpal), in which access to the injection site is not possible with a straight needle. Bending of the needle is essential to success in these cases. As the needle does not enter into soft tissue more than 2 to 4 mm (PDL), or at all (intrapulpal), there is no danger of the needle becoming nonretrievable in the unlikely event that it breaks.

Do not attempt to change the direction of a needle when it is embedded in tissue. If the direction of a needle must be changed, first withdraw the needle almost completely from the tissue and then alter its direction.

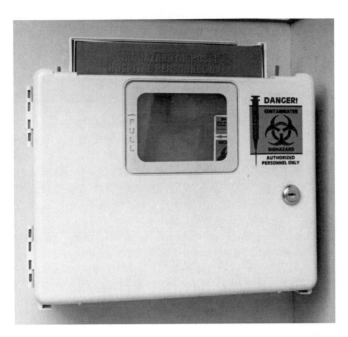

Fig. 6-5 A sharps container is recommended for disposing of contaminated needles.

A

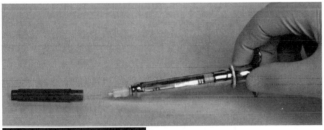

B

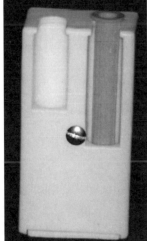

Fig. 6-6 A, "Scoop" technique for recapping used needle. B, Acrylic needle holder.

   c. Where needles are to be reused for subsequent injections, recapping is accomplished using the "scoop" technique or a needle holder (Fig. 6-6).

   d. *Never* discard contaminated needles into open trash containers.

In summary: There need be but one local anesthetic needle available in the dental office, the *25-gauge long,*

Never attempt to force a needle against resistance (needles are not designed to penetrate bone). Smaller (30- and 27-gauge) needles are more likely to break than larger (25-gauge) needles.

Recommended needles for specific injection techniques are presented in the recommendations section to follow.

Pain on Withdrawal

Pain on withdrawal of the needle from tissue can be produced by "fishhook" barbs on the tip. Fishhook barbs may be produced during the manufacturing process, but it is much more likely that they occur when the needle tip forcefully contacts a hard surface (bone). A needle should never be forced against resistance. If in doubt about the presence of barbs, change the needle between insertions.

Injury to the Patient or Administrator

Penetration of areas of the body with the needle can occur unintentionally. A major cause is carelessness and inattention by the administrator, although sudden unexpected movement by the patient is also a frequent cause. The needle should remain capped until it is to be used and should be made safe (sheathed or recapped) immediately after withdrawal from the mouth.

RECOMMENDATIONS

1. Sterile disposable needles should be used.
2. If multiple injections are to be administered, needles should be changed after three or four insertions in a single patient.
3. Needles must *never* be used on more than one patient.
4. Needles should not be inserted into tissue to their hub unless it is absolutely necessary for success of the injection.
5. Do not change a needle's direction while it is still in tissue.
6. Never force a needle against resistance.
7. Needles should remain capped until used and made safe immediately on withdrawal.
8. Needles should be discarded and destroyed after use, to prevent injury or reuse by unauthorized persons.

9. The following injection techniques are listed with their recommended needles (for the average-size adult):
   a. Inferior alveolar nerve block—25-gauge long
   b. Gow-Gates mandibular nerve block—25-gauge long
   c. Vazirani-Akinosi mandibular nerve block—25-gauge long
   d. Buccal nerve block—27-gauge short*
   e. Mental/incisive nerve block—27-gauge short
   f. Supraperiosteal (local infiltration)—27-gauge short
   g. Posterior superior alveolar nerve block—27-gauge short†
   h. Infraorbital nerve block—25-gauge long
   i. Maxillary nerve block—25-gauge long
   j. Infiltration for hemostasis—27-gauge short
   k. Periodontal ligament injection—27-gauge short
   l. Intraseptal injection—27-gauge short
   m. Intrapulpal injection—27-gauge short

*In most clinical situations the 25-gauge long needle, used for the IANB, will be used for the buccal nerve block, which is administered immediately after the IANB.
†In the first edition of this book, I recommended the 25-gauge long needle. As a means of minimizing the risk of hematoma following the posterior superior alveolar injection, a short needle is now recommended. If available, a 25-gauge short needle should be used; where this is not available, the 27-gauge short needle is recommended. (See Chapter 13 for additional discussion.)

REFERENCES

1. Aldous JA: Needle deflection: a factor in the administration of local anesthetics, *J Am Dent Assoc* 77:602-604, 1977.
2. Jeske AH, Boshart BF: Deflection of conventional versus non-deflecting dental needles in vitro, *Anesth Prog* 32:62-64, 1985.
3. Robison SF, Mayhew RB, Cowan RD, Hawley RJ: Comparative study of deflection characteristics and fragility of 25-, 27-, and 30-gauge short dental needles, *J Am Dent Assoc* 109:920-924, 1984.
4. Hamburg HL: Preliminary study of patient reaction to needle gauge, *NY State Dent J* 38:425-426, 1972.
5. Foldes FF, McNall PG: Toxicity of local anesthetics in man, *Dent Clin North Am* 5:257-258, 1961.
6. Harris S: Aspirations before injection of dental local anesthetics, *J Oral Surg* 25:299-303, 1957.
7. Kramer H, Mitton V: Dental emergencies, *Dent Clin North Am* 17:443-460, 1973.
8. McClure DB: Local anesthesia for the preschool child, *J Dent Child* 35:441-448, 1968.
9. Trapp LD, Davies RO: Aspiration as a function of hypodermic needle internal diameter in the in-vivo human upper limb, *Anesth Prog* 27:49-51, 1980.
10. Wittrock JW, Fischer WE: The aspiration of blood through small-gauge needles, *J Am Dent Assoc* 76:79-81, 1968.

CHAPTER

seven

The Cartridge

The dental cartridge is a glass cylinder containing, among other ingredients, the local anesthetic drug. The glass cylinder itself can hold 2 ml of solution; however, as prepared today in the United States the dental cartridge contains 1.8 ml of local anesthetic solution. In other countries, notably Great Britain and Australia, the prefilled dental cartridge contains 2.2 ml of local anesthetic solution.

The dental cartridge is, by common usage, referred to as a "carpule" by dental professionals. The term *Carpule* is actually a registered trade name for the dental cartridge prepared by Cook-Waite Laboratories.

In recent years local anesthetic manufacturers in some countries have introduced a local anesthetic cartridge composed of plastic.[1]

COMPONENTS

The prefilled 1.8 ml dental cartridge consists of four parts (Fig. 7-1):

1. Cylindrical glass tube
2. Stopper
3. Aluminum cap
4. Diaphragm

The *stopper* (plunger) is located at the end of the cartridge that receives the harpoon of the aspirating syringe. The harpoon is embedded in the plunger with gentle finger pressure applied to the thumb ring of the syringe. The plunger occupies a little less than 0.2 ml of the volume of the entire cartridge. In the recent past the stopper was mixed with paraffin (wax) to produce an airtight seal against the glass walls of the cartridge. Glycerine was added in channels around the stopper as a lubricant, permitting it to traverse the glass cylinder more easily. Today most manufacturers of local anesthetics treat the stopper with silicone, eliminating both the paraffin and the glycerine. "Sticky stoppers" (stoppers that do not move smoothly down the glass cartridge) are infrequent today. An additional change in the stopper in recent years has been the move toward a uniform black rubber stopper in all local anesthetic drug combinations. Virtually gone are the red, green, and blue stoppers that aided in identification of the drug. Where black stoppers are used, a color-coding band is found around the glass cartridge.

In an intact dental cartridge (Fig. 7-1) the stopper is slightly indented from the lip of the glass cylinder. Cartridges whose plungers are flush with or extruded beyond the glass of the cylinder should not be used. This problem is discussed later in this chapter. (See "Problems.")

An *aluminum cap* is located at the opposite end of the cartridge from the rubber plunger. It fits snugly around the neck of the glass cartridge, holding the thin diaphragm in position. It is silver colored on all cartridges.

The *diaphragm* is a semipermeable membrane, usually latex rubber, through which the cartridge end of the needle penetrates. When properly prepared, the perforation of the needle is centrically located and round, forming a tight seal around the needle. Improper preparation of the needle and cartridge can produce an eccentric puncture with ovoid holes and leakage of the anesthetic solution during injection. The permeability of the diaphragm allows solutions in which the dental cartridge may be stored to diffuse into the cartridge, contaminating the local anesthetic solution.

Persons with latex allergy may be at increased risk when administered a local anesthetic through a glass cartridge.[2]

A thin plastic label is applied to all cartridges. It protects the patient and administrator in the event the glass should crack and also provides specifications about the enclosed drug. In addition, some manufacturers include a volume indicator on their label, making it easier for the administrator to deposit precise volumes of anesthetic (Figs. 7-2 and 7-3).

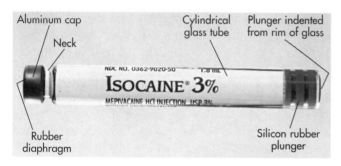

Fig. 7-1 Components of the glass dental cartridge.

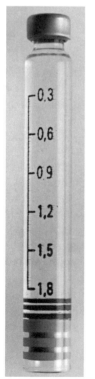

Fig. 7-2 Local anesthetic cartridge. Notice the volume indicators on the glass.

CARTRIDGE CONTENTS

The solution contained within the dental cartridge has several components:

1. Local anesthetic drug
2. Vasopressor drug
   a. Preservative for vasopressor
3. Sodium chloride
4. Distilled water

The *local anesthetic drug* is the raison d' être for the entire dental cartridge. It interrupts the propagated nerve impulse, preventing it from reaching the brain. The drug or drugs contained within the cartridge are listed by their percent concentration. The number of milligrams of the agent can be calculated by multiplying the percent concentration (e.g., 2% = 20 mg/ml) by 1.8 or 2.2 (number of milliliters in the cartridge). Thus a 1.8 ml cartridge of a 2% solution contains 36 mg (Table 7-1). The local anesthetic drug is quite stable, capable of being autoclaved, heated, or boiled without breaking down. However, other components of the cartridge are more labile (i.e., vasopressor drug and cartridge seals) and are destroyed rather handily.

A *vasopressor drug* is included in some anesthetic cartridges to increase the safety and the duration of action of the local anesthetic. The pH of dental cartridges containing vasopressors is lower (more acidic) than that of cartridges not containing vasopressors (pH of 3.3 to 4.0 versus 5.5 to 6.0). Because of this pH difference, plain anesthetics have a somewhat more rapid onset of clinical action and are more comfortable (less "burning" on injection).

Cartridges containing vasopressors also contain a chemical that serves as an *antioxidant.* The antioxidant

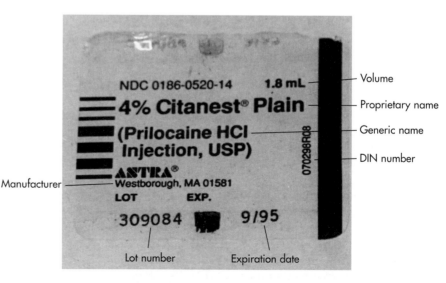

Fig. 7-3 Mylar plastic label.

T A B L E 7 - 1 Calculation of Milligrams per Cartridge

Percent solution		Milligrams per milliliter	Volume of cartridge		Milligrams per cartridge
0.25	=	2.5	× 1.8	=	4.5
0.40	=	4.0	× 1.8	=	7.2
0.50	=	5.0	× 1.8	=	9.0
1.0	=	10.0	× 1.8	=	18.0
1.5	=	15.0	× 1.8	=	27.0
2.0	=	20.0	× 1.8	=	36.0
3.0	=	30.0	× 1.8	=	54.0
4.0	=	40.0	× 1.8	=	72.0

most frequently used is sodium bisulfite. It prevents the biodegradation of the vasopressor by oxygen, which might be present in the cartridge during manufacture or which can diffuse through the semipermeable diaphragm after filling. Sodium bisulfite reacts with oxygen before the oxygen can destroy the vasopressor. The sodium bisulfite is oxidized to sodium bisulfate, a chemical with an even lower pH. The clinical relevance of this lies in the fact that increased burning (discomfort) is experienced by the patient on injection of an "older" cartridge of anesthetic with vasopressor than with a fresher cartridge. Allergy to bisulfites must be considered in the medical evaluation of all patients prior to local anesthetic administration.[3,4] (See Chapter 10.)

Sodium chloride is added to the contents of the cartridge to make the solution isotonic with the tissues of the body. In the past isolated instances have been reported in which local anesthetic solutions containing too much sodium chloride (hypertonic solutions) produced tissue edema or paresthesia, sometimes lasting for several months, following drug administration.[5]

Distilled water is used as the diluent to provide the volume of solution in the cartridge.

A significant change in cartridge composition in the United States and many other countries has been the removal of methylparaben, a bacteriostatic agent. A ruling by the United States Food and Drug Administration mandated the removal of methylparaben from dental local anesthetic cartridges manufactured after January 1, 1984. Methylparaben possesses bacteriostatic, fungistatic, and antioxidant properties. It and related compounds (ethyl-, propyl-, and butylparaben) are commonly used as preservatives in ointments, creams, lotions, and dentifrices. In addition, paraben preservatives are found in all multiple-dose vials of drugs. Methylparaben is commonly used in a 0.1% concentration (1 mg/ml). Its removal from local anesthetic cartridges was predicated on two facts. First, dental local anesthetic cartridges are single-use items meant to be discarded and not reused. Inclusion of a bacteriostatic

agent is therefore unnecessary. Second, repeated exposure to parabens has led to reports of increased allergic reactions in some persons.[6,7] Responses have been limited to localized edema, pruritus, and urticaria. Fortunately, there has not been, to date, a systemic allergic reaction to a paraben. Removal of methylparaben has further decreased an already minimal risk of allergy to local anesthesic drugs.

CARE AND HANDLING

Some local anesthetics are marketed in vacuum-sealed tin containers of 50 cartridges. Although no manufacturer makes any claim of sterility regarding the exterior surface of the cartridge, bacterial cultures taken immediately on opening a container usually fail to produce any growth. It therefore seems obvious that extraordinary measures related to cartridge sterilization are unwarranted. Indeed, the glass dental cartridge should not be autoclaved. The seals on the cartridge cannot withstand the extreme temperatures of autoclaving, and the heat-labile vasopressors will be destroyed in the process. Plastic cartridges cannot be autoclaved.

More and more commonly, local anesthetics are marketed in cardboard boxes of approximately 100 cartridges. Within the box are 10 sealed units of 10 cartridges each (Fig. 7-4), called a blister pack. Kept in this container until use, cartridges remain clean and uncontaminated.

Local anesthetic cartridges should be stored in their original container, preferably at room temperature (i.e., 21° to 22° C [70° to 72° F]) and in a dark place. There is no need to "prepare" a cartridge before use. The doctor or assistant need but insert it into the syringe. However, many doctors feel compelled to somehow "sterilize" the cartridge. When this urge strikes, the doctor should apply an alcohol wipe moistened with undiluted 91% isopropyl alcohol or 70% ethyl alcohol to the rubber diaphragm (Fig. 7-5).

If a clear plastic cartridge dispenser is used, 1 day's supply of cartridges should be placed with the aluminum cap and diaphragm facing downward (Fig. 7-6). Several (two or three) sterile dry 2 × 2 inch gauze wipes are placed in the center of the dispenser (Fig. 7-7) and moistened with (not immersed in) either 91% isopropyl alcohol or 70% ethyl alcohol. There should be no liquid alcohol present around the cartridges. Prior to loading the syringe, the aluminum cap and rubber diaphragm are rubbed against the moistened gauze (Fig. 7-8).

Cartridges should not be permitted to soak in either alcohol or other sterilizing solutions because the semipermeable diaphragm permits diffusion of these solutions into the dental cartridge, contaminating it. It is therefore recommended that cartridges be kept in their original container until they are to be used.

Cartridge warmers are not necessary. Indeed, they may occasionally produce problems. Overheating the local anesthetic solution can lead to discomfort for the patient and destruction of a heat-labile vasopressor (producing a shorter duration of anesthesia). It has been demonstrated that after the warmed glass cartridge is removed from the cartridge warmer and placed in a metal syringe and the solution forced through a fine

metal needle, its temperature has decreased almost to room temperature.[8]

Cartridge warmers, designed to maintain anesthetic solutions at "body temperature," are not needed and cannot be recommended. Local anesthetics in cartridges maintained at room temperature (20° to 22° C) do not cause the patient any discomfort on injection into tissues, nor do patients complain of the solution being too cold.[9] On the other hand, warmed local anesthetic solutions at 27° C (80° F) or above have a much greater incidence of being described as too hot or burning on injection.[9]

Local anesthetic cartridges should not be left exposed to direct sunlight because some contents may undergo accelerated deterioration. The primary clinical effect of this will be destruction of the vasopressor, with a corresponding decrease in the duration of clinical action of the anesthetic solution.

Included in every package of local anesthetic is an important document—the *drug package insert*. It contains valuable information about the product such as dosages, warnings, precautions, and care and handling. All persons involved in the handling or administration of local anesthetics should review this document periodically (Fig. 7-9).

PROBLEMS

Problems occasionally develop with dental cartridges. Although most are minor, producing slight inconvenience to the drug administrator, others are more significant and might prove harmful to the patient:

1. Bubble in the cartridge
2. Extruded stopper

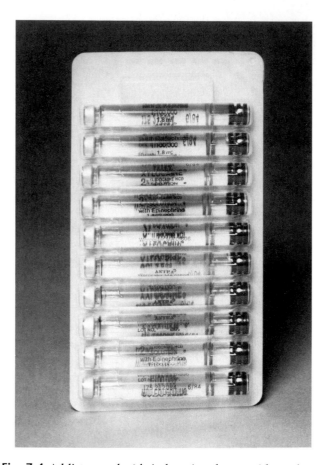

Fig. 7-4 A blister pack aids in keeping the cartridges clean.

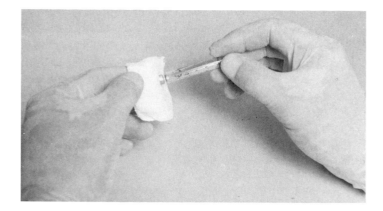

Fig. 7-5 Preparing a dental cartridge by wiping the rubber diaphragm with alcohol.

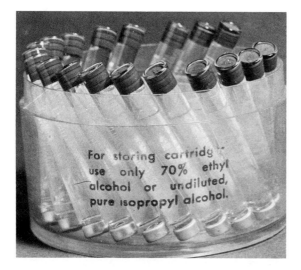

Fig. 7-6 Single day's supply of cartridges in a dispenser.

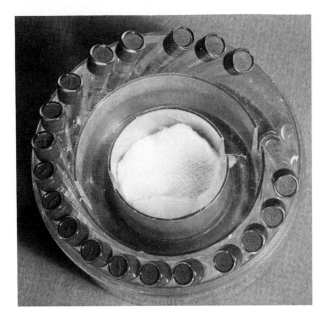

Fig. 7-7 Sterile gauze is placed in the center portion of the dispenser.

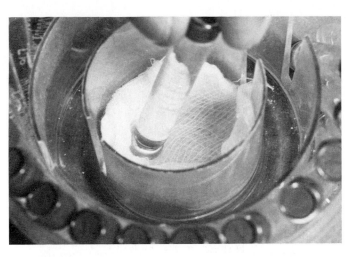

Fig. 7-8 Before loading, moisten the cap end of the cartridge on the gauze.

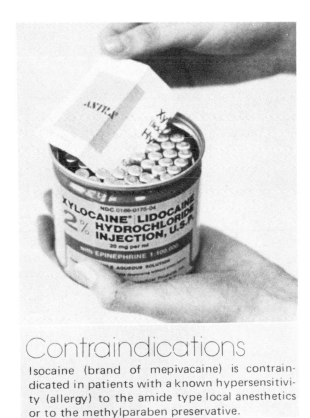

A

Contraindications

Isocaine (brand of mepivacaine) is contraindicated in patients with a known hypersensitivity (allergy) to the amide type local anesthetics or to the methylparaben preservative.

B

WARNINGS

DENTAL PRACTITIONERS WHO EMPLOY LOCAL ANESTHETICS IN THEIR OFFICES SHOULD BE WELL VERSED IN DIAGNOSIS AND MANAGEMENT OF EMERGENCIES WHICH MIGHT ARISE FROM THEIR USE. RESUSCITATIVE EQUIPMENT, OXYGEN AND OTHER RESUSCITATIVE DRUGS SHOULD BE AVAILABLE FOR IMMEDIATE USE.

Reactions resulting in fatality have occurred on rare occasions with the use of local anesthetics, even in the absence of a history of hypersensitivity.

Fig. 7-9 A, All local anesthetic containers have a product identification package insert. Read it! **B,** Important information is contained in all package inserts. *(Courtesy Cook-Waite Laboratories, New York.)*

3. Burning on injection
4. Sticky stopper
5. Corroded cap
6. "Rust" on the cap
7. Leakage during injection
8. Broken cartridge

Bubble in the Cartridge

A small bubble of approximately 1 to 2 mm diameter (described as "BB"-sized) will frequently be found in the dental cartridge (Fig. 7-10, *A*). It is composed of nitrogen gas, which was bubbled into the local anesthetic solution during its manufacture to prevent oxygen from being trapped in the cartridge and potentially destroying the vasopressor. The nitrogen bubble may not always be visible in a normal cartridge (Fig. 7-10, *B*).

A larger bubble, which may be present with a plunger that is extruded beyond the rim of the cartridge, is the result of the freezing of the anesthetic solution (Fig. 7-10, *C*). Such cartridges should not be used, since sterility of the solution cannot be assured, but rather the cartridges should be returned to their manufacturer for replacement.

Extruded Stopper

The stopper can become extruded when a cartridge is frozen and the liquid inside expands. In this case the solution can no longer be considered sterile and should

not be used for injection. Frozen cartridges can be identified by the presence of a large (> 2 mm) air bubble by the extruded stopper (Fig. 7-10, *C*).

An extruded stopper with no bubble (Fig. 7-11) is indicative of prolonged storage in a chemical disinfecting solution and diffusion of the solution into the cartridge. Shannon and Wescott demonstrated that alcohol enters a cartridge through the diaphragm in measurable amounts within 1 day if the diaphragm is immersed in alcohol.[10] Local anesthetic solutions containing alcohol will produce an uncomfortable burning on injection. Alcohol in sufficiently high concentration is a neurolytic agent and can produce long-term paresthesia. The greatest concentration of alcohol reported to date in a dental cartridge has been 8%, which is not likely to produce significant long-term injury.[11]

Antirust tablets should not be used in disinfectant solutions. The sodium nitrate (or similar agent) that they contain is capable of releasing metal ions, which have been related to an increased incidence of edema after local anesthetic administration.[12]

It should be remembered that small quantities of sterilizing solution can diffuse into a dental cartridge without any visible movement of the plunger. Care must always be taken in storage of local anesthetic cartridges.

Burning on Injection

A burning sensation on injection of anesthetic solution may be the result of one of the following:

1. Normal response to the pH of the drug
2. Cartridge containing sterilizing solution
3. Overheated cartridge
4. Cartridge containing a vasopressor

During the few seconds immediately following deposition of a local anesthetic solution the patient may complain of a slight sensation of burning. This normal reac-

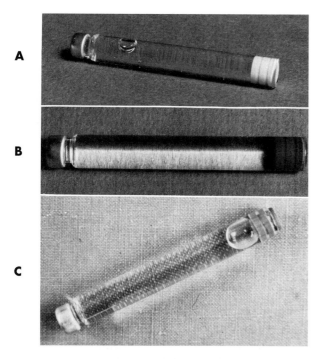

Fig. 7-10 Normal cartridge with a small bubble, **A,** or no bubble, **B.** Notice that the rubber stopper is indented from the glass rim. **C,** Local anesthetic cartridge with an extruded stopper and large bubble caused by freezing.

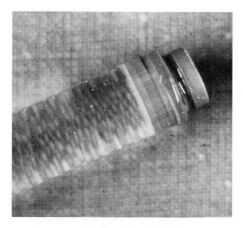

Fig. 7-11 Local anesthetic cartridge with extruded stopper and no bubble, caused by prolonged storage in alcohol.

tion is caused by the pH of the local anesthetic solution; it lasts but a second or two, until the anesthetic takes effect, and will be noted mainly by more sensitive patients.

A more intense burning on injection is usually the result of the diffusion of disinfecting solution into the dental cartridge and its subsequent injection into the oral mucous membranes. Although burning is most often a mere annoyance, the inclusion of disinfecting agents such as alcohol in dental cartridges can lead to more serious sequelae, such as postinjection paresthesia and tissue edema.[10,11]

Overheating of the solution in a cartridge warmer may also produce burning on injection. The (Christmas-tree) bulb-type cartridge warmer is most often at fault in this regard. Unless local anesthetic cartridges are unusually cold, there is little justification for using a cartridge warmer. Local anesthetic solutions injected at room temperature are well tolerated by tissues and patients.

Use of a cartridge containing a vasopressor may also be responsible for the sensation of burning on injection. The addition of a vasopressor and an antioxidant (sodium bisulfite) lowers the pH of the solution to between 3.3 and 4, significantly more acidic than solutions not containing a vasopressor (pH about 5.5).[12] Patients are more likely to feel the burning sensation with these solutions. A further decrease in the pH of the local anesthetic solution results when the sodium bisulfite is oxidized to sodium bisulfate. This response can be minimized by carefully checking the expiration date of all cartridges before use. Conversely, increasing the pH of the anesthetic solution has the effect of making local anesthetic administration more comfortable for the patient.[13]

Sticky Stopper

A sticky stopper has become rare today, with the inclusion of silicone as a lubricant and the removal of paraf-

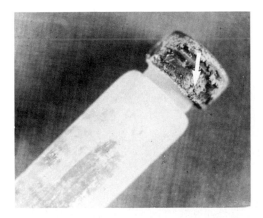

Fig. 7-12 Use of quaternary ammonium compound (e.g., benzalkonium chloride) to *sterilize* local anesthetic cartridges may lead to corrosion of the aluminum cap *(arrow)*.

fin as a sealant in the cartridge. Where paraffin is still used, difficulty in advancing the stopper may occur on colder days as the paraffin hardens. Using cartridges at room temperature minimizes this problem; using silicone-coated stoppers eliminates it. Plastic cartridges appear to suffer from this problem to a greater degree than glass cartridges.

Corroded Cap

The aluminum cap on a local anesthetic cartridge can be corroded if immersed in disinfecting solutions that contain quaternary ammonium salts, such as benzalkonium chloride (i.e., "cold" sterilizing solution). These salts are electrolytically incompatible with aluminum. Aluminum-sealed cartridges should be disinfected in either 91% isopropyl alcohol or 70% ethyl alcohol. Cartridges with corroded caps must not be used. Corrosion (Fig. 7-12) may be easily distinguished from rust, which appears as a red deposit on an intact aluminum cap.

Rust on the Cap

Rust found on a cartridge indicates that at least one cartridge in the tin container has broken or leaked. The "tin" container (actually steel dipped in molten tin) rusts, and the deposit comes off on the cartridges. Cartridges containing rust should not be used. If any cartridge contains rust or a crack, all cartridges in the container must be carefully checked prior to use. With the introduction of nonmetal packaging, rust is now rarely seen.

Leakage during Injection

Leakage of local anesthetic solution into the patient's mouth during injection will occur if the cartridge and needle are prepared improperly, and the needle puncture of the diaphragm is ovoid and eccentric. Properly placed on the syringe after the cartridge is inserted, the needle produces a centric perforation of the diaphragm that tightly seals itself around the needle. When pressure is applied to the plunger during injection, all of the solution will be directed into the lumen of the needle. If the cartridge is placed in a breech-loading syringe *after* the needle, an eccentric ovoid perforation may occur and, with pressure on the plunger, some solution will be directed into the lumen of the needle and some may leak out of the cartridge between the needle and the diaphragm and run into the patient's mouth. (See Fig. 5-15.) When the safety syringe is used, it is necessary to insert the cartridge after the needle has been attached; however, as the cartridge slides directly into the syringe, not from the side, leakage during injection is rarely a problem. Verbal and written communications from doctors using plastic cartridges indicate that the occurrence of leakage appears to be considerably greater with them.

The plastic dental cartridge does not withstand the application of injection pressure as well as the tradition-

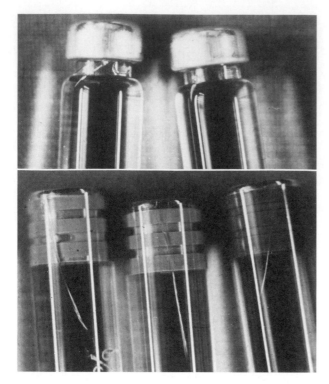

Fig. 7-13 Local anesthetic cartridges with cracks in the neck region, **A,** and around the rubber stopper, **B.**

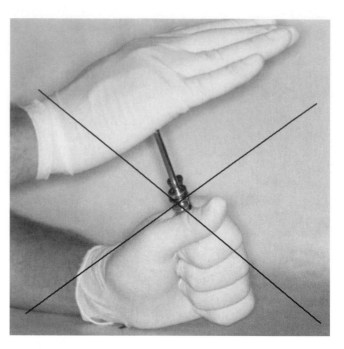

Fig. 7-14 If force is needed to embed the harpoon in the rubber stopper, cover the glass face of the syringe with your hand.

al glass cartridge. Meechan et al applied pressures equal to that achieved during the periodontal ligament (PDL) injection to both glass and plastic local anesthetic cartridges.[1] Leakage of anesthetic occurred in 1.4% of glass cartridges, whereas leakage was noted in 75.1% of plastic cartridges.

Broken Cartridge

The most common cause of cartridge breakage is the use of a cartridge that has been cracked or chipped during shipping. Dented metal containers or damaged boxes should be returned to the supplier immediately for exchange. If a broken cartridge is found in a container, all remaining cartridges must be examined for hairline cracks or chips. Two areas that must be carefully examined are the thin neck of the cartridge where it joins the cap (Fig. 7-13, *A*) and the glass surrounding the plunger (Fig. 7-13, *B*). Subjecting a cracked cartridge to the pressure of injection will often cause the cartridge to shatter or "explode." If this occurs inside the patient's mouth, serious sequelae may result from the ingestion of glass. It is essential to suction the patient's mouth thoroughly and consult with a physician or emergency department regarding follow-up therapy before discharging the patient. The addition of a thin Mylar plastic label to the glass cartridge has minimized such injury.

Plastic cartridges do not fracture when subjected to PDL injection pressures.[1]

Excessive force used to engage the aspirating harpoon in the stopper has resulted in numerous cases of shattered cartridges. Although they have not broken in the patient's mouth, there has been injury to dental personnel. Try to avoid hitting the thumb ring of the syringe in an attempt to engage the harpoon in the rubber stopper. If this technique is essential to embed the harpoon in the rubber plunger (as it is with the plastic safety syringe), use one hand to cover the entire exposed glass face of the cartridge (Fig. 7-14). Proper preparation of the armamentarium (Chapter 9) will minimize this problem.

Breakage can also occur as a result of attempting to use a cartridge with an extruded plunger. Extruded plungers can be forced back into the cartridge only with difficulty, if at all. Do not use cartridges with extruded plungers.

Syringes with bent harpoons may cause cartridges to break. (See Fig. 5-17.) Bent needles that are no longer patent create a pressure buildup within the cartridge during attempted injection. (See Fig. 5-16.) *Never* attempt to force local anesthetic solution from a dental cartridge against significant resistance.

RECOMMENDATIONS

1. Dental cartridges must never be used on more than one patient.

2. Cartridges should be stored at room temperature.
3. Cartridges need not be warmed prior to use.
4. Do not use cartridges beyond their expiration date.
5. Cartridges should be carefully checked for cracks, chips, and the integrity of the stopper and cap prior to use.

REFERENCES

1. Meechan JG, McCabe JF, Carrick TE: Plastic dental anaesthetic cartridges: a laboratory investigation, *Br Dent J* 169(2):54-56, 1990.
2. Sussman GL, Beezhold DH: Allergy to latex rubber, *Ann Intern Med* 122(1):43-46, 1995.
3. Seng GF, Gay BJ: Dangers of sulfites in dental local anesthetic solutions: warning and recommendations, *J Am Dent Assoc* 113:769-770, 1986.
4. Perusse R, Goulet JP, Turcotte JY: Contraindications to vasoconstrictors in dentistry: Part II. Hyperthyroidism, diabetes, sulfite sensitivity, cortico-dependent asthma, and pheochromocytoma, *Oral Surg* 74(5):687-691, 1992.
5. Nickel AA: Paresthesia resulting from local anesthetics, *J Oral Maxillofac Surg* 42(5):279, 1984.
6. Wurbach G, Schubert H, Pillipp I: Contact allergy to benzyl alcohol and benzyl paraben, *Contact Dermatitis* 28(3):187-188, 1993.
7. Klein CE, Gall H: Type IV allergy to amide-type anesthetics, *Contact Dermatitis* 25(1):45-48, 1991.
8. Volk RJ, Gargiulo AV: Local anesthetic cartridge warmer—first in, first out, *Ill Dent J* 53(2):92-94, 1984.
9. Rogers KB, Fielding AF, Markiewicz SW: The effect of warming local anesthetic solutions prior to injection, *Gen Dent* 37(6):496-499, 1989.
10. Shannon IL, Wescott WB: Alcohol contamination of local anesthetic cartridges, *J Acad Gen Dent* 22:20-21, 1974.
11. Oakley J: Personal communications, 1985.
12. Moorthy AP, Moorthy SP, O'Neil R: A study of pH of dental local anesthetic solutions, *Br Dent J* 157(11): 394-395, 1984.
13. Crose VW: Pain reduction in local anesthetic administration through pH buffering, *J Ind Dent Assoc* 70(2):24-25, 1991.

eight

Additional Armamentarium

In previous chapters the three major components of local anesthetic armamentarium—syringe, needle, and cartridge—have been discussed. There are other important items in the local anesthetic armamentarium, however, including the following:

1. Topical antiseptic
2. Topical anesthetic
3. Applicator sticks
4. Cotton gauze (2 × 2 inches)
5. Hemostat

TOPICAL ANTISEPTIC

A topical antiseptic may be used to prepare the tissues at the site of injection prior to the initial needle penetration. Its function is to produce a transient decrease in the bacterial population at the injection site, thereby minimizing any risk of postinjection infection.

The topical antiseptic, on an applicator stick, is placed at the site of injection for 15 to 30 seconds. There is no need to place a large quantity on the applicator stick; it should be sufficient just to moisten the cotton portion of the swab.

Commonly used agents include Betadine (povidone-iodine) and Merthiolate (thimerosal). Topical antiseptics containing alcohol (e.g., *tincture* of iodine or *tincture* of Merthiolate) should not be used because the alcohol will produce tissue irritation. In addition, allergy to iodine-containing compounds is not uncommon.[1] Before any iodine-containing topical antiseptic is applied to tissues,

care should be taken to determine if adverse reactions to iodine have previously developed.

In a survey of local anesthetic techniques in dental practice,[2] 7.9% of the dentists mentioned that they always used topical antiseptics prior to injection, 22.4% sometimes used them, and 69.7% never used them.

Postinjection infections can and do occur, but the regular use of a topical antiseptic can virtually eliminate them. If a topical antiseptic is not available, a sterile gauze wipe may serve to prepare the tissues adequately before injection.

The application of a topical antiseptic is considered an optional step in tissue preparation prior to intraoral injection.

TOPICAL ANESTHETIC

Topical anesthetic preparations are discussed in depth in Chapter 4. Their use prior to initial needle penetration of the mucous membrane is strongly recommended. With proper application I have found that the *initial* penetration of mucous membrane can usually be made anywhere in the oral cavity without the patient being aware of it.

For effectiveness, I recommend that a minimal quantity of topical anesthetic be applied to the end of the applicator stick and placed directly at the site of penetration for approximately 1 minute. Gill and Orr have demonstrated that when topical anesthetics are applied according to the manufacturer's instructions (approximately 10 to 15 seconds) their effectiveness is no greater than that of a placebo, especially for palatal injections.[3]

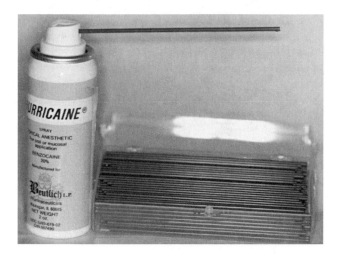

Fig. 8-1 Disposable nozzle for spray topicals.

Stern and Giddon showed that application of the topical anesthetic to mucous membrane for 2 to 3 minutes leads to profound soft tissue analgesia.[4]

A variety of topical anesthetic agents are available for use today. Most contain the ester local anesthetic benzocaine. The occurrence of allergic reactions to esters is greater than that to amide topical anesthetics; however, since benzocaine is not absorbed systemically, allergic reactions are usually localized to the site of application. Of the amides available, only lidocaine possesses topical anesthetic activity in clinically acceptable concentrations. The risk of overdose with amide topical anesthetics is greater than that with the esters and increases with the area of application of the topical anesthetic. Topical forms of lidocaine are available as ointments, gels, pastes, and sprays.

Unmetered topical anesthetic sprays of nonbenzocaine topicals are potentially dangerous and are not recommended for routine use. Because topical anesthetics require greater concentration to penetrate mucous membranes, and because nonbenzocaine topical anesthetics are absorbed rapidly into the cardiovascular system, only small measured doses should be administered. Nonbenzocaine topical anesthetic sprays that deliver a continuous stream of topical anesthetic until being deactivated are capable of delivering overly high doses of the topical anesthetic. If absorbed into the cardiovascular system, the topical anesthetic may induce high local anesthetic blood levels, increasing the risk of an overdose reaction. Metered sprays that deliver a fixed dose with each administration, regardless of the length of time the nozzle is depressed, are preferred for topical formulations that are absorbed systemically. An example of this form of topical anesthetic spray is Xylocaine, which delivers 10 mg per administration.

Yet another potential problem with topical anesthetic sprays is difficulty keeping the spray nozzle sterile. This is a very important consideration when selecting the form

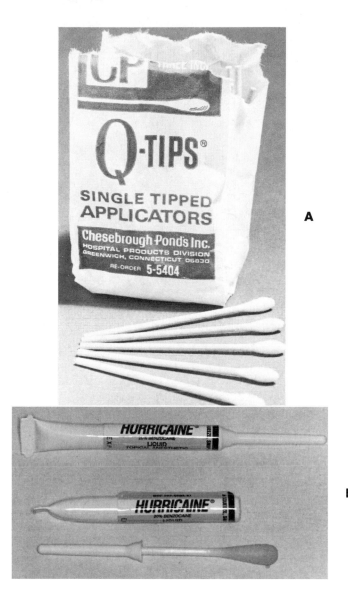

Fig. 8-2 A, Applicator sticks. **B,** Topical anesthetic swab. *(A, Courtesy Chesebrough-Ponds)*

of topical anesthetic to be used. Many topical anesthetic sprays come with disposable applicator nozzles (Fig. 8-1).

It is important to remember that some topical anesthetic formulations contain preservatives, such as methylparaben, that may be significant in instances of allergy to local anesthetics.

APPLICATOR STICKS

Applicators should be available as part of the local anesthetic armamentarium. They are wooden sticks with a cotton swab at one end, and they can be used to apply topical antiseptic and anesthetic solutions to mucous membranes (Fig. 8-2) and to compress tissue during palatal injections.

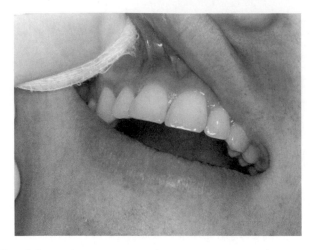

Fig. 8-3 Sterile gauze is used to wipe tissue at the site of needle penetration and to aid in tissue retraction.

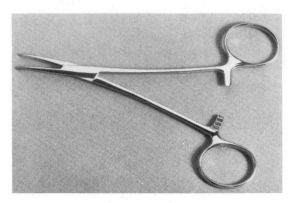

Fig. 8-4 Hemostat.

COTTON GAUZE

Cotton gauze is included in the local anesthetic armamentarium for wiping the area of injection prior to the administration of a local anesthetic and for drying the mucous membrane to aid retraction for increased visibility.

Many dentists select gauze in lieu of topical antiseptic solution for wiping. The gauze effectively dries the injection site and removes any gross debris from the area (Fig. 8-3). It is *not* as effective as the topical antiseptic but can be used in its place.

Retraction of lips and cheeks for improved access and visibility to the injection site is important during all intraoral injections. Quite often this task becomes unnecessarily difficult if these tissues are moist, and it is made even more vexing with the wearing of latex or vinyl gloves. A dry cotton gauze makes the tissues easier to grasp and retract.

A variety of sizes of cotton gauze are available, but the most practical and indeed the most commonly used is the 2 × 2 inch size.

HEMOSTAT

Although not considered an essential element of the local anesthetic armamentarium, a hemostat or pickup forceps should be readily available at all times in the dental office. Its primary function in local anesthesia is the removal of a needle from the soft tissues of the mouth in the unlikely event that the needle breaks off within tissues (Fig. 8-4).

REFERENCES

1. Bennasr S, Magnier S, Hassan M, Jacqz-Aigrain E: Anaphylactic shock and low osmolarity contrast medium, *Arch Pediatr* 1(2):155-157, 1994.
2. Malamed SF: Results of a survey of 209 dentists, Unpublished data, 1975.
3. Gill CJ, Orr DL II: A double blind crossover comparison of topical anesthetics, *J Am Dent Assoc* 98:213-214, 1979.
4. Stern I, Giddon DB: Topical anesthesia for periodontal procedures, *Anesth Prog* 22:105-108, 1975.

nine

Preparation of the Armamentarium

Proper care and handling of the local anesthetic armamentarium can prevent or at least minimize the development of complications associated with the needle, syringe, and cartridge—many of which have been discussed in the preceding chapters. Other complications and minor annoyances may be prevented through proper preparation of the armamentarium.

BREECH-LOADING, METALLIC OR PLASTIC, CARTRIDGE-TYPE SYRINGE*

1. *Remove the sterilized syringe* from its container (Fig. 9-1).
2. *Retract the piston* fully prior to attempting to load the cartridge (Fig. 9-2).
3. *Insert the cartridge,* while the piston is fully retracted, into the syringe. Insert the rubber stopper end of the cartridge first (Fig. 9-3).
4. *Engage the harpoon.* Holding the syringe as if injecting, *gently* push the piston forward until the harpoon is firmly engaged in the plunger (Fig. 9-4). Excessive force is not required. Do *not* hit the piston in an effort to engage the harpoon (Fig. 9-5). This will frequently lead to cracked or shattered glass cartridges.
5. *Attach the needle* to the syringe. Remove the white or clear protective plastic cap from the syringe end of the needle and screw the needle onto the syringe

(Fig. 9-6). Metal-hubbed needles have threading, but plastic-hubbed needles do not, and the needle must be constantly pushed onto the metal hub of the syringe while being turned.
6. *Carefully remove the colored plastic protective cap* from the opposite end of the needle and *expel a few drops of solution* to test for proper flow.
7. The syringe is now ready for use.

Note: It is common practice in dentistry to attach the needle to the syringe *prior* to placing the cartridge. This requires hitting the piston hard to engage the harpoon, a process that can lead to broken cartridges or leakage of anesthetic solution into the patient's mouth during the injection. The recommended sequence, described above, virtually eliminates this possibility and should always be used.

Recapping the Needle

Following removal of the syringe from the patient's mouth, the needle should be recapped immediately. Recapping is *the* time when health professionals are most likely to be stuck with a needle, and probably the most dangerous time to be stuck, for the needle is now contaminated with blood, saliva, and debris. Though a variety of techniques and devices for recapping have been suggested, the technique recommended by most state safety and health agencies is termed the "scoop" technique (Fig. 9-7), in which the uncapped needle is slid into the needle sheath lying on the instrument tray or table. Until a better method is designed, the scoop technique should be used for needle recapping.

*From Astra Pharmaceutical Products, Worcester, Mass. This is a portion of the instructions that Astra encloses with its syringes.

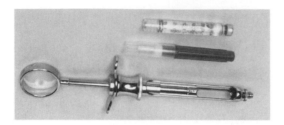

Fig. 9-1 Local anesthetic armamentarium: *(from top)* cartridge, needle, syringe.

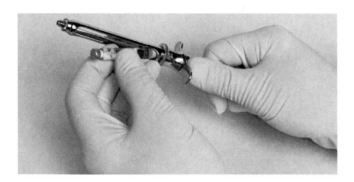

Fig. 9-2 Retract the piston.

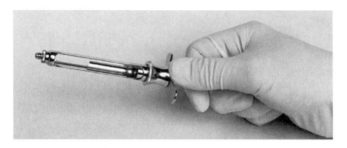

Fig. 9-3 Insert the cartridge.

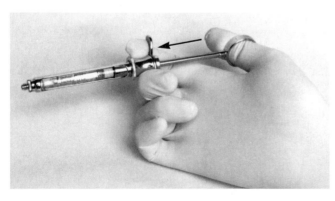

Fig. 9-4 Engage the harpoon with *gentle* finger pressure *(arrow)*.

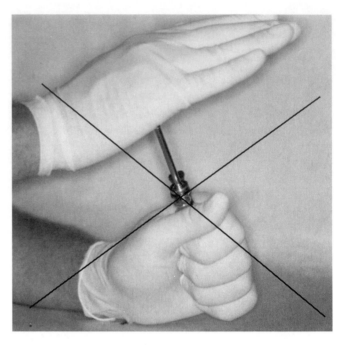

Fig. 9-5 Do *not* exert force on the plunger; the glass may crack.

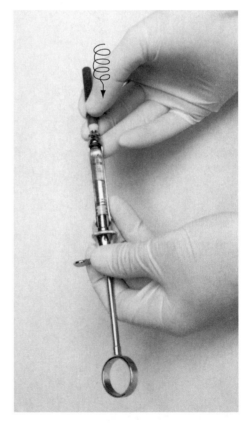

Fig. 9-6 A plastic needle must be screwed onto the syringe while simultaneously being pushed into the metal hub *(arrow)*.

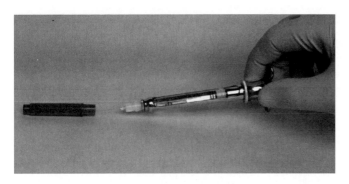

Fig. 9-7 "Scoop" technique for recapping the needle after injection.

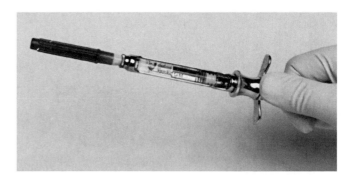

Fig. 9-9 Retract the piston.

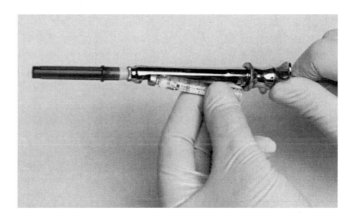

Fig. 9-10 Remove the used cartridge.

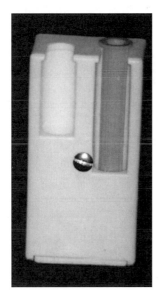

Fig. 9-8 Acrylic needle cap holder.

Various needle cap holders are available, either commercially made or selfmade (from acrylic) (Fig. 9-8) that hold the cap stationary while the needle is being inserted into it, making the recapping somewhat easier to accomplish.

Unloading the Breech-loading, Metallic or Plastic, Cartridge-type Syringe*

After administration of the local anesthetic, the following sequence is suggested for removing the used cartridge:

1. *Retract the piston* and pull the cartridge away from the needle with your thumb and forefinger as you retract the piston (Fig. 9-9), until the harpoon disengages from the plunger.
2. *Remove the cartridge* from the syringe by inverting the syringe, permitting the cartridge to fall free (Fig. 9-10).

*From Astra Pharmaceutical Products, Worcester, Mass. This is a portion of the instructions that Astra encloses with its syringes.

3. *Discard the used needle.* All needles must be discarded following use to prevent injury or intentional misuse by unauthorized persons. Carefully unscrew the now recapped needle, being careful not to accidentally discard the metal needle adaptor (Fig. 9-11). The use of a sharps container is recommended (Fig. 9-12) for needle disposal.

SELF-ASPIRATING SYRINGE*

1. Insert the cartridge (as above).
2. Attach the needle.
3. The syringe is now ready for use.

Because of the absence of a harpoon, loading and unloading the self-aspirating syringe are quite simple procedures.

*From Astra Pharmaceutical Products, Worcester, Mass. This is a portion of the instructions that Astra encloses with its syringes.

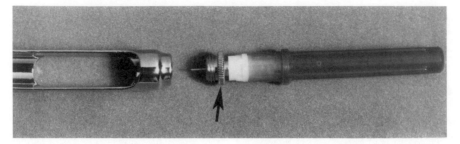

Fig. 9-11 When discarding the needle, check to be sure that the metal needle adaptor is not inadvertently discarded too (*arrow*).

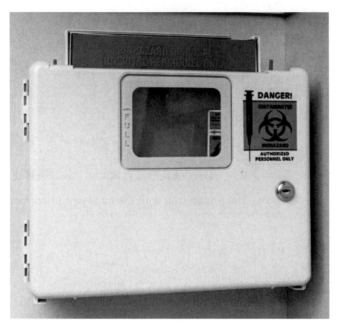

Fig. 9-12 A sharps container is recommended for discarding contaminated needles.

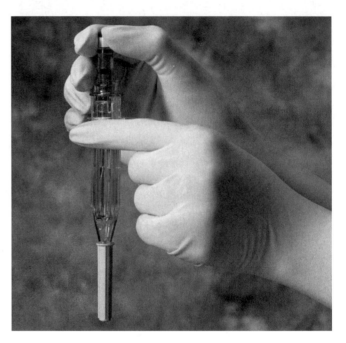

Fig. 9-13 Insert a cartridge into the syringe.

ULTRASAFE ASPIRATING SYRINGE*
Loading the Safety Syringe

1. *Insert the anesthetic cartridge into the body assembly* (Fig. 9-13), making certain that the needle pierces the rubber diaphragm on the cartridge.
2. Grasp the octagonal plug on the body assembly between the thumb and the index finger. *Align the legs with the notches and snap the two sections (body and plunger) together* (Fig. 9-14). A very distinct snapping sound will be heard when the two sections are forced together.
3. Grasp the body assembly below its collar between the thumb and the index finger. Point the needle end of the syringe down (Fig. 9-15).

*From Safety Syringes, Arcadia, Calif. This is a portion of the instructions that Safety Syringes encloses with its syringes.

4. *Engage the harpoon into the stopper of the cartridge* by striking the flat top of the plunger with the palm of the hand (Fig. 9-16).
5. Express several drops of anesthetic solution to ensure proper preparation of the syringe.
6. The syringe is now ready for use (Fig. 9-17).

Unloading the UltraSafe Aspirating Syringe

The syringe is designed for single use. After the last injection, discard the entire device into a sharps container as soon as possible. The UltraSafe aspirating syringe may be reloaded with an additional cartridge as follows:

1. *Release the harpon from the rubber stopper* by pulling back the plunger to its original position.
2. Holding the body assembly in one hand, use the other hand to grasp the plug with the thumb and

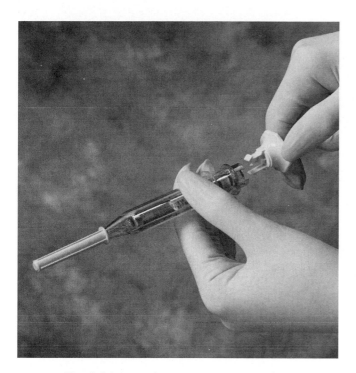

Fig. 9-14 Snap the two sections together.

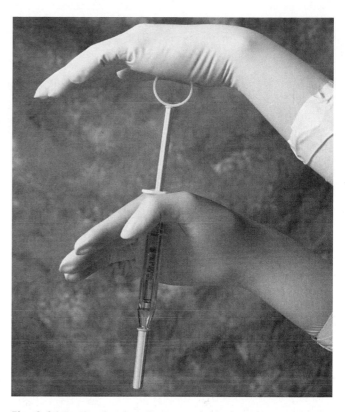

Fig. 9-16 Strike the thumb ring with the hand to embed the plunger into the rubber stopper of the cartridge.

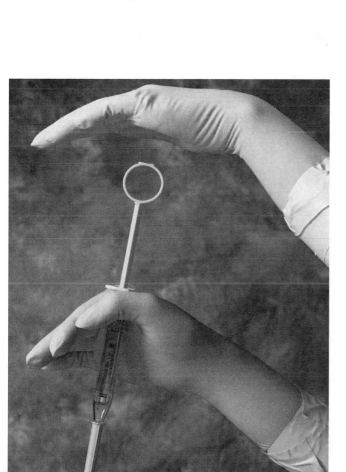

Fig. 9-15 Prepare for harpoon insertion. Hold facing down.

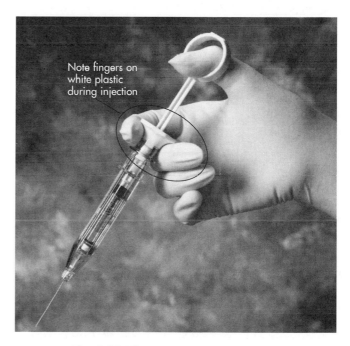

Fig. 9-17 The syringe is ready for use.

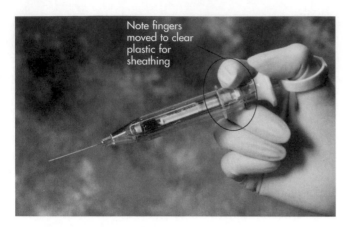

Note fingers moved to clear plastic for sheathing

Fig. 9-18 One-handed guarding technique: place fingers on front of the guard.

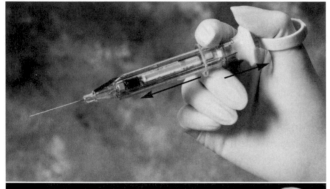

A

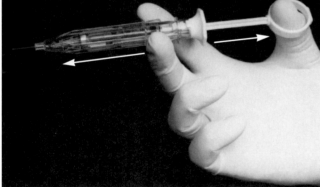

B

Fig. 9-19 One-handed guarding technique: pull back until a click is heard.

the index finger. Twist the plug counter counterclockwise until the plug releases from the body assembly.

3. *Remove the cartridge.*

4a. Holding the guard near the collar, use the thumb and the index finger to release the lock by pinching the walls of the body assembly forward until the needle clears the guard opening.

4b. Load the cartridge and push forward with the thumb until the body and cartridge are fully loaded into their original positions.

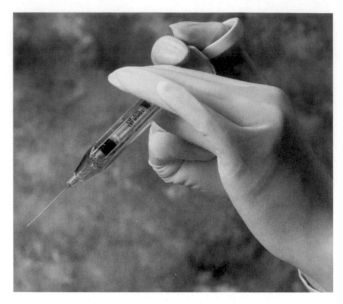

Fig. 9-20 Two-handed guarding technique: grasp guard near its collar with free hand.

5. Grasp the octogonal plug, align the legs with the body notches, and push forward firmly until the sections snap together.

6. *Reengage the harpoon* by striking the flat top of the plunger with the palm of the hand. The syringe is ready for the next injection.

Making the UltraSafe Aspirating Syringe "Safe"

One-handed Guarding Technique*

1. Following completion of the injection, gently move the index and middle fingers against the front collar of the guard (Fig. 9-18).
2. Pull back on the needle (pulling back the plunger) until it is retracted into the guard and the guard legs lock into the body notches (Fig. 9-19).

Two-handed Guarding Technique*

Use of the two-handed guarding technique is suggested when the entire cartridge has not been administered or if the administrator has small or petite glove-size hands.

1. Grasp the guard near its collar with the free hand (Fig. 9-20).
2. Pull the body back until the needle is retracted into the guard and the guard legs lock into the body notches (Fig. 9-21).

The needle is now safe. The entire assembly unit can be discarded in the sharps container.

*From Safety Syringes, Arcadia, Calif. This is a portion of the instructions that Safety Syringes encloses with its syringes.

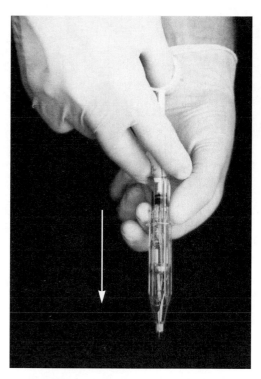

Fig. 9-21 Two-handed guarding technique: pull back the needle until locked (arrow).

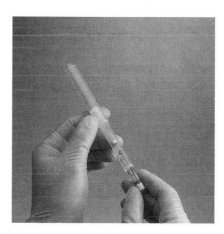

Fig. 9-22 Insert the anesthetic cartridge into the open end of the injection unit. (Courtesy Septodont, New Castle, Del.)

The manufacturer of the UltraSafe aspirating syringe recommends several safety precautions:

1. Hands must remain behind the needle at all times during use and disposal.
2. Do not attempt to override or defeat the locking safety mechanism.
3. Single use only.
4. For aspiration, use standard operating procedures for the administration of an anesthetic.

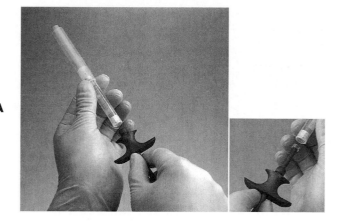

Fig. 9-23 A, With the T-bar pushed all the way forward, snap the injection unit onto the syringe handle. B, Incorrect position. (Courtesy Septodont, New Castle, Del.)

SEPTODONT SAFETY PLUS*

Loading the Safety Plus System

1. Unwrap the color-coded, sterile injection unit and attach the syringe handle onto the empty injection unit to widen the opening slightly; then remove. Insert the anesthetic cartridge into the open end of the injection unit (Fig. 9-22).
   a. The Safety Plus system is available with the following dental needles:
      25 gauge × 1³/₈ inch (long)
      27 gauge × 1³/₈ inch
      30 gauge × 1 inch
      27 gauge × 1 inch (short)
      30 gauge × ³/₈ inch (extra-short)
2. With the T-bar pushed all the way forward, snap the injection unit onto the syringe handle (Fig. 9-23).
3. Pull back on the protective sheath until it is flush with the syringe handle; the capped needle is now visible (Fig. 9-24).
4. Remove and discard the needle cap, exposing the sterile needle (Fig. 9-25).
5. Check to make sure the anesthetic solution is flowing by gently pushing on the syringe handle.
6. The syringe is now ready for use.

Safety Plus: Multiple Injections with the Same Anesthetic Cartridge

7. Following the initial injection, slide the protective sheath forward to the *first* locking level to recover the exposed needle (Fig. 9-26).
8. When ready to reinject the patient, refer to Steps 3, 5, and 6 above. (Disregard Step 4, as needle cap has already been discarded.)

*From Septodont, New Castle, Del. This is a portion of the instructions that Septodont encloses with its syringes.

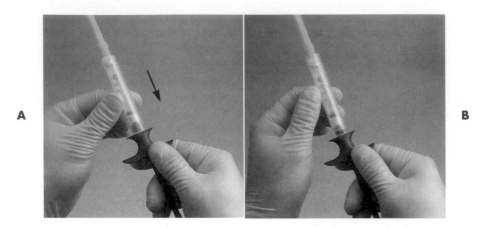

Fig. 9-24 A, Pull back on the protective sheath until it is flush with the syringe handle *(arrow);* the capped needle is now visible. **B,** Incorrect position. *(Courtesy Septodont, New Castle, Del.)*

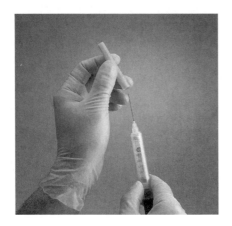

Fig. 9-25 Remove and discard the needle cap, exposing the sterile needle. *(Courtesy Septodont, New Castle, Del.)*

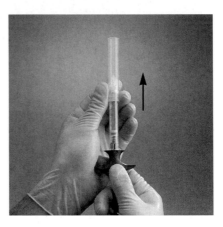

Fig. 9-26 Following the initial injection, slide the protective sheath forward to the *first* locking level to cover the exposed needle *(arrow). (Courtesy Septodont, New Castle, Del.)*

Safety Plus: Multiple Injections Using More Than One Anesthetic Cartridge

9. Following the initial injection, slide the protective sheath forward to the *first* locking level to cover the exposed needle (Fig. 9-26).
10. While holding the middle of the plastic barrel in one hand, use the other hand to pull back on the T-bar only, not the plunger (Fig. 9-27).
    a. The injection unit is now separated from the syringe holder; the empty cartridge is removed (Fig. 9-28).
11. Insert a new cartridge. (Refer to Steps 1 and 2 above.)
12. Reinject the patient. (Refer to Steps 3, 5, and 6 above, disregarding Step 4, as needle cap has already been discarded.)

Safety Plus: Disposal and Sterilization

After completion of the final injection:

13. While holding the plastic barrel in one hand, slide the protective sheath to the second and final locking position (Fig. 9-29).
    a. A "clicking" sound indicates that the sheath is in its final locking position.
14. Hold the T- bar and pull the thumb ring all the way back so that the plunger is completely backed out of the anesthetic cartridge (Fig. 9-30).
15. Hold the T- bar and simply "snap" off the entire injection unit with the anesthetic cartridge still inside (Fig. 9-31).
16. The injection unit/cartridge can now be discarded in the sharps container.

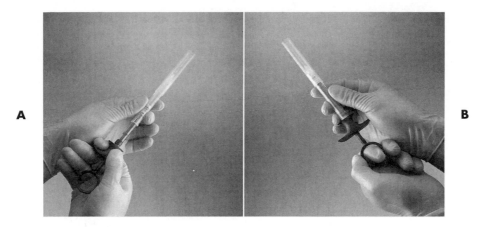

Fig. 9-27 A, While holding the middle of the plastic barrel in one hand, use the other hand to pull back on the T- bar only, not the plunger. **B,** Incorrect position. *(Courtesy Septodont, New Castle, Del.)*

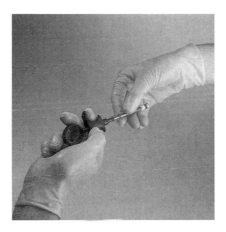

Fig. 9-28 The injection unit is now separated from the syringe holder; the empty cartridge is removed. *(Courtesy Septodont, New Castle, Del.)*

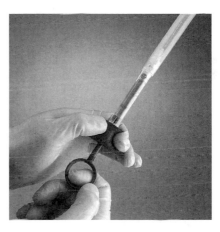

Fig. 9-30 Hold the T- bar and pull the thumb ring all the way back so that the plunger is completely backed out of the anesthetic cartridge. *(Courtesy Septodont, New Castle, Del.)*

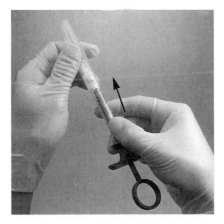

Fig. 9-29 While holding the plastic barrel in one hand, slide the protective sheath to the second and final locking position *(arrow).* A "clicking" sound indicates that the sheath is in its final locking position. *(Courtesy Septodont, New Castle, Del.)*

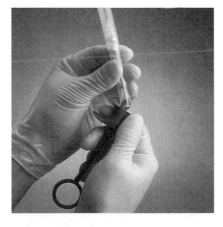

Fig. 9-31 Hold the T- bar and simply "snap" off the entire injection unit with the anesthetic cartridge still inside. *(Courtesy Septodont, New Castle, Del.)*

17. Disinfect the syringe handle following routine disinfection procedures.
18. Follow routine procedures for sterilization of the syringe handle.

PLACING AN ADDITIONAL CARTRIDGE IN A SYRINGE

On occasion it will be necessary to deposit an additional cartridge of local anesthetic solution. To do so, the following sequence is suggested with the metallic or plastic breech-loading syringe.

1. Recap the needle using the scoop (or other appropriate) technique and remove it from the syringe.
2. Retract the piston (which disengages the harpoon from the rubber stopper).
3. Remove the used cartridge.
4. Insert the new cartridge.
5. Embed the harpoon.
6. Reattach the needle.

The approximate time required to complete this procedure is 10 to 15 seconds.

In light of the fact that most doctors do not remove the needle when reloading a syringe, the following is offered as an alternative procedure for reloading a local anesthetic syringe:

1. Recap the needle using the scoop (or other appropriate) technique.
2. Retract the piston (which disengages the harpoon from the rubber stopper).
3. Remove the used cartridge.
4. Fully retract the piston; insert the new local anesthetic cartridge.
   a. It is important to ensure that the piston is fully retracted so that the cartridge is placed into the syringe without bending the needle stylus.
5. Embed the harpoon into the stopper of the cartridge.
   a. This will require the administrator to strike a hard, sharp blow with their hand on the thumb ring of the syringe.
6. Ensure proper placement and lack of glass breakage by expressing a small volume of anesthetic solution before administering the next injection.

in this part

Techniques of regional anesthesia in dentistry

The anatomy of the head, neck, and oral cavity is presented as a prelude to detailed descriptions of the techniques of regional anesthesia. Techniques that are commonly used in dentistry are presented. Although many of the techniques described in these chapters may also be carried out successfully with an extraoral, rather than intraoral, approach, I have limited descriptions to intraoral techniques. This is primarily because of the extremely limited use of extraoral nerve blocks in contemporary dental practice. The interested reader is referred to the many textbooks that describe these extraoral techniques at some length.[1,2] In the second edition of this book, "new" injection techniques were added—the *Akinosi closed-mouth mandibular block* and the *periodontal ligament injection*, both of which had received favorable clinical acceptance since the publication of the first edition in 1980. In this fourth edition, descriptions of these and other techniques of regional anesthesia have been rewritten to take into account subtle changes in procedure that have occurred over the years.

There are usually several variations of each injection technique. Subtle differences are noted when techniques are taught to students by different persons. The reader must always keep in mind that there is never only one "correct" technique. The goals in the administration of local anesthesia are (1) to provide clinically adequate pain control (2) without unnecessarily increasing risk or provoking any immediate or delayed complications in the patient. Any technique meeting these two criteria is acceptable. The techniques presented in this section are those that I find most acceptable in my practice. In several situations alternative approaches to the injection are also described.

After describing these injection techniques, an all too often neglected subject is discussed—the requirements for pain control and local anesthesia within the dental specialties. These vary somewhat, from endodontics to pediatric dentistry to periodontics to prosthodontics to oral and maxillofacial surgery, and require special attention (Chapter 16). The administration of local anesthetics to the geriatric patient, a significant and growing segment of the population, is also reviewed.

The beginning of this section, Chapters 10 and 11, addresses two important subjects relating to all injections—the physical and psychological evaluation of the patient, and basic injection technique (i.e., the preparation of the patient and tissues for administration of any local anesthetic, and the procedure for an atraumatic [painless] injection).

REFERENCES
1. Mulroy MF: *Regional anesthesia: an illustrated procedural guide,* Boston, 1989, Little Brown.
2. Mulroy MF: *Peripheral nerve blocks.* In Rogers MC, Tinker JH, Covino BG, Longnecker DE, editors: *Principles and practice of anesthesiology,* St Louis, 1993, Mosby–Year Book.

CHAPTER

ten

Physical and Psychological Evaluation

Prior to starting any dental therapy, the doctor or hygienist must determine whether the patient can tolerate, both physically and psychologically, the planned dental procedures in relative safety. If this is not the case, it is important to determine the specific treatment modifications that will be necessary to decrease the risk presented by the patient. This is especially important whenever drugs are to be administered during treatment and includes all drugs, such as analgesics, anxiolytics, inhalation sedation, sedative-hypnotics, and local anesthetics. Prior to administering local anesthetics, the administrator must determine the relative risk presented by the patient. This is important because local anesthetics, like all drugs, exert actions on many parts of the body. (See Chapter 2.) Local anesthetics' actions include depressant effects on excitable membranes (e.g., the central nervous system [CNS] and the cardiovascular system [CVS]). Because local anesthetics undergo biotransformation, primarily in the liver (amides) and/or blood (esters), it is important to determine the functional status of these systems prior to drug administration. It is also important to evaluate the kidneys, where a percentage of all local anesthetics is excreted in an active (unmetabolized) form. Other questions should be asked: *Has the patient ever received a local anesthetic for either medical or dental care? If so, were any adverse reactions observed?*

Most undesirable reactions to local anesthetics are produced not by the drugs themselves but as a response to the act of drug administration.[1] These reactions are usually psychogenic and are potentially life threatening. The two most commonly occurring psychogenic reactions are vasodepressor syncope and hyperventilation. Other

psychogenically induced reactions I have noted as a response to local anesthetic administration include tonic-clonic convulsions, bronchospasm, and angina pectoris.

Local anesthetics are not, however, absolutely innocuous drugs, nor is the act of local anesthetic administration entirely benign. The doctor must seek to uncover as much information as possible concerning a patient's physical and mental status prior to administering a local anesthetic. Fortunately the means to do so exists in the form of the patient's completed medical history questionnaire, the dialogue history, and the physical examination of the patient. Adequate use of these safeguards can lead to an accurate determination of a patient's physical status and prevent up to 90% of all life-threatening medical emergencies in dental practice.[2]

• • •

A brief review follows of the procedure of physical evaluation recommended for all dental patients, with emphasis on patients who are to receive local anesthesia.

• • •

MEDICAL HISTORY QUESTIONNAIRE

As a general standard of care,* dentists have their patients complete a medical history questionnaire at the initial office visit. This history should be updated every 6 months or whenever the patient has been absent from the office for an extended time. Although many such questionnaires are available, there exist two basic types

*Standard of care: what a reasonably prudent doctor would do, or would not do, in a given situation

116

MEDICAL HISTORY

CIRCLE

1. Are you having pain or discomfort at this time? . . . . .YES NO
2. Do you feel very nervous about having dentistry treatment? . . . . .YES NO
3. Have you ever had a bad experience in the dentistry office? . . . . .YES NO
4. Have you been a patient in the hospital during the past two years? . . . . .YES NO
5. Have you been under the care of a medical doctor during the past two years? .YES NO
6. Have you taken any medicine or drugs during the past two years? . . . . .YES NO
7. Are you allergic to (i.e., itching, rash, swelling of hands, feet or eyes) or made sick by
   penicillin, aspirin, codeine, or any drugs or medication? . . . . .YES NO
8. Have you ever had any excessive bleeding requiring special treatment? . . . . .YES NO
9. Circle any of the following which you have had or have at present:

Heart failure	Emphysema	AIDS
Heart Disease or Attack	Cough	Hepatitis A (infectious)
Angina Pectoris	Tuberculosis (TB)	Hepatitis B (serum)
High Blood Pressure	Asthma	Liver Disease
Heart Murmur	Hay Fever	Yellow Jaundice
Rheumatic Fever	Sinus Trouble	Blood Transfusion
Congenital Heart Lesions	Allergies or Hives	Drug Addiction
Scarlet Fever	Diabetes	Hemophilia
Artificial Heart Valve	Thyroid Disease	Venereal Disease (Syphilis, Gonorrhea)
Heart Pacemaker	X-ray or Cobalt Treatment	Cold Sores
Heart Surgery	Chemotherapy (Cancer, Leukemia)	Genital Herpes
Artificial Joint	Arthritis	Epilepsy or Seizures
Anemia	Rheumatism	Fainting or Dizzy Spells
Stroke	Cortisone Medicine	Nervousness
Kidney Trouble	Glaucoma	Psychiatric Treatment
Ulcers	Pain in Jaw Joints	Sickle Cell Disease
		Bruise Easily

10. When you walk up stairs or take a walk, do you ever have to stop because of pain in your chest,
    or shortness of breath, or because you are very tired? . . . . .YES NO
11. Do your ankles swell during the day? . . . . .YES NO
12. Do you use more than 2 pillows to sleep? . . . . .YES NO
13. Have you lost or gained more than 10 pounds in the past year? . . . . .YES NO
14. Do you ever wake up from sleep short of breath? . . . . .YES NO
15. Are you on a special diet? . . . . .YES NO
16. Has your medical doctor ever said you have a cancer or tumor? . . . . .YES NO
17. Do you have any disease, condition, or problem not listed?
18. WOMEN: Are you pregnant now? . . . . .YES NO
             Are you practicing birth control? . . . . .YES NO
             Do you anticipate becoming pregnant? . . . . .YES NO

*To the best of my knowledge, all of the preceding answers are true and correct. If I ever have any change
in my health, or if my medicines change, I will inform the doctor of dentistry at the next appointment
without fail.*

_____   _____   _____
Date   *Faculty Signature*   *Signature of Patient, Parent or Guardian*

MEDICAL HISTORY / PHYSICAL EVALUATION DATE

Date   Addition   *Student/Faculty Signatures*

_____ _____ _____ _____

_____ _____ _____ _____

_____ _____ _____ _____

Fig. 10-1 University of Southern California School of Dentistry medical history questionnaire.

from which most others are derived: the short- and long-form medical histories. Both provide a knowledgeable practitioner with adequate information from which to determine a patient's physical status. The University of Southern California (U.S.C.) School of Dentistry medical history questionnaire (short form) is shown in Fig. 10-1.

A long-form medical history questionnaire is especially valuable in teaching institutions and in those situations in which a doctor manages many patients with significant medical disorders. In addition, the long form is valuable for the doctor lacking extensive experience in physical evaluation. The in-depth questions found on this form elicit more information from a patient than those on most short-form histories. The short form is more frequently used by doctors experienced in physical evaluation.

The following questions in the medical history questionnaire (U.S.C.) should be carefully evaluated for any patient who is to receive a local anesthetic.

Question 1: Are you having pain or discomfort at this time?

COMMENT: The requirement for immediate treatment is gathered from this question. Also, the doctor can determine whether any additional steps (i.e., sedation) may be required to achieve pain control. It is more difficult to achieve adequate analgesia when chronic pain or infection is present.

Question 2: Do you feel very nervous about having dental treatment?

Question 3: Have you ever had a bad experience in the dental office?

COMMENT: These represent critical questions that are often not found on the medical history questionnaire. The patient's psychological attitude toward dentistry should be assessed before the start of treatment. A positive response to either question requires the evaluator to pursue a detailed dialogue history and to consider the possible use of psychosedation during treatment. Many patients will state that they have had bad experiences related to injections or "shots" in the dental office.

Question 4: Have you been a patient in the hospital during the past 2 years?

Question 5: Have you been under the care of a medical doctor during the past 2 years?

COMMENT: These questions seek information regarding any medical problems for which the patient required medical intervention and that might be of significance to the planned dental therapy. Question 9 provides somewhat more detail in this area.

Question 6: Have you taken any medicine or drugs during the past 2 years?

COMMENT: Although few, interactions with local anesthetics or vasopressors can occur when certain drugs are taken by patients for medical disorders. These include potential drug-drug interactions between the following:

Cimetidine and lidocaine
Sulfonamides and esters
Nonselective beta blockers and vasopressors
Tricyclic antidepressants (TCAs) and vasopressors
Phenothiazines and vasopressors
Cocaine and vasodepressors

These potential interactions are discussed later in this chapter.

Question 7: Are you allergic to (i.e., experience itching, rash, or swelling of hands, feet, or eyes) or made sick by penicillin, aspirin, codeine, or any medications?

COMMENT: Determine the name of the drug involved and the nature of the adverse reaction that developed. Evaluation of alleged allergy to local anesthetics ("Novocain") is described in depth in Chapter 18. The incidence of true, documented, and reproducible allergy to the amide local anesthetics is virtually nil.[3] However, reports of alleged allergy to local anesthetics are reported frequently.[4] Thorough investigation of such alleged allergy is essential if the patient is not to be condemned to a labeling of "allergic to all caine drugs," thereby precluding dental (and surgical) care in a normal manner. Avoidance of dental care or dental care under general anesthesia are the alternatives in these cases.

Reports of allergy to "epinephrine" should also be evaluated carefully. Most often such reports prove to be simply an exaggerated physiologic response by the patient to either the injected epinephrine or to the endogenous catecholamines released in response to the act of administering the local anesthetic.

Question 8: Have you ever had excessive bleeding that required special treatment?

COMMENT: Prior to inserting a needle into the well-vascularized soft tissues of the oral cavity, it should be determined if the patient is at risk for excessive bleeding. In the presence of coagulopathies or other bleeding disorders, injection techniques with a greater incidence of positive aspiration should be avoided in favor of supraperiosteal, periodontal ligament (PDL), or other techniques less likely to produce bleeding. Techniques that might be avoided when bleeding disorders are present include the maxillary nerve block (high tuberosity approach), posterior superior alveolar nerve block, inferior alveolar nerve block, mental/incisive nerve block, and probably both the Gow-Gates and the Vazirani-Akinosi mandibular nerve blocks. Although both the Gow-Gates and Vazirani-Akinosi nerve blocks have relatively low positive aspiration rates, bleeding occurring following their administration is likely to be deep in the tissues and might therefore be more difficult to manage. Modifications in therapy should be listed on the patient's chart (Fig. 10-2).

Question 9: Have you ever had any of the following conditions or treatments:
Heart failure

COMMENT: The degree of heart failure must be assessed. Ambulatory patients with congestive heart failure (CHF) may be considered as either ASA II, III, or IV risks. CHF patients who demonstrate disability (undue fatigue, shortness of breath) at rest (ASA IV) or who are unable to complete normal functions without disability (ASA III) will probably demonstrate some degree of decreased liver perfusion, leading to an increase in the half-life of amide local anesthetics.[5] Additionally, in more significant heart failure a greater percentage of cardiac stroke volume is delivered to the cerebral circulation (15% normal, up to 30% in more severe heart failure), increasing the risk of an overdose reaction to the local anesthetic. Additionally, ASA III and IV heart failure patients are less tolerant of stress, having a decreased functional reserve. Anxiety must be dealt with, not ignored. Psychosedation is appropriate (inhalation seda-

MODIFICATIONS TO THERAPY:
      – General –   Specific

_____   _____
_____   _____
_____   _____
DENTISTRY DIAGNOSTIC SUMMARY: _____

_____
_____
TREATMENT PLAN SEQUENCE

_____
_____
_____

Fig. 10-2 Possible treatment modifications are listed on the patient's chart.

TABLE 10-1 Adult Blood Pressure Guidelines

Blood pressure (mm Hg) systolic		diastolic	ASA classification	Dental treatment considerations
<140	and	<90	I	Routine dental management Recheck in 6 months
140 to159	and/or	90 to 94	II	Recheck blood pressure prior to dental treatment for three consecutive appointments; if all exceed these guidelines, seek medical consultation
160 to 179	and/or	95 to 104	IIIa	Recheck blood pressure in 5 minutes Routine dental therapy Consider stress reduction protocol
180 to 199	and/or	105 to 114	IIIb	Recheck blood pressure in 5 minutes If still elevated, seek medical consultation prior to dental treatment If all other medical history factors are within normal limits (WNL), routine dental therapy Seriously consider stress reduction protocol
>200	and/or	>115	IV	Recheck blood pressure in 5 minutes Immediate medical consultation if still elevated No dental care, elective or emergent, until blood pressure is decreased (Noninvasive) Emergency care with drugs: analgesics, antibiotics Refer to hospital for invasive dental care

tion preferred). Placement of the patient into the "ideal" position for administering local anesthetics and dental treatment may not prove possible because of the presence of orthopnea. Compromise in patient positioning may be necessary.

Heart disease or heart attack

COMMENT: Recent (< 6 months) or repeated myocardial infarction increases risk to patients during dental care or the administration of local anesthetics. Patients ought not receive elective dental care within 6 months of a myocardial infarction (ASA IV) as reinfarction rates are considerably increased during this time.[6,7] After this period of recuperation, most status post–myocardial infarction patients are treatable (ASA III) with appropriate therapy modification. Administering local anesthetics containing vasopressors in cardiac risk patients is a never-ending question and is discussed fully in Chapter 20. Suffice it to say here that all ASA I and some ASA II and III patients may safely receive the concentrations of vasoconstrictor contained in local anesthetic cartridges. For the more severely cardiovascular compromised ASA III patient, the dose of vasoconstrictor should be limited. The ASA IV cardiovascular risk patient is not a candidate for vasopressors or elective dental care.

Angina pectoris

COMMENT: Angina pectoris is defined as a transient chest pain produced by myocardial ischemia, relieved by rest or the administration of a vasodilator. Stable angina pectoris (angina of exertion) represents an ASA III risk. Any factor, such as anxiety or inadequate pain control, that increases myocardial oxygen requirements may provoke an anginal episode. The judicious use of vasopressors in local anesthetics is not contraindicated in stable angina. Unstable angina (preinfarction angina) represents an ASA IV risk.[8]

High blood pressure

COMMENT: Patients with mild to moderate elevations in systolic or diastolic pressure (Table 10-1) are acceptable risks for dental care, including use of local anesthetics with vasopressors. Hypertensive patients should have their blood pressure monitored at each appointment and be managed according to the most recent reading. It must be remembered that patient noncompliance with antihypertensive drug regimens is epidemic. Patients should be reminded to take these potentially lifesaving medications as prescribed by their physician.

Heart murmur, rheumatic fever, congenital heart lesions, or scarlet fever

COMMENT: Patients with clinical manifestations of heart disease (i.e., valvular defects or murmurs) must undergo a more in-depth evaluation (dialogue history and physical evaluation) to determine whether any degree of disability or stress intolerance exists and whether antibiotic prophylaxis is required prior to dental care, including local anesthetic administration. Patients with mitral valve prolapse are included in this evaluation. Current regimens of the American Heart Association are presented in Table 10-2.[9]

The administration of local anesthetics does not, in and of itself, require antibiotic prophylaxis. The one exception to this is the PDL injection.[10] However, as it is highly unlikely that a local anesthetic would be administered without dental treatment being carried out subsequently, the nature of the dental treatment would dictate whether antibiotic prophylaxis is required.

Artificial heart valve

COMMENT: The presence of a prosthetic heart valve indicates the need for antibiotic prophylaxis prior to any dental care. Specific regimens may be individualized and consultation with the patient's primary care physician is required prior to initiating any form of dental care.

Heart pacemaker

COMMENT: Rhythm disturbances of the heart may necessitate the insertion of a pacemaker. Most current pacemakers are of the demand type (functioning only when needed), and patients usually do not require antibiotic prophylaxis. Although use of certain dental equipment increases the risk of pacemaker failure (i.e., certain ultrasonic scalers and electronic dental anesthesia), local anesthetics with vasoconstrictors may be administered safely.

Heart operation

COMMENT: Determine the nature of the surgical procedure (i.e., valve replacement, insertion of a pacemaker, or coronary artery bypass), the degree of any disability, and whether there is a need for antibiotic prophylaxis. In most cases these patients, with proper treatment modification, may safely receive dental care, including local anesthetics with vasoconstrictors, with little or no increase in risk. Physician consultation may be required.

Anemia

COMMENT: The presence of methemoglobinemia, either congenital or idiopathic, represents a *relative contraindication* to the administration of two amide local anesthetics: articaine and prilocaine.[11] Methemoglobinemia is discussed in depth on p.129.

Other forms of anemia, iron deficiency and sickle cell, do not impact the administration of local anesthetics with or without vasopressors.

Stroke

COMMENT: Patients with a history of cerebrovascular accident (CVA) or transient ischemic attack require therapy modification to decrease risk. Blood pressure should be monitored routinely and treatment modified accordingly.

T A B L E   1 0 - 2   Summary of Recommended Antibiotic Regimens for Dental and Respiratory Tract Procedures

Standard Regimen

For dental procedures that cause gingival bleeding and for oral–respiratory tract surgery	Penicillin V 2.0 g orally 1 hr before, and then 1.0 g 6 hr later
	For patients unable to take oral medications 2 million units of aqueous penicillin G intravenously or intramuscularly 30 to 60 min before procedure and 1 million units 6 hr later may be substituted

Special Regimens

Parenteral, for use when maximum protection desired, as for patients with prosthetic valves	Ampicillin 1.0 to 2.0 g intramuscularly or intravenously, plus gentamicin 1.5 mg/kg intramuscularly or intravenously 1/2 hr before procedure followed by 1.0 g oral penicillin V 6 hr later. Alternatively, parenteral regimen may be repeated once 8 hr later
Oral, for penicillin-allergic patients	Erythromycin 1.0 g orally 1 hr before, and then 500 mg 6 hr later
Parenteral, for penicillin-allergic patients	Vancomycin 1.0 g intravenously slowly over 1 hr, starting 1 hr before procedure; no repeat dose necessary

From Committee on Rheumatic Fever, Endocarditis and Kawazaki Disease of the Council on Cardiovascular Disease in the Young of the American Heart Association: Prevention of bacterial endocarditis: recommendations of the American Heart Association, *JAMA* 264:2219, 1990.
Note: Pediatric doses are as follows: ampicillin 50 mg/kg/dose; erythromycin 20 mg/kg for first dose, then 10 mg/kg; gentamicin 2 mg/kg/dose; penicillin V full adult dose if greater than 60 lb (27 kg), one-half adult dose if less than 60 lb (27 kg); aqueous penicillin G 50,000 units/kg (25,000 units/kg for follow-up); vancomycin 20 mg/kg/dose. The intervals between doses are the same as for adults. Total doses should not exceed the adult doses.

Use of minimal effective doses of local anesthetics with vasoconstrictors is indicated. Intravascular administration of vasopressors should be scrupulously avoided in these patients. Most status post-CVA patients are considered ASA II or III risks 6 months or more after the acute incident.

Kidney trouble

COMMENT: A small percentage of local anesthetic is excreted unmetabolized in the urine. Patients who are functionally anephric (kidney failure) could theoretically attain high levels of local anesthetic in their blood, thereby increasing their risk of local anesthetic overdose. In actual clinical situations, usual doses of local anesthetics do not pose any increased risk in these patients.

Hay fever, sinus trouble, or allergies or hives

COMMENT: A positive response to any of these items, which might indicate the presence of allergy, requires that a more complete dialogue history be performed to elucidate the precise nature of the problem (which is described further in Chapter 18).

Thyroid disease

COMMENT: Patients who are clinically hyperthyroid (i.e., sensitive to heat, sweat easily, and have experienced tachycardia, palpitation, loss of weight, increased body temperature, tremor of extremities, and increased nervousness) are more sensitive to catecholamines and may demonstrate an exaggerated response to vasopressors included in local anesthetic solutions. Although unlikely to be significant, such reactions can be prevented or minimized by the use of minimum concentrations of epinephrine and other vasopressors. Patients with surgically corrected or medication-controlled hyperthyroid or hypothyroid conditions are termed *euthyroid* and respond in a normal manner to catecholamines.

Pain in jaw joints

COMMENT: The patient may be unable to open his or her mouth adequately, thus rendering certain injection techniques useless (e.g., the Gow-Gates and inferior alveolar nerve blocks). If dental care must be completed, alternate techniques should be considered (e.g., the Akinosi closed-mouth mandibular block).

Acquired immunodeficiency syndrome (AIDS), hepatitis A (infectious), hepatitis B (serum), liver disease, jaundice, drug addiction, hemophilia

COMMENT: The unifying bonds among these conditions are an increased risk of infection (AIDS, hepatitis A and B) via blood or saliva and an increased risk of liver dysfunction (hepatitis A and B, liver disease, jaundice, drug addiction, hemophilia). Thorough evaluation of the disorder is strongly needed so the degree of risk to the administrator and to the patient can be ascertained prior to starting dental care. With significant (ASA IV) liver dysfunction (only rarely encountered in ambulatory patients), the half-life of amide local anesthetics may be significantly prolonged, thereby increasing the risk of overdose.

Epilepsy or seizures

COMMENT: Stress may provoke a seizure in even well-controlled epileptics. Appropriate stress reduction procedures should be used to minimize the risk of seizures developing during treatment. Hypoglycemia and hyperventilation are two other causes of seizures in the dental environment. Severe local anesthetic overdose reactions manifest themselves clinically as generalized tonic-clonic convulsions. Local anesthetics, however, are not contraindicated in seizure-prone patients. (Indeed, carefully administered intravenous local anesthetics may be used as anticonvulsants in a patient during grand mal seizures.)

Fainting, dizzy spells, and nervousness

COMMENT: These may indicate the presence of abnormal anxiety, fear, seizures, or possible orthostatic (postural) hypotension. The nature of the problem should be determined prior to starting dental care. Psychosedation and/or other therapy modifications may be required when a psychogenic component is present.

Psychiatric treatment

COMMENT: Patients under psychiatric care can usually receive a local anesthetic with no increased risk. Patients may be taking psychotropic drugs that alter their behavior patterns. Two types of drugs are frequently prescribed: TCAs and MAOIs. These pose a minimal risk to the administration of vasopressor-containing local anesthetics, provided the catecholamine dose is kept minimal (as was also noted for cardiovascular risk patients). See the discussion later in this chapter.

In the recent past MAOIs and TCAs were considered to be relative contraindications to the administration of vasopressors. Recent information has demonstrated that this is *not* the case.[12,13]

Bruise easily

COMMENT: Any potential bleeding disorder must be evaluated prior to administering a local anesthetic, especially with a technique in which the risk of blood vessel penetration is increased, such as with the inferior alveolar nerve block, posterior superior alveolar nerve block, and mental/incisive nerve block.

Questions 10 through 16 provide the patient an opportunity to volunteer the presence of clinical signs and symptoms of diseases or syndromes that may not as yet have been diagnosed by a physician (Fig. 10-1). Questions 10 through 14 pertain to clinical symptoms of various cardiovascular disorders (as well as disorders of other systems). The reader should consult *Medical Emergencies in the Dental Office*[14] for an in-depth discussion of the significance of each of these questions.

Question 17: Do you have any disease, condition, or problem not listed?

COMMENT: This question allows the patient to mention any disease process not noted in Question 9. Two disorders are worthy of additional discussion: *malignant hyperthermia* (MH; hyperpyrexia) and *atypical plasma cholinesterase.* MH poses a *relative contraindication* to dental care. Previously MH was considered to represent an absolute contraindication to the administration of amide local anesthetics.[15] At present it is thought that MH does *not* represent a contraindication to the administration of any local anesthetic.[16] I consider MH a relative contraindication since a medical consultation should be obtained prior to starting any dental care on MH patients. Atypical plasma cholinesterase also represents a *relative contraindication,* but only to the administration of ester local anesthetics. *Idiopathic* or *congenital methemoglobinemia* might also be mentioned here, although its presence will most likely be elicited in response to Question 9. These three entities are evaluated more fully later in this chapter.

> **Question 18: Women: Are you pregnant now? Are you practicing birth control? Do you anticipate becoming pregnant?**

COMMENT: Pregnancy represents a *relative contraindication* to elective dental care, especially during the first trimester (thus the need for the latter two questions). Consultation with the patient's physician prior to starting treatment is indicated, especially if there are any problems with this or prior pregnancies. Local anesthetics and vasopressors are not teratogens and may be safely administered to pregnant patients during any trimester. It is prudent, however, to be conservative in administering any drugs to pregnant women.

Patients are asked to read the statement following Question 18 and to sign (in ink) the questionnaire, attesting that the answers provided are, to the best of their knowledge, true and correct. The doctor or hygienist reviewing the questionnaire should countersign the form.

• • •

The medical history questionnaire should be updated on a regular basis (i.e., every 6 months or whenever a patient has been away from the office for an extended period of time) and any changes or additions noted on the form (bottom of Fig. 10-1) or in the patient's dental record. The patient should be asked two questions:"Has there been any change in your health since your last visit?" and, "Are you now taking any drugs or medications?" The answers should be noted in the record (e.g., medical history update, no change).

DIALOGUE HISTORY

After the patient completes the medical history questionnaire, the doctor must review it for any medical disorders of possible significance. If disorders are present, the doctor next discusses these with the patient to obtain as much information as possible concerning the severity of the problem and its potential impact on the planned dental care. This questioning of the patient is called the *dialogue history,* and it forms an essential part of the physical evaluation process. The doctor must use all available knowledge of the disease entity to assess accurately the degree of risk represented by the patient. Dialogue history related to the administration of local anesthetic in patients with alleged allergy is presented in Chapter 18.

PHYSICAL EXAMINATION

The doctor should next conduct a physical examination of the patient. Although the scope of such an examination is not limited and can include heart and lung auscultation and laboratory and function tests, the following is recommended as a minimum physical examination for dental patients. It includes visual inspection and the recording of vital signs.

Visual Inspection

Visual examination can provide the doctor with valuable information concerning the patient's medical status. Observation of a patient's posture, body movements, speech patterns, and skin can assist in a diagnosis of possibly significant disorders that may have previously gone undetected. The interested reader is referred to textbooks that deal with physical examination in greater depth.[14,17]

Vital Signs

There are six vital signs: blood pressure, heart rate and rhythm (pulse), respiratory rate, temperature, height, and weight. Vital signs should be recorded on the patient's dental chart (Fig. 10-3). For a minimum examination, it is recommended that the blood pressure and heart rate and rhythm be monitored for all patients seeking dental care. Table 10-1 presents guidelines for dental management of adult patients according to their blood pressure. Adherence to these guidelines will minimize the development of acute complications of high blood pressure, such as CVA. A patient with a systolic pressure in excess of 200 mm Hg and/or a diastolic in excess of 115 (ASA IV) is at significant risk and ought not receive any invasive elective dental care until the elevation has been brought under control. Administering local anesthetics can only further elevate the blood pressure of an already anxious patient.

The heart rate, or pulse, can be measured at any readily accessible artery. Most frequently used for routine assessment are the brachial or the radial artery. Three factors should be evaluated when monitoring the pulse: the heart *rate* (recorded as beats per minute), the heart *rhythm* (regular or irregular), and the *quality* of the pulse (thready, bounding, or weak). The normal resting adult heart rate ranges from 60 to 110 beats/min. It is suggested that any adult patient with a heart rate below 60 or above 110 undergo further evaluation. Anxiety is

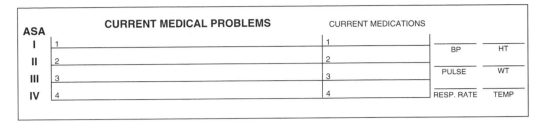

Fig. 10-3 Baseline vital signs are recorded on the patient's chart.

TABLE 10-3 University of Southern California Physical Evaluation System	
ASA physical status classification/definition	**Dental therapy modifications**
I. Normal healthy patient	None (stress reduction protocol [SRP], as indicated)
II. Patient with mild to moderate systemic disease	Possible SRP and other modifications as indicated
IIIab. Patient with a severe systemic disease that limits activity but is not incapacitating	Possible strict modifications; SRP and medical consultations are priorities
IV. Patient with severe systemic disease that limits activity and is a constant threat to life	Elective care contraindicated Noninvasive emergency care in office; hospitalize for invasive emergency care; medical consultation urged
V. Moribund patient not expected to survive 24 hours with or without an operation	Hospitalized; dental care limited to palliative treatment only
VI. Clinically dead (brain dead)	

the most frequent cause of an elevated heart rate in the dental environment. The rhythm of the heart is equally, if not more, important. A normal pulse maintains a relatively regular rhythm. Occasional premature ventricular contractions (PVCs) are not uncommon, produced by smoking, fatigue, stress, various drugs and medications (e.g., epinephrine), and the ingestion of alcohol. A PVC is noted as a "missed beat" when a peripheral pulse is taken. If PVCs occur at a rate of five or more per minute with no obvious cause, medical consultation should be considered. Unusually frequent PVCs in a high-risk cardiovascular patient (ASA III or IV) indicate myocardial irritability (ischemia) and may presage more serious ventricular dysrhythmias (tachycardia and fibrillation).[18] The administration of epinephrine-containing local anesthetics is relatively contraindicated in patients with cardiac dysrhythmias that are unresponsive to medical therapy. Dysrhythmias often indicate an ischemic or irritable myocardium, and epinephrine and other catecholamines are capable of producing further irritability, potentially leading to more serious, possibly lethal, dysrhythmias.

Determination of Medical Risk

Having completed all components of the physical evaluation and a thorough dental examination, the doctor must then gather this information and answer the following questions:

1. Is the patient capable, physiologically and psychologically, of tolerating in relative safety the stresses involved in the proposed treatment?
2. Does the patient represent a greater risk (of morbidity or mortality) than normal during this treatment?
3. If the patient does represent an increased risk, what modifications will be necessary in the planned treatment to minimize this risk?
4. Is the risk too great for the patient to be managed safely as an outpatient in the medical or dental office?

The U.S.C. School of Dentistry developed a physical evaluation system, based on the American Society of Anesthesiologists Physical Status Classification System, that enables the doctor to readily evaluate a patient's risk status prior to starting treatment. This system, presented in Table 10-3, is described in considerable detail in other monographs.[19-21] The steps in the stress reduction protocols (SRPs) for medically compromised ASA categories II, III, and IV are presented in the adjacent column.

Careful consideration of the pretreatment evaluation will enable the doctor to determine accurately a potential patient's ability to withstand the stresses associated with dental care. If there is any doubt concerning a patient's ability to tolerate these stresses, medical consultation should be obtained, leading to possible modifications in the planned dental treatment. Contra-indications, both relative and absolute, to the use of local anesthetic solutions are summarized in Chapter 4.

• • •

Potential drug-drug interactions involving either local anesthetics or vasopressors, and three *relative contraindications* to the administration of local anesthetics—MH, atypical plasma cholinesterase, and idiopathic or congenital methemoglobinemia—are detailed in the following discussion. A fourth—allergy (an *absolute contraindication*)—is discussed in Chapter 18.

DRUG-DRUG INTERACTIONS

Cimetidine and Lidocaine

The H_2-receptor blocker *cimetidine* modifies the biotransformation of lidocaine by competing with it for binding to hepatic oxidative enzymes. Other H_2-receptor blockers, such as ranitidine and famotidine, do not inhibit lidocaine biotransformation.[22,23] The net result of this interaction with cimetidine is for the half-life of the circulating local anesthetic to be increased somewhat. In typical dental practice usage of local anesthetics, this interaction is of little clinical significance. The interaction between amide local anesthetics and cimetidine might be of greater clinical significance in the presence of a history of CHF (ASA III or greater), where the percentage of cardiac output delivered to the liver falls while the percentage of cardiac output delivered to the brain increases.[5] With greater blood levels of lidocaine secondary to cimetidine, and an increased percentage in blood being delivered to the brain, the risk of local anesthetic overdose is increased somewhat. This combination of factors—cimetidine and ASA III + CHF—would represent a *relative contraindication* to the use of amide local anesthetics. Minimal doses of amide anesthetics should be administered.

Sulfonamides and Esters

Ester anesthetics, such as procaine and tetracaine, may inhibit the bacteriostatic action of the sulfonamides. With the uncommon use of sulfonamides today, along with the extremely rare administration of ester local anesthetics in dentistry, this potential drug interaction is unlikely to be noted. As a rule, ester local anesthetics should not be administered to patients receiving sulfonamides.

Nonselective Beta Blockers and Epinephrine

The administration of vasopressors in patients being treated with nonselective beta blockers increases the likelihood of a serious elevation of the blood pressure. This is accompanied by a reflex bradycardia. Several cases have been reported in the medical literature and appear to be dose related.[24,25] Reactions have occurred

TABLE 10-4 Beta Blockers

Nonselective (B_1 and B_2 adrenoreceptors)	Cardioselective (B_1 adrenoreceptors)
Propranolol (Inderal)	Metoprolol
Nadolol (Corgard)	(Lopressor)
Timolol (Blocadren,	Atenolol (Tenormin)
Timoptic, Timoptol)	Acebutolol (Sectral)
Pindolol (Visken)	Betaxolol (Kerlone)
Alprenolol	
Labetalol (Trandate,	
Normodyne)	
Oxprenolol (Trasicor)	
Sotalol (Sotacor)	
Carteolol (Cartrol)	
Penbutolol (Levatol)	

with epinephrine doses ranging from 0.04 to 0.32 mg, the equivalent of the administration of from 4 to 32 ml of local anesthetic with a 1:100,000 epinephrine concentration.[26] Table 10-4 lists both nonselective and cardioselective beta blockers.

Monitoring preoperative vital signs—specifically the blood pressure, heart rate and rhythm—is strongly recommended for all patients, but especially in patients receiving beta blockers. Rerecording these vital signs at 5 to 10 minutes following the administration of a vasopressor-containing local anesthetic is strongly suggested.

Tricyclic Antidepressants and Epinephrine

Tricyclic antidepressants (TCAs) are commonly prescribed in the management of major depression. TCAs may potentially enhance the cardiovascular actions of exogenously administered vasopressors. This enhancement of activity is approximately fivefold to tenfold with levonordefrin and norepinephrine, but is only twofold with epinephrine and phenylephrine.[13] This interaction has been reported to have resulted in a series of hypertensive crises, one of which led to the death of a patient (following a small dose of norepinephrine).[27] *The administration of norepinephrine and levonordefrin should be avoided in patients receiving TCAs.* Patients receiving epinephrine-containing local anesthetics should be administered the smallest effective dose. Yagiela et al recommend limiting the epinephrine dose to patients receiving TCAs in a dental appointment to 0.05 mg or 5.4 ml of a 1:100,000 epinephrine concentration.[28] Commonly prescribed TCAs are listed in Table 10-5.

Monoamine Oxidase Inhibitors and Epinephrine

Monoamine oxidase inhibitors (MAOIs) are prescribed in the management of major depression, certain phobic-

TABLE 10-5 Antidepressant Medications

Tricyclic antidepressants	Monoamine inhibitors
Amitriptyline (Elavil)	Isocarboxazid (Marplan)
Desipramine (Norpramin)	Pargyline (Eutonyl)
Imipramine (Tofranil)	Phenelzine (Nardil)
Nortriptyline (Aventyl)	Tranylcypromine
Protriptyline (Vivactil)	(Parnate)

anxiety states and obsessive-compulsive disorders.[12] They are capable of potentiating the actions of vasopressors used in dental local anesthetics by inhibiting their biodegradation by the enzyme monoamine oxidase (MAO) at the presynaptic neuron level.[29]

Historically the administration of local anesthetics containing vasopressors has been absolutely contraindicated for patients receiving MAOIs because of the increased risk of hypertensive crisis. However, Yagiela et al demonstrated that such an interaction between epinephrine, levonordefrin, norepinephrine, and MAO did not occur.[12,28] Such a response, hypertensive crisis, did develop with phenylephrine—a vasopressor not used at present in dental local anesthetic solutions.

It therefore seems appropriate for it to be stated "that there seems to be no restriction, from a theoretical basis, to use local anesthetic with vasoconstrictor other than phenylephrine in patients currently treated with MAOIs."[12]

Phenothiazines and Epinephrine

Phenothiazines are psychotropic drugs usually prescribed for the management of serious psychotic disorders. The most commonly observed side effect of phenothiazines involving the cardiovascular system is *postural hypotension*. The phenothiazines suppress the vasoconstricting actions of epinephrine, permitting its milder vasodilating actions to work unopposed. This response is not likely to develop when local anesthetics are administered extravascularly; however, the accidental intravascular administration of a vasopressor-containing local anesthetic could lead to hypotension in patients receiving phenothiazines.[12]

Local anesthetics containing vasopressors are not contraindicated in patients receiving phenothiazines; however, it is recommended that *the smallest volume of vasopressor-containing local anesthetic that is compatible with clinically adequate pain control be administered.*

Cocaine and Epinephrine/Local Anesthetics

Cocaine is a local anesthetic drug that also possesses significant stimulatory properties on the CNS and CVS. Cocaine stimulates norepinephrine release and inhibits its reuptake in adrenergic nerve terminals, thus producing a state of catecholamine hypersensitivity.[30,31] Tachycardia and hypertension are frequently observed with cocaine administration, both of which increase cardiac output and myocardial oxygen requirements.[32] When this results in myocardial ischemia, potentially lethal dysrhythmias, anginal pain, myocardial infarction, or cardiac arrest may ensue.[33-35] The risk of such problems is elevated in dentistry when a local anesthetic containing a vasopressor is accidentally administered intravascularly in a patient with already high cocaine blood levels. Following intranasal application of cocaine, peak blood levels develop within 30 minutes and usually disappear after 4 to 6 hours.[36] *Whenever possible, local anesthetics containing vasopressors should not be administered to patients who have used cocaine on the day of their dental appointment.*[37] Unfortunately it is the rare abuser of cocaine who will volunteer this vital information to the dentist. The use of epinephrine-impregnated gingival retraction cord, though not recommended for use in any dental patient, is absolutely contraindicated for use in the cocaine abuser.

The administration of local anesthetics to cocaine abusers can also increase the risk of a local anesthetic overdose reaction. If there is any suspicion about a patient having used cocaine recently, the patient should be questioned directly. *If cocaine has been used within 24 hours of the dental appointment, or it is suspected that cocaine has been used within 24 hours, the planned dental treatment should be postponed.*[12,37]

• • •

Most known drug-drug interactions involving local anesthetics or vasopressors occur with CNS depressants and CVS depressants. Whenever a potential drug-drug interaction exists, doses of local anesthetics should be decreased. There is no formula for the degree of this reduction. Prudence dictates, however, that the smallest dose of local anesthetic or vasopressor that is clinically effective be used.

Knowledge of all drugs and medications being taken by a patient better enables the doctor to evaluate the patient's overall physical and psychological well-being. Current medications should be listed in the dental record (Fig. 10-3).

MALIGNANT HYPERTHERMIA

Malignant hyperthermia (MH; malignant hyperpyrexia) is one of the most intense and life-threatening complications associated with the administration of general anesthesia. It occurs rarely—a 1:15,000 incidence among children receiving general anesthesia and a 1:50,000 incidence among adults.[38] The syndrome is transmitted genetically by an autosomally dominant gene. Reduced penetrance and variable expressivity in siblings of families inheriting the syndrome are also characteristic of its genetic transmission. MH is seen more frequently in males than females, a finding that increases with ascending age. To date, the youngest reported case of MH was in a boy aged 2 months and the oldest in a 78-year-old man.

The reports of MH in North America appear to be clustered in three regions: Toronto (in Canada) and Wisconsin and Nebraska (in the United States). Most persons with MH are functionally normal, the presence of MH becoming known only when the individual is exposed to triggering agents or through specific testing.

For many years it was thought that MH could be triggered when susceptible patients were exposed to amide local anesthetics.[39] Indeed, in both the first and second editions of this textbook MH was considered an absolute contraindication to amide local anesthetics. Recent findings[40-42] and publications by the Malignant Hyperthermia Association of the United States (MHAUS),[43] however, have demonstrated that amide anesthetics are not likely to trigger such episodes; thus the recategorization of MH as a *relative contraindication* in the third and later editions.

Mechanism

Current thinking has it that the mechanism underlying MH is a defect in the distribution of myoplasmic calcium (Ca^{++}). The primary event in the acute episode is a rise in Ca^{++} concentration in the myoplasm, which serves to explain the observed muscular rigidity, metabolic acidosis, and elevated body temperature.

Elevation of Ca^{++} levels occurs in normal muscles as well as in MH-susceptible (MHS) muscles. Increased Ca^{++} concentration acts on the contractile proteins troponin and tropomyosin. Tropomyosin molecules are repositioned as a result of Ca^{++} binding to troponin so the myosin heads can contact the actin molecules. Muscle fibrils shorten and the muscle contracts. When the myoplasmic Ca^{++} level decreases to its initial concentration, muscle relaxation occurs. The strength of muscle contraction is a function of the concentration of free Ca^{++} in the cytoplasm. Kalow et al[44] first demonstrated the increased contractility of MHS muscle using exposure to caffeine. Subsequent studies have shown spontaneous contractures of MHS muscle with exposure to halothane and succinylcholine.[45,46] Halothane increases myoplasmic Ca^{++} concentration by a direct action on the cell membrane. Succinylcholine increases Ca^{++} levels through muscle fasciculation.

Why do Ca^{++} concentrations remain elevated in MHS patients? The reason might be a continuous release of Ca^{++} or a defect in the mechanism of Ca^{++} reuptake. Nelson and Denborough[47] demonstrated that halothane produces a continuous release of Ca^{++} into the myoplasm of MHS muscle. Cheah and Cheah[48] reported a Ca^{++} efflux

rate from mitochondria of MH-sensitive pigs in anaerobic circumstances twice that of stress-resistant animals—a rate that is further enhanced with exposure to halothane.

Lactic acidosis occurring in MH results from the activation of phosphorylase by Ca^{++} so that glycogen is broken down into lactic acid. Phosphorylase activation helps to supply the fructose-1,6-diphosphate for adenosine triphosphate (ATP) production by glycolysis. Heat is generated during the continuous synthesis and utilization of ATP during glycolysis in both muscle and the liver (increased metabolism), a possible explanation for the elevated temperature seen in MH patients.

Clinical Signs and Symptoms

The MH syndrome is characterized by tachycardia, fever (increased body core temperature), tachypnea, cardiac dysrhythmias, muscle rigidity, cyanosis, and death—which occur when the patient is exposed to a triggering agent, usually a drug used to induce or maintain general anesthesia. Most episodes of MH have occurred on the patient's first exposure to general anesthesia; however, some have developed following a prior uneventful exposure to these same drugs.

The initial clinical sign of MH is frequently an unexplained tachycardia, produced by the hypermetabolic state that is starting to manifest itself. Tachypnea and cyanosis also develop in response to the increased production of carbon dioxide and the body's increased demand for oxygen. Muscle rigidity frequently develops, particularly in the masseter, and may occur following the administration of a muscle relaxant such as succinylcholine.

Increased body temperature does not occur immediately in all cases of MH. Pyrexia usually follows muscle rigidity and is a result—not a cause—of the reaction. Increases in body temperature may occur gradually over many hours or may rise abruptly within 10 to 15 minutes. Core temperatures of greater than 110° F (43° C) have been monitored. The mortality associated with MH was 80% but has been reduced to 10% since 1985 through the combination of increased awareness and early recognition and treatment.[49] A syndrome with a mortality of even 10% despite vigorous treatment remains one that all health professionals should respect and seek to prevent.

Etiology

All reported cases of MH (associated with drug administration) have developed during the administration of general anesthesia. There appears to be no association with the type of surgical procedure being performed. Several cases of MH have been reported among anesthetized patients receiving dental care, including one case in a dental office.[50,51]

Anesthetic agents that have been associated with cases of MH are as follows (several of these drugs [e.g., lidocaine, mepivacaine] have been associated with MH only anecdotally):

Succinylcholine (77% of all cases)
Halothane (60% of all cases)
Nitrous oxide with meperidine
Lidocaine
Mepivacaine
Methoxyflurane
Ether
Ethyl chloride
Trichloroethylene
Cyclopropane
Ethylene
Gallamine
d-Tubocurarine
Isoflurane
Enflurane

Two drugs have been associated with a preponderance of MH cases: succinylcholine, a skeletal muscle relaxant (77% of all cases), and halothane (60%).[52] Of significance to dentistry is the fact that the two most commonly used (amide) local anesthetics, lidocaine and mepivacaine, had been administered along with other agents in cases in which MH developed. Initially it was considered that a history of documented MH or a high risk of MH should be considered an absolute contraindication to the administration of all amide local anesthetics. However, *recent findings indicate that MH is not a likely occurrence with amide local anesthetics as used in dentistry and as such should only be considered a relative contraindication.* The MHAUS published a policy statement on the use of local anesthetics[43]: "Based on limited clinical and laboratory evidence, all local anesthetic drugs appear to be safe for MH susceptible individuals." This statement followed several reports in the literature, including one by Adragna,[53] which stated that: "After an extensive search of the literature, I have been unable to find any reports of any malignant hyperthermic crisis caused solely by the use of amide local anesthetics without epinephrine. . . . In fact, lidocaine has been used successfully to treat the arrhythmias of a severe MH reaction and, in fact, lidocaine has been used routinely as a local anesthetic without problems on MHS patients in at least one institution . . . The question I am posing is clear. Is there any evidence that amide local anesthetics are contraindicated in MHS patients, or is our habit of avoiding them just a habit?" Since the MH syndrome has yet to be reported in a situation in which local anesthetic alone was administered, it is reasonable for the dentist to manage the dental needs of such patients using either amide or ester local anesthetics. I strongly suggest consulting the patient's physician prior to starting any treatment.

Adriani and Sundin reported that in susceptible patients MH may be precipitated by factors other than the drugs just listed.[54] These would include emotional factors (excitement, stress) and physical factors (mild infection, muscle injury, vigorous exercise, elevated environmental temperatures). It appears, then, that the dental office could be a site where the susceptible patient, exposed to excessive stresses such as pain and fear, might exhibit symptoms of MH.

Recognition of the High-risk Malignant Hyperthermia Patient

There are no questions on medical history questionnaires currently being used in dental practice that specifically address MH. The only one on the U.S.C. health history questionnaire that might elicit this information is Question 17: *Do you have any disease, condition, or problem not listed?* The patient with MH or a family member at risk will have to volunteer this information to the doctor at an early visit.

Following the occurrence of MH, family members are usually evaluated for their risk. Initial evaluation involves determination of the blood levels of creatinine phosphokinase (CPK).[55] Elevated CPK levels are seen when muscle damage has occurred. With an elevated CPK, a second phase of evaluation is required, involving the histological examination of a biopsy specimen taken from the quadriceps muscle (with the patient under a type of anesthesia known to be safe) and testing of the specimen for an increased contracture response to halothane and caffeine.

Dental Management of the Malignant Hyperthermia Patient

On disclosure of the presence of MH, or when there is a high risk of its occurrence, it is recommended that the dentist contact the patient's primary care physician to discuss treatment options.

Dental management on an outpatient basis is possible in most cases, but with higher-risk patients it might be prudent to conduct such treatment within the confines of a hospital, where immediate emergency care is available should the syndrome be triggered. "Normal" doses of amide local anesthetics may be used with little increase in risk.[43] Ester anesthetics may also be used for nerve block or infiltration anesthesia. Esters include chloroprocaine and procaine/propoxycaine. Vasoconstrictors may be included with either the esters or the amides to provide longer periods of pain control or hemostasis.

General anesthesia may be used when it is absolutely necessary, although with great care and preparation. Agents that may be administered safely to MHS patients include the following:

1. Amide and ester local anesthetics
2. Diazepam, midazolam

3. Droperidol
4. Barbiturates (e.g., thiopental)
5. Propofol
6. Pancuronium (for muscle paralysis)

The ultra–short-acting barbiturates methohexital, thiopental, and thiamylal, as well as narcotics, may be administered along with nondepolarizing muscle relaxants such as pancuronium. Nitrous oxide with oxygen is frequently included in lists of "safe" drugs; however, Ellis et al reported a case of MH induced by nitrous oxide.[56] Because of these conflicting reports, I have elected to omit nitrous oxide–oxygen from this list. Unfortunately, even with this list of "safe" drugs, risk is still present, because triggering agents may have been administered to the patient uneventfully on prior occasions but may now produce the syndrome. The potential risk of drug administration must always be carefully weighed against the benefit.

The development and use of dantrolene sodium (Dantrium), a long-acting hydantoin-type muscle relaxant (it is the only direct-acting skeletal muscle relaxant), has greatly benefited both the prevention and the treatment of MH. Dantrolene effectively blocks the release of Ca^{++} from the sarcoplasmic reticulum. It became available in oral form in 1972 and as an injectable in 1978 and has been used extensively in the treatment of MH. Its use prophylactically decreases the potential risk from MH. Dantrolene is started 24 hours prior to the proposed exposure to anesthesia and given in a dosage of 4 to 7 mg/kg/day in divided doses.[57,58]

Management of Acute Episodes

MHAUS guidelines (modified for this edition) for emergency treatment of patients with MH follow:

1. Discontinue all inhalation anesthetics and hyperventilate with 100% oxygen.
2. In the absence of blood gas analysis to treat acidosis, administer sodium bicarbonate (1 to 2 mEq/kg).
3. Mix dantrolene with distilled water and administer 1 mg/kg intravenously (a vial contains 20 mg as a lyophilized preparation).
4. Simultaneously begin cooling via all available routes:
   a. Skin
   b. Nasogastric lavage
   c. Cold intravenous solutions
   d. Wound
   e. Rectally
5. Change both the anesthetic tubing and, if possible, the soda-lime canister.
6. Dysrhythmias usually respond to management of acidosis and hyperkalemia. Administer procainamide intravenously if dysrhythmias persist or are life threatening.

Note: Procainamide is recommended for dysrhythmias because it prevents halothane-potentiated caffeine contractures in skeletal muscle; by contrast, lidocaine potentiates halothane contractures.

7. Administer additional dantrolene as necessary. Response to intravenous dantrolene occurs within minutes, indicated by muscle relaxation. Tachycardia and elevated blood pressure may decrease over several hours. Additional doses of dantrolene (2 mg/kg) may be administered until a total of 10 mg/kg has been reached.
8. Determine and closely monitor urine output, clotting, and serum potassium, calcium, and arterial blood gas levels.
9. Closely observe the patient in an intensive care unit setting for at least 24 hours, since a recurrence may develop.
10. Monitor CPK, calcium, and potassium concentrations until such time as they return to baseline levels.
11. Initiate electrocardiographic monitoring and continue it during the postoperative period.
12. Monitor body temperature closely, since hypothermia may result from overvigorous treatment of MH. Core temperatures of 106° F (41° to 42° C) are compatible with survival and normal brain function if recognized and treated promptly.
13. Ensure adequate output of urine (>2 ml/kg/hr).
14. Convert from intravenous to oral dantrolene when the condition permits. It is currently recommended that 4 mg/kg/day in divided doses be given orally for 48 hours after operation.

Summary

As these guidelines for treatment indicate, MH is a life-threatening event. Drugs, equipment, techniques, and facilities are required for its management that are available only in a well-equipped medical center. Prevention is therefore the key to successful dental management of the MHS patient. Immediate medical consultation with the patient's primary care physician, the anesthesiology department of a local medical center, or MHAUS is important. When the patient is well prepared and well monitored, prophylaxis with dantrolene sodium and the use of "safe" drugs can lead to a successful dental experience.

ATYPICAL PLASMA CHOLINESTERASE

Choline-ester substrates, such as the depolarizing muscle relaxant succinylcholine and the ester local anesthetics, are hydrolyzed in the blood by the enzyme plasma cholinesterase, which is produced in the liver. Hydrolysis of these chemicals is usually quite rapid, their blood levels decreasing rapidly and thereby terminating the agent's action (succinylcholine) or minimizing the risk of overdose (ester local anesthetics).

Approximately 1 out of every 2820 persons possesses an atypical form of plasma cholinesterase, transmitted as an inherited autosomal recessive trait.[59] Although a number of genetic variations of atypical plasma cholinesterase are identifiable, not all produce clinically significant signs and symptoms.

Determination

In most cases the presence of atypical plasma cholinesterase is determined through the patient's response to succinylcholine, a depolarizing skeletal muscle relaxant. Succinylcholine is commonly administered to facilitate intubation of the trachea following the induction of general anesthesia. Apnea is produced for a brief time, with spontaneous ventilation returning as the succinylcholine is hydrolyzed by plasma cholinesterase. When atypical plasma cholinesterase is present, the apneic period is prolonged—from minutes to many hours. Management simply involves the maintenance of controlled ventilation until effective spontaneous respiratory efforts return. After recovery the patient and family members are tested for a serum cholinesterase survey. The dibucaine number is determined from a sample of blood. Normal patients have dibucaine numbers between 66 and 86. Atypical plasma cholinesterase patients exhibiting prolonged response to succinylcholine have dibucaine numbers as low as 20, with other genetic variants exhibiting intermediate values. Patients with low dibucaine numbers are more likely to exhibit prolonged succinylcholine-induced apnea.[60]

Significance in Dentistry

The presence of atypical plasma cholinesterase should alert the doctor to the increased risk of prolonged apnea in patients receiving succinylcholine during general anesthesia. Additionally, and of greater significance in the typical ambulatory dental patient not receiving general anesthesia or succinylcholine, is the increased risk of developing elevated blood levels of ester local anesthetics. Signs and symptoms of local anesthetic overdose are more apt to be noted in these patients, even following "normal" dosages.

Atypical plasma cholinesterase represents a *relative contraindication* to the administration of ester local anesthetics. Whenever possible, amide local anesthetics should be administered. Because they undergo biotransformation in the liver, amide anesthetics do not present the increased risk of overly high blood levels in these patients. Ester anesthetics may be administered, if deemed necessary by the doctor, but their doses should be minimized.

METHEMOGLOBINEMIA

Methemoglobinemia is a condition in which a cyanosis-like state develops in the absence of cardiac or respiratory abnormalities. When the condition is severe, the blood appears chocolate brown, and clinical signs and symptoms, including respiratory depression and syncope, may be noted; death, though unlikely, can result. Methemoglobinemia may occur through inborn errors of metabolism or may be acquired through the administration of drugs or chemicals that are able to increase the formation of methemoglobin. Two injectable local anesthetics, articaine and prilocaine, when administered in large doses, can produce methemoglobinemia in patients with subclinical methemoglobinemia.[61,62] Administration of these two local anesthetics to patients with congenital methemoglobinemia or other clinical syndromes in which the oxygen-carrying capacity of blood is reduced should be avoided because of the increased risk of producing clinically significant methemoglobinemia. The topical anesthetic benzocaine can also induce methemoglobinemia—however, only when administered in very large doses.[63,64]

Etiology

In the hemoglobin molecule, iron is normally present in the reduced or ferrous state (Fe^{++}). Each hemoglobin molecule contains four ferrous atoms, each loosely bound to a molecule of oxygen. In the ferrous state, hemoglobin can carry oxygen that is available to the tissues. Because hemoglobin in the erythrocyte is inherently unstable, it is continuously being oxidized to the ferric form (Fe^{+++}), in which state the oxygen molecule is more firmly attached and cannot be released to the tissues. This form of hemoglobin is called methemoglobin. To permit an adequate oxygen-carrying capacity in the blood, an enzyme system is present that continually reduces the ferric form to the ferrous form. In usual clinical situations approximately 97% to 99% of hemoglobin is found in the more functional ferrous state, and 1% to 3% is found in the ferric state. This enzyme system is known commonly as methemoglobin reductase (erythrocyte nucleotide diaphorase), and it acts to reconvert the iron from the ferric to the ferrous state at a rate of 0.5 g/dl/hr, thus maintaining a level of less than 1% methemoglobin (0.15 g/dl) in the blood at any given time. As blood levels of methemoglobin increase, clinical signs and symptoms of cyanosis and resiratory distress may become noticeable. In most instances they will not be observed until a methemoglobin blood level of 1.5 to 3.0 g/dl (10% to 20% methemoglobin) is reached.[65]

Acquired Methemoglobinemia

Although articaine and prilocaine can produce elevated methemoglobin levels, other chemicals and substances also do this—including acetanilid, aniline derivatives (e.g., crayons, ink, shoe polish, and dermatologicals), benzene derivatives, cyanides, methylene blue in large doses, nitrates (antianginals), para-aminosalicylic acid, and the sulfonamides. Sarangi and Kumar reported the case of a fatality that occurred due to a chemically-induced methemoglobinemia from writing ink.[66] Daly et al reported the case of a child born with 16% (2.3 g/dl) methemoglobin that supposedly resulted because the mother, while still pregnant, had stood with wet bare feet on a bath mat colored with aniline dye.[67] In these situations the nitrates in the pen and dye were absorbed and converted to nitrites, which oxidized the ferrous atoms to ferric atoms and thus produced methemoglobinemia.

The production of methemoglobin by articaine and prilocaine is dose related. Toluene is present in the prilocaine molecule, which as the drug is biotransformed becomes o-toluidine, a compound capable of oxidizing ferrous iron to ferric iron and of blocking the methemoglobin reductase pathways. Peak blood levels of methemoglobin develop approximately 3 to 4 hours following drug administration and persist for 12 to 14 hours.

Clinical Signs and Symptoms and Management

The signs and symptoms of methemoglobinemia usually appear 3 to 4 hours after administration of large doses of articaine or prilocaine in healthy patients, or of smaller doses in patients with the congenital disorder. Most dental patients will have left the office, thus provoking a worried telephone call to the doctor. Although the signs and symptoms vary with blood levels of methemoglobin, typically the patient will appear lethargic and in respiratory distress; mucous membranes and nail beds will be cyanotic, and the skin will appear pale gray (ashen). Diagnosis of methemoglobinemia is made on the presentation of cyanosis unresponsive to oxygen administration and a distinctive arterial blood brown color.[64] Administration of 100% oxygen does not lead to significant improvement (ferric atoms cannot surrender oxygen to tissues). Venous blood (gingival puncture) may appear chocolate brown and will not turn more red when exposed to oxygen. Definitive treatment of this situation requires the slow intravenous administration of 1% methylene blue (1.5 mg/kg or 0.7 mg/lb). This dose may be repeated every 4 hours if cyanosis persists or returns. Methylene blue acts as an electron acceptor in the transfer of electrons to methemoglobin, thus hastening the conversion of ferric to ferrous atoms. It is interesting to note that methylene blue administered to excess can itself cause methemoglobinemia.

Another treatment, although not as rapid acting as methylene blue and therefore not as popular, is the intravenous or intramuscular administration of ascorbic acid (100 to 200 mg/day). Ascorbic acid accelerates the metabolic pathways that produce ferrous atoms.

Methemoglobinemia ought not develop in a healthy ambulatory dental patient, provided the doses of local anesthetic remain within recommended limits. The presence of congenital methemoglobinemia remains a *relative contraindication* to the administration of either articaine or prilocaine. Although these agents may be administered if absolutely necessary, their doses must be minimized. Whenever possible, alternate local anesthetics should be used.

The maximum recommended dose of prilocaine is 8.0 mg/kg. Methemoglobinemia is unlikely to develop at doses below this level.

REFERENCES

1. Aldrete JA, Johnson DA: Evaluation of intracutaneous testing for investigation of allergy to local anesthetic agents, *Anesth Analg* 49:173-183, 1970.
2. McCarthy FM: *Essentials of safe dentistry for the medically compromised patient,* Philadelphia, 1989, WB Saunders.
3. Sindel LJ, deShazo RD: Accidents resulting from local anesthetics. True or false allergy? *Clin Rev Allergy* 9(3-4):379-395, 1991.
4. Jackson D, Chen AH, Bennett CR: Identifying true lidocaine allergy, *J Am Dent Assoc* 125(10):1362-1366, 1994.
5. Wu FL, Razzaghi A, Souney PF: Seizure after lidocaine for bronchoscopy: case report and review of the use of lidocaine in airway anesthesia, *Pharmacotherapy* 13(1):72-78, 1993.
6. Tarhan S, Giuliani ER: General anesthesia and myocardial infarction, *Am Heart J* 87:137, 1974.
7. Weinblatt E, Shapiro S, Frank CW, et al: Prognosis of men after first myocardial infarction: mortality and first recurrence in relation to selected parameters, *Am J Public Health* 58:1329, 1968.
8. Gottlieb SO, Flaherty JT: Medical therapy of unstable angina pectoris, *Cardiol Clin* 9(1):89-98, 1991.
9. Committee on Rheumatic Fever, Endocarditis, and Kawasaki Disease of the Council on Cardiovascular Disease in the Young of the American Heart Association: Prevention of bacterial endocarditis: recommendations of the American Heart Association, *JAMA* 264:2219, 1990.
10. Quilici DL: Contraindications in the use of the periodontal ligament injection, *Compendium* 11(2):96, 100, 1990.
11. Bardoczky GI, Wathieu M, Dhollander A: Prilocaine-induced methemoglobinemia evidenced by pulse oximetry, *Acta Anaesthesiol Scand* 34(2):162-164, 1990.
12. Perusse R, Goulet J-P, Turcotte J-Y: Contraindications to vasoconstrictors in dentistry, *Oral Surg* 74:679-697, 1992.
13. Jastak JT, Yagiela JA: Vasoconstrictors and local anesthesia: a review and rational use, *J Am Dent Assoc* 107:623-630, 1983.
14. Malamed SF: *Medical emergencies in the dental office,* ed 4, St Louis, 1994, Mosby–Year Book.
15. Strazis KP, Fox AW: Malignant hyperthermia: a review of published cases, *Anesth Analg* 77(2):297-304, 1993.
16. Monaghan A, Hindle I: Malignant hyperthermia in oral surgery: case report and literature review, *Br J Oral Maxillofac Surg* 32(3):190-193, 1994.
17. Bates B, Bickley LS, Hoekelman RA, editors: *A guide to physical examination and history taking,* ed 6, Philadelphia, 1995, JB Lippincott.
18. Dhurandhar RW, MacMillan RL, Brown KW: Primary ventricular fibrillation complicating myocardial infarction, *Am J Cardiol* 27:347-351, 1971.

19. American Society of Anesthesiologists: New classification of physical status, *Anesthesiology* 24:111, 1963.

20. Wong CA: Preoperative patient preparation, *J Post Anesth Nurs* 5(3):149-156, 1990.

21. Malamed SF: *Sedation: a guide to patient management,* ed 3, St Louis, 1995, Mosby–Year Book.

22. Kishikawa K, Namiki A, Miyashita K, Saitoh K: Effects of famotidine and cimetidine on plasma levels of epidurally administered lignocaine, *Anaesthesia* 45(9):719-721, 1990.

23. Wood M: Pharmacokinetic drug interactions in anaesthetic practice, *Clin Pharmacokinet* 21(4):285-307, 1991.

24. Hansbrough JF, Near A: Propanolol-epinephrine antagonism with hypertension and stroke, *Ann Intern Med* 92:717, 1980 (letter).

25. Kram J, Bourne HR, Melmon KL, Maibach H: Propanolol, *Ann Intern Med* 80:282, 1974 (letter).

26. Foster CA, Aston SJ: Propanolol-epinephrine interaction: a potential disaster, *Reconstr Surg* 72:74-78, 1983.

27. Boakes AJ, Laurence DR, Lovel KW, et al: Adverse reactions to local anesthetic vasoconstrictor preparations: a study of the cardiovascular responses to xylestesin and hostcain with noradrenalin, *Br Dent J* 133:137-140, 1972.

28. Yagiela JA, Duffin SR, Hunt LM: Drug interactions and vasoconstrictors used in local anesthetic solutions, *Oral Surg* 59:565-571, 1985.

29. Gilman AG, Goodman LS, Rall TW, Murad F: *Goodman and Gilman's the pharmacological basis of therapeutics.* ed 7, New York, 1985, Macmillan.

30. Hoffman BB, Lefkowitz RJ, Taylor P: *Neurotransmission: the autonomic and somatic motor nervous systems.* In *Goodman and Gilman's the pharmacological basis of therapeutics,* ed 9, New York, 1996, McGraw-Hill.

31. Hueter DC: Cardiovascular effects of cocaine, *JAMA* 257:979-980, 1987.

32. Gradman AH: Cardiac effects of cocaine. a review, *Biol Med* 61:137-141, 1988.

33. Pasternack PF, Colvin SB, Baumann FG: Cocaine-induced angina pectoris and acute myocardial infarction in patients younger than 40 years, *Am J Cardiol* 55:847, 1985.

34. Rollingher IM, Belzberg AS, Macdonald IL: Cocaine-induced myocardial infarction, *Can Med Assoc J* 135:45-46, 1986.

35. Nanji AA, Filipenko JD: Asystole and ventricular fibrillation associated with cocaine intoxication, *Chest* 85:132-133, 1984.

36. Van Dyke D, Barash PG, Jatlow P, Byck R: Cocaine: plasma concentrations after intranasal application in man, *Science* 191:859-861, 1976.

37. Friedlander AH, Gorelick DA: Dental management of the cocaine addict, *Oral Surg* 65:45-48, 1988.

38. Rosenberg H, Fletcher JE: An update on the malignant hyperthermia syndrome, *Ann Acad Med Singapore* 23(suppl 6):84-97, 1994.

39. Carson JM, Van Sickels JE: Preoperative determination of susceptibility to malignant hyperthermia, *J Oral Maxillofac Surg* 40(7):432-435, 1982.

40. Gielen M, Viering W: 3-in-1 lumbar plexus block for muscle biopsy in malignant hyperthermia patients: amide local anaesthetics may be used safely, *Acta Anaesthesiol Scand* 30:581-583, 1986.

41. Paasuke RT, Brownell AKW: Amine local anaesthetics and malignant hyperthermia, *Can Anaesth Soc J* 33:126-129, 1986 (editorial).

42. Ording H: Incidence of malignant hyperthermia in Denmark, *Anesth Analg* 64:700-704, 1985.

43. Malignant Hyperthermia Association of the United States: MHAUS Professional Advisory Council adopts new policy statement on local anesthetics, *Communicator* 3(4):1, 1985.

44. Kalow W, Britt BA, Terreau ME, Haist C: Metabolic error of muscle metabolism after recovery from malignant hyperthermia, *Lancet* 2:895-898, 1970.

45. Donnelly AJ: Malignant hyperthermia: epidemiology, pathophysiology, treatment, *AORN J* 59(2):393-395, 398-400, 403-405, 1994.

46. Mastaglia FL: Adverse effects of drugs on muscles, *Drugs* 24(4):304-321, 1982.

47. Nelson TE, Denborough MA: Studies on normal human skeletal muscle in relation to the pH and pathopharmacology of malignant hyperpyrexia, *Clin Exp Pharmacol Physiol* 4:315-322, 1977.

48. Cheah KS, Cheah AM: Mitochondrial calcium transport and calcium-activated phospholipase in porcine malignant hyperthermia, *Biochim Biophys Acta* 634:70-84, 1981.

49. Kolb ME, Horne ML, Martz R: Dantrolene in human malignant hyperthermia, *Anesthesiology* 56(4):254-262, 1982.

50. Steelman R, Holmes D: Outpatient dental treatment of pediatric patients with malignant hyperthermia: report of three cases, *ASDC J Dent Child* 59(1):62-65, 1992.

51. Amato R, Giordano A, Patrignani F, Segatore I: Malignant hyperthermia in the course of general anesthesia in oral surgery: a case report, *J Int Assoc Dent Child* 12(1):25-28, 1981.

52. The European Malignant Hyperpyrexia Group: A protocol for the investigation of malignant hyperpyrexia (MH) susceptibility, *Br J Anaesthes* 56(11):1267-1269, 1984.

53. Adragna MG: Medical protocol by habit: avoidance of amide local anesthetics in malignant hyperthermia susceptible patients, *Anesthesiology* 62:99-100, 1985 (letter).

54. Adriani J, Sundin R: Malignant hyperthermia in dental patients, *J Am Dent Assoc* 108:180-184, 1984.

55. Kaus SJ, Rockoff MA: Malignant hyperthermia, *Pediatr Clin North Am* 41(1):221-237, 1994.

56. Ellis ER, Clarke IMC, Appleyard TN, et al: Proceedings: malignant hyperpyrexia induced by nitrous oxide and treated with dexamethrone, *Br Med J* 47:632, 1974.

57. Free CW, Jaimon MPC: Pre-anesthetic administration of dantrolene sodium to a patient at risk from malignant hyperthermia: case report, *N Z Med J* 88:493-494, 1978.

58. Pandit SK, Kothary SP, Cohen PJ: Orally administered dantrolene for prophylaxis of malignant hyperthermia, *Anesthesiology* 50:156-158, 1979.

59. Williams FM: Clinical significance of esterases in man, *Clin Pharmacokinet* 10(5):392-403, 1985.

60. Abernethy MH, George PM, Herron JL, Evans RT: Plasma cholinesterase phenotyping with use of visible-region spectrophotometry, *Clin Chem* 32(1 pt 1):194-197, 1986.

61. Prilocaine-induced methemoglobinemia—Wisconsin, 1993, *MMWR Morb Mortal Wkly Rep* 43(35):655-657, 1994.

62. Bellamy MC, Hopkins PM, Hallsall PJ, Ellis FR. A study into the incidence of methaemoglobinaemia after "three-in-one" block with prilocaine, *Anaesthesia* 47(12):1084-1085, 1992.

63. Guertler AT, Pearce WA: A prospective evaluation of benzocaine-associated methemoglobinemia in human beings, *Ann Emerg Med* 24(4):626-630, 1994.

64. Rodriguez LF, Smolik LM, Zbehlik AJ: Benzocaine-induced methemoglobinemia: a report of a severe reaction and review of the literature, *Ann Pharmacother* 28(5):643-649, 1994.

65. Eilers MA, Garrison TE: *General management principles.* In Rosen P, Barkin RM, editors: *Emergency medicine: concepts and clinical practice,* ed 3, St Louis, 1992, Mosby–Year Book.

66. Sarangi MP, Kumar B: Poisoning with writing ink, *Indian Pediatr* 31(7):856-857, 1994.

67. Daly DJ, Davenport J, Newland MC: Methemoglobinemia following the use of prilocaine, *Br J Anaesth* 36:737-739, 1964.

CHAPTER
eleven

Basic Injection Technique

Nothing that is done by a dentist for a patient is of greater importance than the administration of a drug for the prevention of pain during dental treatment. Yet the act of administering a local anesthetic frequently induces great anxiety or is associated with pain in the recipient. Patients frequently mention that they would prefer anything to the injection, or "shot" (to use the patients' term for injection). Not only can the injection of local anesthetics be fear- and pain-producing, it may also be a factor in the occurrence of emergency medical situations. In a review of medical emergencies developing in Japanese dental offices, Matsuura determined that 54.9% of the emergency situations arose either during the administration of the local anesthetic or in the 5 minutes immediately following its administration.[1] Most of these emergency situations were directly related to the increased stress associated with the receipt of the anesthetic (the injection) and not to the drug being used. Additionally, in a survey on the occurrence of medical emergencies in dental practices in North America, 4,309 dentists responded that a total of over 30,000 emergency situations had developed in their offices over the previous 10 years.[2] Ninety-five percent of the respondents stated that they had experienced a medical emergency in their office in this time period. Over half of the emergencies, 15,407, were vasodepressor syncope (common faint), the overwhelming majority of which occurred during or immediately following the administration of the local anesthetic.

Local anesthetics can be and should be administered in a nonpainful, or atraumatic, manner. Recall your first injection in dental school. Most likely your "patient" was a classmate who, on completion of the injection, would give the same injection to you. Wouldn't you go out of your way to make *his* or *her* injection painless in this situation? At the University of Southern California School of Dentistry these first injections are usually absolutely atraumatic. Students are uniformly surprised at this, many having experienced the more usual (painful) injection at some time in the past when they were "real" dental patients. Why should there be a difference in dental injections and pain between those administered by the inexperienced beginning student and those given by the more experienced practitioner? All too often, local anesthetic administration becomes increasingly traumatic to the patient the longer a dentist has been out of school. Can this discouraging situation be corrected?

Local anesthetic administration need not be painful. Every one of the techniques presented in the following chapters can be done atraumatically, including the administration of local anesthetics on the palate (normally the most sensitive area in the oral cavity). Required from the drug administrator are several skills and attitudes, the most important of which is probably *empathy*. If the administrator truly believes that local anesthetic injections need not be painful, then through a conscious or subconscious effort it is possible to make minor changes in technique that will lead to making formerly traumatic procedures less painful for the patient.

There are two components to an atraumatic injection: a technical aspect and a communicative aspect.*

*The atraumatic injection technique was developed over many years by Dr. Nathan Friedman and the Department of Human Behavior of the University of Southern California School of Dentistry. These principles are incorporated into this section.

Step 1: Use a sterilized sharp needle The stainless steel disposable needles currently used in dentistry are quite sharp and rarely produce any pain on insertion or withdrawal. However, because these needles are machine manufactured, occasionally (exceedingly rare) a fishhook-type barb may appear on the tip. This leads to an atraumatic insertion of the needle that is followed by painful withdrawal as the tip tears the unanesthetized tissue. This may be avoided by use of a sterile 2 × 2 inch gauze. Place the needle tip against the gauze and draw the needle backward. If the gauze is snagged, a barb is present and the needle should be discarded. *(This procedure is optional and may be omitted if fear of needle contamination is great.)*

Disposable needles are sharp on first use. With each succeeding penetration, however, their sharpness diminishes. By the third or fourth penetration the operator can sense increased tissue resistance to needle penetration. Clinically this is evidenced by increased pain on penetration and increased postanesthetic tissue discomfort. It is recommended therefore that stainless steel disposable needles be changed after every three or four tissue penetrations.

The increasing use of disposable safety syringes precludes reuse of the needle, minimizing the problem of dulling needles.

The gauge of the needle should be determined solely by the injection to be administered. Pain caused by needle penetration in the absence of adequate topical anesthesia can be eliminated in dentistry through the use of needles not larger than 25-gauge. Studies have demonstrated that patients cannot differentiate among 25-, 27-, and 30-gauge needles inserted into mucous membranes without the benefit of topical anesthesia.[3] Twenty-three-gauge and larger needles are associated with increased pain on initial insertion.

Step 2: Check the flow of local anesthetic solution After properly loading the cartridge into the syringe, and with the aspirator tip (harpoon) embedded into the rubber stopper (if appropriate), expel a few drops of local anesthetic from the cartridge. This ensures a free flow of solution when it is deposited at the target area. The stoppers on the anesthetic cartridge are made of a silicon rubber in order to ensure ease of administration. Only a few drops of solution should be expelled from the needle to determine if a free flow of solution exists.

Step 3: Determine whether or not to warm the anesthetic cartridge and/or syringe There is no reason for a cartridge of local anesthetic solution to be warmed prior to its injection into soft tissues, if the cartridge is stored at room temperature (approximately 72° F, 22° C). The patient will not perceive local anesthetic solution stored at room temperature as too cold or too hot when it is injected.

Most complaints concerning overly warm local anesthetic cartridges come from those stored in cartridge warmers heated by a (Christmas tree–type) light bulb. Temperatures within these cartridges frequently become excessive, leading to patient discomfort and adverse effects on the contents of the cartridge.[4] (See Chapter 7.)

Cartridges stored in refrigerators or other cool areas should be brought to room temperature before use.

Some persons advocate a slight warming of the *metal syringe* prior to its use. The rationale is that a cold metal object is psychologically more disturbing to the patient than is the same object at room temperature. It is recommended that both the local anesthetic cartridge and the metal syringe be as close to room temperature as possible, preferably without the use of any mechanical devices to achieve these temperatures. Holding the loaded metal syringe in the palm of one's hand for half a minute prior to injection will warm the metal. Plastic syringes do not pose this problem.

Step 4: Position the patient Any patient receiving local anesthetic injections should be in a physiologically sound position prior to and during the injection.

Vasodepressor syncope (common faint) is not infrequently reported before, during, and on occasion after local anesthetic administration. The primary pathophysiological component of this situation is cerebral ischemia secondary to an inability of the heart to supply the brain with an adequate volume of oxygenated blood. When a patient is seated in an upright position the effect of gravity is such that the blood pressure in cerebral arteries is decreased by 2 mm Hg for each inch above the level of the heart.

In the presence of anxiety, blood flow is increasingly directed toward the skeletal muscles at the expense of other organ systems such as the gastrointestinal tract. In the absence of muscular movement ("I can take it like a man!"), the increased volume of blood in the skeletal muscles remains there, decreasing venous return to the heart and decreasing the volume of blood available to be pumped by the heart (uphill) to the brain. A slight decrease in cerebral blood flow is evidenced by the signs and symptoms of vasodepressor syncope (i.e., light-headedness, dizziness, tachycardia, and palpitation). If this situation continues, cerebral blood flow declines still further and the patient ultimately loses consciousness.

To prevent this occurrence, it is recommended that during the administration of a local anesthetic the patient be placed with head and heart parallel to the floor and the feet elevated slightly (Fig. 11-1). Although this position may vary according to the dentist's preference, the patient's medical status, and the specific injection technique, all techniques of regional block anesthesia can be carried out successfully with the patient positioned thus.

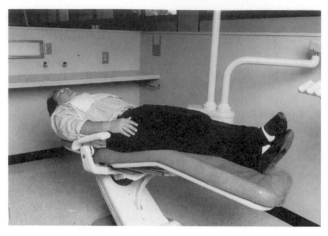

Fig. 11-1 Physiological position for the administration of nerve block anesthesia: patient supine (feet elevated slightly).

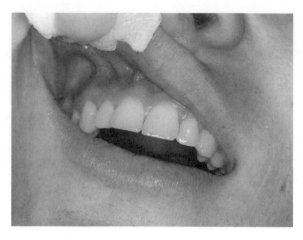

Fig. 11-3 Sterilized gauze is used as an aid in tissue retraction.

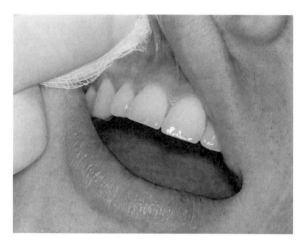

Fig. 11-2 Sterilized gauze is used to wipe tissue at the site of needle penetration.

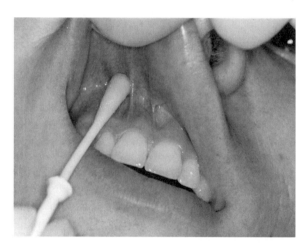

Fig. 11-4 A small quantity of topical anesthetic is placed at the site of needle penetration and permitted to remain for at least 1 minute.

Step 5: Dry the tissue　Use a 2 × 2 inch gauze to dry the tissue in and around the site of needle penetration and to remove any gross debris (Fig. 11-2). In addition, if the lip must be retracted to obtain adequate visibility during the injection, it too should be dried to make retraction easier (Fig. 11-3).

Step 6: Apply topical antiseptic (optional)　After drying the tissues, apply a suitable topical antiseptic at the site of injection. This will further decrease the risk of introducing septic materials into the soft tissues, producing either inflammation or infection. Antiseptics include Betadine (povidone-iodine) and Merthiolate (thimerosal). Alcohol-containing antiseptics can cause burning of the soft tissue and should be avoided. (*This step is optional*; however, the preceding step (no. 5) of drying the tissue must *not* be eliminated.)

Step 7a: Apply topical anesthetic　A topical anesthetic is applied after the topical antiseptic. As with the topical antiseptic, it need be applied only at the site of needle penetration. All too often excessive amounts of topical anesthetic are used on large areas of soft tissues, producing undesirably wide areas of anesthesia (e.g., the soft palate and pharynx), an unpleasant taste, and, perhaps even more importantly, with some topical anesthetics (such as lidocaine), a rapid absorption into the cardiovascular system (CVS), leading to higher local anesthetic blood levels with an increased risk of overdose reaction. Only a small quantity of topical anesthetic need be placed on the cotton applicator stick and applied directly at the injection site (Fig. 11-4).

Topical anesthetics produce anesthesia of the outermost 1 or 2 mm of mucous membrane, tissue that is quite sensitive. The topical anesthetic should remain in contact with the tissue for 2 minutes to ensure effectiveness.[5] A minimum application of 1 minute is recommended.

Step 7b: Communicate with the patient During the application of a topical anesthetic it is desirable for the operator to speak to the patient about the reasons for its use. I tell the patient that "I'm applying a topical anesthetic to the tissue so the remainder of the procedure will be much more comfortable." This statement places a positive idea in the patient's mind concerning the upcoming injection.

Note that the words "injection," "shot," "pain," or "hurt" are not used. These words have a negative connotation; they tend to increase a patient's fears. Their use should, if at all possible, be avoided. More positive words can be substituted in their place. "Administer the local anesthetic" is used in place of "give an injection" or "give a shot." The latter is a particularly poor choice of words and should be avoided. A statement such as "this will not hurt" should also be avoided. Patients hear only the word "hurt," ignoring the rest of the statement. The same is true for the word "pain." An alternative to this is the word "discomfort." Although their meanings are similar, "discomfort" is much less threatening and produces less fear.

Step 8: Establish a firm hand rest After removing the topical anesthetic from the tissue, prepare the syringe. (See Chapter 9.) It is essential to maintain complete control over it at all times. To do so requires a steady hand so tissue penetration can be accomplished readily, accurately, and without inadvertent nicking of tissues. A firm hand rest is necessary. The types of hand rest vary according to the practitioner's likes, dislikes, and physical abilities. Persons with long fingers will be able to use finger rests on the patient's face for many injections; those with shorter fingers may need elbow rests. Figures 11-5 to 11-7 illustrate a variety of hand and finger rests that can be used to stabilize syringes.

Any finger and/or hand rest that permits the anesthetic syringe to be stabilized without increasing risk to a patient is acceptable. Two techniques to be avoided are (1) using no syringe stabilization of any kind and (2) placing the arm holding the syringe directly on the patient's arm or shoulder (Fig. 11-8). In the first situation it is highly unlikely that a needle can be adequately stabilized without the use of some form of rest. The operator has less control over the syringe, thereby increasing the possibility of inadvertent needle movement and injury. Resting on a patient's arm or shoulder is also dangerous and can lead to patient or administrator needle-stick injury. If the patient inadvertently moves during the injection, damage can occur as the needle tip moves around within the mouth. Apprehensive patients, and especially children, frequently move their arms during local anesthetic administration.

Step 9: Make the tissue taut The tissues at the site of needle penetration should be stretched prior to inserting the needle (Fig. 11-9). This can be accomplished in all areas of the mouth except the palate (where the tissues are naturally quite taut). Stretching of the tissues permits the sharp stainless steel needle to *cut* through the mucous membrane with minimum resistance. Loose tissues, on the other hand, are pushed and *torn* by the needle as it is inserted, producing more discomfort on injection and more postoperative soreness.

Techniques of distraction are also effective in this regard. Some dentists advocate jiggling the lip as the needle is inserted; others recommend leaving the needle tip stationary and pulling the soft tissues over the needle tip (Fig. 11-10). Though there is nothing inherently wrong with these distraction techniques, I find that there is no need for either. I believe that the operator should maintain sight of the needle tip at all times. Needles should not be inserted blindly into tissues, as is required in many distraction techniques.

Proper application of topical anesthetic, taut tissues, and a firm hand rest can produce an unnoticed initial penetration of tissues virtually 100% of the time.

Step 10: Keep the syringe out of the patient's line of sight With the tissue prepared and the patient positioned, the assistant should pass the syringe to the administrator either behind the patient's head or across, in front of the patient but below the patient's line of sight. A right-handed administrator doing a right-side injection can sit facing the patient (Fig. 11-11) or, if doing a left-side injection, facing in the same direction as the patient (Fig. 11-12). In all cases it is better that the syringe not be visible to the patient. Proper positioning for left-handed operators is a mirror image of that for right-handed ones. (Specific recommendations for administrator positioning during local anesthetic injections are discussed in Chapters 13 and 14.)

Step 11a: Insert the needle into the mucosa With the needle bevel properly oriented (see specific injection technique for bevel orientation—however, as a general rule *the bevel of the needle should be oriented toward bone*), insert the needle *gently* into the tissue at the injection site to the depth of the bevel. With a firm hand rest and adequate tissue preparation this potentially traumatic procedure can be accomplished without the patient's ever being aware of it.

Step 11b: Watch and communicate with the patient During Step 11a watch and communicate with the patient, observing the patient's face for evidence of discomfort during needle penetration. Signs such as furrowing of the brow or forehead and blinking of the eyes may indicate discomfort (Fig. 11-13). More frequently you will not notice any change in the patient's facial expression at this time (indicating a painless, or atraumatic, needle insertion).

Communicate with the patient as Step 11a is being carried out. State to the patient in a positive manner, "I don't expect you to feel this," as the needle penetrates the tissues. Do not say, "This will not hurt"; of this negative statement, the patient hears only the word "hurt."

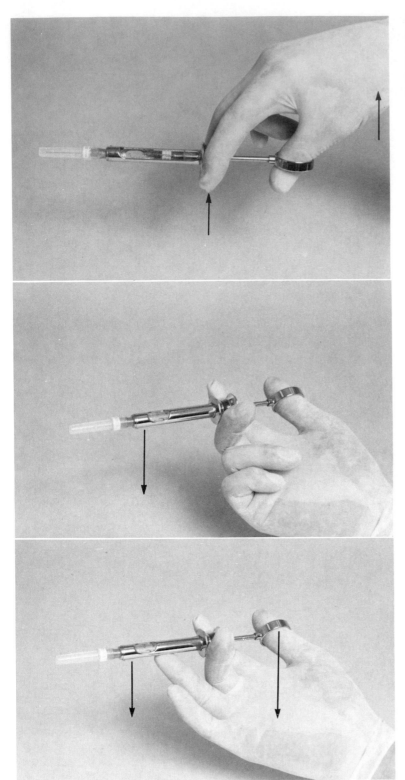

A

B

C

Fig. 11-5 Hand positions for injections. **A,** Palm down: poor control over the syringe; *not recommended.* **B,** Palm up: better control over the syringe because it is supported by the wrist; *recommended.* **C,** Palm up and finger support: greatest stabilization; *highly recommended.*

Step 12: Inject several drops of local anesthetic solution (optional)

Step 13: Slowly advance the needle toward the target Steps 12 and 13 are carried out together. The soft tissue in front of the needle may be anesthetized with a few drops of local anesthetic solution. After waiting 2 or 3 seconds for anesthesia to develop, advance the needle into this area and deposit more. Then advance the needle once again. These procedures may be repeated until the needle reaches the target area.

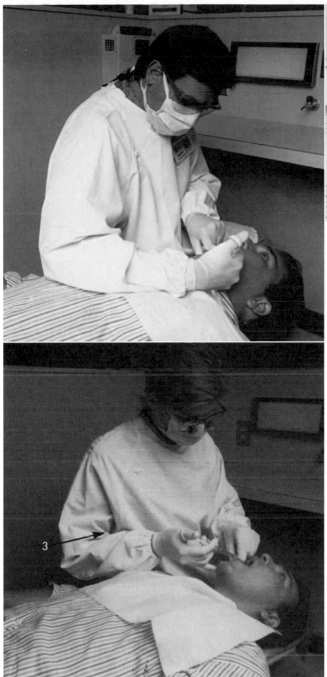

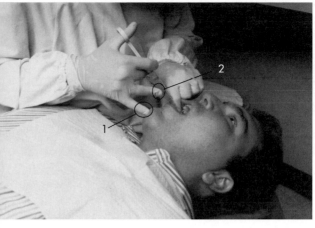

Fig. 11-6 A, Use of the patient's chest for stabilization of the syringe during a right inferior alveolar nerve block. *Do not use the arm of the patient to stabilize a syringe.* **B,** Use of the chin *(1)* as a finger rest, with the syringe barrel stabilized by the lip of the patient *(2)*. **C,** When necessary, stabilization may be increased by drawing the administrator's arm in against his or her chest *(3)*.

In most patients the injection of local anesthetic during insertion of the needle toward the target area is entirely unnecessary. Pain is rarely encountered between the surface mucosa and the mucoperiosteum. If patients are asked what they feel as a needle is being advanced through soft tissue (as in an inferior alveolar or posterior superior alveolar nerve block), the usual reply is that they are aware that something is there but it does not hurt them at all.

On the other hand, patients who are apprehensive about injections of local anesthetics are more likely to react to any sensation as though it were painful. These patients are said to have a lowered pain reaction threshold. Communicate with these patients: "To make you more comfortable I will deposit a little anesthetic as I advance (the needle) toward the target." Inject minimal amounts of anesthetic as you proceed. In an injection such as the inferior alveolar nerve block, for which the average depth of needle insertion is 20 to 25 mm, deposit not more than one eighth of a cartridge of local anesthetic as you penetrate the soft tissues. Aspiration need *not* be performed at this stage because of the small

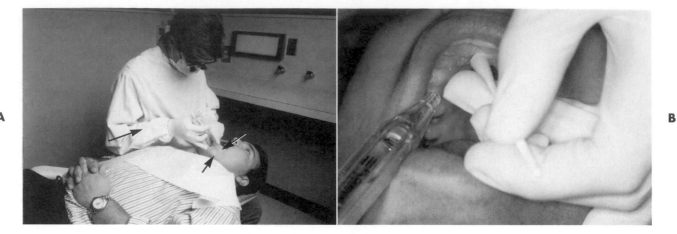

Fig. 11-7 A, Syringe stabilization for a right posterior superior alveolar nerve block: syringe barrel on the patient's lip, one finger resting on the chin and one on the syringe barrel (*arrows*), upper arm kept close to the administrator's chest to maximize stability. **B,** Syringe stabilization for a nasopalatine nerve block: index finger used to stabilize the needle, syringe barrel resting in the corner of the patient's mouth.

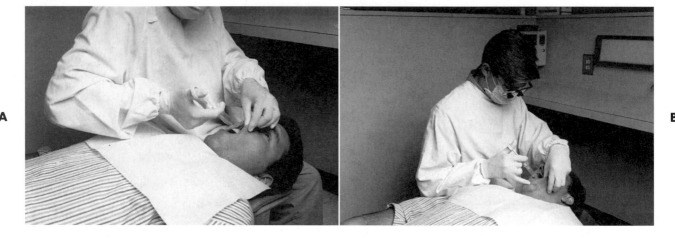

Fig. 11-8 A, Incorrect position: no hand or finger rest. **B,** Incorrect position: administrator resting on the patient's arm.

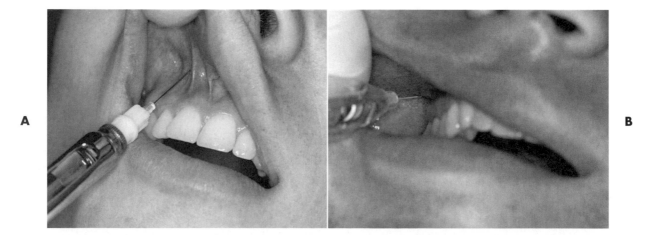

Fig. 11-9 A, Tissue at the penetration site is pulled taut, aiding both an atraumatic needle insertion and visibility. **B,** Taut tissue provides excellent visibility of the penetration site for a right posterior superior alveolar nerve block.

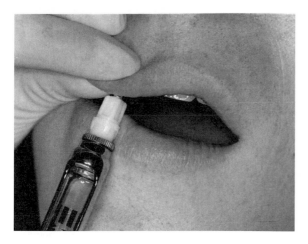

Fig. 11-10 When the soft tissues are pulled over the needle, visibility of the injection site is impaired.

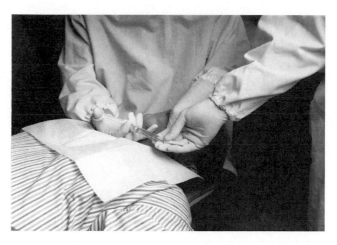

Fig. 11-12 Passing the syringe from the assistant to the administrator for a left-sided injection below the patient's line of sight.

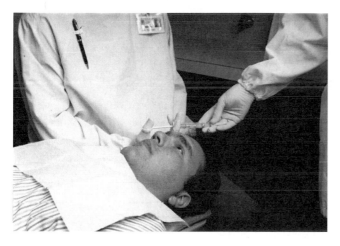

Fig. 11-11 Passing the syringe from the assistant to the administrator behind the patient and out of the patient's line of sight.

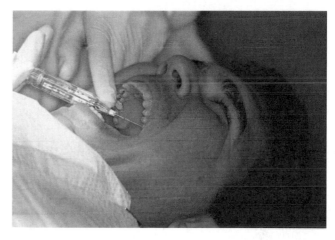

Fig. 11-13 Watch the patient's face during administration of the local anesthetic for squinting of the eyes and/or furrowing of the brows, indicating discomfort.

amount of anesthetic solution that is being continually deposited over a changing injection site. If a vessel is penetrated during this procedure, only a drop or two (< 1 mg) of anesthetic will be deposited intravascularly. As the needle is advanced further, it leaves the vessel. Aspiration must always be carried out, however, prior to depositing any significant volume of solution (Steps 15 and 16).

Step 14: Deposit several drops of local anesthetic before touching periosteum In techniques of regional block anesthesia in which the needle touches or approximates the periosteum, deposit several drops of solution just prior to contact. Periosteum is richly innervated, and contact with the needle tip produces pain (discomfort). Anesthetizing the periosteum allows atraumatic contact. Regional block injection techniques that require this are the inferior alveolar, Gow-Gates mandibular, and infraorbital nerve blocks.

Knowledge of when to deposit the anesthetic solution comes with experience. The depth of penetration of soft tissue at any injection site varies from patient to patient; therefore periosteum may be contacted inadvertently. However, with repetition a keen tactile sense is developed, enabling the needle to be used gently as a probe. This enables the administrator to detect subtle changes in tissue density as the needle approaches bone. With experience and development of this tactile sense, a small volume of local anesthetic solution may be deposited just prior to gently contacting the periosteum.

Step 15: Aspirate Aspiration must always be carried out prior to deposing a volume of local anesthetic at any site. Aspiration minimizes the possibility of an intravascular injection. The goal of aspiration is to determine whether the needle tip lies within a blood vessel. To aspirate, you must create a negative pressure within the dental cartridge. The self-aspirating syringe does this

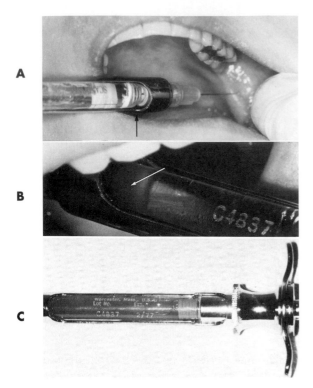

Fig. 11-14 A, Negative aspiration. With the needle in position at the injection site, the administrator pulls the thumb ring of the harpoon aspirator syringe 1 or 2 mm. The needle tip should *not* move. Check the cartridge at the site where the needle penetrates the diaphragm (*arrow*) for a bubble or blood. **B,** Positive aspiration. A slight reddish discoloration at the diaphragm end of the cartridge (*arrow*) on aspiration usually indicates venous penetration. Reposition the needle, reaspirate, and if negative, deposit the solution. **C,** Positive aspiration. Bright red blood rapidly filling the cartridge usually indicates arterial penetration. Remove the syringe from the mouth, change the cartridge, and repeat the procedure.

whenever the operator stops applying positive pressure to the thumb ring (plunger). With the more commonly used harpoon-type syringe the administrator must make a conscious effort to create this negative pressure within the cartridge.

Adequate aspiration requires that the tip of the needle remain unmoved, neither pushed further into nor pulled out of the tissues during aspiration. Adequate stabilization is mandatory. Beginners have a tendency to pull the syringe from the tissues while attempting to aspirate.

Pull back gently on the thumb ring. Movement of only 1 or 2 mm is needed. This produces a negative pressure within the cartridge, which then translates to the tip of the needle. Whatever is lying in the soft tissues around the needle tip (e.g., blood, tissue, or air) will be drawn back into the anesthetic cartridge. By observing the needle end within the cartridge for signs of blood return,

you can determine if a positive aspiration has occurred. *Any sign of blood is a positive aspiration*, and local anesthetic solution should not be deposited at that site (Fig. 11-14). No return at all, or an air bubble, indicates a negative aspiration. Aspiration should be performed at least twice prior to administering local anesthetic, with the orientation of the bevel changed (rotate barrel of syringe about 45 degrees for second aspiration test) to ensure that the bevel of the needle is not located inside a blood vessel but abutting against the wall of the vessel, providing a false-negative aspiration. Several additional aspiration tests are suggested during the administration of the anesthetic drug. This will serve two functions: (1) to slow down the rate of anesthetic administration and (2) to preclude the deposition of large volumes of anesthetic into the cardiovascular system.

The major factor determining whether aspiration can be reliably performed is the needle gauge. Larger-gauge needles (e.g., 25) are recommended over smaller gauges (e.g., 27 and 30) whenever a greater risk of positive aspiration exists.

Step 16a: Slowly deposit the local anesthetic solution With the needle in position at the target area and aspirations completed and *negative,* begin pressing gently on the plunger to start administering the predetermined (for the technique) volume of anesthetic. Slow injection is vital for two reasons: (1) of utmost significance is the safety factor (discussed in greater detail in Chapter 18); (2) slow injection also prevents the solution from tearing the tissue into which it is deposited. Rapid injection results in immediate discomfort (for a few seconds) followed by a prolonged soreness when the action of the local anesthetic is terminated.

Slow injection is defined as the deposition of 1 ml of local anesthetic solution in not less than 60 seconds. A full 1.8-ml cartridge therefore requires approximately 2 minutes. Through slow deposition the solution is able to diffuse along normal tissue planes without producing postoperative discomfort.

Most local anesthetic administrators tend to administer these drugs too rapidly. In a survey completed several years ago,[6] 84% of over 200 respondents stated that the average time spent to deposit 1.8-ml of local anesthetic solution was less than 20 seconds.

In actual clinical practice it therefore seems highly improbable to expect doctors to change their rate of injection from less than 20 seconds to a safe and comfortable 2 minutes per cartridge. *A more realistic time span in a clinical situation is 60 seconds for a full 1.8-ml cartridge.* This rate of deposition of solution will not produce tissue damage either during or after anesthesia and, in the event of accidental intravascular injection, will not produce a serious reaction. There are very few injection techniques requiring the administration of 1.8 ml for success.

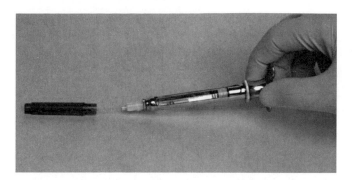

Fig. 11-15 Scoop technique for recapping used needle.

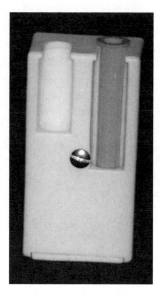

Fig. 11-16 Acrylic needle holder.

For many years I have used one particular method for slowing down my rate of injection. After two negative aspirations, I deposit a volume of solution (approximately one fourth of the total to be deposited) and then aspirate again. If the aspiration is negative, I deposit another fourth of the solution, reaspirate, and continue this process until the total volume of solution for the given injection is deposited. This enables me to do two positive things during injection: (1) to reaffirm through multiple negative aspirations that the solution is, in fact, being deposited extravascularly and (2) to stop the injection for aspiration, which automatically slows down the rate of deposit and thereby minimizes patient discomfort. In the first situation, if positive aspiration occurs following deposition of a fourth of a cartridge, only 9 mg of a 2% solution or 13.5 mg of a 3% solution or 18 mg of a 4% solution will have been deposited intravascularly—doses unlikely to provoke a serious adverse reaction, if, in fact, any reaction develops at all. The needle tip should be repositioned, a negative aspiration achieved, and the injection continued. The incidence of adverse reactions due to intravascular injection is greatly minimized in this manner.

Step 16b: Communicate with the patient During deposition of the local anesthetic it is important to communicate with the patient. Most patients are accustomed to receiving local anesthetic injections rapidly. Statements such as *"I'm depositing the solution (or I'm doing this) slowly so it will be more comfortable for you, but you're not receiving any more than is usual"* go far to allay a patient's apprehension at this time. The second part of the statement is important, since patients might not realize that there is a fixed volume of anesthetic solution in the syringe. A reminder that they are not receiving any more than is usual is a comfort to the patient.

Step 17: Slowly withdraw the syringe Following completion of the injection, the syringe should be slowly withdrawn from the soft tissues and the needle made safe by drawing its protective sheath over it (safety syringe) or by capping it immediately with its plastic sheath via the scoop technique.

Recent concerns over the possibility of needle-stick injuries and the spread of infection due to inadvertent sticking with contaminated needles have led to the formulation of guidelines for the recapping of needles.[7] It has been demonstrated that the time health professionals are most apt to be injured with needles is when recapping following the administration of an injection.[8,9] At this time the needle is contaminated with blood, tissue, and (after intraoral injection) saliva. A number of devices have been marketed to aid the health professional in recapping the needle safely. Needle guards, placed over the needle cap *prior* to injection, prevent fingers from being stuck during recapping. Though no guidelines are yet in effect, the following are most often mentioned for preventing accidental needle stick: (1) *Do not reuse needles.* After their use, immediately discard needles into a sharps container. This policy, though applicable in most nondental hospital situations in which but one injection is administered, is impractical in dentistry, where multiple injections are commonplace. (2) *The "scoop" technique* (Fig. 11-15)—in which the needle cap has been placed on the instrument tray and following injection the administrator simply slides the needle tip into the cap (without touching the cap), scooping up the needle cap—can be used for multiple injections without increased risk. The now capped needle is discarded in a sharps container. (3) An acrylic needle holder can be purchased or fabricated that holds the cap upright during injection. The needle can then be reinserted into the cap without difficulty following injection (Fig. 11-16).

Step 18: Observe the patient After completion of the injection the doctor, hygienist, or assistant should remain with the patient while the anesthetic begins to take effect (and its blood level increases). Most adverse drug reactions, especially those to intraorally administered local anesthetics, will develop either during the injection or within 5 to 10 minutes of completion of the injection. All too often reports are heard of situations in which a local anesthetic was administered and the doctor left the patient alone for a few minutes only to return to find the patient in convulsions or unconscious. Matsuura reported that 54.9% of all medical emergencies arising in Japanese dental offices developed either during the injection of local anesthetics or in the 5 minutes immediately following their administration.[1] *Patients should never be left unattended following administration of a local anesthetic.*

Step 19: Record the injection on the patient's chart An entry should be made of (1) the local anesthetic used, (2) the vasoconstrictor used (if any), (3) the volume (in milligrams) of the solution(s) used, (4) the needle(s) used, (5) the injection(s) given, and (6) the patient's reaction. For example, on the patient's dental progress notes the following might be inscribed: *R-IANB, 25-long, 2% lido + 1:100,000 epi, 36 mgs. Tolerated procedure well.*

Following is a summary of the atraumatic injection technique:

1. Use a sterilized sharp needle.
2. Check the flow of local anesthetic solution.
3. Determine whether to warm the anesthetic cartridge and/or syringe.
4. Position the patient.
5. Dry the tissue.
6. Apply topical antiseptic (optional).
7a. Apply topical anesthetic.
7b. Communicate with the patient.
8. Establish a firm hand rest.
9. Make the tissue taut.
10. Keep the syringe out of the patient's line of sight.
11a. Insert the needle into the mucosa.
11b. Watch and communicate with the patient.
12. Inject several drops of local anesthetic solution (optional).

13. Slowly advance the needle toward the target.
14. Deposit several drops of local anesthetic before touching the periosteum.
15. Aspirate.
16a. Slowly deposit the local anesthetic solution.
16b. Communicate with the patient.
17. Slowly withdraw the syringe. Cap the needle and discard.
18. Observe the patient after the injection.
19. Record the injection on the patient's chart.

The administrator of local anesthetics who adheres to these steps will develop a reputation as a "painless doctor." It is not possible to guarantee that every injection will be absolutely atraumatic, since the reactions of both patients and doctors are far too variable. However, even when they feel some discomfort, patients will invariably state that the injection was better than any other they had previously experienced. This should be the goal sought with every local anesthetic injection.

REFERENCES

1. Matsuura H: Analysis of systemic complications and deaths during dental treatment in Japan, *Anesth Prog* 36:219-228, 1989.
2. Malamed SF: Managing medical emergencies, *J Am Dent Assoc* 124(8):40-53, 1993.
3. Mollen AJ, Ficara AJ, Provant DR: Needles—25 gauge versus 27 gauge—can patients really tell? *Gen Dent* 29(5):417-418, 1981.
4. Rogers KB, Fielding AF, Markiewicz SW: The effect of warming local anesthetic solutions prior to injection, *Gen Dent* 37(6):496-499, 1989.
5. Gill CJ, Orr DL: A double blind crossover comparison of topical anesthetics, *J Am Dent Assoc* 98:213, 1979.
6. Malamed SF: Results of a survey of 209 dentists. Unpublished data, 1975.
7. Goldwater PN, Law R, Nixon AD, et al: Impact of a recapping device on venipuncture-related needlestick injury, *Infect Control Hosp Epidemiol* 10(1):21-25, 1989.
8. McCormick RD, Maki DG: Epidemiology of needle-stick injuries in hospital personnel, *Am J Med* 70(4):928-932, 1981.
9. Berry AJ, Greene ES: The risk of needlestick injuries and needlestick-transmitted diseases in the practice of anesthesiology, *Anesthesiology* 77(5):1007-1021, 1992.

Anatomical Considerations

TRIGEMINAL NERVE

The management of pain in dentistry requires a thorough knowledge of the fifth cranial nerve (Fig. 12-1). The right and left trigeminal nerves provide, among other functions, the overwhelming majority of sensory innervation from the teeth, bone, and soft tissues of the oral cavity. The trigeminal nerve is also the largest cranial nerve. It is composed of a small motor root and a considerably larger (tripartite) sensory root. The motor root supplies the muscles of mastication and other muscles in the region. The three branches of the sensory root supply the skin of the entire face and the mucous membrane of the cranial viscera and oral cavity, except for the pharynx and the base of the tongue. Table 12-1 summarizes the functions of the trigeminal and the 11 other cranial nerves.

Motor Root

The motor root of the trigeminal nerve arises separately from the sensory root, originating in the motor nucleus within the pons and medulla oblongata (Fig. 12-2). Its fibers, forming a small nerve root, travel anteriorly along with, but entirely separate from, the larger sensory root to the region of the semilunar (or gasserian) ganglion. At the semilunar ganglion the motor root passes in a lateral and inferior direction under the ganglion toward the foramen ovale, through which it leaves the middle cranial fossa along with the third division of the sensory root, the mandibular nerve (Figs. 12-3 and 12-4). Just after leaving the skull, the motor root unites with the sensory root of the mandibular division to form a single nerve trunk.

Motor fibers of the trigeminal nerve supply the following muscles:

1. Masticatory
   a. Masseter
   b. Temporalis
   c. Pterygoideus medialis
   d. Pterygoideus lateralis
2. Mylohyoid
3. Anterior belly of the digastric
4. Tensor tympani
5. Tensor veli palatini

Sensory Root

Sensory root fibers of the trigeminal nerve comprise the central processes of ganglion cells located in the trigeminal (semilunar or gasserian) ganglion. There are two ganglia, one innervating each side of the face. They are located in Meckel's cavity, on the anterior surface of the petrous portion of the temporal bone (Fig. 12-3). The ganglia are flat and crescent shaped, their convexities facing anteriorly and downward, and they measure approximately 1.0×2.0 cm. Sensory root fibers enter the concave portion of each crescent, and the three sensory divisions of the trigeminal nerve exit from the convexity:

1. The *ophthalmic division (V₁)* travels anteriorly in the lateral wall of the cavernous sinus to the medial part of the superior orbital fissure, through which it exits the skull into the orbit.
2. The *maxillary division (V₂)* travels anteriorly and downward to exit the cranium through the foramen

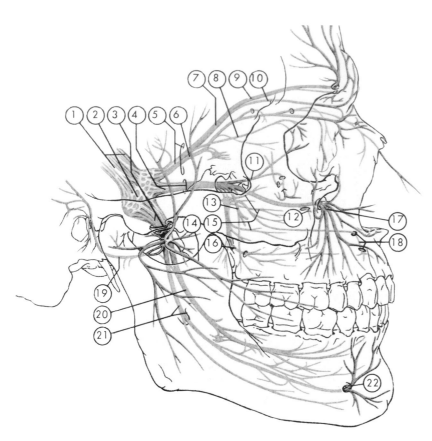

Fig. 12-1 Distribution of the trigeminal nerve. *1,* The branches are as follows: *2,* gasserian ganglion; *3,* mandibular nerve and foramen ovale; *4,* maxillary nerve and foramen rotundum; *5,* ophthalmic nerve and superior orbital fissure; *6,* nasociliary nerve; *7,* frontal nerve; *8,* lacrimal nerve; *9,* supraorbital nerve; *10,* supratrochlear nerve; *11,* zygomatic nerve; *12,* anterior superior alveolar branches; *13,* posterior superior alveolar branches; *14,* buccal nerve; *15,* posterior nasal branches; *16,* greater palatine nerve; *17,* infraorbital nerve; *18,* nasopalatine nerve; *19,* auriculotemporal nerve; *20,* lingual nerve; *21,* inferior alveolar nerve; *22,* mental nerve. *(From Haglund J, Evers H:* Local anaesthesia in dentistry, *ed 2, Södertälje, Sweden, 1975, Astra Läkemedel.)*

TABLE 12-1   Cranial Nerves

Number	Name	Type
I	Olfactory	Sensory
II	Optic	Sensory
III	Oculomotor	Motor
IV	Trochlear	Motor
V	Trigeminal	Mixed
		V_1: sensory
		V_2: sensory
		V_3: sensory, motor
VI	Abducens	Motor
VII	Facial	Motor
VIII	Auditory	Sensory
IX	Glossopharyngeal	Mixed
X	Vagus	Mixed
XI	Accesory	Motor
XII	Hypoglossal	Motor

rotundum into the upper portion of the pterygopalatine fossa.

3. The *mandibular division(V_3)* travels almost directly downward to exit the skull, along with the motor root, through the foramen ovale. These two roots then intermingle, forming one nerve trunk that enters the infratemporal fossa.

On exiting the cranium through their respective foramina,* the three divisions of the trigeminal nerve divide into a multitude of sensory branches.

• • •

Each of the three divisions of the trigeminal nerve is described, but more attention will be devoted to the maxillary and mandibular divisions because of their greater importance in pain control in dentistry. Figure 12-5 illustrates the sensory distribution of the trigeminal nerve.

Ophthalmic Division (V_1)

The ophthalmic division is the first branch of the trigeminal nerve. It is exclusively sensory and is the smallest of the three divisions. It leaves the cranium and enters the orbit through the superior orbital fissure (Fig. 12-6). The nerve trunk is approximately 2.5 cm long. It supplies the eyeball, conjunctiva, lacrimal gland, parts of the mucous membrane of the nose and paranasal sinuses, and the skin of the forehead, eyelids, and nose. When the ophthalmic nerve (V_1) is paralyzed, the ocular conjunctiva becomes insensitive to touch.

*To be somewhat more precise, since the three branches of the trigeminal nerve are almost exclusively sensory, they do not *exit from* the cranium but rather *enter into* the cranium, carrying nerve impulses from the periphery toward the brain.

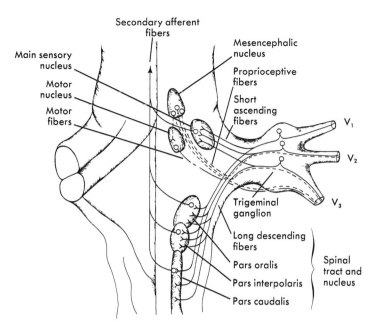

Fig. 12-2 Intracranial distribution of the trigeminal nerve. *(From Jastak JT, Yagiela JA: Regional anesthesia of the oral cavity, St Louis, 1981, Mosby–Year Book.)*

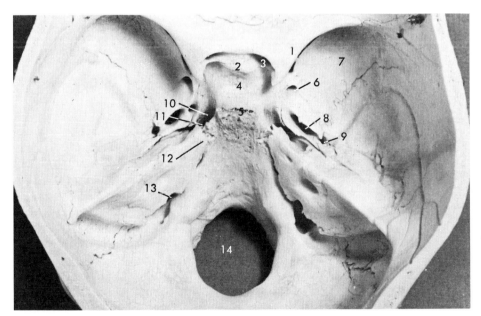

Fig. 12-3 Internal surface of the base of the skull. *1,* Lesser wing of the sphenoid bone; *2,* chiasmatic sulcus; *3,* optic canal; *4,* sella turcica; *5,* dorsum sellae; *6,* foramen rotundum; *7,* greater wing of the sphenoid; *8,* foramen ovale; *9,* foramen spinosum; *10,* carotid groove; *11,* foramen lacerum; *12,* depression for the semilunar ganglion; *13,* jugular foramen; *14,* foramen magnum.

Just before the ophthalmic nerve passes through the superior orbital fissure, it divides into its three main branches—the nasociliary, the frontal, and the lacrimal nerves.

Nasociliary nerve The nasociliary nerve travels along the medial border of the orbital roof, giving off branches to the nasal cavity and ending in the skin at the root of the nose. It then branches into the *anterior ethmoidal* and *external nasal nerves.* The *internal nasal nerve* (from the anterior ethmoidal) supplies the mucous membrane of the anterior part of the nasal septum and the lateral wall of the nasal cavity. The *ciliary ganglion* contains sensory fibers that travel to the eyeball via the *short ciliary nerves.* There are two or three *long ciliary nerves* supplying the iris and cornea. The *infratrochlear nerve* supplies the skin of the lacrimal sac and the lacrimal caruncle; the *posterior ethmoidal nerve* supplies the ethmoidal and sphenoidal sinuses; and the *external nasal nerve* supplies the skin over the apex (tip) and the ala of the nose.

Frontal nerve The frontal nerve travels anteriorly in the orbit—dividing into two branches: the *supratrochlear* and the *supraorbital.* The frontal is the largest branch of the ophthalmic division. The supratrochlear

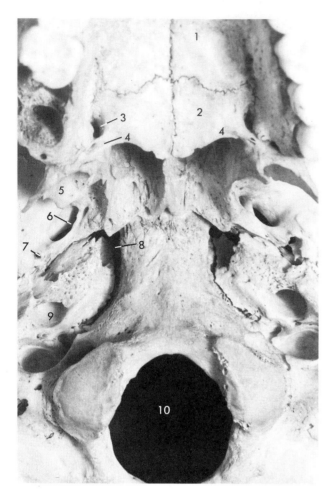

Fig. 12-4 Inferior surface of the base of the skull. *1,* Palatal process of the maxilla; *2,* horizontal process of the palate; *3,* greater palatine foramen; *4,* lesser palatine foramina; *5,* lateral pterygoid plate; *6,* foramen ovale; *7,* foramen spinosum; *8,* foramen lacerum; *9,* carotid canal; *10,* foramen magnum.

nerve supplies the conjunctiva and skin of the medial aspect of the upper eyelid and the skin over the lower and mesial aspects of the forehead. The supraorbital nerve is sensory to the upper eyelid, to the scalp as far back as the parietal bone, and to the lambdoidal suture.

Lacrimal nerve The lacrimal nerve is the smallest branch of the ophthalmic division. It supplies the lateral part of the upper eyelid and a small adjacent area of skin.

Maxillary Division (V₂)

The maxillary division of the trigeminal nerve arises from the middle of the trigeminal ganglion. Intermediate in size between the ophthalmic and mandibular divisions, it is purely sensory in function.

Origins The maxillary nerve passes horizontally forward, leaving the cranium through the foramen rotundum (Fig. 12-3). The foramen rotundum is located in the

greater wing of the sphenoid bone. Once outside the cranium, the maxillary nerve crosses the uppermost part of the pterygopalatine fossa, between the pterygoid plates of the sphenoid bone and the palatine bone. As it crosses the pterygopalatine fossa, it gives off branches to the sphenopalatine ganglion, the posterior superior alveolar nerve, and the zygomatic branches. It then angles laterally in a groove on the posterior surface of the maxilla, entering the orbit through the inferior orbital fissure. Within the orbit it occupies the infraorbital groove and becomes the infraorbital nerve, which courses anteriorly into the infraorbital canal.

The maxillary division emerges on the anterior surface of the face through the infraorbital foramen, where it divides into its terminal branches, supplying the skin of the face, nose, lower eyelid, and upper lip (Fig. 12-7). Following is a breakdown of maxillary division innervation:

1. Skin of
    a. Middle portion of the face
    b. Lower eyelid
    c. Side of the nose
    d. Upper lip
2. Mucous membrane of
    a. Nasopharynx
    b. Maxillary sinus
    c. Soft palate
    d. Tonsil
    e. Hard palate
3. Maxillary teeth and periodontal tissues

Branches The maxillary division gives off branches in four regions—within the cranium, in the pterygopalatine fossa, in the infraorbital canal, and on the face.

Branch within the cranium Immediately after separating from the trigeminal ganglion, the maxillary division gives off a small branch, the *middle meningeal nerve,* that travels with the middle meningeal artery to provide sensory innervation to the dura mater.

Branches in the pterygopalatine fossa After exiting the cranium through the foramen rotundum, the maxillary division crosses the pterygopalatine fossa. In this fossa several branches are given off (Fig. 12-8)—the zygomatic nerve, the pterygopalatine nerves, and the posterior superior alveolar nerve.

The *zygomatic nerve* comes off the maxillary division in the pterygopalatine fossa and travels anteriorly, entering the orbit through the inferior orbital fissure, where it divides into the zygomaticotemporal and zygomaticofacial nerves—the *zygomaticotemporal* supplying sensory innervation to the skin on the side of the forehead, and the *zygomaticofacial* supplying the skin on the prominence of the cheek. Just before leaving the orbit the zygomatic nerve sends a branch that communicates with the lacrimal nerve of the ophthalmic division. This

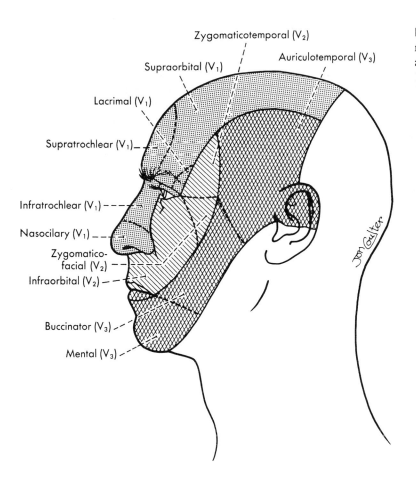

Zygomaticotemporal (V₂)

Supraorbital (V₁)

Auriculotemporal (V₃)

Lacrimal (V₁)

Supratrochlear (V₁) —

Infratrochlear (V₁) — ---

Nasocilary (V₁) — --

Zygomatico-
facial (V₂) — --

Infraorbital (V₂) — --

Buccinator (V₃) --

Mental (V₃) --

Fig. 12-5 Superficial sensory nerves of head and neck regions. *(From Bennett CR: Monheim's local anesthesia and pain control in dental practice, ed 7, St Louis, 1984, Mosby-Year Book.)*

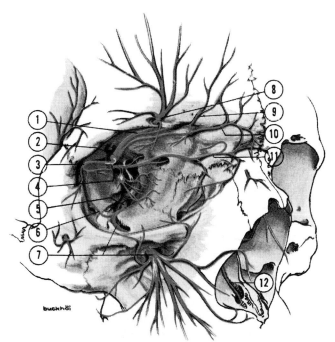

Fig. 12-6 Distribution of the ophthalmic division (V₁). *1,* Supraorbital nerve; *2,* frontal nerve; *3,* lacrimal nerve; *4,* nasociliary nerve; *5,* maxillary nerve; *6,* zygomatic nerve; *7,* infraorbital nerve; *8,* lateral branch of the frontal nerve; *9,* medial branch of the frontal nerve; *10,* supratrochlear nerve; *11,* infratrochlear nerve; *12,* nasopalatine nerve. *(From Haglund J, Evers H: Local anaesthesia in dentistry, ed 2, Södertälje, Sweden, 1975, Astra Läkemedel.)*

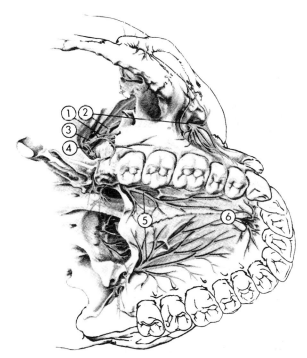

Fig. 12-7 Distribution of the maxillary division (V₂). *1,* Posterior superior alveolar branches; *2,* infraorbital nerve; *3,* maxillary nerve; *4,* foramen rotundum; *5,* greater palatine nerve; *6,* nasopalatine nerve. *(From Haglund J, Evers H: Local anaesthesia in dentistry, ed 2, Södertälje, Sweden, 1975, Astra Läkemedel.)*

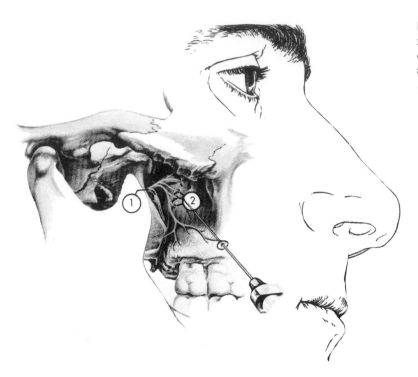

Fig. 12-8 Branches of V₂ in the pterygopalatine fossa. *1,* Maxillary nerve; *2,* posterior superior alveolar branches. *(From Haglund J, Evers H: Local anaesthesia in dentistry, ed 2, Södertälje, Sweden, 1975, Astra Läkemedel.)*

branch carries secretory fibers from the sphenopalatine ganglion to the lacrimal gland.

The *pterygopalatine nerves* are two short trunks that unite in the pterygopalatine ganglion and are then redistributed into several branches. They also serve as a communication between the pterygopalatine ganglion and the maxillary nerve (V₂). Postganglionic secretomotor fibers from the pterygopalatine ganglion pass through these nerves and back along V₂ to the zygomatic nerve, through which they are routed to the lacrimal nerve and lacrimal gland.

Branches of the pterygopalatine nerves include those that supply four areas—the orbit, the nose, the palate, and the pharynx.

1. The orbital branches supply the periosteum of the orbit.
2. The nasal branches supply the mucous membranes of the superior and middle conchae, the lining of the posterior ethmoidal sinuses, and the posterior portion of the nasal septum. One branch is significant in dentistry, the *nasopalatine nerve,* which passes across the roof of the nasal cavity downward and forward, where it lies between the mucous membrane and the periosteum of the nasal septum. The nasopalatine nerve continues downward, reaching the floor of the nasal cavity and giving branches to the anterior part of the nasal septum and the floor of the nose. It then enters the incisive canal, through which it passes into the oral cavity via the incisive foramen, located in the midline of the palate about 1 cm posterior to the maxillary central incisors. The

right and left nasopalatine nerves emerge together through this foramen and provide sensation to the palatal mucosa in the region of the premaxilla (canines through central incisors) (Fig. 12-9).
3. The palatine branches are the greater (or anterior) palatine nerve and the lesser (middle and posterior) palatine nerves (Fig. 12-10). The *greater (or anterior) palatine nerve* descends through the pterygopalatine canal, emerging on the hard palate through the greater palatine foramen (which is usually located about 1 cm toward the palatal midline, just distal to the second molar). Sicher and DuBrul have stated that the greater palatine foramen may be located 3 to 4 mm in front of the posterior border of the hard palate.[1] The nerve courses anteriorly between mucoperiosteum and the osseous hard palate, supplying sensory innervation to the palatal soft tissues and bone anterior to the first premolar, where it communicates with terminal fibers of the nasopalatine nerve (Fig. 12-10). It also provides sensory innervation to some parts of the soft palate. The *middle palatine nerve* emerges from the lesser palatine foramen, along with the *posterior palatine nerve.* The middle palatine nerve provides sensory innervation to the mucous membrane of the soft palate; the tonsillar region is innervated, in part, by the posterior palatine nerve.
4. The pharyngeal branch is a small nerve that leaves the posterior part of the pterygopalatine ganglion, passes through the pharyngeal canal, and is distributed to the mucous membrane of the nasal part of the pharynx, posterior to the auditory (eustachian) tube.

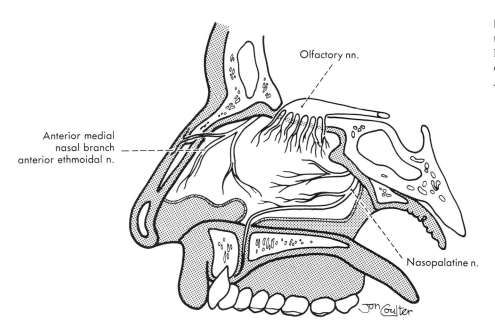

Olfactory nn.

Anterior medial
nasal branch
anterior ethmoidal n.

Nasopalatine n.

Fig. 12-9 Nerves of the nasal septum. *(From Bennett CR:* Monheim's local anesthesia and pain control in dental practice, *ed 7, St Louis, 1984, Mosby–Year Book.)*

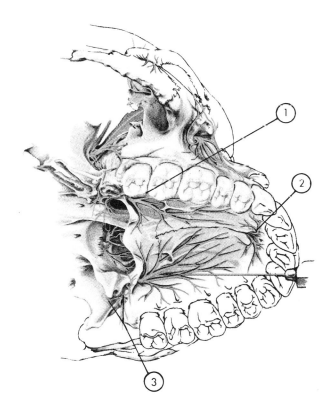

Fig. 12-10 Palatal branches of V_2. *1,* Greater (anterior) palatine nerve; *2,* nasopalatine nerve; *3,* lesser (posterior) palatine nerves. *(From Haglund J, Evers H:* Local anaesthesia in dentistry, *ed 2, Södertälje, Sweden, 1975, Astra Läkemedel.)*

The *posterior superior alveolar (PSA) nerve* descends from the main trunk of the maxillary division in the pterygopalatine fossa just before the maxillary division enters the infraorbital canal (Fig. 12-11). Commonly there are two PSA branches, but on occasion

a single trunk will arise. Passing downward through the pterygopalatine fossa they reach the inferior temporal (posterior) surface of the maxilla. When two trunks are present, one remains external to the bone, continuing downward on the posterior surface of the maxilla to provide sensory innervation to the buccal gingiva in the maxillary molar region and adjacent facial mucosal surfaces, while the other branch enters into the maxilla (along with a branch of the internal maxillary artery) through the posterior superior alveolar canal to travel down the posterior or posterolateral wall of the maxillary sinus and provide sensory innervation to the mucous membrane of the sinus. Continuing downward, this second branch of the PSA provides sensory innervation to the alveoli, periodontal ligaments, and pulpal tissues of the maxillary third, second, and first molars (with the exception [in 28% of patients[2]] of the mesiobuccal root of the first molar).

Branches in the infraorbital canal Within the infraorbital canal the maxillary division (V_2) gives off two branches of significance in dentistry, the middle superior and anterior superior alveolar nerves. While in the infraorbital groove and canal, the maxillary division is known as the infraorbital nerve.

The *middle superior alveolar (MSA) nerve* branches off the main nerve trunk (V_2) within the infraorbital canal to form a part of the superior dental plexus,[1] composed of the posterior, middle, and anterior superior alveolar nerves. The site of origin of the MSA nerve varies, from the posterior portion of the infraorbital canal to the anterior portion, near the infraorbital foramen. The MSA nerve provides sensory innervation to the two maxillary premolars and, perhaps, to the mesiobuccal root of the first molar as well as the periodontal tissues, buccal soft tissue, and bone in the pre-

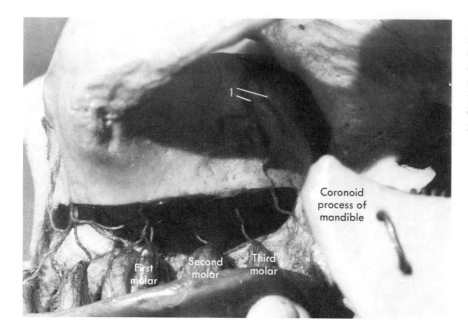

Fig. 12-11 Posterolateral view of the maxilla illustrating the posterior superior alveolar (PSA) nerves on the posterior aspect of the maxillary tuberosity (*1*). Injecting the PSA nerves provides pulpal anesthesia to the first, second, and third molars (except the mesiobuccal root of the first molar).

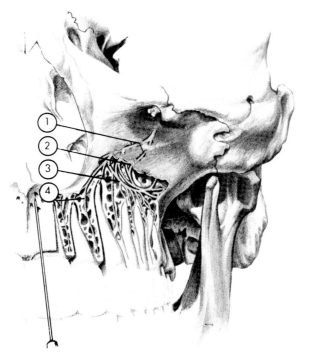

Fig. 12-12 Anterior superior alveolar (ASA) nerve (bone over the nerves removed). *1*, Branches of the ASA nerve; *2*, superior dental plexus; *3*, dental branches; *4*, interdental and interradicular branches. *(From Haglund J, Evers H: Local anaesthesia in dentistry, ed 2, Södertälje, Sweden, 1975, Astra Läkemedel.)*

molar region. Traditionally it has been stated that the MSA nerve is absent in 30%[3] to 54%[4] of individuals. In a more recent dissection study Loetscher and Walton[2] found the MSA nerve to be present in 72% of the specimens examined. In its absence its usual innervations

are provided by either the PSA or the ASA nerves, most frequently the latter.[1]

The *anterior superior alveolar (ASA) nerve,* a relatively large branch, is given off the infraorbital nerve (V_2) approximately 6 to 10 mm before the latter's exit from the infraorbital foramen. Descending *within* the anterior wall of the maxillary sinus, it provides pulpal innervation to the central and lateral incisors and the canine as well as sensory innervation to the periodontal tissues, buccal bone, and mucous membranes of these teeth (Fig. 12-12).

The ASA nerve communicates with the MSA and gives off a small nasal branch that innervates the anterior part of the nasal cavity, along with branches of the pterygopalatine nerves. In persons without an MSA nerve the ASA frequently provides sensory innervation to the premolars and occasionally the mesiobuccal root of the first molar.

The actual innervation of individual roots of all teeth, bone, and periodontal structures in both the maxilla and the mandible derives from terminal branches of larger nerves in the region. These nerve networks are termed the *dental plexus.*

The superior dental plexus is composed of smaller nerve fibers from the three superior alveolar nerves (and in the mandible, from the inferior alveolar nerve). Three types of nerves emerge from these plexuses—dental nerves, interdental branches, and interradicular branches—and each is accompanied along its pathway by a corresponding artery.

The *dental nerves* are those that enter a tooth through the apical foramen, dividing into many small branches within the pulp. Pulpal innervation of all teeth is derived from dental nerves. Although in most instances one easily identifiable nerve is responsible, in some cases (usually the maxillary first molar) more than one nerve will be.

The *interdental branches* (also termed *perforating branches*) travel through the entire height of the interradicular septum, providing sensory innervation to the periodontal ligaments of adjacent teeth through the alveolar bone. They emerge at the height of the crest of the interalveolar septum and enter the gingiva to innervate the interdental papillae and buccal gingiva.

The *interradicular branches* traverse the entire height of the interradicular or interalveolar septum, providing sensory innervation to the periodontal ligaments of adjacent roots. They terminate in the periodontal ligament (PDL) at the root furcations.

Branches on the face   Through the infraorbital foramen the infraorbital nerve emerges onto the face to divide into its terminal branches—the inferior palpebral, the external nasal, and the superior labial. The *inferior palpebral branches* supply the skin of the lower eyelid with sensory innervation, the *external nasal branches* provide sensory innervation to the skin on the lateral aspect of the nose, and the *superior labial branches* provide sensory innervation to the skin and mucous membranes of the upper lip.

Although anesthesia of these nerves is not necessary for adequate pain control during dental treatment, they are frequently blocked in the process of carrying out other anesthetic procedures.

Summary   Following is a summary of the branches of the maxillary division (italicized nerves denote those of special significance in dental pain control):

1. Branches within the cranium
   a. Middle meningeal nerve
2. Branches within the pterygopalatine fossa
   a. Zygomatic nerve
      (1) Zygomaticotemporal nerve
      (2) Zygomaticofacial nerve
   b. Pterygopalatine nerves
      (1) Orbital branches
      (2) Nasal branches
         (a) Nasopalatine nerve
      (3) Palatine branches
         (a) Greater (anterior) palatine nerve
         (b) Lesser (middle and posterior) palatine nerves
      (4) Pharyngeal branch
   c. Posterior superior alveolar nerve
3. Branches within the infraorbital canal
   a. Middle superior alveolar nerve
   b. Anterior superior alveolar nerve
4. Branches on the face
   a. Inferior palpebral branches
   b. External nasal branches
   c. Superior labial branches

Mandibular Division (V₃)

Mandibular Division (V$_3$)

The mandibular division is the largest branch of the trigeminal nerve. It is a mixed nerve with two roots—a large sensory root and a smaller motor root (the latter representing the entire motor component of the trigeminal nerve). The sensory root of the mandibular division originates at the inferior angle of the trigeminal ganglion, whereas the motor root arises in motor cells located in the pons and medulla oblongata. The two roots emerge from the cranium separately through the foramen ovale, the motor root lying medial to the sensory. They unite just outside the skull and form the main trunk of the third division. This trunk remains undivided for only 2 to 3 mm before it splits into a small anterior and a large posterior division (Fig. 12-13).

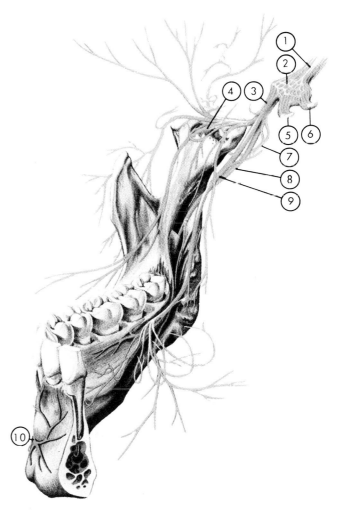

Fig. 12-13 Distribution of the mandibular division (V$_3$). *1,* Trigeminal nerve; *2,* gasserian ganglion; *3,* mandibular nerve; *4,* buccal nerve; *5,* maxillary nerve; *6,* ophthalmic nerve; *7,* auriculotemporal nerve; *8,* inferior alveolar nerve; *9,* lingual nerve; *10,* mental nerve. *(From Haglund J, Evers H:* Local anaesthesia in dentistry, *ed 2, Södertälje, Sweden, 1975, Astra Läkemedel.)*

The areas innervated by V_3 are included in the following outline:

1. Sensory root
   a. Skin of
      (1) Temporal region
      (2) Auricula
      (3) External auditory meatus
      (4) Cheek
      (5) Lower lip
      (6) Lower part of the face (chin region)
   b. Mucous membrane of
      (1) Cheek
      (2) Tongue (anterior two thirds)
      (3) Mastoid cells
   c. Mandibular teeth and periodontal tissues
   d. Bone of the mandible
   e. Temporomandibular joint
   f. Parotid gland
2. Motor root
   a. Masticatory muscles
      (1) Masseter
      (2) Temporalis
      (3) Pterygoideus medialis
      (4) Pterygoideus lateralis
   b. Mylohyoid
   c. Anterior belly of the digastric
   d. Tensor tympani
   e. Tensor veli palatini

Branches The third division of the trigeminal nerve gives off branches in three areas—from the undivided nerve, and from the anterior and posterior divisions.

Branches from the undivided nerve On leaving the foramen ovale the main undivided nerve trunk gives off two branches during its 2 to 3 mm course. These are the nervus spinosus (meningeal branch of the mandibular nerve) and the medial pterygoid nerve. The *nervus spinosus* reenters the cranium through the foramen spinosum along with the middle meningeal artery to supply the dura mater and mastoid air cells. The *medial pterygoid nerve* is a motor nerve to the medial (internal) pterygoid muscle. It gives off small branches that are motor to the tensor veli palatini and tensor tympani.

Branches from the anterior division Branches from the anterior division of V_3 provide motor innervation to the muscles of mastication and sensory innervation to the mucous membrane of the cheek and buccal mucous membrane of the mandibular molars.

The anterior division is significantly smaller than the posterior. It runs forward under the lateral (external) pterygoid muscle for a short distance and then reaches the external surface of that muscle by either passing between its two heads or, less frequently, winding over its upper border. From this point it is known as the *buccal nerve*. While under the lateral pterygoid muscle, the buccal nerve gives off several branches—the *deep temporal nerves* (to the temporal muscle) and the *masseter* and *lateral pterygoid nerves* (providing motor innervation to the respective muscles).

The buccal nerve, also known as the buccinator nerve and the long buccal nerve, usually passes between the two heads of the lateral pterygoid to reach the external surface of that muscle (Fig. 12-13). It then follows the inferior part of the temporal muscle and emerges under the anterior border of the masseter muscle, continuing in an anterolateral direction. At the level of the occlusal plane of the mandibular third or second molar it crosses in front of the anterior border of the ramus and enters the cheek through the buccinator muscle. Sensory fibers are distributed to the skin of the cheek. Other fibers pass into the retromolar triangle, providing sensory innervation to the buccal gingiva of the mandibular molars and the mucobuccal fold in that region. The buccal nerve does *not* innervate the buccinator muscle; the facial nerve does. Nor does it provide sensory innervation to the lower lip or corner of the mouth. This is significant, because some doctors do not administer the "long" buccal injection following inferior alveolar nerve block until the lower lip has become numb. Their thinking is that the long buccal nerve block will provide anesthesia of the lower lip and therefore might falsely lead them to believe that their inferior alveolar nerve block has been successful, when in fact it has been missed. Such concern is unwarranted. *The long buccal nerve block should be administered immediately following inferior alveolar nerve block.*

Anesthesia of the buccal nerve is important for dental procedures requiring soft tissue manipulation on the buccal surface of the mandibular molars.

Branches of the posterior division The posterior division of V_3 is primarily sensory, with a small motor component. It descends for a short distance, downward and medially to the lateral pterygoid muscle, at which point it branches into the auriculotemporal, lingual, and inferior alveolar nerves.

The *auriculotemporal nerve* is not profoundly significant in dentistry. It traverses the upper part of the parotid gland and then crosses the posterior portion of the zygomatic arch. It gives off a number of branches, all of which are sensory. These include (1) a communication with the facial nerve, providing sensory fibers to the skin over the areas of innervation of the following motor branches of the facial nerve: the zygomatic, the buccal, and the mandibular; (2) a communication with the otic ganglion, providing sensory, secretory, and vasomotor fibers to the parotid gland; (3) the anterior auricular branches, supplying the skin over the helix and tragus of the ear; (4) branches to the external auditory meatus, innervating the skin over the meatus and the tympanic membrane; (5) articular branches to the posterior portion of the temporomandibular joint; and (6)

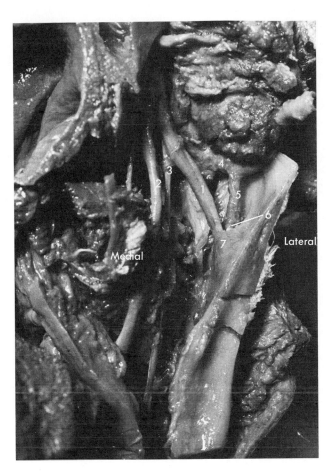

Fig. 12-14 Posterior division of V$_3$. Dissection in the region of the mandibular foramen. *1*, Inferior alveolar nerve; *2*, lingual nerve; *3*, mylohyoid nerve; *4*, maxillary artery; *5*, inferior alveolar artery; *6*, mandibular foramen; *7*, lingula.

the superficial temporal branches, supplying the skin over the temporal region.

The *lingual nerve* is the second branch of the posterior division of V$_3$. It passes downward medial to the lateral pterygoid muscle and, as it descends, lies between the ramus and the medial pterygoid muscle in the pterygomandibular space. It runs anterior and medial to the inferior alveolar nerve, whose path it parallels. It then continues downward and forward, deep to the pterygomandibular raphe and below the attachment of the superior constrictor of the pharynx, to reach the side of the base of the tongue slightly below and behind the mandibular third molar (Figs. 12-13 and 12-14). Here it lies just below the mucous membrane in the lateral lingual sulcus, where it is so superficial in some persons that it may be seen just below the mucous membrane. It then proceeds anteriorly across the muscles of the tongue, looping downward and medial to the submandibular (Wharton's) duct to the deep surface of the sublingual gland, where it breaks up into its terminal branches.

The lingual nerve is the sensory tract to the anterior two thirds of the tongue. It provides both general sensation and gustation (taste) for this region. It is the nerve that supplies fibers for general sensation, whereas the chorda tympani (a branch of the facial nerve) supplies fibers for taste. In addition, the lingual nerve provides sensory innervation to the mucous membranes of the floor of the mouth and the gingiva on the lingual of the mandible.

The *inferior alveolar nerve* is the largest branch of the mandibular division (Fig. 12-14). It descends, medial to the lateral pterygoid muscle and lateroposterior to the lingual nerve, to the region between the sphenomandibular ligament and the medial surface of the mandibular ramus, where it enters the mandibular canal at the level of the mandibular foramen. Throughout its path it is accompanied by the inferior alveolar artery (a branch of the internal maxillary artery) and the inferior alveolar vein. The artery lies just anterior to the nerve. The nerve, the artery, and the vein travel anteriorly in the mandibular canal as far forward as the mental foramen, where the nerve divides into terminal branches: the incisive nerve and the mental nerve.

Bifid (from the Latin meaning "cleft into two parts") inferior alveolar nerves and mandibular canals have been observed radiographically and categorized by Langlais et al.[5] In 6000 panoramic radiographs studied, bifid mandibular canals were evident in 0.95%. The bifid mandibular canal is clinically significant in that it increases the difficulty of achieving adequate anesthesia in the mandible with conventional techniques. This is especially so in the Type 4 variation (Fig. 12-15), in which two separate mandibular foramina are present on each side of the mouth.

The *mylohyoid nerve* branches from the inferior alveolar nerve prior to the latter's entry into the mandibular canal (Figs. 12-14 and 12-16). It runs downward and forward in the mylohyoid groove on the medial surface of the ramus and along the body of the mandible to reach the mylohyoid muscle. The mylohyoid is a mixed nerve, being motor to the mylohyoid muscle and the anterior belly of the digastric. It is thought to contain sensory fibers that supply the skin on the inferior and anterior surfaces of the mental protuberance. It may also provide sensory innervation to the mandibular incisors. There is evidence[6] that the mylohyoid may also in some persons be involved in supplying pulpal innervation to portions of the mandibular molars, usually the mesial root of the mandibular first molar.

Once the inferior alveolar nerve enters the mandibular canal, it travels anteriorly along with the inferior alveolar artery and vein. The *dental plexus* serves the mandibular posterior teeth, entering through their apices and providing pulpal innervation. Other fibers supply sensory innervation to the buccal periodontal tissues of these same teeth.

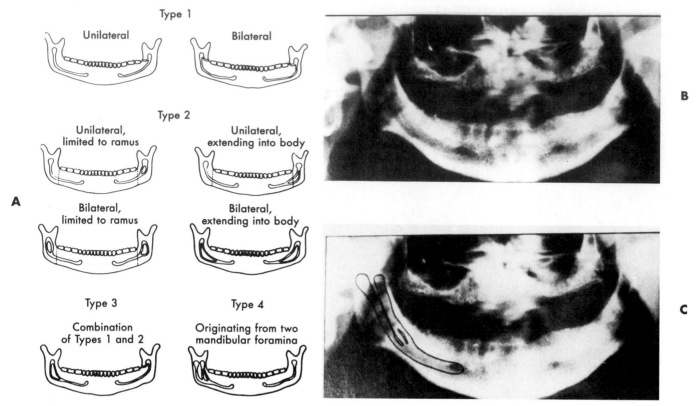

Fig. 12-15 **A,** Variations of bifid mandibular canals. **B** and **C,** Radiographs of a Type 4 bifid mandibular canal (on the patient's right, **B,** outlined in **C**). *(From Langlais RP, Broadus R, Glass BJ: Bifid mandibular canals in panoramic radiographs, J Am Dent Assoc 110:923-926, 1985. Copyright the American Dental Association. Reprinted by permission.)*

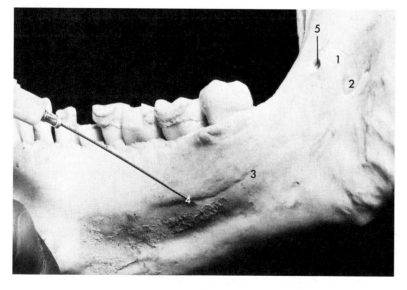

Fig. 12-16 Lingual aspect of the mandible illustrates the mylohyoid nerve and position of the needle for anesthesia of that nerve when partial anesthesia exists in the mandibular molars. *1,* Lingula; *2,* mandibular foramen; *3,* mylohyoid groove; *4,* injection site (below second molar); *5,* artifact.

At the mental foramen the inferior alveolar nerve divides into its two terminal branches, the incisive nerve and the mental nerve (Fig. 12-17). The *incisive nerve* remains within the mandibular canal and forms a nerve plexus that innervates the pulpal tissues of the mandibular first premolar, canine, and incisors via the dental branches. The *mental nerve* exits the canal through the mental foramen and divides into three branches that innervate the skin of the chin and the skin and mucous membrane of the lower lip.

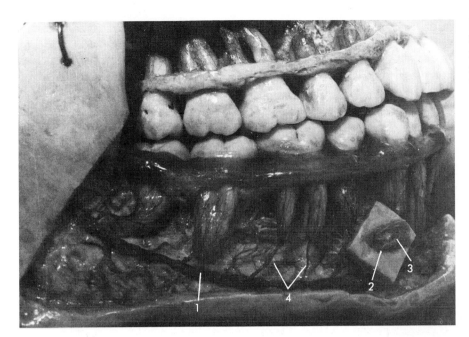

Fig. 12-17 Branches of V_3 within the mandibular canal (lateral plate of bone removed). *1,* Inferior alveolar nerve; *2,* mental foramen; *3,* mental nerve; *4,* dental branches.

Summary The following outline summarizes the branches of the mandibular division (italicized nerves denote those especially significant in dental pain control):

1. Undivided nerve
   a. Nervus spinosus
   b. Nerve to the medial pterygoid muscle
2. Divided nerve
   a. Anterior division
      (1) Nerve to the lateral pterygoid muscle
      (2) Nerve to the masseter muscle
      (3) Nerve to the temporal muscle
      (4) Buccal nerve
   b. Posterior division
      (1) Auriculotemporal nerve
      (2) Lingual nerve
      (3) Mylohyoid nerve
      (4) Inferior alveolar nerve: dental branches
      (5) Incisive branch: dental branches
      (6) Mental nerve

OSTEOLOGY: MAXILLA

In addition to the neuroanatomy of pain control in dentistry, it is important to be aware of the relationship of these nerves to the osseous and soft tissues through which they course.

The maxilla (more properly, the right and left maxillae) is the largest bone of the face, excluding the mandible. Its anterior (or facial) surface (Fig. 12-18) is directed both forward and laterally. At its inferior borders are a series of eminences that correspond to the roots of the maxillary teeth. The most prominent is usually found

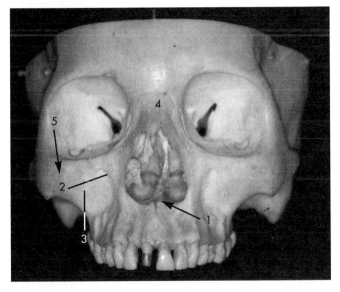

Fig. 12-18 Skull with the mandible removed. Notice in particular the root eminences of the maxillary teeth. *1,* Anterior nasal spine; *2,* infraorbital foramen; *3,* maxilla; *4,* nasal bone; *5,* zygomatic bone.

over the canine tooth, often referred to as the *canine eminence.* Superior to the canine fossa (located just distal to the canine eminence) is the infraorbital foramen, through which blood vessels and terminal branches of the infraorbital nerve emerge. Bone in the region of the maxillary teeth is quite commonly of the more porous cancellous variety, leading to a significantly greater incidence of clinically adequate anesthesia than in areas where more dense cortical bone is present, such as in the mandible. In many areas bone over the apices of the maxillary teeth either is paper thin or shows evidence of dehiscence (Fig. 12-19).

The inferior temporal surface of the maxilla is directed backward and laterally (Fig. 12-20). Its posterior surface is pierced by several alveolar canals that transmit the posterior superior alveolar nerves and blood vessels. The maxillary tuberosity, a rounded eminence, is found on the inferior posterior surface. On the superior surface is a groove, directed laterally and slightly superiorly, through which the maxillary nerve passes. This groove is continuous with the infraorbital groove.

The palatal processes of the maxilla are thick horizontal projections that form a large portion of the floor of the nose and the roof of the mouth. The bone here is considerably thicker anteriorly than posteriorly. Its inferior (or palatal) surface constitutes the anterior three fourths of the hard palate (Fig. 12-21). Many foramina (passages for nutrient blood vessels) perforate it. Along its lateral border, at the junction with the alveolar process, is a groove through which the anterior palatine nerve passes from the greater palatine foramen. In the midline in the anterior region is the funnel-shaped opening of the incisive foramen. In this opening four canals are located—two for the descending palatine arteries, and two for the nasopalatine nerves. In many skulls, especially those of younger persons, a fine suture line extends laterally from the incisive foramen to the border of the palatine process by the canine teeth. The small area anterior to this suture is termed the *premaxilla*.

The horizontal plate of the palatine bone forms the posterior fourth of the hard palate. Its anterior border articulates with the palatine process of the maxilla, and its posterior border serves as the attachment for the soft palate. Foramina are present on its surface, representing the lower end of the pterygopalatine canal, through which descending palatine blood vessels and the anterior palatine nerve run.

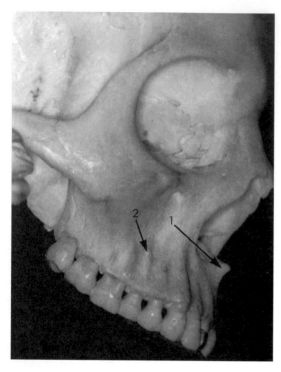

Fig. 12-19 Maxilla. *1*, Anterior nasal spine; *2*, dehiscence over the root of the first premolar.

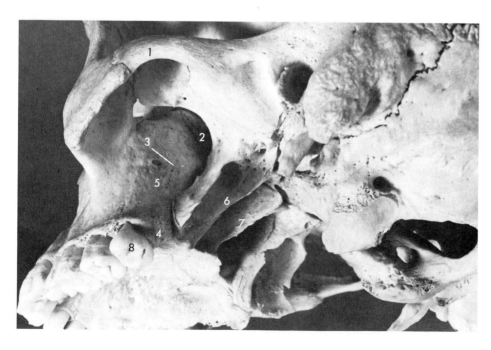

Fig. 12-20 Inferior temporal aspect of the maxilla. *1*, Zygomatic arch; *2*, pterygomaxillary fissure and pterygopalatine fossa; *3*, foramina for the posterior superior alveolar nerve; *4*, maxillary tuberosity; *5*, inferior temporal (posterior) surface; *6*, lateral pterygoid plate; *7*, medial pterygoid plate; *8*, maxillary third molar.

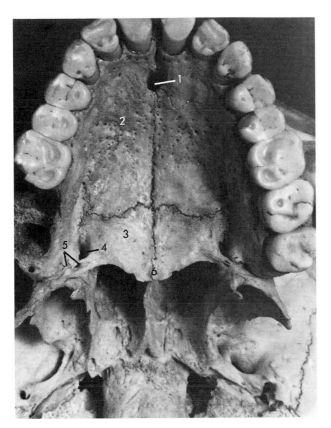

Fig. 12-21 Palate. *1,* Incisive foramen; *2,* palatal process of the maxilla; *3,* horizontal process of the palatal bone; *4,* greater palatine foramen; *5,* lesser palatine foramen; *6,* posterior nasal spine.

OSTEOLOGY: MANDIBLE

The mandible is the largest and strongest bone of the face. It consists of a curved horizontal portion (the body) and two perpendicular portions (the rami).

The external (lateral) surface of the *body* of the mandible is marked in the midline by a faint ridge, an indication of the symphysis of the two pieces of bone from which the mandible is created (Figs. 12-22 and 12-23). The bone forming the buccal alveolar processes in the anterior region (incisors) is usually less dense than that over the posterior teeth, permitting infiltration (supraperiosteal) anesthesia to be employed with some expectation of success (in adults usually in the area of the lateral incisor only). In the region of the second premolar on each side, midway between the upper and lower borders of the body, lies the mental foramen. Phillips et al, in an evaluation of 75 dry, adult human mandibles, determined that the usual position of the mental foramen is below the crown of the second premolar.[7] The mental nerve, artery, and vein exit the mandibular canal here. Bone along this external surface of the mandible is commonly quite thick cortical bone.

The lingual border of the body of the mandible is concave from side to side (Fig. 12-24). Extending upward and backward is the mylohyoid line, giving origin to the mylohyoid muscle. Bone along the lingual of the mandible is usually quite thick; however, in approximately 68% of mandibles there are lingual foramina located in the posterior (molar) region.[8] The function of

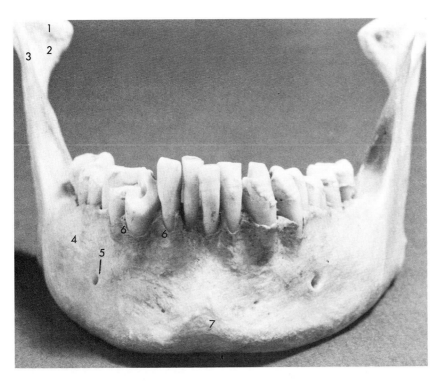

Fig. 12-22 Mandible. *1,* Condylar head; *2,* condylar neck; *3,* coronoid process; *4,* body; *5,* mental foramen; *6,* alveolar process; *7,* mental protuberance.

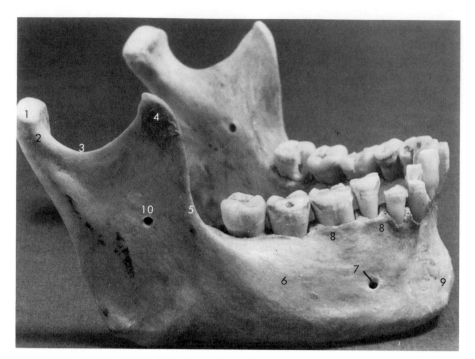

Fig. 12-23 Mandible. Notice the density of bone compared with that of the maxilla (Fig. 12-19). *1*, Head of the condyle; *2*, neck of the condyle; *3*, sigmoid (mandibular) notch; *4*, coronoid process; *5*, coronoid notch; *6*, body; *7*, mental foramen; *8*, alveolar process; *9*, mental protuberance; *10*, artifact.

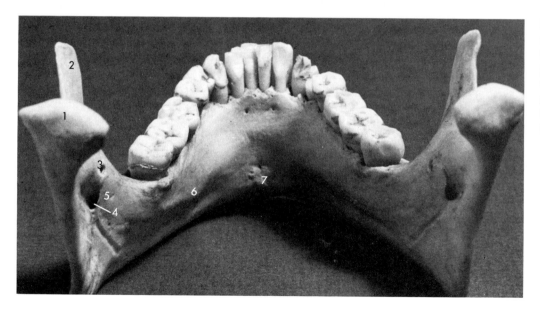

Fig. 12-24 Lingual border of the mandible. *1*, Head of the condyle; *2*, coronoid process; *3*, artifact; *4*, mandibular foramen; *5*, lingula; *6*, mylohyoid line; *7*, superior and inferior mental spines.

these foramina is as yet unclear, but some may contain sensory fibers from the mylohyoid nerve that innervate portions of mandibular molars.[3]

The lateral surface of each *ramus* is flat, composed of quite dense cortical bone and providing attachment for the masseter muscle along most of its surface (Fig. 12-23). The medial surface (Fig. 12-24) contains the mandibular foramen, located approximately halfway between the superior and inferior borders and two thirds to three fourths the distance from the anterior border of the ramus to its posterior border.[9] Other studies of the anteroposterior location of the mandibular foramen

have provided differing locations. Hayward et al.[10] found the foramen most often in the third quadrant from the anterior part of the ramus, Monheim[11] found it at the midpoint of the ramus, whereas Hetson et al[12] located it at 55% distal to the anterior ramus (a range of 44.4% to 65.5%). The mandibular canal extends obliquely downward and anteriorly within the ramus. It then courses horizontally forward in the body, distributing small dental branches to the mandibular teeth posterior to the mental foramen. The mandibular foramen is the entrance through which the inferior alveolar nerve, artery, and vein enter the mandibular canal. The height of this fora-

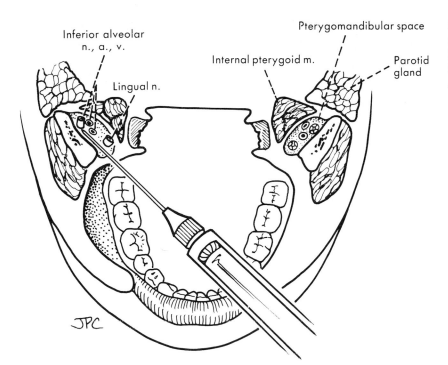

Inferior alveolar
n., a., v.

Lingual n.

Pterygomandibular space

Internal pterygoid m.

Parotid gland

JPC

Fig. 12-25 Pathway of needle in inferior alveolar nerve block. *(From Bennett CR: Monheim's local anesthesia and pain control in dental practice, ed 7, 1984, St Louis, Mosby–Year Book.)*

men varies greatly, ranging from 1 to 19 mm or more above the level of the occlusal plane.[10] A prominent ridge, the lingula mandibulae, lies on the anterior margin of the foramen. The lingula serves as an attachment for the sphenomandibular ligament. At the lower end of the mandibular foramen the mylohyoid groove begins, coursing obliquely downward and anteriorly. In this groove lie the mylohyoid nerve and vessels.

Bone along the lingual surface of the mandible is usually quite dense. On very rare occasions bone over the lingual aspect of the third molar roots will be less dense, permitting a greater chance of supraperiosteal anesthesia.

The superior border of the ramus has two processes: the coronoid anteriorly and the condylar posteriorly. Between these two processes is a deep concavity, the mandibular (sigmoid) notch. The coronoid process is thinner than the condylar. Its anterior border is concave, the coronoid notch. The coronoid notch represents a landmark for determining the height of needle penetration in the inferior alveolar nerve block technique. The condylar process is thicker than the coronoid. The condylar head, the thickened articular portion of the condyle, sits atop the constricted neck of the condyle. The condylar neck is flattened front to back. On its anterior surface is the attachment for the external pterygoid muscle.

When cut horizontally at the level of the mandibular foramen, the ramus of the mandible can be seen to be thicker in its anterior region than it is posteriorly (Fig. 12-25). This is of clinical importance during the inferior alveolar nerve block. The thickness of soft tissues between needle penetration and the osseous tissues of the ramus at

the level of the mandibular foramen averages about 20 to 25 mm. Because of the increased thickness of bone in the anterior third of the ramus, the thickness of soft tissue is decreased accordingly (approximately 10 mm). Knowing the depth of penetration of soft tissue before contacting osseous tissues can aid the administrator in determining correct positioning of the needle tip.

REFERENCES

1. DuBrul EL: *Sicher's oral anatomy,* ed 7, St Louis, 1980, Mosby–Year Book.
2. Loetscher CA, Walton RE: Patterns of innervation of the maxillary first molar: a dissection study, *Oral Surg* 65:86-90, 1988.
3. Heasman PA: Clinical anatomy of the superior alveolar nerves, *Br J Oral Maxillofac Surg* 22:439-447, 1984.
4. McDaniel WL: Variations in nerve distributions of the maxillary teeth, *J Dent Res* 35:916-921, 1956.
5. Langlais RP, Broadus R, Glass BJ: Bifid mandibular canals in panoramic radiographs, *J Am Dent Assoc* 110:923-926, 1985.
6. Frommer J, Mele FA, Monroe CW: The possible role of the mylohyoid nerve in mandibular posterior tooth sensation, *J Am Dent Assoc* 85:113-117, 1972.
7. Phillips JL, Weller N, Kulild JC: The mental foramen: Part III. Size and position on panoramic radiographs, *J Endodont* 18(8):383-386, 1992.
8. Shiller WR, Wiswell OB: Lingual foramina of the mandible, *Anat Rec* 119:387-390, 1954.
9. Bremer G: Measurements of special significance in connection with anesthesia of the inferior alveolar nerve, *Oral Surg* 5:966-988, 1952.
10. Hayward J, Richardson ER, Malhotra SK: The mandibular foramen: its anteroposterior position, *Oral Surg* 44:837-843, 1977.
11. Monheim LM: Local anesthesia and pain control in dental practice, ed 4, St Louis, 1969, Mosby–Year Book, p 49.
12. Hetson G, Share J, Frommer J, Kronman JH: Statistical evaluation of the position of the mandibular ramus, *Oral Surg* 65:32-34, 1988.

thirteen

Techniques of Maxillary Anesthesia

There are several general methods of obtaining pain control with local anesthetics. The site of deposition of the drug relative to the area of operative intervention determines the type of injection administered. Three major types of local anesthetic injection can be differentiated—local infiltration, field block, and nerve block.

Local infiltration Small terminal nerve endings *in the area* of the dental treatment are flooded with local anesthetic solution. Incision (or treatment) is then made *into the same area* in which the solution has been deposited (Fig. 13-1). An example of local infiltration would be the administration of a local anesthetic into an interproximal papilla prior to root planing.

Field block Local anesthetic solution is deposited near the larger terminal nerve branches so the anesthetized area will be circumscribed, to prevent the passage of impulses from the tooth to the central nervous system (CNS). Incision (or treatment) is then made into an area *away from* the site of injection of the anesthetic (Fig. 13-2). Maxillary injections administered above the apex of the tooth to be treated are properly termed field blocks (although common usage identifies them as infiltration or supraperiosteal).

Nerve block Local anesthetic is deposited close to a main nerve trunk, usually *at a distance* from the site of operative intervention (Fig. 13-3). Posterior superior alveolar, inferior alveolar, and nasopalatine injections are examples of nerve blocks.

Discussion Technically, the injection commonly referred to in dentistry as a local infiltration is a field block, since anesthetic solution is deposited at or above the apex of the tooth to be treated. Terminal nerve branches to the pulpal and soft tissues distal to the injection site are anesthetized.

Field block and nerve block may be distinguished by the extent of anesthesia achieved. In general, field blocks are more circumscribed, involving the tissues in and around one or two teeth, whereas nerve blocks affect a larger area (e.g., that observed following inferior alveolar or infraorbital nerve block).

The type of injection administered for a given treatment will be determined by the extent of the operative area. For management of small, isolated areas, *infiltration anesthesia* may suffice. When two or three teeth are being restored, *field block* is indicated, while for pain control in quadrant dentistry, *regional block anesthesia* is recommended.

MAXILLARY INJECTION TECHNIQUES

A number of injection techniques are available to aid in providing clinically adequate anesthesia of the teeth and soft and hard tissues in the maxilla. Selection of the specific technique to be used is determined, in large part, by the nature of the treatment to be provided. The available techniques are as follows:

1. *Supraperiosteal* (infiltration), recommended for limited treatment protocols
2. *Periodontal ligament* (PDL, intraligamentary) *injection,* recommended as an adjunct to other techniques or for limited treatment protocols

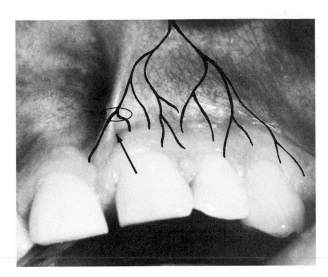

Fig. 13-1 Local infiltration. The area of treatment is flooded with local anesthetic. An incision is made into the same area

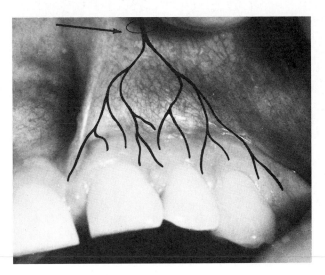

Fig. 13-3 Nerve block. Local anesthetic is deposited close to the main nerve trunk, located at a distance from the site of incision (*arrow*).

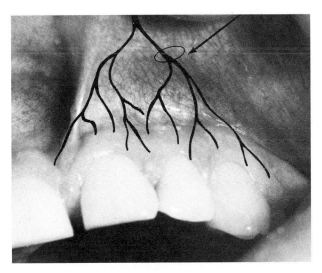

Fig. 13-2 Field block. Local anesthetic is deposited near the larger terminal nerve endings (*arrow*). An incision is made away from the site of injection.

3. *Intraseptal injection,* recommended primarily for periodontal surgical techniques
4. *Intraosseous injection,* recommended for single teeth (primarily mandibular molars) when other techniques have failed
5. *Posterior superior alveolar nerve block,* recommended for management of several molar teeth in one quadrant
6. *Middle superior alveolar nerve block,* recommended for management of premolars in one quadrant
7. *Anterior superior alveolar* (infraorbital) *nerve block,* recommended for management of anterior teeth in one quadrant

8. *Maxillary* (second division) *nerve block,* recommended for extensive buccal, palatal, and pulpal management in one quadrant
9. *Greater* (anterior) *palatine nerve block,* recommended for palatal soft and osseous tissue treatment distal to the canine in one quadrant
10. *Nasopalatine nerve block,* recommended for palatal soft and osseous tissue management from canine to canine bilaterally

The supraperiosteal, periodontal ligament, intraseptal, and intraosseous injections are appropriate for administration in either the maxilla or the mandible. Because of the great success of the supraperiosteal injection in the maxillary arch, it will be discussed in this chapter. The periodontal ligament, intraseptal, and intraosseous injections are supplemental injections that are of somewhat greater importance in the mandible and are described in Chapter 15.

TEETH AND BUCCAL SOFT AND HARD TISSUES
Supraperiosteal Injection

The supraperiosteal injection, more commonly (but incorrectly) called local infiltration, is the most frequently used local anesthetic technique for obtaining pulpal anesthesia in maxillary teeth. Although it is a rather simple procedure to accomplish successfully, there are several valid reasons for using other techniques (e.g., regional nerve blocks) whenever more than two or three teeth are involved in treatment.

Multiple supraperiosteal injections require numerous needle penetrations of the tissue, each with the potential for producing pain, either during the procedure or after the anesthetic effect has resolved. In addition, and perhaps even more important, using supraperiosteal injections for pulpal anesthesia on multiple teeth leads to the administration of a larger volume of local anesthetic solution, with an attendant increase in the risk of systemic and local complications.

The supraperiosteal injection is indicated whenever dental procedures are confined to a relatively circumscribed area in either the maxilla or the mandible.

Other common names Local infiltration, paraperiosteal injection

Nerves anesthetized Large terminal branches of the dental plexus

Areas anesthetized The entire region innervated by the large terminal branches of this plexus: pulp and root area of the tooth, buccal periosteum, connective tissue, mucous membrane (Fig. 13-4)

Indications

1. Pulpal anesthesia of the maxillary teeth when treatment is limited to one or two teeth
2. Soft tissue anesthesia when indicated for surgical procedures in a circumscribed area

Contraindications

1. Infection or acute inflammation in the area of injection.
2. Dense bone covering the apices of teeth (can be determined only by trial and error; most likely over

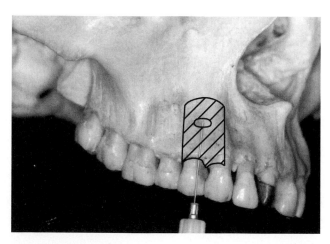

Fig. 13-4 Supraperiosteal injection in the anterior region of the maxilla. Notice the placement of the needle and the area anesthetized.

the permanent maxillary first molar in children because the apex of this tooth lies beneath the zygomatic bone, which is relatively dense). The central incisor apex may also be located beneath denser bone (i.e., of the nose), thereby increasing the failure rate (though not significantly).

Advantages
1. High success rate (> 95%)
2. Technically easy injection
3. Usually entirely atraumatic

Disadvantages Not recommended for large areas, because of the need for multiple needle insertions and the necessity to administer larger total volumes of anesthetic solution

Positive aspiration Negligible, but possible (< 1%)

Alternatives PDL injection, regional nerve block

Technique
1. A 25- or 27-gauge short needle recommended
2. Area of insertion: height of the mucobuccal fold above the apex of the tooth to be anesthetized
3. Target area: apical region of the tooth to be anesthetized
4. Landmarks
   a. Mucobuccal fold
   b. Crown of the tooth
   c. Root contour of the tooth
5. Orientation of the bevel*: *toward* bone
6. Procedure
   a. Prepare the tissue at the injection site.
      (1) Clean with sterile dry gauze.
      (2) Apply topical antiseptic (optional).
      (3) Apply topical anesthetic.
   b. Orient the needle bevel so it faces the bone.
   c. Lift the lip, pulling the tissue taut.
   d. Hold the syringe parallel with the long axis of the tooth (Fig. 13-5).
   e. Insert the needle into the height of the mucobuccal fold over the target tooth.

---

*Bevel orientations are specified for all injection techniques in Chapters 13 and 14. The orientation of the needle bevel is *not* a significant factor in the success or failure of an injection technique, and these recommendations need not be rigidly adhered to; yet there will be a fuller expectation of successful anesthesia if they are followed, provided all other technical and anatomical principles are maintained. In general, whenever possible, the bevel of the needle is to be facing toward bone; then, in the unlikely event that the needle comes into contact with bone, the bevel will slide over periosteum, provoking minor discomfort, but not tearing the periosteum. If the bevel faces away from bone, the sharp point of the needle would contact periosteum, tearing it and leading to a more painful (subperiosteal) injection. Postinjection discomfort is considerably greater with subperiosteal than with supraperiosteal injections.

f. Advance it until the bevel is at or above the apical region of the tooth (Table 13-1); in most instances the depth of penetration will be only a few millimeters. Since the needle is in soft tissue (not touching bone), there should be *no* resistance to its advancement, nor should there be any patient discomfort with this injection.

g. Aspirate.
   (1) If negative, deposit approximately 0.6 ml (one third of a cartridge) slowly over 20 seconds. (Do not permit the tissues to balloon.)

h. Slowly withdraw the syringe.

i. Make the needle safe.

j. Wait 2 to 3 minutes before commencing the dental procedure.

Signs and symptoms
1. Feeling of numbness in the area of administration
2. Absence of pain during treatment

Safety features
1. Minimum opportunity for intravascular administration.
2. Slowness of injection, aspiration

TABLE 13-1 Average Tooth Length				
	Length of crown (mm)	+	Length of root (mm)	=	Length of tooth
Maxillary				
Central incisors	11.6		12.4		24.0
Lateral incisors	9.0 to 10.2		12.3 to 13.5		22.5
Canines	10.9		16.1		27.0
First premolars	8.7		13.0		21.7
Second premolars	7.9		13.6		21.5
First molars	7.7		13.6		21.3
Second molars	7.7		13.4		21.1
Third molars	Extremely variable		Extremely variable		Extremely variable
Mandibular				
Central incisors	9.4		12.0		21.4
Lateral incisors	9.9		13.3		23.2
Canines	11.4		14.0		25.4
First premolars	7.5 to 11.0		11.0 to 16.0		18.5 to 27.0
Second premolars	8.5		14.7		23.2
First molars	8.3		14.5		22.8
Second molars	8.1		14.7		22.8
Third molars	Extremely variable		Extremely variable		Extremely variable

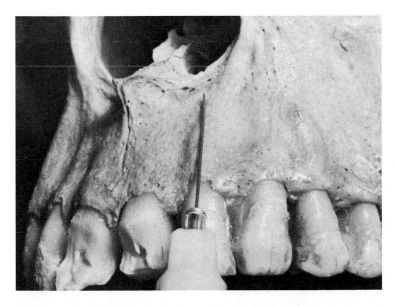

Fig. 13-5 The syringe should be held parallel with the long axis of the tooth and inserted at the height of the mucobuccal fold over the tooth.

Precautions Do not use for larger areas. A greater number of tissue penetrations increases the possibility of pain both during and after the injection, and the larger volume of solution administered increases the possibility of local anesthetic overdose and postinjection pain.

Failures of anesthesia

1. Needle tip lies below the apex (along the root) of the tooth (Table 13-1). Depositing anesthetic solution below the apex of a maxillary tooth will result in excellent soft tissue anesthesia but poor or absent pulpal anesthesia.
2. Needle tip lies too far from the bone (solution deposited in the buccal soft tissues). To correct: Redirect the needle toward the periosteum.

Complications Pain on needle insertion with the needle tip against periosteum. To correct: Withdraw the needle and reinsert it farther from the periosteum.

Posterior Superior Alveolar Nerve Block

The posterior superior alveolar (PSA) nerve block is a commonly used dental nerve block. Although it is a highly successful technique (> 90%), there are several issues to weigh when considering its use. These include the extent of anesthesia produced and the potential for hematoma formation.

When used to achieve pulpal anesthesia, the PSA nerve block is effective for the maxillary third, second, and first molars in 77% to 100% of patients.[1] However, the mesiobuccal root of the maxillary first molar is not consistently innervated by the PSA nerve. In a dissection study by Loetscher et al[2] the middle superior alveolar nerve provided sensory innervation to the mesiobuccal root of the maxillary first molar in 28% of the specimens examined. Therefore a second injection, usually a supraperiosteal, is indicated following the PSA nerve block when effective anesthesia of the first molar does not develop after the PSA. Loetscher et al concluded by stating that the PSA nerve *usually* provides sole pulpal innervation to the maxillary first molar and that a single PSA nerve block usually provides clinically adequate pulpal anesthesia.

The risk of a potential complication must also be considered whenever the PSA block is used. Penetration of the needle too far distally may lead to a temporarily unaesthetic hematoma. When the PSA is to be administered, one must always consider the patient's (skull) size in determining the depth of soft tissue penetration. An "average" depth of penetration in a patient who has a smaller than average skull may produce a hematoma, whereas a needle inserted "too far" in a larger-skulled patient might not provide anesthesia of any teeth. As a means of decreasing the risk of hematoma formation following a PSA nerve block, the use of a "short" dental needle is recommended for all but the largest of patients (the 25-gauge

long needle was previously recommended for use in the PSA). Since the average depth of soft tissue penetration from the insertion site (the mucobuccal fold over the maxillary second molar) to the area of the PSA nerves is 16 mm, the short dental needle (approximately 20 mm in length) can be successfully and safely used. Overinsertion of the needle is less likely to occur, thereby minimizing the risk of hematoma formation. The 25-gauge short needle is preferred, but in its absence a 27-gauge short needle may be used as long as aspiration is performed carefully and the anesthetic solution is injected slowly. One must remember to aspirate several times before and during drug deposition during a PSA nerve block, in order to avoid inadvertent intravascular injection.

Other common names Tuberosity block, zygomatic block

Nerves anesthetized Posterior superior alveolar and branches

Areas anesthetized

1. Pulps of the maxillary third, second, and first molars (entire tooth = 72%; mesiobuccal root of the maxillary first molar not anesthetized = 28%)
2. Buccal periodontium and bone overlying these teeth (Fig. 13-6)

Indications

1. Treatment involving two or more maxillary molars
2. When supraperiosteal injection is contraindicated (e.g., with infection or acute inflammation)
3. When supraperiosteal injection has proved ineffective

Contraindication When the risk of hemorrhage is too great—as with a hemophiliac—in which case a supraperiosteal or PDL injection is recommended

Advantages

1. Atraumatic; with the PSA block administered properly, there is usually no pain experienced by the patient because of the relatively large area of soft tissue into which the anesthetic is deposited and the fact that bone is not contacted
2. High success rate (> 95%)
3. Minimum number of injections required
   a. One injection compared with option of three infiltrations
4. Minimizes the total volume of anesthetic solution injected
   a. Equivalent volume of anesthetic solution required for three supraperiosteal injections = 1.8 ml

Disadvantages

1. Risk of hematoma, which is usually diffuse; also quite discomfiting and embarrassing to the patient

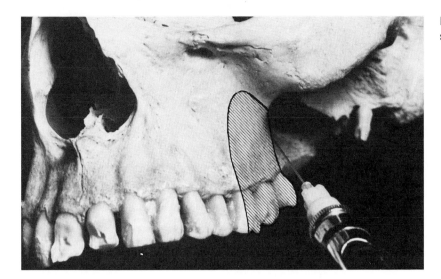

Fig. 13-6 Area anesthetized by a posterior superior alveolar (PSA) nerve block.

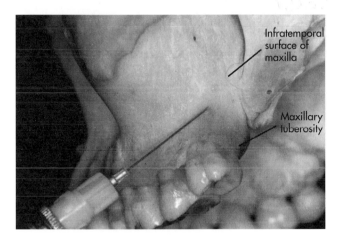

Fig. 13-7 Needle at the target area for a PSA nerve block.

2. Technique somewhat arbitrary: no bony landmarks during insertion
3. Second injection required for treatment of the first molar (mesiobuccal root) in 28% of patients

Positive aspiration   Approximately 3.1%

Alternatives
1. Supraperiosteal or PDL injections for pulpal and root anesthesia
2. Infiltrations for the buccal periodontium and hard tissues
3. Maxillary nerve block

Technique
1. A 25-gauge short needle recommended, though the 27-gauge short is more likely to be available and is also acceptable
2. Area of insertion: height of the mucobuccal fold above the maxillary second molar

3. Target area: PSA nerve—posterior, superior, and medial to the posterior border of the maxilla (Fig. 13-7)
4. Landmarks
   a. Mucobuccal fold
   b. Maxillary tuberosity
   c. Zygomatic process of the maxilla
5. Orientation of the bevel: *toward* bone during the injection. If bone is accidentally touched, the sensation will be less unpleasant.
6. Procedure
   a. Assume the correct position (Fig. 13-8).
      (1) For a left PSA nerve block and a right-handed administrator, sit at the 10 o'clock position facing the patient.
      (2) For a right PSA block and a right-handed administrator, sit at the 8 o'clock position facing the patient.
   b. Prepare the tissues at the height of the mucobuccal fold for penetration.
      (1) Dry with sterile gauze.
      (2) Apply topical antiseptic (optional).
      (3) Apply topical anesthetic.
   c. Orient the bevel of the needle *toward* bone.
   d. Partially open the patient's mouth, pulling the mandible to the side of injection.
   e. Retract the patient's cheek with your finger (for visibility).
   f. Pull the tissues at the injection site taut.
   g. Insert the needle into the height of the mucobuccal fold over the second molar (Fig. 13-9).
   h. Advance it slowly in an upward, inward, and backward direction (Fig. 13-10) *in one movement* (not three).
      (1) *Upward:* superiorly at a 45-degree angle to the occlusal plane
      (2) *Inward:* medially toward the midline at a 45-degree angle to the occlusal plane (Fig. 13-11)

Fig. 13-8 Position of the administrator for a right, **A**, and left, **B**, PSA nerve block.

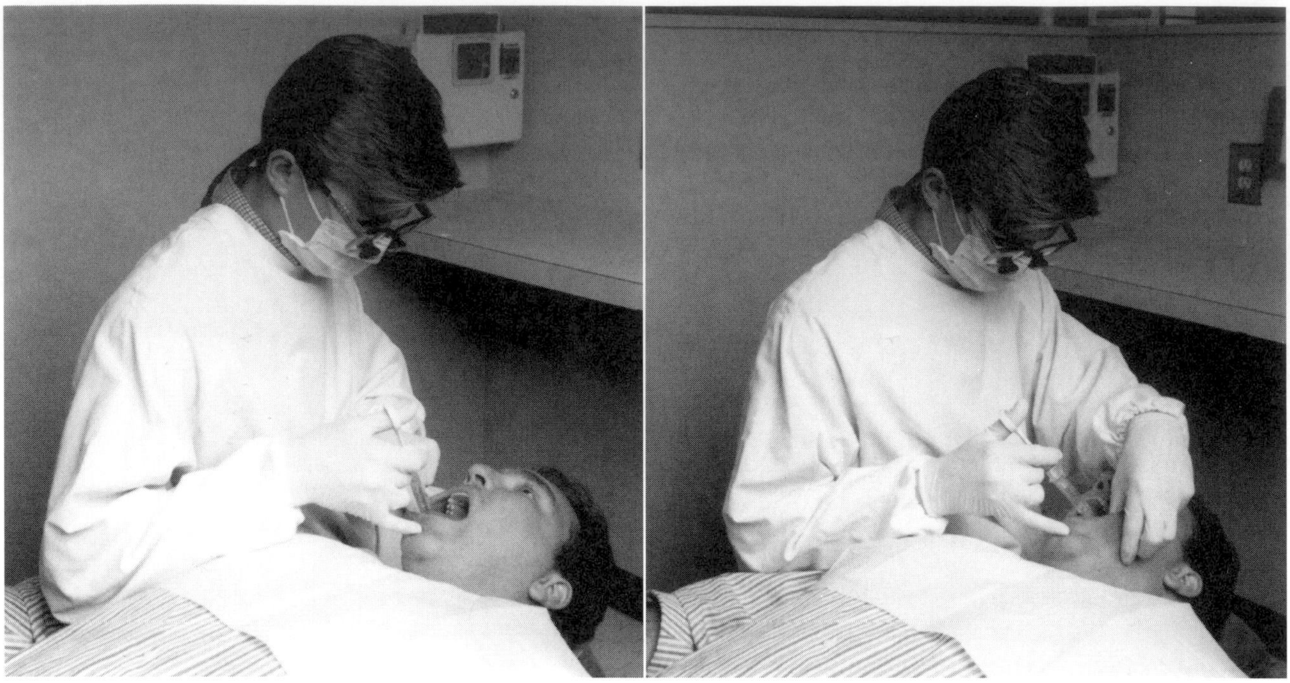

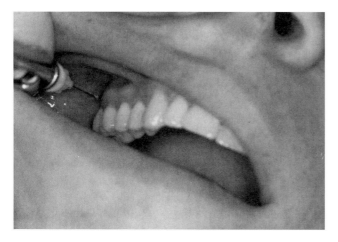

Fig. 13-9 PSA nerve block. Tissue retracted at the site of penetration. Notice the orientation of the needle toward the midline.

(3) *Backward:* posteriorly at a 45-degree angle to the long axis of the second molar
i. Slowly advance the needle through soft tissue.
   (1) There should be no resistance and therefore no discomfort to the patient.
   (2) If resistance (bone) is felt, the angle of the needle in toward the midline is too great; then
      (a) Withdraw the needle slightly (but do not remove it entirely from the tissues) and bring the syringe barrel closer to the occlusal plane.

(b) Readvance the needle.
j. Advance the needle to the desired depth (Fig. 13-11).
   (1) In an adult of normal size, penetration to a depth of 16 mm will place the needle tip in the immediate vicinity of the foramina through which the PSA nerves enter the posterior face of the maxilla. When a long needle is used (average length 32 mm), it is inserted half its length into the tissue. With a short needle (average length 20 mm), 4 mm should remain visible.
   (2) For smaller adults and children it is prudent to halt the advance of the needle short of its usual depth of penetration, to avoid a possible hematoma caused by overpenetration. Penetrating to a depth of 10 to 14 mm will place the needle tip in the target area in most small-skulled patients.
   (3) Halting the advance of the needle slightly short of 16 mm depth in all patients will usually provide adequate anesthesia of the PSA nerves because of the relative porosity of bone in this region, although solution is *not* deposited on the posterior surface of the maxilla.
   (4) *Note:* The goal is to deposit local anesthetic close to the PSA nerves, located posterosuperior and medial to the maxillary tuberosity.
k. Aspirate in two planes.
l. Rotate the syringe barrel (needle bevel) one-fourth turn and reaspirate.
m. If *both* aspirations are negative

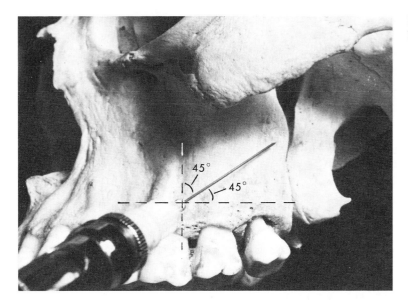

Fig. 13-10 Advance the needle upward, inward, and backward.

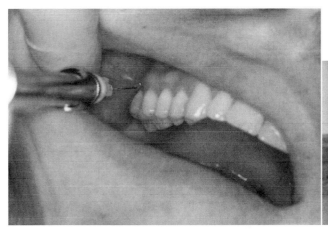

A

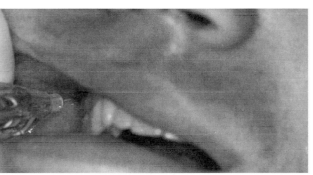

B

Fig. 13-11 A, With a "long" dental needle in an average-sized adult, the depth of penetration is half its length and the risk of overinsertion and hematoma is increased. **B,** The depth of penetration for an average-sized adult is 16 mm. With a "short" dental needle (25- or 27-gauge) 4 mm will remain visible in the oral cavity.

(1) Slowly, over 30 to 60 seconds, deposit 0.9 to 1.8 ml of anesthetic solution.
(2) Aspirate several times during the procedure.
(3) The PSA injection is usually atraumatic because of the large tissue space available to accommodate the anesthetic solution and the fact that bone is not touched.
n. Slowly withdraw the syringe.
o. Make the needle safe.
p. Wait 3 to 5 minutes before commencing the dental procedure.

Signs and symptoms
1. Usually no symptoms; the patient has difficulty reaching this region to determine the extent of anesthesia

2. Absence of pain during therapy

Safety features
1. Slow injection, repeated aspirations
2. No anatomical safety features to prevent overinsertion of the needle; therefore careful observation is required

Precaution Check the depth of needle penetration: overinsertion (too deep) increases the risk of hematoma; too shallow may still provide adequate anesthesia

Failures of anesthesia
1. Needle too lateral. To correct: Redirect the needle tip medially. (See complication *2*, below.)

2. Needle not high enough. To correct: Redirect the needle tip superiorly.
3. Needle too far posterior. To correct: Withdraw it to the proper depth.

Complications
1. Hematoma
   a. This is commonly produced by inserting the needle too far posteriorly into the pterygoid plexus of veins. Additionally, the maxillary artery may be perforated. Use of a short needle minimizes the risk of pterygoid plexus puncture.
   b. A visible hematoma develops within several minutes, usually noted in the buccal tissues of the mandibular region. (See Chapter 17.)
      (1) There is no easily accessible area to which pressure can be applied to stop the hemorrhage.
      (2) Bleeding continues until the pressure of the extravascular blood is equal to or greater than that of intravascular blood.
2. Mandibular anesthesia
   a. The mandibular division of the fifth cranial nerve (V_3) is located lateral to the PSA nerves. Deposition of local anesthetic lateral to the desired location can produce varying degrees of mandibular anesthesia. Most often, when this occurs, patients will mention that their tongue and perhaps their lower lip are anesthetized.

Middle Superior Alveolar Nerve Block

The MSA nerve is present in only about 28% of the population. Therefore this block has limited clinical usefulness. However, when the infraorbital nerve block fails to achieve pulpal anesthesia distal to the maxillary canine, the MSA block is indicated for procedures on premolars and for the mesiobuccal root of the maxillary first molar. The success rate of the MSA nerve block is high.

Nerves anesthetized Middle superior alveolar and terminal branches

Areas anesthetized
1. Pulps of the maxillary first and second premolars, mesiobuccal root of the first molar
2. Buccal periodontal tissues and bone over these same teeth (Fig. 13-12)

Indications
1. When infraorbital nerve block fails to provide pulpal anesthesia distal to the maxillary canine
2. Dental procedures involving both maxillary premolars only

Contraindications
1. Infection or inflammation in the area of injection or needle insertion or drug deposition

2. Where the MSA nerve is absent, innervation is through the anterior superior alveolar (ASA) nerve; branches of the ASA innervating the premolars and mesiobuccal root of the first molar can be anesthetized by means of the MSA technique

Advantages Minimizes the number of injections and volume of solution

Disadvantages None

Positive aspiration Negligible ($< 3\%$)

Alternatives
1. Local infiltration (supraperiosteal), PDL injection
2. Infraorbital nerve block for the first and second premolar and mesiobuccal root of the first molar

Technique
1. A 25-gauge short or long needle recommended, though the 27-gauge short is more likely to be used and is perfectly acceptable
2. Area of insertion: height of the mucobuccal fold above the maxillary second premolar
3. Target area: maxillary bone above the apex of the maxillary second premolar (Fig. 13-13)
4. Landmark: mucobuccal fold above the maxillary second premolar
5. Orientation of the bevel: *toward* bone
6. Procedure
   a. Assume the correct position (Fig. 13-14).
      (1) For a right MSA nerve block and right-handed administrator, face the patient from the 10 o'clock position.
      (2) For a left MSA block, face the patient directly from the 8 or 9 o'clock position.
   b. Prepare the tissues at the site of injection.

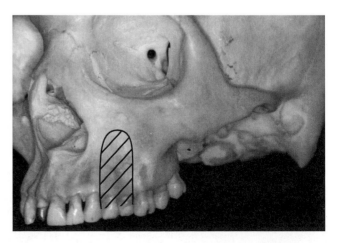

Fig. 13-12 Area anesthetized by a middle superior alveolar (MSA) nerve block.

(1) Dry with sterile gauze.

(2) Apply topical antiseptic (optional).

(3) Apply topical anesthetic.

c. Stretch the patient's upper lip to make the tissues taut and to gain visibility.

d. Insert the needle into the height of the mucobuccal fold above the second premolar with the bevel directed toward bone.

e. Penetrate the mucous membrane and slowly advance the needle until its tip is located well above the apex of the second premolar (Fig. 13-15).

f. Aspirate.

g. Slowly deposit 0.9 to 1.2 ml (half to two-thirds cartridge) of solution (approximately 30 to 45 sec).

h. Withdraw the syringe and make the needle safe.

i. Wait 2 to 3 minutes before commencing dental therapy.

Signs and symptoms

1. Upper lip numb
2. No pain during dental therapy

Safety features   Relatively avascular area, anatomically safe

Precautions   To avoid pain, do not insert too close to the periosteum and do not inject too rapidly; the MSA should be an atraumatic injection

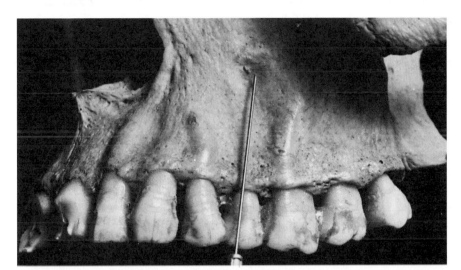

Fig. 13-13 Needle in position above the second premolar for an MSA nerve block.

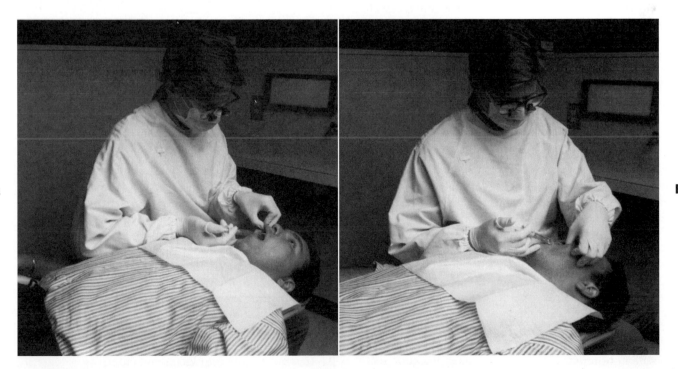

Fig. 13-14 Position of the administrator for a right, **A**, and left, **B**, MSA nerve block.

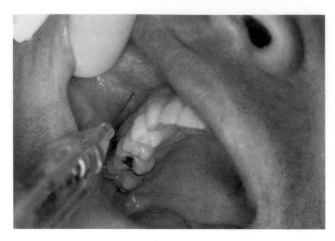

Fig. 13-15 Needle penetration for an MSA nerve block.

Failures of anesthesia

1. Anesthetic solution not deposited high above the apex of the second premolar
   a. To correct: Check radiographs and increase the depth of penetration.
2. Deposition of solution too far from the maxillary bone with the needle placed in tissues lateral to the height of the mucobuccal fold
   a. To correct: Reinsert at the height of the mucobuccal fold.
3. Bone of the zygomatic arch at the site of injection preventing the diffusion of anesthetic
   a. To correct: Use the supraperiosteal, infraorbital, or PSA injection in place of the MSA.

Complications   Quite rare. A hematoma may develop at the site of injection. Apply pressure with a sterile gauze over the site of swelling and discoloration for a minimum of 60 seconds.

Anterior Superior Alveolar Nerve Block (Infraorbital Nerve Block)

The anterior superior alveolar (ASA) nerve block does not enjoy the popularity of the PSA block, primarily because there is a general lack of experience with this highly successful and extremely safe technique. It provides profound pulpal and buccal soft tissue anesthesia from the maxillary central incisor through the premolars in about 72% of patients.

Used in place of supraperiosteal injections, the ASA nerve block requires a smaller volume of local anesthetic solution to achieve equivalent anesthesia—0.9 to 1.2 ml versus 3.0 ml for supraperiosteal injections of the same teeth.

It has been my experience that the major factor inhibiting dentists from using the ASA nerve block is fear of injury to the patient's eye. Fortunately this fear is unfounded. Adherence to the following protocol will produce a high success rate devoid of complications and adverse side effects.

Other common name   Infraorbital nerve block

Nerves anesthetized

1. Anterior superior alveolar
2. Middle superior alveolar
3. Infraorbital nerve
   a. Inferior palpebral
   b. Lateral nasal
   c. Superior labial

Areas anesthetized

1. Pulps of the maxillary central incisor through the canine on the injected side
2. In about 72% of patients, pulps of the maxillary premolars and mesiobuccal root of the first molar
3. Buccal (labial) periodontium and bone of these same teeth
4. Lower eyelid, lateral aspect of the nose, upper lip (Fig. 13-16)

Indications

1. Dental procedures involving more than two maxillary teeth and their overlying buccal tissues
2. Inflammation or infection (which contraindicates supraperiosteal injection); if a cellulitis is present, the maxillary nerve block may be indicated in lieu of the infraorbital nerve block
3. When supraperiosteal injections have been ineffective because of dense cortical bone

Contraindications

1. Discrete treatment areas (one or two teeth only—supraperiosteal preferred)
2. Hemostasis of localized areas, when desirable, cannot be adequately achieved with this injection; local infiltration into the treatment area is indicated

Advantages

1. Comparatively simple technique
2. Comparatively safe; minimizes the volume of solution used and the number of needle punctures required to achieve anesthesia

Disadvantages

1. Psychological
   a. Administrator: there may be an initial fear of injury to the patient's eye. (Experience with the technique leads to confidence.)
   b. Patient: an *extraoral* approach to the infraorbital nerve may prove disturbing; however, intraoral techniques are rarely a problem.
2. Anatomical: difficulty defining landmarks

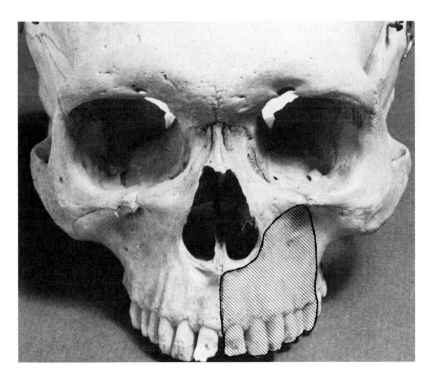

Fig. 13-16 Infraorbital nerve block, showing the area anesthetized in 72% of patients.

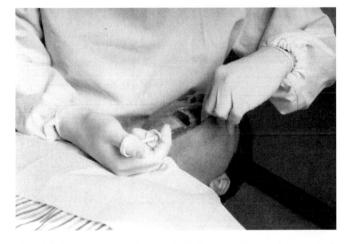

Fig. 13-17 Position of the administrator for a right or left infraorbital nerve block. The patient's head should be turned slightly to improve visibility.

Positive aspiration 0.7%

Alternatives
1. Supraperiosteal or PDL injection for each tooth
2. Infiltration for the periodontium and hard tissues
3. Maxillary nerve block

Technique
1. A 25-gauge long needle recommended, though the 25-gauge short may also be used, especially for children and smaller adults

2. Area of insertion: height of the mucobuccal fold directly over first premolar
   Note: The needle may be inserted into the height of the mucobuccal fold over any tooth from the second premolar anteriorly to the central incisor. The ensuing path of penetration is to the target area, the infraorbital foramen. The first premolar usually provides the shortest route to this target area.
3. Target area: infraorbital foramen (below the infraorbital notch)
4. Landmarks
   a. Mucobuccal fold
   b. Infraorbital notch
   c. Infraorbital foramen
5. Orientation of the bevel: *toward* bone
6. Procedure
   a. Assume the correct position (Fig. 13-17). For a right or left infraorbital nerve block and right-handed administrator, sit at the 10 o'clock position, directly facing the patient *or* facing in the same direction as the patient.
   b. Position the patient supine (much preferred) or semisupine with the neck extended slightly. If the patient's neck is not extended, the patient's chest may interfere with the syringe barrel.
   c. Prepare the tissues at the injection site (height of the mucobuccal fold) for penetration.
      (1) Dry with sterile gauze.
      (2) Apply topical antiseptic (optional).
      (3) Apply topical anesthetic.
   d. Locate the infraorbital foramen (Fig. 13-18).

(1) Feel the infraorbital notch.
(2) Move your finger downward from the notch, applying gentle pressure to the tissues.
(3) The bone immediately inferior to the notch will be convex (feeling as a bulge outward). This represents the lower border of the orbit and the roof of the infraorbital foramen (Fig. 13-18, *B*).
(4) As your finger continues inferiorly, a concavity will be felt; this is the infraorbital foramen.
(5) Applying pressure, feel the outlines of the infraorbital foramen at this site. The patient will sense a mild aching when the foramen is palpated.
e. Maintain your finger on the foramen or mark the skin at the site (Fig. 13-19).

f. Retract the lip, pulling the tissues in the mucobuccal fold taut and increasing visibility. A 2 × 2 inch sterile gauze placed beneath your gloved finger aids in retraction of the lip during the ASA injection.
g. Insert the needle into the height of the mucobuccal fold over the first premolar with the bevel facing bone (Fig. 13-20).
h. Orient the syringe *toward* the infraorbital foramen.
i. The needle should be held parallel with the long axis of the tooth as it is advanced, to avoid premature contact with bone (Fig. 13-21).
j. Advance the needle *slowly* until bone is gently contacted.
(1) The point of contact should be the upper rim of the infraorbital foramen.

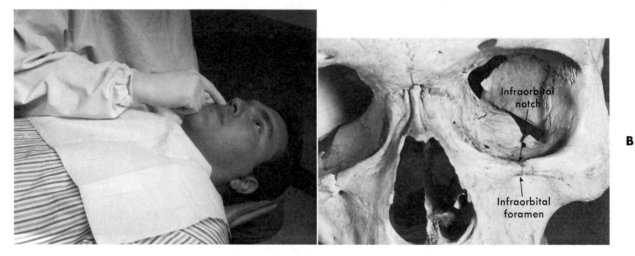

A

B

Infraorbital notch

Infraorbital foramen

Fig. 13-18 A, Palpating the infraorbital notch. **B,** Location of the infraorbital foramen in relation to the infraorbital notch.

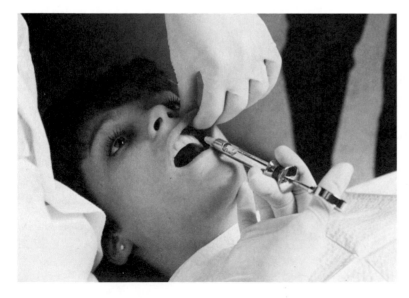

Fig. 13-19 Using a finger over the foramen, lift the lip and hold the tissues in the mucobuccal fold taut.

(2) The approximate depth of needle penetration will be 16 mm for an adult of average height (equivalent to approximately half the length of a long needle).

(3) The depth of penetration will, of course, vary. In a patient with a high (deep) mucobuccal fold or a low infraorbital foramen, less tissue penetration will be required than in one with a shallow mucobuccal fold or high infraorbital foramen.

(4) A preinjection approximation of the depth of penetration can be made by placing one finger on the infraorbital foramen and another on the injection site in the mucobuccal fold and estimating the distance between them.

k. Prior to injecting the anesthetic solution, check for the following:

(1) Depth of needle penetration (adequate to reach the foramen)

(2) Any lateral deviation of the needle from the infraorbital foramen; correct before injecting solution

(3) Orientation of the bevel (facing bone)

l. Position the needle tip during injection with the bevel facing into the infraorbital foramen and the needle tip touching the roof of the foramen (Fig. 13-22).

m. Aspirate.

n. Slowly deposit 0.9 to 1.2 ml (half to two thirds cartridge). Little or no swelling should be visible as the solution is deposited. If the needle tip is properly inserted at the opening of the foramen, solution will be directed toward the foramen.

(1) The administrator will be able to "feel" the anesthetic solution as it is deposited beneath their finger on the foramen if the needle tip is

in the correct position. At the conclusion of the injection the foramen should no longer be palpable (because of the volume of anesthetic in this position).

The *infraorbital nerve block,* providing anesthesia to the soft tissues on the anterior portion of the face and

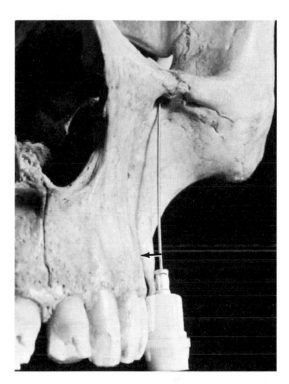

Fig. 13-21 Advance the needle parallel with the long axis of the tooth to preclude prematurely contacting bone. Notice how the bone of the maxilla becomes concave between the root eminence and the infraorbital foramen (*arrow* and *shadow*).

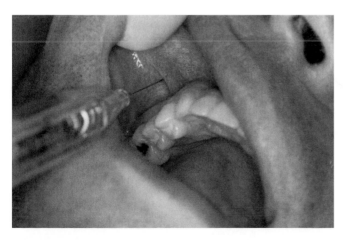

Fig. 13-20 Insert the needle for an infraorbital nerve block into the mucobuccal fold adjacent to the first premolar.

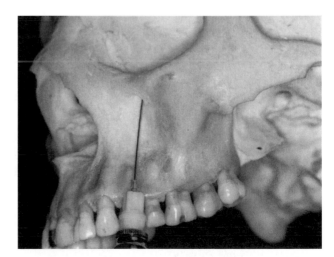

Fig. 13-22 Position of the needle tip prior to deposition of local anesthetic at the infraorbital foramen.

lateral aspect of the nose, is complete. To complete the *anterior superior alveolar nerve block,* providing anesthesia to the teeth and their supporting structures:

o. Maintain firm pressure with your finger over the injection site both during and for at least 1 minute after the injection (to increase the diffusion of anesthetic solution into the infraorbital foramen).

p. Withdraw the syringe slowly and immediately make the needle safe.

q. Maintain direct finger pressure over the injection site for a minimum of 1 minute, preferably 2 minutes, following injection.

r. Wait 3 to 5 minutes after completion of the injection before commencing the dental procedure.

Signs and symptoms

1. Tingling and numbness of the lower eyelid, side of the nose, and upper lip indicate anesthesia of the infraorbital nerve, not the ASA or MSA nerve (develops almost instantly as the anesthetic is being administered)
2. Numbness in the teeth and soft tissues along the distribution of the ASA and MSA nerves (developing within 3 to 5 minutes if pressure is maintained over the injection site)
3. No pain during dental therapy

Safety features

1. Needle contact with bone at the roof of the infraorbital foramen prevents inadvertent overinsertion and possible puncture of the orbit.
2. A finger over the infraorbital foramen helps direct the needle toward the foramen.
   a. The needle may be palpable if its path is too superficial (away from the bone). If this occurs, withdraw it slightly and redirect it toward the target area.
   b. In most patients it will not be possible to palpate the needle through soft tissues over the foramen unless it is too superficial. However, in some patients with less well-developed facial musculature a properly positioned needle may be palpable.

Precautions

1. For *pain on insertion* of the needle and *tearing* of the periosteum, reinsert the needle in a more lateral (away from bone) position and/or deposit solution as the needle advances through soft tissue.
2. For *overinsertion* of the needle, estimate the depth of penetration before injection (review procedure) and exert finger pressure over the infraorbital foramen.
   a. Overinsertion is unlikely because of the rim of bone that forms the superior rim of the infraorbital foramen. The needle tip will contact this rim.

Failures of anesthesia

1. Needle contacting bone *below* (inferior to) the infraorbital foramen; anesthesia of the lower eyelid, lateral side of the nose, and upper lip develop, with little or no dental anesthesia; a bolus of solution may be felt beneath the skin in the area of deposition, which lies at a distance from the infraorbital foramen (which is still palpable after the injection). These are, by far, the most common causes of anesthetic failure within the distribution of the ASA nerve. In essence a failed ASA is a supraperiosteal injection over the first premolar. To correct:
   a. Keep the needle in line with the infraorbital foramen during penetration. Do not direct the needle toward bone.
   b. Estimate the depth of penetration before injecting.
2. Needle deviation medial or lateral to the infraorbital foramen. To correct:
   a. Direct the needle toward the foramen immediately after inserting and before advancing it through the tissue.
   b. Recheck needle placement prior to aspirating and depositing the anesthetic solution.

Complications   Hematoma (rare) may develop across the lower eyelid and the tissues between it and the infraorbital foramen. To manage, apply pressure on the soft tissue over the foramen for 2 to 3 minutes. Hematoma is extremely rare because pressure is routinely applied to the injection site both during and after the ASA nerve block.

PALATAL ANESTHESIA

Anesthesia of the hard palate is necessary for dental procedures involving manipulation of palatal soft or hard tissues. For many dental patients palatal injections prove to be a very traumatic experience. For many dentists the administration of palatal anesthesia is one of the most traumatic procedures they perform in dentistry.[3] Indeed, many dentists and dental hygienists advise their patients that they expect them to feel pain (dental professionals usually use the term "discomfort" rather than "pain" in describing uncomfortable procedures) during palatal injections! Forewarning the patient about procedural pain does permit the patient to become more prepared psychologically, and it also relieves the administrator of responsibility when the pain occurs. When the patient acknowledges the existence of pain, the administrator can console the patient with a shrug of the shoulders and a kind word, once again confirming to both the patient and the administrator that palatal injections hurt—always!

Palatal anesthesia, however, can be achieved atraumatically. At best, patients will be unaware of the needle penetration of soft tissues and deposition of the local anesthetic solution (they won't even feel it!). At worst, when the following techniques are adhered to, patients will state that although they still were somewhat uncomfortable, *this* palatal injection was the least painful they had ever received.

The steps in the atraumatic administration of palatal anesthesia are as follows:

1. Provide adequate topical anesthesia at the injection site.
2. Use pressure anesthesia at the site both before and during needle insertion and the deposition of solution.
3. Maintain control over the needle.
4. Deposit the anesthetic solution slowly.
5. Trust yourself . . . that you can complete the procedure atraumatically.

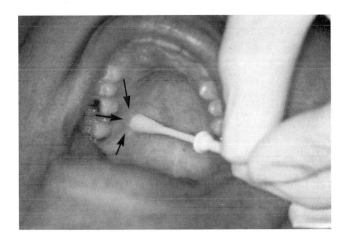

Fig. 13-23 Notice the ischemia of palatal tissues (*arrows*) under pressure from the applicator stick.

Adequate topical anesthesia at the injection site can be provided by allowing topical anesthetic to remain in contact with the soft tissues for at least 2 minutes. The palate is the one area in the mouth where the cotton swab must be held in position by the administrator for the full time.

Pressure anesthesia can be produced at the site of injection by applying considerable pressure to the tissues adjacent to the injection site with a firm object. I prefer the cotton applicator stick previously used to apply the topical anesthetic. Other objects, such as the handle of a mouth mirror, are used by some, but being metal are more likely to hurt the patient. The goal is to produce anesthesia of the soft tissues through the gate control theory of pain.[4] The applicator stick should be pressed firmly enough to produce blanching (ischemia) of the normally pink tissues at the penetration site and a feeling of intense pressure (dull and tolerable, not sharp and painful) (Fig. 13-23). Pressure anesthesia should be maintained during penetration of the soft tissues with the needle and must be maintained throughout the time that the needle remains in the palatal soft tissues.

Control over the needle is probably of greater importance in palatal anesthesia than in other intraoral injections. To achieve this, the administrator must secure a firm hand rest. Several positions were illustrated in Chapter 11. When palatal anesthesia is administered, it is also possible on occasion to stabilize the needle with *both hands* (Fig. 13-24). Perfection of this technique will develop only with experience.

Slow deposition of the local anesthetic is important in all injection techniques, not only as a safety feature but also as a means of providing an atraumatic injection. Because of the density of the palatal soft tissues and their firm adherence to the underlying palatal bone, slow deposition is of even greater importance here. Rapid

A 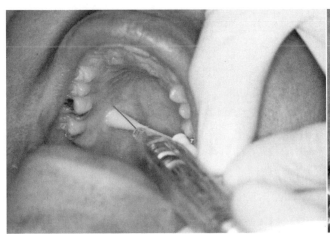 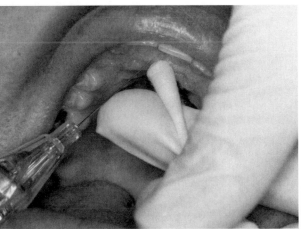 B

Fig. 13-24 Stabilization of the needle for a greater palatine, **A**, and nasopalatine, **B**, nerve block. With both injections the barrel of the syringe should rest against the patient's lower lip.

injection of the solution produces high tissue pressure, which tears the palatal soft tissues and leads to pain on injection and to localized soreness when the anesthetic actions are terminated. Slow injection of the anesthetic does not produce discomfort.

Probably the most important factor in providing an atraumatic palatal injection is the *belief by the administrator that it can be done painlessly;* special care will then be taken to minimize discomfort to the patient, and this generally results in a more atraumatic palatal injection.

• • •

Of the three palatal injections to be described—the anterior (or greater) palatine nerve block, providing anesthesia of the posterior portions of the hard palate; the nasopalatine nerve block, producing anesthesia of the anterior hard palate; and local infiltration of the hard palate, used primarily to achieve hemostasis prior to surgical procedures—none provides any pulpal anesthesia to the maxillary teeth.

Greater Palatine Nerve Block

The greater palatine nerve block is quite useful during dental procedures involving the palatal soft tissues distal to the canine. Minimum volumes of solution (0.45 to 0.6 ml) provide profound hard and soft tissue anesthesia. Although potentially traumatic, the greater palatine nerve block is less so than the nasopalatine nerve block because the tissues surrounding the greater palatine foramen are better able to accommodate the volume of solution deposited.

Other common name   Anterior palatine nerve block

Nerve anesthetized   Greater palatine

Areas anesthetized   The posterior portion of the hard palate and its overlying soft tissues, anteriorly as far as the first premolar and medially to the midline (Fig. 13-25)

Indications

1. When palatal soft tissue anesthesia is required for restorative therapy on more than two teeth (e.g., with subgingival restorations and insertion of matrix bands subgingivally)
2. For *pain* control during periodontal or oral surgical procedures involving the palatal soft and hard tissues

Contraindications

1. Inflammation or infection at the injection site
2. Smaller areas of therapy (one or two teeth)

Advantages

1. Minimizes needle penetrations and volume of solution
2. Minimal patient discomfort

Disadvantages

1. No hemostasis except in the immediate area of injection
2. Potentially traumatic

Positive aspiration   Less than 1%

Alternatives

1. Local infiltration into specific regions
2. Maxillary nerve block

Technique

1. A 27-gauge short needle recommended (though the 25-gauge short may also be used)
2. Area of insertion: soft tissue slightly anterior to the greater palatine foramen
3. Target area: greater (anterior) palatine nerve as it passes anteriorly between the soft tissues and bone of the hard palate (Fig. 13-26)
4. Landmarks: greater palatine foramen and junction of the maxillary alveolar process and palatine bone
5. Path of insertion: advance the syringe from the

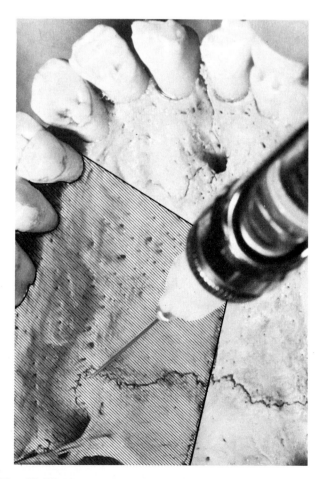

Fig. 13-25 Placement of the needle in the area to be anesthetized by a greater palatine nerve block.

opposite side of the mouth at a right angle to the target area.

6. Orientation of the bevel: *toward* the palatal soft tissues (Steps g and h on p. 178)
7. Procedure
   a. Assume the correct position (Fig. 13-27).
      (1) For a right greater palatine nerve block and a right-handed administrator, sit *facing* the patient at the 7 or 8 o'clock position.
      (2) For a left greater palatine block and a right-handed administrator, sit facing in the *same direction* as the patient at 11 o'clock
   b. Request the patient, who is in a supine position (Fig. 13-28, A), to
      (1) Open wide.
      (2) Extend the neck.
      (3) Turn the head to the left or right (for improved visibility).
   c. Locate the greater palatine foramen (Fig. 13-28, B) (Table 13-2).
      (1) Place a cotton swab at the junction of the maxillary alveolar process and the hard palate.
      (2) Start in the region of the maxillary first molar and palpate posteriorly by pressing firmly into the tissues with the swab.
      (3) The swab will "fall" into the depression created by the greater palatine foramen (Fig. 13-29).
      (4) The foramen is most frequently located distal to the maxillary second molar, but it may be either anterior or posterior to its usual position. (See "Maxillary nerve block," p. 189.)

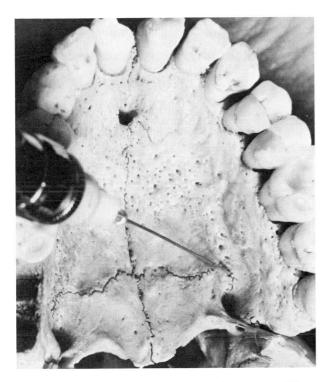

Fig. 13-26 Target area for a greater palatine nerve block.

TABLE 13-2 Location of the Greater Palatine Foramen*

Location	No.	Percent
Anterior half 2nd molar	0	0
Posterior half 2nd molar	63	39.87
Anterior half 3rd molar	80	50.63
Posterior half 3rd molar	15	9.49

From Malamed SF, Trieger N: Intraoral maxillary nerve block: an anatomical and clinical study, *Anesth Prog* 30:44-48, 1983.
*Measurements from 158 skulls with the maxillary second and third molars present.

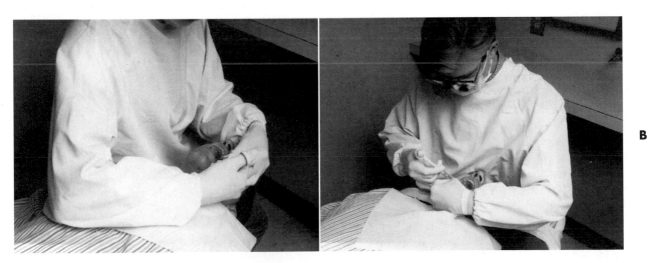

A

B

Fig. 13-27 Position of the administrator for a right, **A**, and left, **B**, greater palatine nerve block.

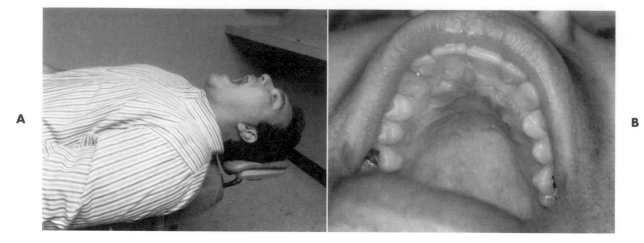

Fig. 13-28 **A**, Patient position for a greater palatine nerve block. **B**, Hard palate when the patient is positioned properly.

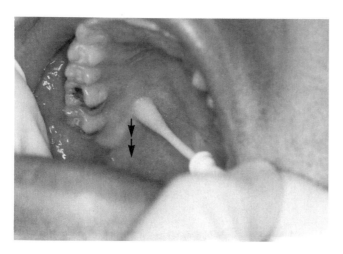

Fig. 13-29 A cotton swab is pressed against the hard palate at the junction of the maxillary alveolar process and palatal bone. The swab is slowly moved distally (*arrows*) until a depression in the tissue is felt. This is the greater (anterior) palatine foramen.

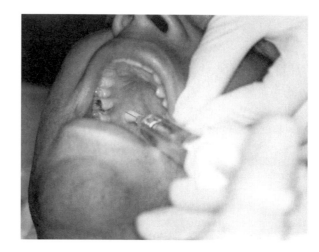

Fig. 13-30 Notice the angle of needle entry into the mouth. The insertion is into ischemic tissues slightly anterior to the applicator stick. The barrel of the syringe is stabilized by the corner of the mouth and the teeth.

d. Prepare the tissue at the injection site, just 1 to 2 mm *anterior* to the greater palatine foramen.
   (1) Clean and dry with sterile gauze.
   (2) Apply topical antiseptic (optional).
   (3) Apply topical anesthetic.
e. After 2 minutes of topical anesthetic application, move the swab posteriorly so it is *directly over* the greater palatine foramen.
   (1) Apply considerable pressure at the area of the foramen with the swab in the left hand (if right-handed).
   (2) Note the ischemia (whitening of the soft tissues) at the injection site.
   (3) Apply pressure for a minimum of 30 seconds, and while doing this proceed to

f. Direct the syringe into the mouth from the opposite side with the needle approaching the injection site at a right angle (Fig. 13-30).
g. Place the bevel (not the point) of the needle gently against the previously blanched (ischemic) soft tissue at the injection site. It must be well stabilized to prevent accidental penetration of the tissues.
h. With the bevel lying against the tissue
   (1) Apply enough pressure to bow the needle slightly.
   (2) Deposit a *small* volume of anesthetic. The solution will be forced against the mucous membrane, and a droplet will form.
i. Straighten the needle and permit the bevel to penetrate mucosa.

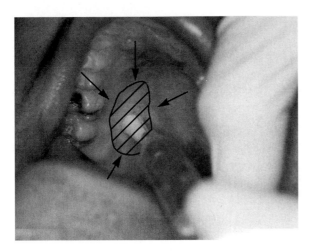

Fig. 13-31 Notice the spread of ischemia (*arrows*) as the anesthetic is deposited.

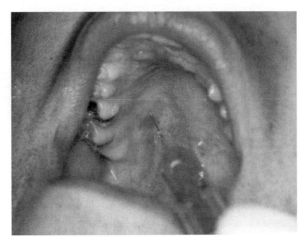

Fig 13-32 The cotton swab is removed when the deposition of solution ceases.

(1) Continue to deposit small volumes of anesthetic throughout the procedure.

(2) Ischemia will spread into the adjacent tissues as the anesthetic (usually with a vasoconstrictor) is deposited (Figs. 13-31 and 13-32).

j. Continue to apply pressure anesthesia throughout the deposition of the anesthetic solution (Fig. 13-31). Ischemia will spread as the vasoconstrictor decreases tissue perfusion.

k. Slowly advance the needle until palatine bone is gently contacted.

(1) The depth of penetration will usually be less than 10 mm.

(2) Continue to deposit small volumes of anesthetic. As the tissue is entered, there will be increased resistance to the deposition of solution, which is entirely normal in the greater palatine nerve block.

l. Aspirate.

m. If negative, *slowly* deposit (30 sec minimum) not more than one fourth to one third of a cartridge (0.45 to 0.6 ml).

n. Withdraw the syringe.

o. Make the needle safe.

p. Wait 2 to 3 minutes before commencing the dental procedure.

Signs and symptoms
1. Numbness in the posterior portion of the palate
2. No pain during dental therapy

Safety features
1. Contact with bone
2. Aspiration

Precautions Do not enter the greater palatine

canal. Although this is not hazardous, there is no reason to enter the canal for this technique to be successful.

Failures of anesthesia
1. The greater palatine nerve block is not a technically difficult injection to administer. Its incidence of success is well above 95%.
2. If local anesthetic is deposited too far anterior to the foramen, adequate soft tissue anesthesia may not develop in the palatal tissues posterior to the site of injection (partial success).
3. Anesthesia on the palate in the area of the maxillary first premolar may prove inadequate because of overlapping fibers from the nasopalatine nerve (partial success).
   a. To correct: local infiltration may be necessary as a supplement in the area of inadequate anesthesia.

Complications
1. Few of significance
2. Ischemia and necrosis of soft tissues when highly concentrated vasoconstricting solution used for hemostasis over a prolonged period
   a. Norepinephrine should never be used for hemostasis on the palatal soft tissues.
3. Hematoma possible but quite rare because of the density and firm adherence of the palatal tissues to underlying bone
4. Some patients may be uncomfortable if their soft palate becomes anesthetized, a distinct possibility when the middle palatine nerve exits near the injection site.

Nasopalatine Nerve Block
The nasopalatine nerve block is an invaluable technique for palatal pain control in that, with the administration of

a minimum volume of anesthetic solution (maximally, one quarter of a cartridge), a wide area of palatal soft tissue anesthesia is achieved, thereby minimizing the need for multiple palatal injections. Unfortunately, the nasopalatine nerve block has the distinction of being a potentially highly traumatic (i.e., painful) injection. With no other injection technique is the need for strict adherence to the protocol of atraumatic injection more important than with the nasopalatine nerve block. Two approaches to this injection are presented. Readers should become familiar with both techniques and then use the one with which they feel more comfortable (i.e., that works best in their hands).

The original technique involves but one tissue penetration, just lateral to the incisive papilla on the palatal aspect of the maxillary central incisors. The soft tissue in this area is dense, firmly adherent to underlying bone, and quite sensitive—three factors that combine to increase patient discomfort during the injection. The second technique was recommended to me by a number of readers of earlier editions of this book. It involves two or three needle punctures but, when carried out properly, is somewhat less traumatic than the more direct single puncture technique. In it the labial soft tissues between the maxillary central incisors are anesthetized (injection no. 1), and then a needle is directed from the labial aspect through the interproximal papilla between the centrals toward the incisive papilla to anesthetize the nasopalatine nerves (injection no. 2). In some cases these two injections suffice to provide acceptable nasopalatine nerve block; in others a third injection, directly into the now partially anesthetized palatal soft tissues overlying the nasopalatine nerve, is necessary. Although I prefer a single-needle

puncture technique whenever possible, I have found that the second technique can produce effective nasopalatine anesthesia with a minimum of discomfort.

Other common names   Incisive nerve block, sphenopalatine nerve block

Nerves anesthetized   Nasopalatine nerves bilaterally

Areas anesthetized   Anterior portion of the hard palate (soft and hard tissues) from the mesial of the right first premolar to the mesial of the left first premolar (Fig. 13-33)

Indications
1. When palatal soft tissue anesthesia is required for restorative therapy on more than two teeth (e.g., subgingival restorations and insertion of matrix bands subgingivally)
2. For pain control during periodontal or oral surgical procedures involving palatal soft and hard tissues

Contraindications
1. Inflammation or infection at the injection site
2. Smaller area of therapy (one or two teeth)

Advantages
1. Minimizes needle penetrations and volume of solution
2. Minimal patient discomfort from multiple needle penetrations

Disadvantages
1. No hemostasis except in the immediate area of injection
2. Potentially the most traumatic intraoral injection; however, the protocol for an atraumatic injection can minimize or entirely eliminate discomfort

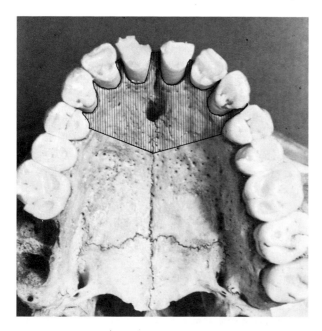

Fig. 13-33 Area anesthetized by a nasopalatine nerve block.

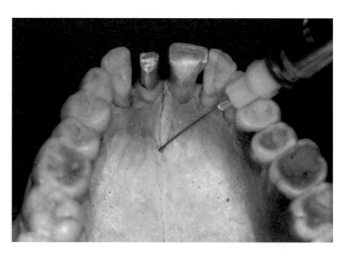

Fig. 13-34 Target area for a nasopalatine nerve block.

Positive aspiration Less than 1%

Alternatives
1. Local infiltration into specific regions
2. Maxillary nerve block

Technique (single needle penetration of the palate)
1. A 27-gauge short needle recommended (though a 25-gauge short may be used)
2. Area of insertion: palatal mucosa just *lateral* to the incisive papilla (located in the midline behind the central incisors); the tissue here is more sensitive than other palatal mucosa
3. Target area: incisive foramen, beneath the incisive papilla (Fig. 13-34)
4. Landmarks: central incisors and incisive papilla
5. Path of insertion: approach the injection site at a 45-degree angle toward the incisive papilla
6. Orientation of the bevel: *toward* the palatal soft tissues (review procedure for the basic palatal injection)
7. Procedure
   a. Sit at the 9 or 10 o'clock position facing in the *same direction* as the patient (Fig. 13-35).
   b. Request the patient to
      (1) Open wide.
      (2) Extend the neck.
      (3) Turn the head to the left or right for improved visibility (Fig. 13-36).
   c. Prepare the tissue just lateral to the incisive papilla (Fig. 13-37).
      (1) Clean and dry with sterile gauze.
      (2) Apply topical antiseptic (optional).
      (3) Apply topical anesthetic.
   d. After 1 to 2 minutes of topical anesthetic application, move the swab *directly onto* the incisive papilla (Figs. 13-37 and 13-38).
      (1) Apply pressure to the area of the papilla with the swab in your left hand (if right-handed).
      (2) Note ischemia at the injection site.
   e. Place the bevel against the ischemic soft tissues at the injection site. The needle must be well stabilized to prevent accidental penetration of tissues (Fig. 13-38).
   f. With the bevel lying against the tissue
      (1) Apply enough pressure to bow the needle slightly.

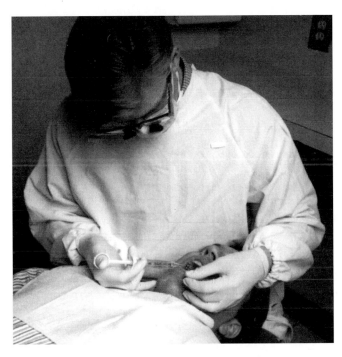

Fig. 13-35 Position of the administrator for a nasopalatine nerve block.

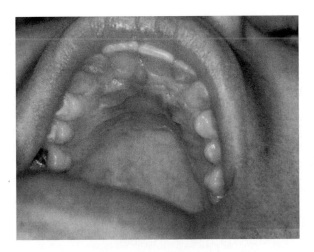

Fig. 13-36 Palate when the patient is positioned properly.

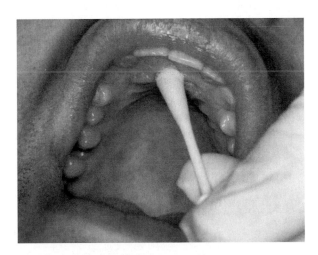

Fig. 13-37 Topical anesthetic is applied lateral to the incisive papilla for 2 minutes, and then pressure is applied directly to the incisive papilla.

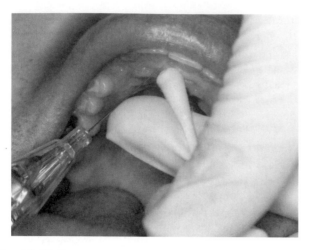

Fig. 13-38 Pressure is maintained until the deposition of solution is completed. Needle penetration is just lateral to the incisive papilla. Notice that the syringe is stabilized by a finger resting on the cheek and that the barrel of the syringe lies against the corner of the mouth.

      (2) Deposit a *small* volume of anesthetic. The solution will be forced against the mucous membrane.
   g. Straighten the needle and permit the bevel to penetrate mucosa.
      (1) Continue to deposit small volumes of anesthetic throughout the procedure.
      (2) Observe ischemia spreading into the adjacent tissues as solution is deposited.
   h. Continue to apply pressure with the cotton applicator stick while injecting the anesthetic.
   i. Slowly advance the needle toward the incisive foramen until bone is gently contacted (Fig. 13-34).
      (1) The depth of penetration will be 6 to 10 mm.
      (2) Deposit small volumes of anesthetic while advancing the needle. As the tissue is entered, there will be increased resistance to the deposition of solution, which is normal with the nasopalatine nerve block.
   j. Withdraw the needle 1 mm (to prevent subperiosteal injection). The bevel now lies over the center of the incisive foramen.
   k. Aspirate.
   l. If negative, deposit slowly (15 to 30 sec minimum) not more than one fourth of a cartridge (0.45 ml).
      (1) It is difficult in some patients to deposit 0.45 ml of anesthetic solution in this injection. Injection of anesthetic can cease when the area of ischemia noted at the injection site has increased from that produced by the application of pressure alone.
   m. Slowly withdraw the syringe.
   n. Make the needle safe.
   o. Wait 2 to 3 minutes before commencing the dental procedure.

Signs and symptoms
1. Numbness in the anterior portion of the palate
2. No pain during dental therapy

Safety features
1. Contact with bone
2. Aspiration

Precautions
1. Against pain
   a. Do not insert directly into the incisive papilla (extremely painful).
   b. Do not deposit solution too rapidly.
   c. Do not deposit too much solution.
2. Against infection
   a. If the needle is advanced more than 5 mm into the incisive canal and the floor of the nose is entered, infection may result. There is no reason for the needle to enter the incisive canal during a nasopalatine nerve block.

Failures of anesthesia
1. Highly successful injection (> 95% incidence of success)
2. Unilateral anesthesia
   a. If solution is deposited to one side of the incisive canal, unilateral anesthesia may develop.
   b. To correct: Reinsert the needle into the already anesthetized tissue and reinject solution into the unanesthetized area.
3. Inadequate palatal soft tissue anesthesia in the area of the maxillary canine and first premolar
   a. If fibers from the greater palatine nerve overlap those of the nasopalatine nerve, anesthesia of the soft tissues palatal to the canine and first premolar could be inadequate.
   b. To correct: Local infiltration may be necessary as a supplement in the area inadequately anesthetized.

Complications
1. Few of significance
2. Hematoma possible but quite rare because of the density and firm adherence of palatal soft tissues to bone
3. Necrosis of soft tissues possible when highly concentrated vasoconstricting solution (e.g., norepinephrine) is used for hemostasis over a prolonged period
4. Because of the density of soft tissues, anesthetic solution may "squirt" back out the needle puncture site either during administration or after needle withdrawal. (This is of no clinical significance. However, do not let it surprise you into uttering a statement such as "whoops!" that might frighten the patient.)

Technique (multiple needle penetrations)

1. A 27-gauge short needle recommended
2. Areas of insertion
   a. Labial frenum in the midline between the maxillary central incisors (Fig. 13-39, *B*)
   b. Interdental papilla between the maxillary central incisors (Fig. 13-39, *C*)
   c. If needed, palatal soft tissues lateral to the incisive papilla (Fig. 13-39, *D*)
3. Target area: incisive foramen, beneath the incisive papilla
4. Landmarks: central incisors and incisive papilla
5. Path of insertion
   a. First injection: infiltration into the labial frenum
   b. Second injection: needle held at a right angle to the interdental papilla
   c. Third injection: needle held at a 45-degree angle to the incisive papilla
6. Orientation of the bevel
   a. First injection: *toward* bone

b. Second injection: not relevant
c. Third injection: not relevant

7. Procedure
   a. *First injection:* infiltration of 0.3 ml into the labial frenum (Fig. 13-39, *B*)
      (1) Prepare the tissue at the injection site.
          (a) Clean and dry with sterile gauze.
          (b) Apply topical antiseptic (optional).
          (c) Apply topical anesthetic for 1 minute (Fig. 13-39, *A*).
      (2) Retract the upper lip to stretch tissues and improve visibility. (Be careful not to overstretch the frenum.)
      (3) Gently insert the needle into the frenum and deposit 0.3 ml of anesthetic in approximately 15 seconds. (The tissue may balloon as solution is injected.)
      (4) Anesthesia of soft tissue will develop immediately.
   b. *Second injection:* penetration through the labial

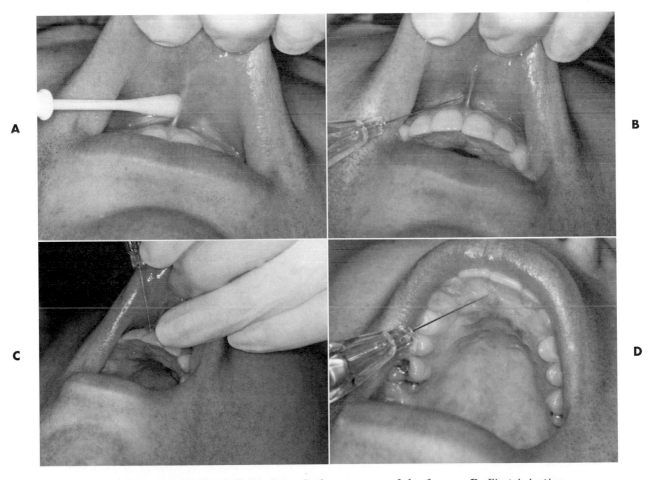

Fig. 13-39 A, Topical anesthetic is applied to mucosa of the frenum. **B,** *First injection,* into the labial frenum. **C,** *Second injection,* into the interdental papilla between the central incisors. **D,** *Third injection,* when anesthesia of the nasopalatine area is inadequate following the first two injections.

aspect of the papilla between the maxillary central incisors toward the incisive papilla (Fig. 13-39, C)

(1) Retract the upper lip gently to increase visibility. (Do not overstretch the labial frenum.)

(2) If a right-handed administrator, sit at 11 or 12 o'clock facing in the same direction as the patient. Tilt the patient's head toward the right to provide a proper angle for needle penetration.

(3) Holding the needle at a right angle to the interdental papilla, insert it into the papilla just above the level of crestal bone.

   (a) Direct it toward the incisive papilla (on the palatal side of the interdental papilla).

   (b) Soft tissues on the labial surface have previously been anesthetized so there will be no discomfort. However, as the needle penetrates toward the unanesthetized palatal side it will become necessary to administer minute amounts of solution to prevent discomfort.

   (c) With the patient's head extended backward, you can see the ischemia produced by the anesthetic and see the needle tip as it approaches the palatal aspect of the incisive papilla. Care must be taken to avoid needle puncture through the papilla into the oral cavity on the palatal side.

(4) When ischemia occurs in the incisive papilla or the needle tip becomes visible just beneath the tissue surface, aspirate. If negative, administer not more than 0.3 ml of anesthetic solution in approximately 15 seconds. There will be considerable resistance to the deposition of solution but no patient discomfort.

(5) Stabilization of the syringe in this second injection is somewhat awkward, but critical. Use of a finger from the other hand to stabilize the needle is recommended (Fig. 13-40). However, the syringe barrel must be held such that it will remain within the patient's line of sight, and this is potentially disconcerting.

(6) Slowly withdraw the syringe.

(7) Make the needle safe.

(8) Anesthesia within the distribution of the right and left nasopalatine nerves usually develops in 2 to 3 minutes.

(9) If the area of clinically effective anesthesia proves to be less than adequate, proceed to the third injection.

c. *Third injection:* used only if the second injection has failed to provide adequate palatal anesthesia

  (1) Dry the tissue just lateral to the incisive papilla.

  (2) Request the patient to open wide.

  (3) Extend the patient's neck.

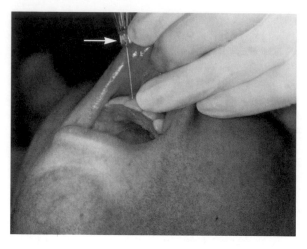

Fig. 13-40 Use a finger of the opposite hand to stabilize the syringe during the second injection *(arrow).*

(4) Place the needle into soft tissue adjacent to the (diamond-shaped) incisive papilla, aiming toward the most distal portion of the papilla.

(5) Advance needle until contact is made with bone.

(6) Withdraw needle 1 mm to prevent a subperiosteal injection.

(7) Aspirate.

(8) If negative, slowly deposit not more than 0.3 ml of anesthetic in approximately 15 seconds. *Note:* Use of topical and pressure anesthesia is unnecessary in the second and third injections because the tissues that the needle penetrates have already been anesthetized (by the first and second injections, respectively).

(9) Withdraw the syringe.

(10) Make the needle safe.

(11) Wait 2 to 3 minutes for the onset of anesthesia before beginning dental treatment.

Signs and symptoms
1. Numbness of the upper lip (in the midline) and anterior portion of the palate
2. No pain during dental therapy

Safety features
1. Aspiration
2. Contact with bone (third injection)

Advantage
Relatively or entirely atraumatic injection

Disadvantages
1. Requires multiple injections (two or three)
2. Difficult to stabilize the syringe during the second injection

3. Syringe barrel usually within the patient's line of sight during the second injection

Precautions

1. Against pain: If each injection is performed as recommended, the entire technique should be atraumatic.
2. Against infection: If a third injection is required, do not advance the needle into the incisive canal. With penetration of the nasal floor, the risk of infection is increased.

Failures of anesthesia

1. A highly successful (> 95%) injection
2. Incomplete palatal anesthesia after the second injection
   a. To correct: A third injection may be required.
3. Inadequate anesthesia around the canine and first premolar because of overlapping fibers from the greater palatine nerve
   a. To correct: Local infiltration may be necessary as a supplement in the area.

Complications

1. Few of significance
2. Necrosis of soft tissues is possible when a highly concentrated vasoconstrictor solution is used for hemostasis over a prolonged period
3. Interdental papilla between the maxillary incisors sometimes quite tender for several days after injection

Local Infiltration of the Palate

Other common names   None

Nerves anesthetized   Terminal branches of the nasopalatine and greater palatine

Areas anesthetized   Soft tissues in the immediate vicinity of injection (Fig. 13-41)

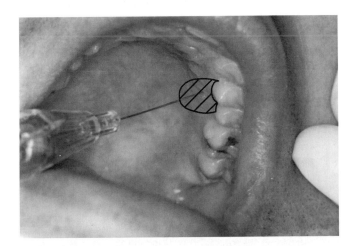

Fig. 13-41 Area anesthetized by a palatal infiltration.

Indications

1. Primarily for achieving hemostasis during surgical procedures
2. Palatogingival pain control when limited areas of anesthesia are required for application of a rubber dam clamp, for packing retraction cord in the gingival sulcus, or for operative procedures on not more than two teeth

Contraindications

1. Inflammation or infection at the injection site
2. Pain control in areas involving more than two teeth

Advantages

1. Provides acceptable hemostasis when a vasoconstrictor is used
2. Provides a minimum area of numbness, thereby minimizing patient discomfort

Disadvantage   Potentially highly traumatic injection

Positive aspiration   Negligible

Alternatives

1. For hemostasis: none
2. For pain control: nasopalatine or greater palatine nerve block, maxillary nerve block

Technique

1. A 27-gauge short needle recommended, though the 25-gauge short may also be used
2. Area of insertion: the attached gingiva 5 to 10 mm from the free gingival margin (Fig. 13-42)
3. Target area: gingival tissues 5 to 10 mm from the free gingival margin
4. Landmark: gingival tissue in the approximate center of the treatment area
5. Pathway of insertion: approaching the injection site at a 45-degree angle
6. Orientation of the bevel: *toward* palatal soft tissues
7. Procedure
   a. If a right-handed administrator, sit at the 10 o'clock position.
      (1) Face *toward* the patient for palatal infiltration on the right side.
      (2) Face in the *same* direction as the patient for palatal infiltration on the left side.
   b. Request the patient to
      (1) Open wide.
      (2) Extend the neck.
      (3) Turn the head to the left or right for improved visibilty.
   c. Prepare the tissue at the site of injection.
      (1) Clean and dry with sterile gauze.
      (2) Apply topical antiseptic (optional).

(3) Apply topical anesthetic.

d. After 1 minute of topical anesthetic application, place the swab on the tissue immediately adjacent to the injection site.

   (1) With the swab in your left hand (if right-handed) apply pressure to the palatal soft tissues.

   (2) Observe the ischemia at the injection site.

e. Place the bevel of the needle against the ischemic soft tissue at the injection site. The needle must be well stabilized to prevent accidental penetration of tissues.

f. With the bevel lying against tissue

   (1) Apply enough pressure to bow the needle slightly.

   (2) Deposit a small volume of local anesthetic. The solution will be forced against mucous membrane, forming a droplet.

g. Straighten the needle and permit the bevel to penetrate mucosa.

   (1) Continue to deposit small volumes of anesthetic throughout this procedure.

   (2) Ischemia of the tissues will spread as additional anesthetic is deposited. (When this injection is used to achieve hemostasis, vasoconstrictor within the solution will produce intense ischemia of tissues.)

h. Continue to apply pressure with the cotton applicator stick throughout the injection.

i. Continue to advance the needle and to deposit anesthetic until bone is gently contacted. Tissue thickness is only 2 to 4 mm in most areas.

j. If hemostasis is the goal in this technique, continue to administer solution until ischemia encompasses the surgical site. In usual practice, 0.2 to 0.3 ml of solution will prove adequate.

k. For hemostasis of larger surgical sites

   (1) Remove the needle from the first injection site.

   (2) Place it in the new injection site at the periphery of the previously anesthetized tissue (Fig. 13-43).

   (3) Penetrate the tissues and deposit anesthetic as in Step *j*. Topical anesthetic may be omitted for subsequent injections since the tissue is anesthetized.

   (4) Continue this overlapping procedure until adequate hemostasis develops over the entire surgical area.

l. Withdraw the syringe.

m. Make the needle safe.

n. Commence the dental procedure immediately.

Signs and symptoms

1. Numbness, ischemia of the palatal soft tissues
2. No pain during dental therapy

Safety feature   Anatomically safe area for injection

Precaution   Highly traumatic procedure if performed improperly

Failures of hemostasis

1. There will be a higher percentage of success if vasoconstrictor is included in the anesthetic solution.
2. However, inflamed tissues may continue to hemorrhage despite the use of vasoconstrictor.

Complications

1. Few of significance.
2. Necrosis of soft tissues may be observed when a highly concentrated vasoconstricting solution is

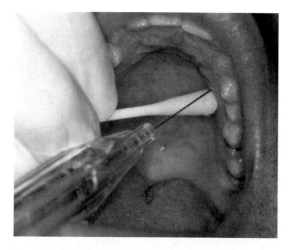

Fig. 13-42 Area of insertion and target area for a palatal infiltration.

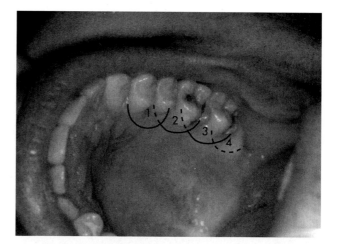

Fig. 13-43 Overlapping of sequential palatal infiltrations and needle penetration sites.

used for hemostasis over a prolonged period (e.g., norepinephrine).

MAXILLARY NERVE BLOCK

The *maxillary* (or *second division*) *nerve block* is an effective method of achieving profound anesthesia of a hemimaxilla. It is useful in procedures involving quadrant dentistry or in extensive surgical procedures. Two approaches are presented here. Both are effective, and I do not maintain a preference for either one. The major difficulties in the *greater palatine canal* approach occur in locating the canal and negotiating it successfully. The major difficulty in the *high tuberosity* approach is the higher incidence of hematoma.

Other common names Second division block, V_2 nerve block

Nerve anesthetized Maxillary division of the trigeminal nerve

Areas anesthetized (Fig. 13-44)
1. Pulpal anesthesia of the maxillary teeth on the side of the block
2. Buccal periodontium and bone overlying these teeth
3. Soft tissues and bone of the hard palate and part of the soft palate, medially to the midline
4. Skin of the lower eyelid, side of the nose, cheek, and upper lip

Indications
1. Pain control prior to extensive oral surgical, periodontal, or restorative procedures requiring anesthesia of the entire maxillary division
2. When tissue inflammation or infection precludes the use of other regional nerve blocks (e.g., PSA, ASA) or supraperiosteal injection
3. Diagnostic or therapeutic procedures for neuralgias or tics of the second division of the trigeminal nerve

Contraindications
1. Inexperienced administrator
2. Pediatric patients
   a. More difficult because of smaller anatomical dimensions
   b. Need a cooperative patient
   c. Usually unnecessary in children because of the high success rate of other regional block techniques
3. Uncooperative patients
4. Inflammation or infection of tissues overlying the injection site
5. When hemorrhage is risky (e.g., in a hemophiliac)

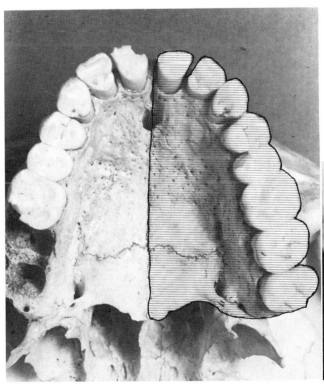
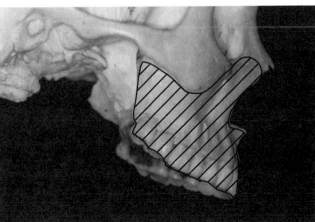

Fig. 13-44 A and **B,** Areas anesthetized by a maxillary nerve block.

6. In the greater palatine canal approach: inability to gain access to the canal; bony obstructions may be present in 5% to 15% of canals

Advantages

1. Atraumatic injection via the high tuberosity approach
2. High success rate (> 95%)
3. Minimizes the number of needle penetrations necessary for successful anesthesia of the hemimaxilla (minimum of four via PSA, infraorbital, greater palatine, and nasopalatine)
4. Minimizes total volume of local anesthetic solution injected
   a. 1.8 ml versus 2.7 ml
5. Neither high tuberosity nor greater palatine canal approach is usually traumatic

Disadvantages

1. Risk of hematoma, primarily with the high tuberosity approach.
2. High tuberosity approach is relatively arbitrary. Overinsertion is possible because of the absence of bony landmarks if proper technique is not followed.
3. Lack of hemostasis. If required, this necessitates infiltration with vasoconstrictor-containing local anesthetic at the surgical site.
4. Pain. The greater palatine canal approach is potentially (though not usually) traumatic.

Positive aspiration Less than 1% (greater palatine canal approach)

Alternatives To achieve the same distribution of anesthesia present with a maxillary nerve block, *all of the following* must be administered:

1. PSA nerve block
2. ASA nerve block
3. Greater palatine nerve block
4. Nasopalatine nerve block

Technique (high tuberosity approach) (Fig. 13-45)

1. A 25-gauge long needle is recommended.
2. Area of insertion: height of the mucobuccal fold above the distal aspect of the maxillary second molar
3. Target area
   a. Maxillary nerve as it passes through the pterygopalatine fossa
   b. Superior and medial to the target area of the PSA nerve block
4. Landmarks
   a. Mucobuccal fold at the distal aspect of the maxillary second molar
   b. Maxillary tuberosity

   c. Zygomatic process of the maxilla
5. Orientation of the bevel: *toward* bone
6. Procedure
   a. Measure the length of a long needle from the tip to the hub (average 32 mm, but varies by manufacturer).
   b. Assume the correct position.
      (1) For a left–high tuberosity injection and a right-handed administrator, sit at the 10 o'clock position facing the patient (Fig. 13-8, *A*).
      (2) For a right–high tuberosity injection and a right-handed administrator, sit at the 8 o'clock position facing the patient (Fig. 13-8, *B*).
   c. Position the patient supine or semisupine for the right or left block.
   d. Prepare the tissue in the height of the mucobuccal fold at the distal of the maxillary second molar.
      (1) Dry with sterile gauze.
      (2) Apply topical antiseptic (optional).
      (3) Apply topical anesthetic.
   e. Partially open the patient's mouth; pull the mandible toward the side of injection.
   f. Retract the cheek in the injection area with your index finger to increase visibility.
   g. Pull the tissues taut with this finger.
   h. Place the needle into the height of the mucobuccal fold over the maxillary second molar.
   i. Advance the needle slowly in an upward, inward, and backward direction as previously described for the PSA nerve block (p. 164).
   j. Advance the needle to a depth of 30 mm.
      (1) No resistance to needle penetration should be felt; if resistance is felt, the angle of the needle in toward the midline is too great.
      (2) At this depth (30 mm) the needle tip should

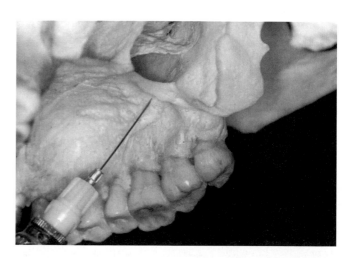

Fig. 13-45 Maxillary nerve block, high tuberosity approach.

lie in the pterygopalatine fossa in proximity to the maxillary division of the trigeminal nerve.

  k. Aspirate.
    (1) Rotate the syringe (needle bevel) one-fourth turn and reaspirate.
    (2) If negative
      (a) Slowly (over 60 sec) deposit 1.8 ml.
      (b) Aspirate several times during injection.
  l. Withdraw the syringe.
  m. Make the needle safe.
  n. Wait 3 to 5 minutes before commencing the dental procedure.

Technique (greater palatine canal approach)
(Fig. 13-46)
1. A 25-gauge long needle recommended
2. Area of insertion: palatal soft tissue directly over the greater palatine foramen
3. Target area: the maxillary nerve as it passes through the pterygopalatine fossa; the needle passes through the greater palatine canal to reach the pterygopalatine fossa
4. Landmark: greater palatine foramen, junction of the maxillary alveolar process and palatine bone
5. Orientation of the bevel: *toward* palatal soft tissues
6. Procedure
  a. Measure the length of a long needle from the tip to the hub (average 32 mm but varies by manufacturer).

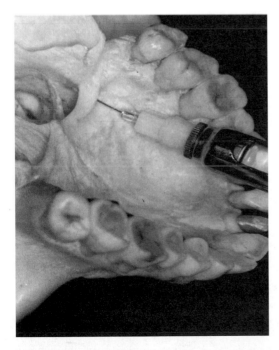

Fig. 13-46 Maxillary nerve block, greater palatine canal approach. Notice the direction of the needle and syringe barrel into the canal.

  b. Assume the correct position.
    (1) For a right greater palatine canal maxillary block, sit facing *toward* the patient at 7 or 8 o'clock.
    (2) For a left greater palatine canal maxillary block, sit facing in the *same direction* as the patient at 10 or 11 o'clock.
  c. Request the patient, who is supine, to
    (1) Open wide.
    (2) Extend the neck.
    (3) Turn the head to the left or right (to improve visibility).
  d. Locate the greater palatine foramen.
    (1) Place a cotton swab at the junction of the maxillary alveolar process and hard palate.
    (2) Start in the region of the second molar and palpate by pressing posteriorly into the tissues with the swab.
    (3) The swab will "fall" into the depression created by the greater palatine foramen.
    (4) The foramen is most frequently located at the distal aspect of the maxillary second molar (Table 13-2).
  e. Prepare the tissues *directly over* the greater palatine foramen.
    (1) Clean and dry with sterile gauze.
    (2) Apply topical antiseptic (optional).
    (3) Apply topical anesthetic.
  f. After 1 minute of topical anesthetic application move the swab posteriorly so it lies just *posterior* to the greater palatine foramen.
    (1) Apply pressure to the tissue with the cotton swab, held in the left hand (if right-handed).
    (2) Note ischemia at the injection site.
  g. Direct the syringe into the mouth from the opposite side with the needle approaching the injection site at a right angle (Fig. 13-47).
  h. Place the bevel against the ischemic soft tissue at the injection site. The needle must be well stabilized to prevent accidental penetration of the tissues.
  i. With the bevel lying against the tissue
    (1) Apply enough pressure to bow the needle slightly.
    (2) Deposit a *small* volume of local anesthetic. The solution will be forced against mucous membrane, forming a droplet.
  j. Straighten the needle and permit the bevel to penetrate mucosa.
    (1) Continue to deposit small volumes of anesthetic throughout the procedure.
    (2) Ischemia will spread into the adjacent tissues as anesthetic is deposited.
  k. Continue to apply pressure with the cotton applicator stick during this part of the procedure.

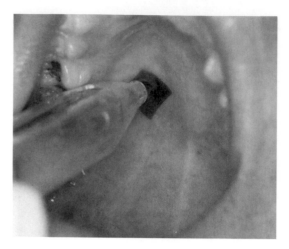

Fig. 13-47 Maxillary nerve block, greater palatine canal approach.

TABLE 13-3 Angle of the Greater Palatine Foramen to the Hard Palate

Angle (°)	n=199	Percent
20 to 22.5	2	1.005
25 to 27.5	4	2.01
30 to 32.5	18	9.045
35 to 37.5	28	14.07
40 to 42.5	25	12.56
45 to 47.5	34	17.08
50 to 52.5	34	17.08
55 to 57.5	29	14.57
60 to 62.5	17	8.54
65 to 67.5	7	3.51
70	1	0.50

From Malamed SF, Trieger N: Intraoral maxillary nerve block: an anatomical and clinical study, *Anesth Prog* 30:44-48, 1983.

The greater palatine nerve block is now complete.

l. Probe gently for the greater palatine foramen.
   (1) The patient will *not* feel discomfort because of the previously deposited anesthetic solution.
   (2) The angle of the needle and syringe may be changed if needed.
   (3) The needle must usually be held at a 45-degree angle to facilitate entry into the greater palatine foramen (Table 13-3).
m. After locating the foramen, very slowly advance the needle into the greater palatine canal to a depth of 30 mm; approximately 5% to 15% of greater palatine canals will have bony obstructions that prevent passage of the needle.
   (1) *Never attempt to force the needle against resistance.*
   (2) If resistance is felt, withdraw the needle slightly and slowly attempt to advance it at a different angle.
   (3) If the needle cannot be advanced further and the depth of penetration is almost adequate, continue with the next steps; however, if the depth is considerably deficient, withdraw the needle and discontinue the attempt.
n. Aspirate.
   (1) Rotate the needle one-fourth turn and reaspirate.
   (2) If negative, slowly deposit 1.8 ml of solution over a minimum of 1 minute.
o. Withdraw the syringe.
p. Make the needle safe.
q. Wait 3 to 5 minutes before commencing the dental procedure.

Signs and symptoms
1. Pressure behind the upper jaw on the side being injected; this usually subsides rapidly, progressing to tingling and numbness of the lower eyelid, side of the nose, and upper lip
2. Sensation of numbness in the teeth and buccal and palatal soft tissues on the side of injection
3. No pain during dental therapy

Safety feature Careful adherence to technique

Precautions
1. *Pain on insertion of the needle*, primarily with the greater palatine canal approach; prevent by using atraumatic palatal injection protocol
2. *Overinsertion of the needle*; can occur in both approaches (though much less likely with the greater palatine canal approach); prevent through careful adherence to protocol
3. *Resistance to needle insertion* in the greater palatine canal approach; never try to advance the needle against resistance

Failures of anesthesia
1. Partial anesthesia; may be due to *underpenetration* by needle. To correct: Reinsert the needle to proper depth and reinject.
2. Inability to negotiate the greater palatine canal. To correct:
   a. Withdraw the needle slightly and reangle.
   b. Reinsert carefully to the proper depth.
   c. If unable to bypass the obstruction *easily*, withdraw the needle and terminate the injection.
      (1) High tuberosity approach may prove more successful in this situation.
   d. The greater palatine canal approach will usually be successful if the needle has been advanced at least two thirds of its length into the canal.

TABLE 13-4 Maxillary Teeth and Available Local Anesthetic Techniques

| Teeth | Pulpal | Soft tissue | |
		Buccal	Palatal
Incisors	Infraorbital (IO)	IO	Nasopalatine
	Infiltration (Inf)	Inf	Inf
Canine	Infraorbital	IO	Nasopalatine
	Infiltration	Inf	Inf
Premolars	Infraorbital	IO	Greater palatine
	Middle superior alveolar (MSA)	MSA	Inf
	Infiltration	Inf	
Molars	Posterior superior alveolar (PSA)	PSA	Greater palatine
	Infiltration	Inf	Inf

TABLE 13-5 Recommended Volumes of Local Anesthetic for Maxillary Techniques

Technique	Volume (ml)
Supraperiosteal (infiltration)	0.6
Posterior superior alveolar	0.9 to 1.8
Middle superior alveolar	0.9 to 1.2
Anterior superior alveolar	0.9 to 1.2
Greater palatine	0.45 to 0.6
Nasopalatine	0.45
Palatal infiltration	0.2 to 0.3
Maxillary nerve block	1.8

Complications

1. Hematoma will develop rapidly if the maxillary artery is punctured during maxillary nerve block via the high tuberosity approach. (Refer to "PSA nerve block, complications," on p. 168.)
2. Penetration of the orbit may occur during a greater palatine foramen approach if the needle goes in too far; more likely to occur in the smaller-than-average skull; complications produced by injection of local anesthetic into the orbit include*
   a. Volume displacement of the orbital structures, producing periorbital swelling and proptosis
   b. Regional block of the sixth cranial nerve (abducens), producing diplopia
   c. Classic retrobulbar block, producing mydriasis, corneal anesthesia, and ophthalmoplegia
   d. Possible optic nerve block with transient loss of vision
   e. Possible retrobulbar hemorrhage
   f. To prevent intraorbital injection: Strictly adhere to protocol and modify your technique for the smaller patient.
3. Penetration of the nasal cavity
   a. If the needle deviates *medially* during insertion through the greater palatine canal, the paper-thin medial wall of the pterygopalatine fossa will be penetrated and the needle will enter into the nasal cavity.
      (1) On aspiration, large amounts of air appear in the cartridge.
      (2) On injection, the patient complains that local anesthetic solution is running down the throat.
      (3) To prevent: Keep the patient's mouth wide open and take care during penetration that the advancing needle stays in the correct plane.

• • •

Table 13-4 summarizes the indications for maxillary local anesthesia. Table 13-5 includes volumes of solutions recommended for maxillary injections.

SUMMARY

Providing clinically adequate anesthesia in the maxilla is seldom a problem. The rather thin maxillary bone permits the ready diffusion of local anesthetic to the apex of the tooth to be treated. For this reason many dentists rely solely on supraperiosteal (or "infiltration") anesthesia for most treatment in the maxilla.

It is only on rare occasion that difficulty arises with maxillary pain control. Most notable, of course, is the pulpally involved tooth, for which, because of infection and/or inflammation, the use of supraperiosteal anesthesia is contraindicated or ineffective. In nonpulpally

*It has been reported[5,6] that complications *a, b,* and *c* were most common after intraorbital injection; complications *d* and *e* were never encountered.

involved teeth the most often observed problems in obtaining adequate pulpal anesthesia via supraperiosteal injection develop in the *central incisor* (whose apex may lie beneath the denser bone and cartilage of the nose), the *canine* (whose root length may be considerable with the anesthetic solution deposited below the apex), and the maxillary *molars* (whose buccal root apices may be covered by denser bone of the zygomatic arch, a problem more often noted in patients 6 to 8 years of age, and whose palatal root may flare toward the palate, making the distance that local anesthetic must diffuse too great). In such situations the use of regional nerve block anesthesia is essential to clinical success in pain control. In reality, two rather safe and simple nerve blocks—the posterior superior alveolar and the anterior superior alveolar—enable dental care to be provided painlessly in virtually all patients.

Palatal anesthesia, though commonly thought of as being highly traumatic, can in most cases be provided with little or no discomfort to the patient.

REFERENCES

1. Adatia AK: Effects of cytotoxic chemotherapy on dental development, *J R Soc Med* 80:784-785, 1987 (letter).
2. Loetscher CA, Melton DC, Walton RE: Injection regimen for anesthesia of the maxillary first molar, *J Am Dent Assoc* 117:337-340, 1988.
3. Frazer M: Contributing factors and symptoms of stress in dental practice, *Br Dent J* 173(3):111, 1992
4. Melzack R: *The puzzle of pain,* New York, 1973, Basic Books.
5. Malamed SF, Trieger N: Intraoral maxillary nerve block: an anatomical and clinical study, *Anesth Prog* 30:44-48, 1983.
6. Poore TE, Carney FMT: Maxillary nerve block: a useful technique, *J Oral Surg* 31:749-755, 1973.

CHAPTER
fourteen

Techniques of Mandibular Anesthesia

Any practicing dentist or dental hygienist is well aware that a major clinical difference exists in the success rates for maxillary nerve blocks (i.e., posterior superior alveolar and infraorbital) and those for mandibular blocks.

Achieving clinically acceptable anesthesia in the maxilla is rarely a problem, except in instances of anatomical anomalies or pathological conditions. Less dense bone covers the apices of maxillary teeth, and the relatively easy access to large nerve trunks provides the well-trained administrator with success rates of 95% or higher.

Not so in the adult mandible. Successful pulpal anesthesia of mandibular teeth is quite a bit more difficult to achieve on a consistently reliable basis. Success rates of 80% to 85% for the inferior alveolar nerve block, the most frequently administered mandibular injection, attest to this fact.[1] Reasons for these lower success rates include the greater density of the buccal alveolar plate (which precludes supraperiosteal injection), limited accessibility to the inferior alveolar nerve, and the wide variation in anatomy. Although an 80% rate of success does not seem particularly low, consider that one out of every five patients will require reinjection to achieve clinically adequate anesthesia.

Six nerve blocks are described in this chapter. Two of these—involving the mental and buccal nerves—provide regional anesthesia to soft tissues only and have exceedingly high success rates. In both instances the nerves anesthetized lie directly beneath the soft tissues, not encased in bone. The four remaining blocks—the inferior alveolar, incisive, Gow-Gates mandibular, and Vazirani-Akinosi (closed-mouth) mandibular—pro-vide regional anesthesia to the pulps of some or all of the mandibular teeth in a quadrant. Three other injections that are of importance in mandibular anesthesia—the periodontal ligament, intraosseous, and the intraseptal—are described in Chapter 15. Although these techniques can be used successfully in either the maxilla or the mandible, their greatest utility lies in the mandible, for in the mandible they can produce pulpal anesthesia of a single tooth without the lingual and buccal soft tissue anesthesia that occurs with other nerve block techniques.

The success rate of the *inferior alveolar* nerve block is lower than for most other (maxillary) nerve blocks. Because of anatomical considerations in the mandible (primarily the density of bone), the administrator must accurately deposit local anesthetic solution to within 1 mm of the target nerve. The inferior alveolar nerve block has a significantly lower success rate because of two factors—(1) anatomical variation in the height of the mandibular foramen on the lingual side of the ramus and (2) the greater depth of soft tissue penetration required—that consistently lead to greater inaccuracy. Fortunately, the *incisive nerve block* provides pulpal anesthesia to the teeth anterior to the mental foramen (i.e., the incisors, canines, first premolars, and [most of the time] second premolars). The incisive nerve block is a valuable alternative to the inferior alveolar nerve block when treatment is limited to these teeth. To achieve anesthesia of the mandibular molars, however, the inferior alveolar nerve must be anesthetized, and this frequently entails (with all its attendant disadvantages) a lower incidence of successful anesthesia.

The third injection technique that provides pulpal anesthesia to the mandibular teeth, the *Gow-Gates mandibular* nerve block, is a true mandibular block injection because it provides regional anesthesia to virtually all the sensory branches of V_3. In actual fact, the Gow-Gates may be termed a high inferior alveolar nerve block. When it is used, two beneficial effects are noted: (1) the problems associated with anatomical variations in the height of the mandibular foramen are obviated and (2) anesthesia of the other sensory branches of V_3 (e.g., the lingual, buccal, and mylohyoid nerves) is usually obtained along with that of the inferior alveolar nerve. With proper adherence to protocol (and with experience using this technique), a success rate in excess of 95% can be achieved.

Another V_3 nerve block, the *closed-mouth mandibular nerve block*, is included in this discussion, mainly because it allows the doctor to achieve clinically adequate anesthesia in an extremely difficult situation—one in which a patient has limited mandibular opening as a result of infection, trauma, or postinjection trismus. It is also known as the Vazirani-Akinosi technique (after the doctors who developed it). Some practitioners use it routinely for anesthesia in the mandibular arch. I describe the closed-mouth technique mainly because with experience it can provide a success rate of better than 80% in situations (extreme trismus) in which the inferior alveolar and Gow-Gates blocks have little or no likelihood of success.

In ideal circumstances the individual who is to administer the local anesthetic should become familiar with each of these techniques. The greater the number of techniques at one's disposal with which to attain mandibular anesthesia, the less likely it is that a patient will be dismissed from an office because adequate anesthesia could not be achieved. More realistically, however, the administrator should become proficient with at least one of these procedures and have a working knowledge of the others to be able to use them with a good expectation of success should the appropriate situation arise.

INFERIOR ALVEOLAR NERVE BLOCK

The inferior alveolar nerve block, commonly (but inaccurately) referred to as the mandibular nerve block, is the most frequently used and quite possibly the most important injection technique in dentistry. Unfortunately, it also proves to be the most frustrating, the one with the highest percentage of clinical failures (approximately 15% to 20%) even when properly administered.[1]

It is an especially useful technique for quadrant dentistry. A supplemental block (buccal nerve) is needed only if soft tissue anesthesia in the buccal posterior region is required. On rare occasion a supraperiosteal injection (infiltration) may be needed in the lower incisor region to correct partial anesthesia caused by the overlap of sensory fibers from the contralateral side. A periodontal ligament (PDL) injection might be required when isolated portions of mandibular teeth (usually the mesial root of a first mandibular molar) remain sensitive following an otherwise successful inferior alveolar nerve block.

The administration of bilateral inferior alveolar nerve blocks is, in my opinion, rarely called for in dental treatments other than bilateral mandibular surgeries. They produce considerable discomfiture, primarily from the lingual soft tissue anesthesia, which usually persists for several hours after injection (the duration, of course, being dependent upon the particular anesthetic used). The patient feels unable to swallow and, because of the lack of all sensation, is more likely to self-injure the anesthetized soft tissues, as well as being unable to enunciate well. I prefer to treat, whenever possible, the entire right or the entire left side of a patient's oral cavity (maxillary and mandibular) at one appointment rather than administer a bilateral inferior alveolar nerve block. Patients are much more able to handle the posttreatment discomfort (e.g., feeling of anesthesia) associated with bilateral maxillary than with bilateral mandibular anesthesia.

One situation in which bilateral mandibular anesthesia is frequently used involves the patient who presents with six or eight lower anterior teeth (e.g., canine to canine) requiring restorative or soft tissue procedures. Two excellent alternatives to *bilateral* inferior alveolar nerve blocks are either bilateral incisive nerve blocks (where lingual soft tissue anesthesia is not required) or a *unilateral* inferior alveolar block on the side that (1) has the greater number of teeth requiring restoration or (2) requires the greater amount of lingual intervention, combined with an *incisive nerve* block on the opposite side. It must be remembered that the incisive nerve block does *not* provide lingual soft tissue anesthesia; thus lingual infiltration may be required.

In the following description of the inferior alveolar nerve block, the injection site will be noted to be slightly higher than that usually depicted. The success rate of this technique, used for many years at the University of Southern California School of Dentistry, approaches 85% to 90% and higher with experience.[2]

Other common name   Mandibular block

Nerves anesthetized
1. Inferior alveolar, a branch of the posterior division of the mandibular
2. Incisive ⎱ Terminal branches of
3. Mental ⎰ the inferior alveolar
4. Lingual (quite commonly)

Areas anesthetized (Fig. 14-1)
1. Mandibular teeth to the midline

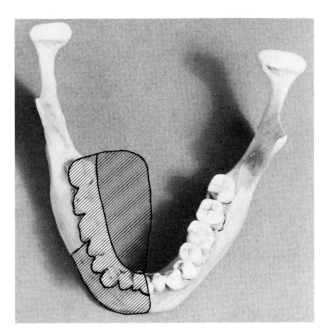

Fig. 14-1 Area anesthetized by an inferior alveolar nerve block.

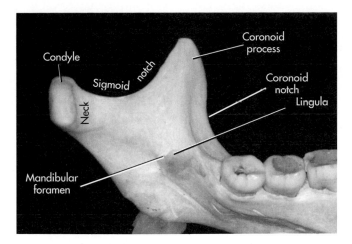

Fig. 14-2 Osseous landmarks for inferior alveolar nerve block.

2. Body of the mandible, inferior portion of the ramus
3. Buccal mucoperiosteum, mucous membrane anterior to the mandibular first molar (mental nerve)
4. Anterior two thirds of the tongue and floor of the oral cavity (lingual nerve)
5. Lingual soft tissues and periosteum (lingual nerve)

Indications
1. Procedures on multiple mandibular teeth in one quadrant
2. When buccal soft tissue anesthesia (anterior to the first molar) is required
3. When lingual soft tissue anesthesia is required

Contraindications
1. Infection or acute inflammation in the area of injection
2. Patients who might bite either the lip or the tongue—for instance, a very young child or a physically or mentally handicapped adult or child

Advantages One injection provides a wide area of anesthesia (useful for quadrant dentistry)

Disadvantages
1. Wide area of anesthesia (not necessary for localized procedures)
2. Rate of inadequate anesthesia (15% to 20%)
3. Intraoral landmarks not consistently reliable
4. Positive aspiration (10% to 15%, highest of all intraoral injection techniques)

5. Lingual and lower lip anesthesia, discomfiting to many patients and possibly dangerous for certain individuals
6. Partial anesthesia possible where a bifid inferior alveolar nerve and bifid mandibular canals are present

Positive aspiration 10% to 15%

Alternatives
1. Mental nerve block, for buccal soft tissue anesthesia anterior to the first molar
2. Incisive nerve block, for pulpal and buccal soft tissue anesthesia of teeth anterior to the mental foramen
3. Supraperiosteal injection, for pulpal anesthesia of the central and lateral incisors, and sometimes the premolars
4. Gow-Gates mandibular nerve block
5. Vazirani-Akinosi mandibular nerve block
6. PDL injection for pulpal anesthesia of any mandibular tooth
7. Intraosseous injection for osseous and soft tissue anesthesia of any mandibular region
8. Intraseptal injection for osseous and soft tissue anesthesia of any mandibular region

Technique
1. A 25-gauge long needle recommended for the adult patient
2. Area of insertion: mucous membrane on the medial side of the mandibular ramus, at the intersection of two lines—one horizontal, representing the height of injection, and the other vertical, representing the anteroposterior plane of injection
3. Target area: inferior alveolar nerve as it passes downward toward the mandibular foramen but before it enters into the foramen
4. Landmarks (Figs. 14-2 and 14-3)

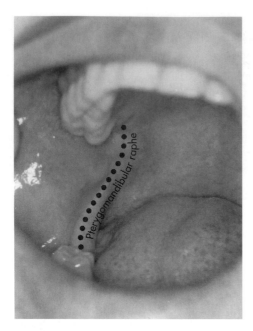

Pterygomandibular raphe

Fig. 14-3 The posterior border of the mandibular ramus can be approximated intraorally by using the pterygomandibular raphe as it turns superiorly toward the maxilla.

a. Coronoid notch (greatest concavity on the anterior border of the ramus)
b. Pterygomandibular raphe
c. Occlusal plane of the mandibular posterior teeth
5. Orientation of the bevel: less critical than with other nerve blocks, because the needle approaches the inferior alveolar nerve at an approximately right angle
6. Procedure
   a. Assume the correct position.
      (1) For a right inferior alveolar nerve block and a right-handed administrator, sit at the 8 o'clock position *facing* the patient (Fig. 14-4, *A*).
      (2) For a left inferior alveolar nerve block and a right-handed administrator, sit at the 10 o'clock position facing in the *same direction* as the patient (Fig. 14-4, *B*).
   b. Position the patient supine (recommended) or semisupine. The mouth should be opened wide to permit greater visibility of and access to the injection site.
   c. Locate the needle penetration (injection) site.

   There are three parameters that must be considered during the administration of the inferior alveolar nerve block (IANB)—the *height* of the injection, the *anteroposterior* placement of the needle (which helps to locate a precise needle entry point), and the *depth* of penetration (which determines the location of the inferior alveolar nerve).

   (1) HEIGHT OF INJECTION: Place the index finger or thumb of your left hand in the coronoid notch.
      (a) An imaginary line extends posteriorly from the finger tip in the coronoid notch to the pterygomandibular raphe (as it turns upward toward the maxilla) and determines the height of injection. This imaginary line should be parallel with the occlusal plane of the mandibular molar teeth. In the majority of patients this line will be 6 to 10 mm above the occlusal plane.
      (b) The finger on the coronoid notch is used to pull the tissues laterally, stretching them over the injection site, making them taut; this will enable the needle insertion to be less traumatic and will provide better visibility.
      (c) The needle insertion point lies three fourths the anteroposterior distance from the coronoid notch back to the pterygomandibular raphe (Fig. 14-5). *Note:* the line should begin at the midpoint of the notch and terminate at the deepest (most posterior) portion of the pterygomandibular raphe as the raphe bends upward toward the palate.
      (d) The posterior border of the mandibular ramus can be approximated intraorally by using the pterygomandibular raphe as it bends superiorly toward the maxilla* (Fig. 14-3).
      (e) An alternative method of approximating the length of the ramus is to place your thumb on the coronoid notch and your index finger extraorally on the posterior ramal border and estimate the distance between these points. However, many practitioners have difficulty envisioning the thickness of the ramus in this manner.
   Prepare tissue at the injection site.
   Dry with sterile gauze.
   Apply topical antiseptic (optional).
   Apply topical anesthetic.
   Place the barrel of the syringe in the corner of the mouth on the contralateral side (Fig. 14-6)
   (2) ANTEROPOSTERIOR SITE OF INJECTION: Needle penetration occurs at the intersection of two points.
      (a) Point 1 falls along the line from the coronoid notch just described for the height of injection.
      (b) Point 2 is on a vertical line through point 1 (about three fourths the distance from the anterior border of the ramus).
      This determines the anteroposterior site of the injection.
   (3) PENETRATION DEPTH: In the third parameter of the inferior alveolar nerve block, *bone must be contacted.* Slowly advance the needle until you can feel it meet bony resistance.
      (a) For most patients it is not necessary to inject any local anesthetic solution as soft tissue is penetrated.

*The pterygomandibular raphe continues posteriorly in a horizontal plane from the retromolar pad before turning upward toward the palate; *only that portion of the pterygomandibular raphe turning upward is used as an indicator of the posterior border of the ramus.*

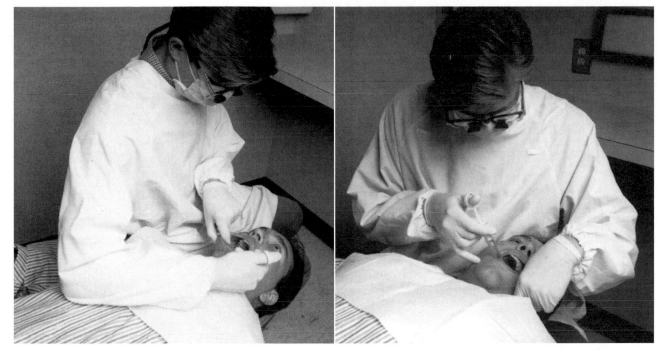

Fig. 14-4 Position of the administrator for a right, **A,** and left, **B,** inferior alveolar nerve block.

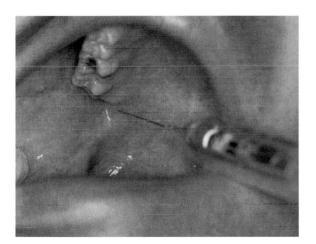

Fig. 14-5 Notice the placement of the syringe barrel at the corner of the mouth, usually corresponding to the premolars. The needle tip gently touches the most distal end of the pterygomandibular raphe.

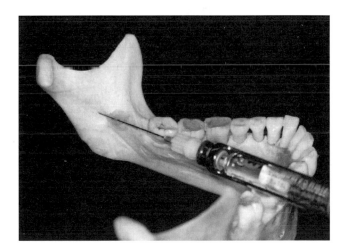

Fig. 14-6 Placement of the needle and syringe for an inferior alveolar nerve block.

(b) For anxious or sensitive patients it may be advisable to deposit small volumes as the needle is advanced.

(c) The average depth of penetration to bony contact will be 20 to 25 mm, approximately two thirds to three fourths the length of a long dental needle (Fig. 14-7).

(d) The needle tip should be located slightly superior to the mandibular foramen (which the inferior alveolar nerve enters). The foramen cannot be seen clinically.

(e) If *bone is contacted too soon* (one half needle depth or less), the needle tip is usually located too far *anteriorly* (laterally) on the ramus (Fig. 14-8). To correct:

(i) Withdraw the needle slightly but do *not* remove it from the tissue.

(ii) Bring the syringe barrel around toward the front of the mouth, over the canine or lateral incisor on the contralateral side.

(iii) Redirect the needle until a more appropriate depth of insertion has been reached. The needle tip will now be located *posterior* to the mandibular sulcus.

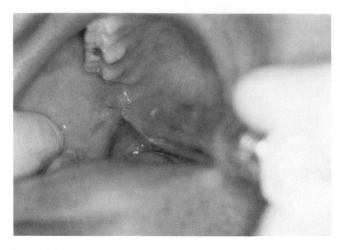

Fig. 14-7 Inferior alveolar nerve block. The depth of penetration is 20 to 25 mm (two thirds to three fourths the length of a long needle).

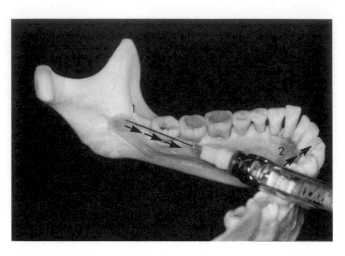

Fig. 14-8 The needle is located too far anteriorly (laterally) on the ramus. To correct: Withdraw it slightly from the tissues (*1*) and bring the syringe barrel anteriorly toward the lateral incisor or canine (*2*); reinsert to proper depth.

A
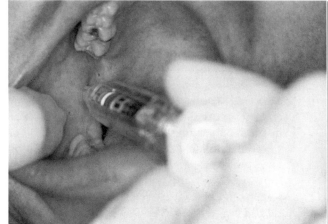

B
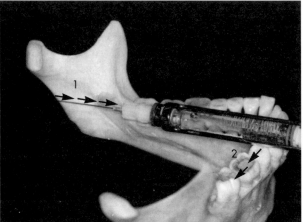

Fig. 14-9 A, Overinsertion with no contact of bone. The needle is usually posterior (medial) to the ramus. **B,** To correct: Withdraw it slightly from the tissues (*1*) and reposition the syringe barrel over the premolars (*2*); reinsert.

(iv) Reposition the syringe barrel over the premolars and continue insertion until bone is again contacted.
(f) If *bone is not contacted,* the needle tip is usually located too far *posterior* (medial) (Fig. 14-9). To correct
   (i) Withdraw it slightly in tissue (leaving approximately one fourth its length in tissue) and reposition the syringe barrel more posteriorly (over the mandibular molars).
   (ii) Continue the insertion until contact with bone is made.

d. Insert the needle. When bone is contacted, withdraw approximately 1 mm to prevent subperiosteal injection.

e. Aspirate. If negative, slowly deposit 1.5 ml of anesthetic over a minimum of 60 seconds. (Because of the high incidence of positive aspiration and the natural tendency to deposit solution too rapidly, the sequence of slow injection, reaspiration, slow injection, reaspiration is strongly recommended.)

f. Slowly withdraw the syringe—and when approximately half its length remains within tissues—reaspirate. If negative, deposit a portion of the remaining solution (0.1 ml) to anesthetize the *lingual nerve.*
   (1) In most patients this deliberate injection for lingual nerve anesthesia *will not be necessary,* since local anesthetic from the inferior alveolar nerve block will diffuse to the lingual nerve.

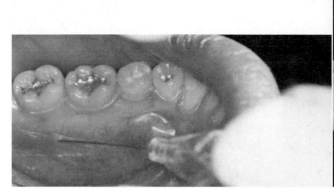
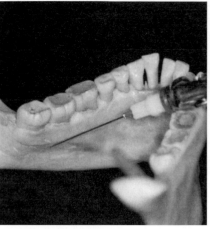

Fig. 14-10 A, Retract the tongue to gain access to, and increase the visibility of, the lingual border of the mandible. **B,** Direct the needle tip below the apical region of the tooth immediately posterior to the tooth in question.

g. Withdraw the syringe slowly and make the needle safe.

h. After approximately 20 seconds, return the patient to the upright or semiupright position.

i. Wait 3 to 5 minutes before commencing the dental procedure.

Signs and symptoms

1. Tingling or numbness of the lower lip indicates anesthesia of the mental nerve, a terminal branch of the inferior alveolar nerve. It is a good indication that the inferior alveolar nerve is anesthetized, although *not* a reliable indicator of the depth of anesthesia.

2. Tingling or numbness of the tongue indicates anesthesia of the lingual nerve, a branch of the posterior division of V_3. It usually accompanies inferior alveolar nerve block but may be present without anesthesia of the inferior alveolar nerve.

3. No pain is felt during dental therapy.

Safety feature   The needle contacts bone and prevents overinsertion, with its attendant complications.

Precautions

1. Do *not* deposit local anesthetic if bone is not contacted. The needle tip may be resting within the parotid gland near the facial nerve (cranial nerve VII), and a transient paralysis of the facial nerve will be produced if solution is deposited.

2. Avoid pain by not contacting bone too forcefully.

Failures of anesthesia   The most common causes of absent or incomplete inferior alveolar nerve block follow:

1. Deposition of anesthetic *too low* (below the mandibular foramen). To correct: Reinject at a higher site.

2. Deposition of anesthetic *too far anteriorly* (laterally) on the ramus. This is diagnosed by a lack of anesthesia except at the injection site and by the minimum depth of penetration prior to contact with bone (i.e., the needle is usually less than halfway into tissue). To correct: Redirect the needle tip posteriorly.

3. Accessory innervation to the mandibular teeth

   a. The primary symptom is isolated areas of incomplete pulpal anesthesia encountered on the mandibular molars (most commonly the mesial portion of the mandibular first molar) or premolars.

   b. Although it has been postulated that several nerves provide the mandibular teeth with accessory sensory innervation (e.g., the cervical accessory and mylohyoid nerves), current thinking supports the mylohyoid nerve as the prime candidate.[3-5] The Gow-Gates mandibular block, which routinely blocks the mylohyoid nerve, is *not* associated with problems of accessory innervation (unlike the inferior alveolar nerve block, which normally *does not* block the mylohyoid nerve).

   c. To correct:

      (1) Primary technique

         (a) Use a 25-gauge long needle.

         (b) Retract the tongue toward the midline with a mirror handle or tongue depressor to provide access and visibility to the lingual border of the body of the mandible (Fig. 14-10).

         (c) Place the syringe in the corner of mouth on the opposite side and direct the needle tip to the apical region of the tooth immediately *posterior* to the tooth in question (e.g., the apex of the second molar if the first molar is causing a problem).

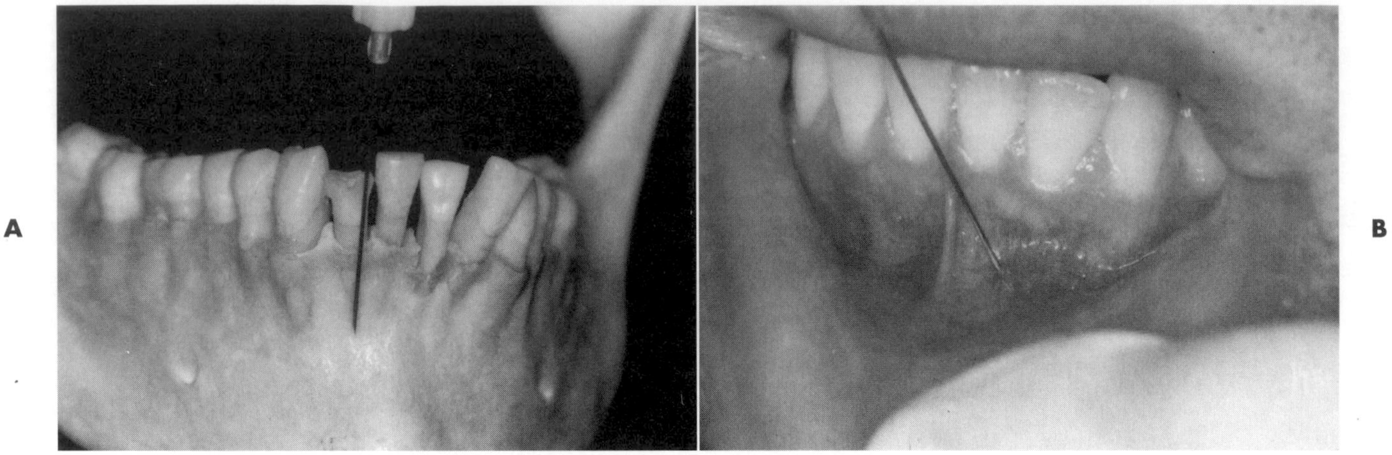

Fig. 14-11 With supraperiosteal injection the needle tip is directed toward the apical region of the tooth in question. **A,** On a skull. **B,** In the mouth.

(d) Penetrate the soft tissues and advance the needle until bone (i.e., the lingual border of the body of the mandible) is contacted. Topical anesthesia will be unnecessary if lingual anesthesia is already present. The depth of penetration is 3 to 5 mm.

(e) Aspirate. If negative, slowly deposit approximately 0.6 ml (one third cartridge) of anesthetic (in about 20 seconds).

(f) Withdraw the syringe and make the needle safe.

(2) Alternate technique. In any situation in which partial anesthesia of a tooth occurs, the periodontal ligament (PDL) injection may be administered; the PDL has a high expectation of success.

d. Whenever a bifid inferior alveolar nerve is detected on the radiograph, incomplete anesthesia of the mandible may develop following an inferior alveolar nerve block. In many such cases a second mandibular foramen, located more inferiorly, exists. To correct: Deposit a volume of solution *inferior* to the normal anatomical landmark.

4. Incomplete anesthesia of the central or lateral incisors

a. This may comprise isolated areas of incomplete pulpal anesthesia.

b. Often it is due to innervation from the mylohyoid nerve, though it also may arise from overlapping fibers of the contralateral inferior alveolar nerve.

c. To correct:

(1) Primary technique

(a) Infiltrate supraperiosteally into the mucobuccal fold below the apex of the tooth in question (Fig. 14-11). This will generally be effective in the lateral incisor and (less often) central incisor region of

the mandible because of the many small nutrient canals in cortical bone near the region of the incisive fossa.

(b) A 27-gauge short needle is recommended.

(c) Direct the needle tip toward the apical region of the tooth in question. Topical anesthesia will not be necessary if mental nerve anesthesia is present

(d) Aspirate.

(e) If negative, slowly deposit not more than 0.6 ml of local anesthetic solution in approximately 20 seconds.

(f) Wait 2 to 3 minutes before starting the dental procedure.

(2) As an alternate technique the PDL injection may be used. The PDL has great success in the mandibular anterior region.

Complications

1. Hematoma (rare)

a. Swelling of tissues on the medial side of the mandibular ramus following the deposition of anesthetic

b. Management: pressure and cold (i.e., ice) to the area for a minimum of 2 minutes

2. Trismus

a. Muscle soreness or limited movement

(1) A slight degree of soreness when opening the mandible is extremely common following IANB.

(2) More severe soreness associated with limited mandibular opening is quite rare.

b. Causes and management discussed in Chapter 17

3. Transient facial paralysis (facial nerve anesthesia)

a. Produced by the deposition of local anesthetic into the body of the parotid gland. Signs and symptoms include the inability to close the lower eyelid and drooping of the upper lip on the affected side.

b. Management of transient facial nerve paralysis is discussed in Chapter 17.

BUCCAL NERVE BLOCK

The buccal nerve is a branch of the anterior division of V_3 and consequently is not anesthetized during the inferior alveolar nerve block. Nor is anesthesia of this nerve required for most restorative dental procedures. The buccal nerve provides sensory innervation to the buccal soft tissues adjacent to the mandibular molars only. The sole indication for administration of a buccal nerve block, therefore, is when manipulation of these tissues is contemplated (e.g., with scaling or curettage, the use of a rubber dam clamp on soft tissues, the removal of subgingival caries, subgingival tooth preparation, placement of gingival retraction cord, and the placement of matrix bands).

Commonly the buccal nerve is blocked routinely following an inferior alveolar nerve block, even when buccal soft tissue anesthesia in the molar region is not required. There is absolutely no indication for this injection in such a situation.

The buccal nerve block, commonly referred to as the long buccal injection, has a success rate approaching 100%. The reason for this is the buccal nerve's readily accessible location immediately beneath mucous membrane and not hidden within bone.

Other common names   Long buccal nerve block, buccinator nerve block

Nerve anesthetized   Buccal (a branch of the anterior division of the mandibular)

Area anesthetized   Soft tissues and periosteum buccal to the mandibular molar teeth (Fig. 14-12)

Indication   When buccal soft tissue anesthesia is required for dental procedures in the mandibular molar region

Contraindication   Infection or acute inflammation in the area of injection

Advantages
1. High success rate
2. Technically easy

Disadvantages   Potential for pain if the needle contacts periosteum during injection

Positive aspiration   0.7%

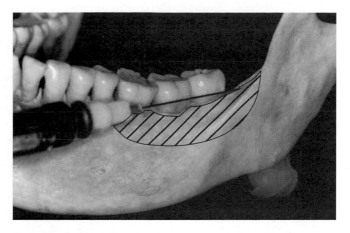

Fig. 14-12 Placement of the needle for, and the area anesthetized by, a buccal nerve block.

Alternatives
1. Buccal infiltration
2. Gow-Gates mandibular nerve block
3. Vazirani-Akinosi mandibular nerve block
4. PDL injection
5. Intraosseous injection
6. Intraseptal injection

Technique
1. A 25-gauge long needle is recommended.
   This is most often used because the buccal nerve block is usually administered immediately following an inferior alveolar nerve block. A 27-gauge long may also be used. The long needle is recommended because of the posterior deposition site, not the depth of tissue insertion (which is minimal).
2. Area of insertion: mucous membrane distal and buccal to the most distal molar tooth in the arch
3. Target area: buccal nerve as it passes over the anterior border of the ramus
4. Landmarks: mandibular molars, mucobuccal fold
5. Orientation of the bevel: *toward* bone during the injection
6. Procedure
   a. Assume the correct position.
      (1) For a right buccal nerve block and a right-handed administrator, sit at the 8 o'clock position directly facing the patient (Fig. 14-13, *A*).
      (2) For a left buccal nerve block and a right-handed administrator, sit at 10 o'clock facing in the same direction as the patient (Fig. 14-13, *B*).
   b. Position the patient supine (recommended) or semisupine.
   c. Prepare the tissues for penetration distal and buccal to the most posterior molar.*

*Because the buccal nerve block most often immediately follows an inferior alveolar nerve block, Steps (1), (2), and (3) of tissue preparation are usually completed prior to the inferior alveolar block.

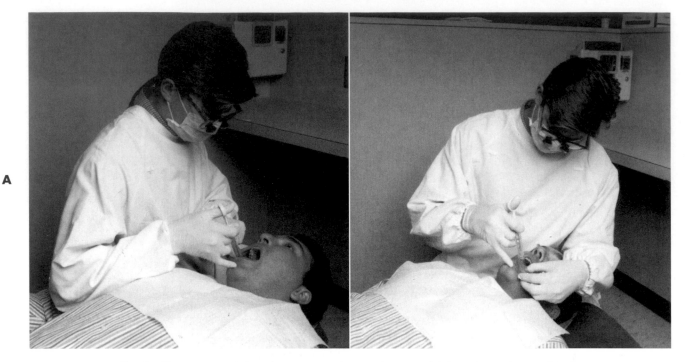

Fig. 14-13 Position of the administrator for a right, **A,** and left, **B,** buccal nerve block.

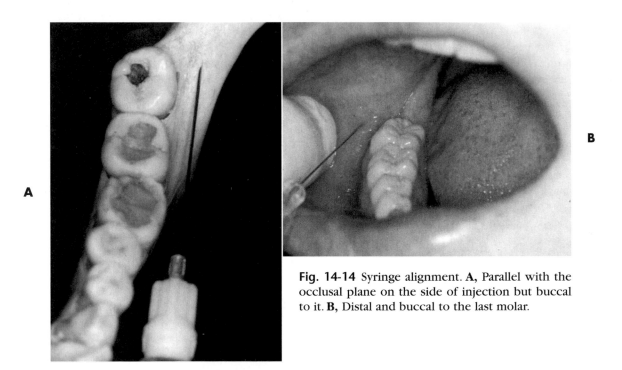

Fig. 14-14 Syringe alignment. **A,** Parallel with the occlusal plane on the side of injection but buccal to it. **B,** Distal and buccal to the last molar.

(1) Dry with sterile gauze.
(2) Apply topical antiseptic (optional).
(3) Apply topical anesthetic.
d. With your left index finger (if right-handed), pull the buccal soft tissues in the area of injection laterally so that visibility will be improved. Taut tissues permit an atraumatic needle penetration.

e. Direct the syringe toward the injection site with the bevel facing down toward bone and the syringe aligned parallel with the occlusal plane on the side of injection but buccal to the teeth (Fig. 14-14, *A*).
f. Penetrate mucous membrane at the injection site, *distal* and *buccal* to the last molar (Fig. 14-14, *B*).

g. Advance the needle slowly until mucoperiosteum is gently contacted.
  (1) To avoid pain when the needle contacts mucoperiosteum, deposit a few drops of local anesthetic just prior to contact.
  (2) The depth of penetration is seldom more than 2 to 4 mm, and usually only 1 or 2 mm.
h. Aspirate.
i. If negative, slowly deposit 0.3 ml (approximately one eighth of a cartridge) over 10 seconds.
  (1) If tissue at the injection site balloons (becomes swollen during injection), stop depositing solution.
  (2) If solution runs out the injection site (back into the patient's mouth) during deposition
    (a) Stop the injection.
    (b) Advance the needle deeper into the tissue.*
    (c) Reaspirate.
    (d) Continue the injection.
j. Withdraw the syringe slowly and immediately make the needle safe.
k. Wait approximately 1 minute before commencing the planned dental procedure.

Signs and symptoms

1. Because of the location and small size of the anesthetized area, the patient rarely experiences any subjective symptoms.
2. Instrumentation in the anesthetized area without pain indicates satisfactory pain control.

Safety features

1. Needle contacting bone and preventing overinsertion
2. Minimum positive aspiration

Precautions

1. Pain on insertion from striking unanesthetized periosteum. This can be prevented by depositing a few drops of local anesthetic before contacting the periosteum.
2. Local anesthetic solution not being retained at the injection site. This generally means that needle penetration is not deep enough, the bevel of the needle is only partially in tissues, and solution is escaping during the injection.
  a. To correct:
    (1) Stop the injection.
    (2) Insert the needle to a greater depth.*
    (3) Reaspirate.
    (4) Continue the injection.

*If an inadequate volume of solution remains in the cartridge, it may be necessary to remove the syringe from the patient's mouth and reload it with a new cartridge.

Failures of anesthesia Rare with the buccal nerve block

1. Inadequate volume of anesthetic retained in the tissues

Complications

1. Few of any consequence
2. Hematoma (bluish discoloration and tissue swelling at the injection site). Blood may exit the needle puncture point into the buccal vestibule. To treat: Apply pressure with gauze directly to the area of bleeding for a minimum of 2 minutes.

MANDIBULAR NERVE BLOCK: THE GOW-GATES TECHNIQUE

Successful anesthesia of the mandibular teeth and soft tissues is more difficult to achieve than anesthesia of maxillary structures. Failure rates of up to 20% are not uncommon with the inferior alveolar nerve block technique previously described. Primary factors for this failure rate are the greater anatomical variation in the mandible and the need for deeper soft tissue penetration. In 1973 George Gow-Gates,[6] a general practitioner of dentistry in Australia, described a new approach to mandibular anesthesia. He had used this technique in his practice for approximately 30 years, with an astonishingly high success rate (approximately 99% *in his experienced hands*).

The Gow-Gates technique is a true mandibular nerve block since it provides sensory anesthesia to virtually the entire distribution of V_3. The inferior alveolar, lingual, mylohyoid, mental, incisive, auriculotemporal, and buccal nerves are all blocked in the Gow-Gates injection.

Significant advantages of the Gow-Gates technique over the inferior alveolar nerve block include its higher success rate, its lower incidence of positive aspiration (approximately 2% versus 10% to 15% with the inferior alveolar nerve block),[6,7] and the absence of problems with accessory sensory innervation to the mandibular teeth.

The only disadvantage I have found is a relatively minor one: the administrator experienced with the inferior alveolar nerve block may feel uncomfortable while learning the Gow-Gates mandibular block. Indeed, the incidence of unsuccessful anesthesia may be as high as (if not higher than) that for the inferior alveolar nerve block until the administrator gains clinical experience with it. Thereafter, success rates of over 95% are common. A new student of local anesthesia usually does not encounter the same difficulty as the more experienced administrator does. This is the result of the strong bias of the experienced administrator to deposit the anesthetic drug "lower" (e.g., in the "usual" place). I suggest two approaches for becoming accustomed to the Gow-Gates technique. The first is to begin to use the technique on all patients requiring mandibular anesthesia. Allow at least 1 to 2 weeks to gain clinical experience. The second is to continue using the conventional inferior alveolar nerve block but to use the Gow-Gates whenever clinically inadequate anesthesia occurs. Reanesthetize the patient using the Gow-Gates technique. Although experience will be accumulated more slowly with this latter approach, its effectiveness will be more dramatic since patients previously difficult to anesthetize will usually now be more easily managed.

Other common names   Gow-Gates technique, third division nerve block, V$_3$ nerve block

Nerves anesthetized
1. Inferior alveolar
2. Mental
3. Incisive
4. Lingual
5. Mylohyoid
6. Auriculotemporal
7. Buccal (in 75% of patients)

Areas anesthetized (Fig. 14-15)
1. Mandibular teeth to the midline
2. Buccal mucoperiosteum and mucous membranes on the side of injection
3. Anterior two thirds of the tongue and floor of the oral cavity
4. Lingual soft tissues and periosteum
5. Body of the mandible, inferior portion of the ramus

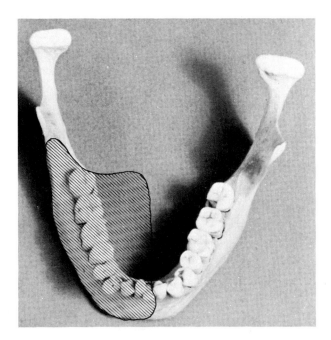

Fig. 14-15 Area anesthetized by a mandibular nerve block (Gow-Gates).

6. Skin over the zygoma, posterior portion of the cheek, and temporal regions

Indications
1. Multiple procedures on mandibular teeth
2. When buccal soft tissue anesthesia, from the third molar to the midline, is required
3. When lingual soft tissue anesthesia is required
4. When a conventional inferior alveolar nerve block is unsuccessful

Contraindications
1. Infection or acute inflammation in the area of injection
2. Patients who might bite either their lip or their tongue, such as young children and physically or mentally handicapped adults
3. Patients who are unable to open their mouth wide

Advantages
1. Requires only one injection; a buccal nerve block not usually necessary (accessory innervation has been blocked)
2. High success rate (> 95%), with experience
3. Minimum aspiration rate
4. Few postinjection complications (i.e., trismus)
5. Provides successful anesthesia where a bifid inferior alveolar nerve and bifid mandibular canals are present

Disadvantages
1. Lingual and lower lip anesthesia is uncomfortable for many patients and possibly dangerous for certain individuals.
2. The time to onset of anesthesia is somewhat longer (5 min) than with an inferior alveolar nerve block (3 to 5 min), primarily because of the size of the nerve trunk being anesthetized and the distance of the nerve trunk from the deposition site (approximately 5 to 10 mm).
3. There is a learning curve with the Gow-Gates technique. Clinical experience is required in order to learn the technique and to fully take advantage of its greater success rate. This learning curve may prove to be frustrating for some persons.

Positive aspiration   2%

Alternatives
1. Inferior alveolar nerve block and buccal nerve block
2. Vazirani-Akinosi closed-mouth mandibular block
3. Incisive nerve block: pulpal and buccal soft tissue anterior to the mental foramen
4. Mental nerve block: buccal soft tissue anterior to the first molar
5. Buccal nerve block: buccal soft tissue from the third to the first molar region

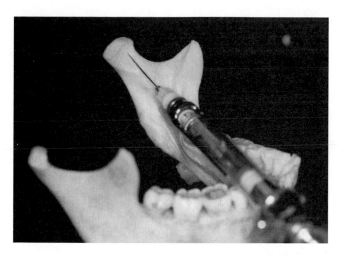

Fig. 14-16 Target area for a Gow-Gates mandibular nerve block—neck of the condyle.

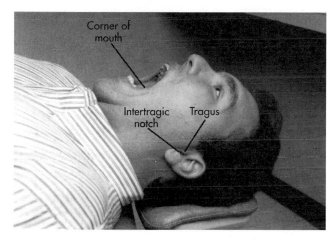

Fig. 14-17 Extraoral landmarks for a Gow-Gates mandibular nerve block.

6. Supraperiosteal injection: for pulpal anesthesia of the central and lateral incisors, and in some instances the canine

Technique

1. 25-gauge long needle recommended
2. Area of insertion: mucous membrane on the mesial of the mandibular ramus, on a line from the intertragic notch to the corner of the mouth, just distal to the maxillary second molar
3. Target area: lateral side of the condylar neck, just below the insertion of the lateral pterygoid muscle (Fig. 14-16)
4. Landmarks
   a. Extraoral
      (1) Lower border of the tragus (intertragic notch); the correct landmark is the center of the external auditory meatus, which is concealed by the tragus; its lower border is therefore adopted as a visual aid (Fig. 14-17)
      (2) Corner of the mouth
   b. Intraoral
      (1) Height of injection established by placement of the needle tip just below the mesiolingual (mesiopalatal) cusp of the maxillary second molar (Fig. 14-18, *A*)
      (2) Penetration of soft tissues just distal to the maxillary second molar at the height established in the preceding step (Fig. 14-18, *B*)
5. Orientation of the bevel: not critical
6. Procedure
   a. Assume the correct position.
      (1) For a right Gow-Gates and right-handed administrator, sit in the 8 o'clock position *facing* the patient.

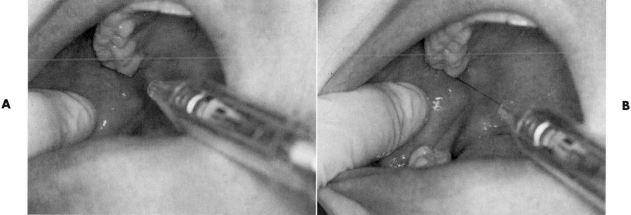

Fig. 14-18 Intraoral landmarks for a Gow-Gates mandibular block. The tip of the needle is placed just below the mesiolingual cusp of the maxillary second molar, **A,** and is moved to a point just distal to the molar, **B,** maintaining the height established in the preceding step. This is the insertion point for the Gow-Gates mandibular nerve block.

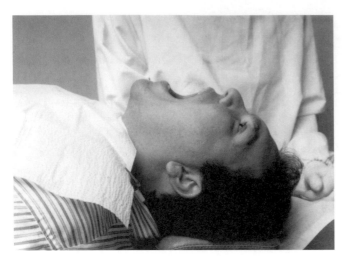

Fig. 14-19 Position of the patient for a Gow-Gates mandibular nerve block.

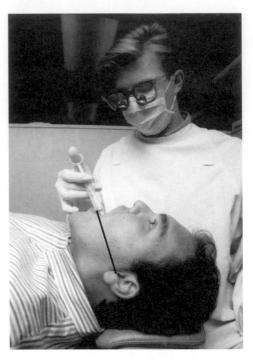

Fig. 14-20 The barrel of the syringe and the needle are held parallel with a line connecting the corner of the mouth and the intertragic notch.

   (2) For a left Gow-Gates and right-handed administrator, sit in the 10 o'clock position facing the *same direction* as the patient.
   (3) These are the same positions used for a right and a left inferior alveolar nerve block.
b. Position the patient (Fig. 14-19).
   (1) Supine is recommended, although semisupine may also be used.
   (2) Request the patient to extend his neck and to open wide for the duration of the technique. The condyle will then assume a more frontal position and be closer to the mandibular nerve trunk.
c. Locate the extraoral landmarks.
   (1) Intertragic notch
   (2) Corner of the mouth
d. Place your left index finger or thumb on the coronoid notch; determination of the coronoid notch is *not* essential to the success of Gow-Gates, but in my experience palpation of this familiar intraoral landmark provides a sense of security besides enabling the tissues to be retracted, and it aids in determining the site of needle penetration.
e. Visualize the intraoral landmarks.
   (1) Mesiolingual (mesiopalatal) cusp of the maxillary second molar
   (2) Needle penetration site is just distal to the maxillary second molar
f. Prepare tissues at the site of penetration.
   (1) Dry tissue with sterile gauze.
   (2) Apply topical antiseptic (optional).
   (3) Apply topical anesthetic.
g. Direct the syringe (held in your right hand) toward the site of injection from the corner of the mouth on the opposite side.
h. Insert the needle gently into tissues at the injection

site just distal to the maxillary second molar at the height of its mesiolingual (mesiopalatal) cusp.
i. Align the needle with the plane extending from the corner of the mouth to the intertragic notch on the side of injection. It should be parallel with the angle between the ear and the face (Fig. 14-20).
j. Direct the syringe toward the target area on the tragus.
   (1) The syringe barrel lies in the corner of the mouth over the premolars, but its position may vary from molars to incisors depending on the divergence of the ramus as assessed by the angle of the ear to the side of the face (Fig. 14-21).
   (2) The height of insertion above the mandibular occlusal plane will be considerably greater (10 to 25 mm, depending on the patient's size) than that noted with the inferior alveolar nerve block.
   (3) When a maxillary third molar is present in a normal occlusion, the site of needle penetration will be just distal to that tooth.
k. Slowly advance the needle until bone is contacted.
   (1) Bone contacted is the neck of the condyle.
   (2) The average depth of soft tissue penetration to bone will be 25 mm, although considerable variation is observed. For a given patient the depth of soft tissue penetration with the Gow-Gates will approximate that with the inferior alveolar nerve block.

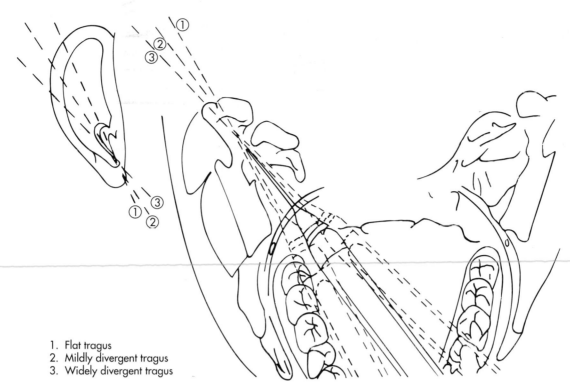

1. Flat tragus
2. Mildly divergent tragus
3. Widely divergent tragus

Fig. 14-21 The location of the syringe barrel depends on the divergence of the tragus. *(Courtesy Dr. George Gow-Gates.)*

(3) If bone is not contacted, withdraw the needle slightly and redirect. (Experience with the Gow-Gates has demonstrated that medial deflection of the needle is the most common cause of failure to contact bone.) Move the barrel of the syringe somewhat more distally, thereby angulating the needle tip anteriorly, and readvance the needle until bony contact is made.

  (a) A second cause of failure to contact bone is a partial closure of the patient's mouth. Once the patient closes even slightly, two negatives occur: (1) the thickness of soft tissue increases and (2) the condyle moves in a distal direction. Both of these make it more difficult to locate the condylar neck with the needle.

(4) *Do not deposit* any local anesthetic if bone has not been contacted.

l. Withdraw the needle 1 mm.

m. Aspirate.

n. If positive, withdraw the needle slightly, angle it superiorly, reinsert, reaspirate, and, if now negative, deposit the solution. Positive aspiration usually occurs in the internal maxillary artery, which is *inferior* to the target area. The positive aspiration rate with the Gow-Gates technique is aproximately 2%.[6,7]

o. If negative, slowly deposit 1.8 ml of solution over 60 to 90 seconds. Gow-Gates originally recommended that 3 ml of anesthetic be deposited.[6] However, I have found (after 20 years of experience with the technique) that 1.8 ml is usually quite adequate to provide clinically acceptable anesthesia in virtually all cases. When partial anesthesia develops following administration of 1.8 ml, a second injection of approximately 1.2 ml is recommended.

p. Withdraw the syringe and make the needle safe.

q. Request that the patient keep the mouth open for 1 to 2 minutes after the injection to permit diffusion of the anesthetic solution.

  (1) Use of a rubber bite block may assist the patient in keeping the mouth open

r. After completion of the injection, return the patient to the upright or semiupright position.

s. Wait minimally 3 to 5 minutes before commencing the dental procedure. The onset of anesthesia with the Gow-Gates may be somewhat slower, requiring 5 to 7 minutes, for the following reasons:

  (1) Greater diameter of the nerve trunk at the site of injection

  (2) Distance (5 to 10 mm) from the anesthetic deposition site to the nerve trunk

Signs and symptoms

1. Tingling or numbness of the lower lip indicates anesthesia of the mental nerve, a terminal branch of the inferior alveolar nerve. It is also a good indication that the inferior alveolar nerve may be anesthetized.

2. Tingling or numbness of the tongue indicates anesthesia of the lingual nerve, a branch of the posterior division of the mandibular nerve. It is always present in a successful Gow-Gates mandibular block.
3. No pain is felt during dental therapy.

Safety features
1. Needle contacting bone and preventing overinsertion
2. Very low positive aspiration rate; minimizes the risk of intravascular injection (the internal maxillary artery lies *inferior* to the injection site)

Precautions   Do not deposit anesthetic solution if bone is not contacted; the needle tip will usually be distal and medial to the desired site.

1. Withdraw slightly.
2. Redirect the needle laterally.
3. Reinsert the needle. Make gentle contact with bone.
4. Withdraw 1 mm and aspirate.
5. Inject if aspiration is negative.

Failures of anesthesia   Rare with the Gow-Gates mandibular block, once the administrator becomes familiar with the technique

1. *Too little volume.* The greater diameter of the mandibular nerve may require a larger volume of anesthetic solution. Deposit up to 1.2 ml in the second injection if the depth of anesthesia is inadequate following the initial 1.8 ml.
2. *Anatomical difficulties. Do not* deposit anesthetic unless bone is contacted.

Complications
1. Hematoma (< 2% incidence of positive aspiration)
2. Trismus (extremely rare)
3. Temporary paralysis of cranial nerves III, IV, and VI
   In a case of cranial nerve paralysis following a right Gow-Gates mandibular block, diplopia, right-sided blepharoptosis, and complete paralysis of the right eye persisted for 20 minutes after the injection. This has occurred following the accidental rapid intravenous administration of local anesthetic.[8] The recommendations of Dr. Gow-Gates include placing the needle on the lateral side of the anterior surface of the condyle, aspirating carefully, and depositing slowly.[6,7] If bone is not contacted, anesthetic solution should not be administered.

VAZIRANI-AKINOSI CLOSED-MOUTH MANDIBULAR BLOCK

The introduction of the Gow-Gates mandibular nerve block in 1973 spurred interest in alternative methods of achieving anesthesia in the lower jaw. In 1977 Dr. Joseph Akinosi reported on a closed-mouth approach to mandibular anesthesia.[9] Although this technique can be used whenever mandibular anesthesia is desired, its primary indication remains those situations in which limited mandibular opening precludes the use of other mandibular injection techniques. Such situations include the presence of spasm of the muscles of mastication (trismus) on one side of the mandible following numerous attempts at inferior alveolar nerve block, as might occur with a "hot" mandibular molar. In this instance, multiple injections have been required to provide anesthesia adequate to extirpate the pulpal tissues of the involved mandibular molar. When the anesthetic effect resolves hours later, the muscles into which the anesthetic solution was deposited become tender, producing some discomfort upon opening the jaw. During a period of sleep, when the muscles are not in use, the muscles go into spasm (the same way one's leg muscles go into spasm following strenuous exercise, making it difficult to stand or walk the next morning), leaving the patient with significantly reduced occlusal opening in the morning.

The management of trismus is reviewed in Chapter 17.

If it is necessary to continue with dental care in the patient with significant trismus, the options for providing mandibular anesthesia are extremely limited. The inferior alveolar and Gow-Gates mandibular blocks cannot be attempted when significant trismus is present. Extraoral mandibular nerve blocks can be attempted and, indeed, possess a significantly high success rate in experienced hands. Extraoral mandibular blocks can be administered either through the sigmoid notch or inferiorly from the chin (Fig. 14-22).[10,11] As the mandibular division of the trigeminal nerve provides motor innervation to the muscles of mastication, a third division block will alleviate trismus that is produced secondary to muscle spasm. Though dentists are permitted to administer extraoral nerve blocks, few actually do so in clinical practice. The Vazirani-Akinosi technique is an intraoral approach to providing both anesthesia and motor blockade in cases of severe unilateral trismus.

In previous editions of this textbook the technique described below was termed the Akinosi closed-mouth mandibular block. However, it appears that a very similar technique was initially described in 1960 by Vazirani.[12] The name Vazirani-Akinosi closed-mouth mandibular block has been adopted in this fourth edition, giving recognition to both of the doctors who devised and publicized this closed-mouth approach to mandibular anesthesia.

In 1992 Wolfe described a modification of the original Vazirani-Akinosi technique.[13] The technique described was identical to the original technique except that the author recommended bending the needle at a 45-degree angle in order to enable it to remain in close proximity to the medial (lingual) side of the mandibular

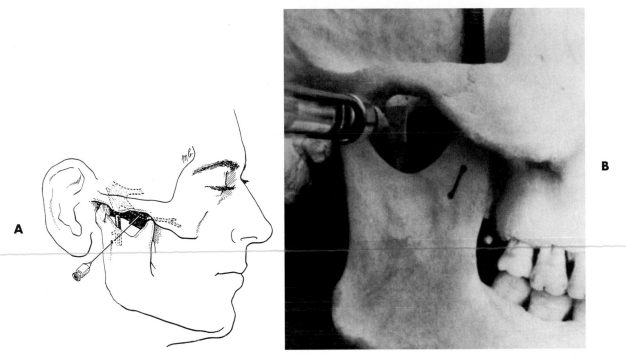

Fig. 14-22 A and **B,** Extraoral mandibular block using lateral approach through the sigmoid notch. *(From Bennett CR:* Monheim's local anesthesia and pain control in dental practice, *ed 6, St Louis, 1978, Mosby–Year Book.)*

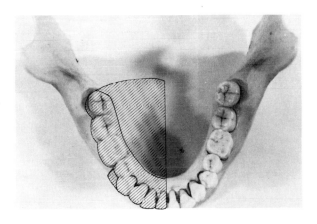

Fig. 14-23 Area anesthetized by a Vazirani-Akinosi closed-mouth mandibular nerve block.

ramus as the needle is advanced through the tissues. I, however, do not feel comfortable recommending the bending of needles when that needle is to be inserted into tissues to any significant depth. The potential for needle breakage is increased when it is bent. The Vazirani-Akinosi closed-mouth mandibular block can be administered quite successfully without the need for bending of the needle.

Other common names   Akinosi technique, closed-mouth mandibular nerve block, tuberosity technique

Nerves anesthetized
1. Inferior alveolar
2. Incisive
3. Mental
4. Lingual
5. Mylohyoid

Areas anesthetized (Fig. 14-23)
1. Mandibular teeth to the midline
2. Body of the mandible and inferior portion of the ramus
3. Buccal mucoperiosteum and mucous membrane in front of the mental foramen
4. Anterior two thirds of the tongue and floor of the oral cavity (lingual nerve)
5. Lingual soft tissues and periosteum (lingual nerve)

Indications
1. Limited mandibular opening
2. Multiple procedures on mandibular teeth
3. Inability to visualize landmarks for IANB

Contraindications
1. Infection or acute inflammation in the area of injection
2. Patients who might bite either their lip or their tongue, such as young children and physically or mentally handicapped adults
3. Inability to visualize or gain access to the lingual aspect of the ramus

Advantages

1. Relatively atraumatic
2. Patient need not be able to open the mouth
3. Fewer postoperative complications (i.e., trismus)
4. Lower aspiration rate (< 10%) than with the inferior alveolar nerve block
5. Provides successful anesthesia where a bifid inferior alveolar nerve and bifid mandibular canals are present

Disadvantages

1. Difficult to visualize the path of the needle and the depth of insertion
2. No bony contact; depth of penetration somewhat arbitrary
3. Potentially traumatic if the needle is too close to periosteum

Alternatives   No intraoral nerve blocks are available. If a patient is unable to open his mouth because of trauma, infection, or postinjection trismus, there are no other suitable intraoral techniques available. The extraoral mandibular nerve block may be used whenever the doctor is well versed in the procedure.

Technique

1. A 25-gauge long needle recommended (although a 27-gauge long may be preferred in patients whose ramus flares laterally more than usual)
2. Area of insertion: soft tissue overlying the medial (lingual) border of the mandibular ramus directly adjacent to the maxillary tuberosity at the height of the mucogingival junction adjacent to the maxillary third molar (Fig. 14-24)
3. Target area: soft tissue on the medial (lingual) border of the ramus in the region of the inferior alveolar, lin-

gual, and mylohyoid nerves as they run inferiorly from the foramen ovale toward the mandibular foramen (the height of injection with the Vazirani-Akinosi being *below* that with the Gow-Gates but *above* that with the inferior alveolar nerve block)
4. Landmarks
   a. Mucogingival junction of the maxillary third (or second) molar
   b. Maxillary tuberosity
   c. Coronoid notch on the mandibular ramus
5. Orientation of the bevel (bevel orientation in the closed-mouth mandibular block is *very significant*): the bevel must be oriented *away* from the bone of the mandibular ramus (i.e., bevel faces toward the midline)
6. Procedure
   a. Assume the correct position. For either a right or a left Vazirani-Akinosi and a right-handed administrator, sit at the 8 o'clock position *facing* the patient.
   b. Position the patient supine (recommended) or semisupine.
   c. Place your left index finger or thumb on the coronoid notch, reflecting the tissues on the medial aspect of the ramus laterally. Reflecting the soft tissues aids in visualization of the injection site and decreases trauma during needle insertion.
   d. Visualize landmarks.
      (1) Mucogingival junction of the maxillary third or second molar
      (2) Maxillary tuberosity
   e. Prepare the tissues at the site of penetration.
      (1) Dry with sterile gauze.
      (2) Apply topical antiseptic (optional).
      (3) Apply topical anesthetic.

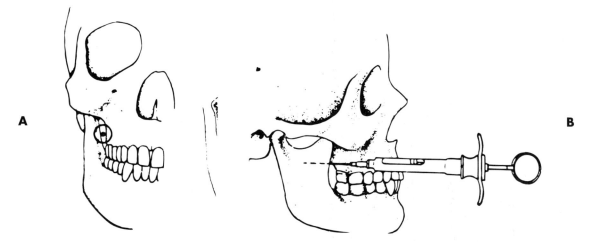

Fig. 14-24 A, Area of needle insertion for a Vazirani-Akinosi block. **B,** Hold the syringe and needle at the height of the mucogingival junction above the maxillary third molar. *(From Gustanis JF, Peterson LJ: An alternative method of mandibular nerve block, J Am Dent Assoc 103:33-36, 1981. Copyright the American Dental Association. Reprinted by permission.)*

f. Ask the patient to occlude gently with the cheeks and muscles of mastication relaxed.

g. Reflect the soft tissues on the medial border of the ramus laterally (Fig. 14-24, *A*).

h. The barrel of the syringe is held parallel with the maxillary occlusal plane, the needle at the level of the mucogingival junction of the maxillary third (or second) molar (Fig. 14-24, *B*).

i. Direct the needle posteriorly and slightly laterally, so it advances at a tangent to the posterior maxillary alveolar process and parallel with the maxillary occlusal plane.

j. Orient the bevel *away* from the mandibular ramus; thus as the needle advances through tissues, needle deflection will occur *toward* the ramus and the needle will remain in close proximity to the inferior alveolar nerve (Fig. 14-25)

k. Advance the needle 25 mm into tissue (for an average-sized adult). This distance is measured from the maxillary tuberosity. The tip of the needle should be in the midportion of the pterygomandibular space, close to the branches of V_3.

l. Aspirate.

m. If negative, deposit 1.5 to 1.8 ml of anesthetic solution in approximately 60 seconds.

n. Withdraw the syringe slowly and immediately make the needle safe.

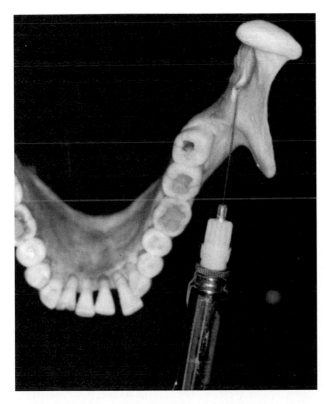

Fig. 14-25 Advance the needle posteriorly into tissues on the medial side of the mandibular ramus.

o. After the injection, return the patient to an upright or semiupright position.

p. Motor nerve paralysis will develop as quickly as or more quickly than sensory anesthesia. The patient with trismus will begin to notice increased ability to open the jaws shortly after the deposition of anesthetic.

q. Anesthesia of the lip and tongue will be noted in 40 to 90 seconds; the dental procedure can usually start within 5 minutes.

r. When motor paralysis is present but sensory anesthesia is inadequate to permit the dental procedure to begin, readminister the Vazirani-Akinosi block or, since the patient can now open the jaws, perform the standard inferior alveolar, Gow-Gates, or incisive nerve block, or a PDL injection.

Signs and symptoms

1. Tingling or numbness of the lower lip indicates anesthesia of the mental nerve, a terminal branch of the inferior alveolar nerve, which is a good sign that the inferior alveolar nerve has been anesthetized.

2. Tingling or numbness of the tongue indicates anesthesia of the lingual nerve, a branch of the posterior division of the mandibular nerve.

3. No pain is felt during dental treatment.

Safety feature Decreased risk of positive aspiration (compared with the inferior alveolar nerve block)

Precaution Do not overinsert the needle (> 25 mm). Decrease the depth of penetration in smaller patients; the depth of insertion will vary with the anteroposterior size of the patient's ramus.

Failures of anesthesia

1. Almost always due to failure to appreciate the flaring nature of the ramus. If the needle is directed medially, it will rest medial to the sphenomandibular ligament in the pterygomandibular space, and the injection will fail. This is more common when a right-handed administrator uses the left-side Vazirani-Akinosi injection (or a left-handed administrator uses the right-side Vazirani-Akinosi injection). It may be prevented by directing the needle tip parallel with the lateral flare of the ramus and by using a 27-gauge needle in place of the 25-gauge.

2. Needle insertion point too low. To correct: Insert the needle at or slightly above the level of the mucogingival junction of the last maxillary molar. The needle must also remain parallel with the occlusal plane as it advances through the soft tissues.

3. Underinsertion or overinsertion of the needle. As no bone is contacted in the Vazirani-Akinosi technique, the depth of soft tissue penetration is somewhat

arbitrary. Akinosi recommended a penetration depth of 25 mm in the *average-sized* adult, measuring from the maxillary tuberosity. In smaller or larger patients this depth of penetration should be altered.

Complications
1. Hematoma (<10%)
2. Trismus (rare)
3. Transient facial nerve (VII) paralysis
   a. This is caused by overinsertion and injection of the local anesthetic solution into the body of the parotid gland.
   b. It can be prevented by modifying the depth of needle penetration based on the length of the mandibular ramus. The 25 mm depth of penetration is the average for a normal-sized adult.

MENTAL NERVE BLOCK

The mental nerve is a terminal branch of the inferior alveolar nerve. Exiting the mental foramen at or near the apices of the mandibular premolars, it provides sensory innervation to the buccal soft tissues lying anterior to the foramen and the soft tissues of the lower lip and chin on the side of injection.

For most dental procedures there is very little indication for use of the mental nerve block. Indeed, of the techniques described in this section, the mental nerve block is the least frequently employed. It is used primarily for buccal soft tissue procedures, such as suturing of lacerations or biopsies. Its success rate approaches 100% because of the ease of accessibility to the nerve.

Other common names   None

Nerve anesthetized   Mental, a terminal branch of the inferior alveolar

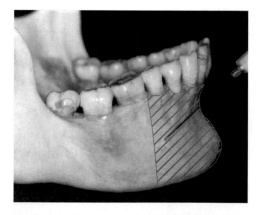

Fig. 14-26 Placement of the needle and the area anesthetized by a mental nerve block.

Areas anesthetized   Buccal mucous membranes anterior to the mental foramen (around the second premolar) to the midline and skin of the lower lip (Fig. 14-26) and chin

Indication   When buccal soft tissue anesthesia is required for procedures in the mandible anterior to the mental foramen, such as

1. Soft tissue biopsies
2. Suturing of soft tissues

Contraindication   Infection or acute inflammation in the area of injection

Advantages
1. High success rate
2. Technically easy
3. Usually entirely atraumatic

Disadvantage   Hematoma

Positive aspiration   5.7%

Alternatives
1. Local infiltration
2. Inferior alveolar nerve block
3. Gow-Gates mandibular nerve block

Technique
1. A 25- or 27-gauge short needle recommended
2. Area of insertion: mucobuccal fold at or just anterior to the mental foramen
3. Target area: mental nerve as it exits the mental foramen (usually located between the apices of the first and second premolars)
4. Landmarks: mandibular premolars and mucobuccal fold
5. Orientation of the bevel: *toward* bone during the injection
   a. Assume the correct position.
      (1) For a right or left incisive nerve block and a right-handed administrator, sit comfortably in front of the patient so that the syringe may be placed into the mouth below the patient's line of sight (Fig. 14-27).
      (2) The recommended position for this injection has been changed in this edition. I received many comments from doctors using this injection mentioning that the "old" position of choice—sitting behind the patient—was psychologically quite traumatic for the patient. The syringe was always in the patient's line of sight (Fig. 14.28)
   b. Position the patient.

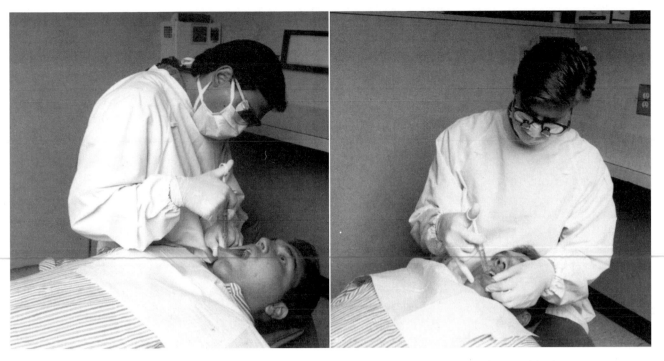

Fig. 14-27 Position of the administrator for a right, **A,** and left, **B,** mental nerve block.

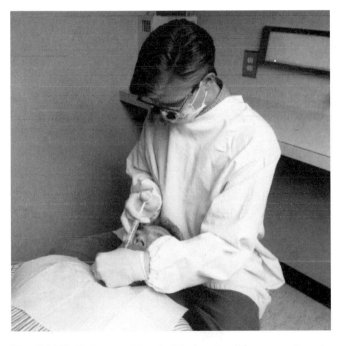

Fig. 14-28 Sitting position behind patient keeps syringe in line of sight.

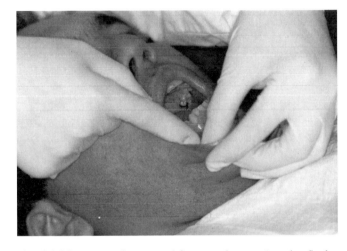

Fig. 14-29 Locate the mental foramen by moving the fleshy pad of your finger anteriorly until the bone beneath becomes irregular and somewhat concave.

   (1) Supine is recommended, but semisupine is acceptable.

   (2) Have the patient partially close. This will permit greater access to the injection site.

 c. Locate the mental foramen.

   (1) Place your index finger in the mucobuccal fold and press against the body of the mandible in the first molar area.

   (2) Move your finger slowly anteriorly until the bone beneath your finger feels irregular and somewhat concave (Fig. 14-29).

     (a) The bone posterior and anterior to the mental foramen will feel smooth; however, the bone immediately around the foramen will feel rougher to the touch.

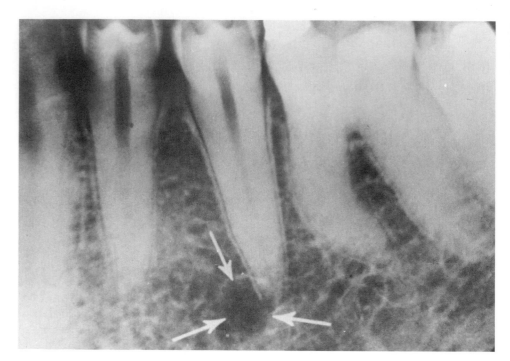

Fig. 14-30 Radiographs can assist in locating the mental foramen (*arrows*). (*Courtesy Dr. Robert Ziehm.*)

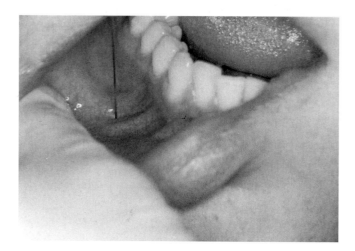

Fig. 14-31 Mental nerve block—needle penetration site.

(b) The mental foramen is usually found between the apices of the two premolars. However, it may be found either anterior or posterior to this site.

(c) The patient will comment that finger pressure in this area produces soreness as the mental nerve is compressed against bone.

(3) If radiographs are available, the mental foramen may easily be located (Fig. 14-30).

d. Prepare tissue at the site of penetration.
(1) Dry with sterile gauze.
(2) Apply topical antiseptic (optional).
(3) Apply topical anesthetic.

e. With your left index finger pull the lower lip and buccal soft tissues laterally.

(1) Visibility will be improved.
(2) Taut tissues permit an atraumatic penetration.

f. Orient the syringe with the bevel directed *toward* bone.

g. Penetrate the mucous membrane at the injection site, at the canine or first premolar, directing the syringe toward the mental foramen (Fig. 14-31).

h. Advance the needle slowly until the foramen is reached. The depth of penetration will be 5 to 6 mm. For the mental nerve block to be successful, there is no need to enter the mental foramen.

i. Aspirate.

j. If negative, slowly deposit 0.6 ml (approximately one-third cartridge) over 20 seconds. If tissue at the injection site balloons (swells as the anesthetic is injected), stop the deposition and remove the syringe.

k. Withdraw the syringe and immediately make the needle safe.

l. Wait 2 to 3 minutes before commencing the procedure.

Signs and symptoms
1. Tingling or numbness of the lower lip
2. No pain during treatment

Safety feature   The region is anatomically "safe."

Precautions   Striking periosteum will produce discomfort. To prevent: Avoid contact with the periosteum *or* deposit a small amount of solution prior to contacting periosteum.

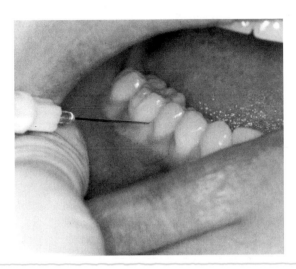

Fig. 14-32 To obtain lingual anesthesia, following the incisive nerve block, insert needle interproximally from buccal and deposit anesthetic as the needle is advanced toward lingual.

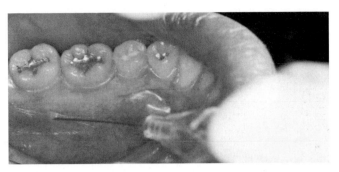

Fig. 14-33 Retract the tongue to gain access to, and increase the visibility of, the lingual border of the mandible.

Failures of anesthesia Rare with the mental nerve block

Complications
1. Few of consequence
2. Hematoma (bluish discoloration and tissue swelling at the injection site). Blood may exit the needle puncture point into the buccal fold. To treat: Apply pressure with gauze directly to the area of bleeding for a minimum of 2 minutes. (See Fig. 17-2.)

INCISIVE NERVE BLOCK

The incisive nerve is a terminal branch of the inferior alveolar nerve. Originating as a direct continuation of the inferior alveolar nerve at the mental foramen, the incisive nerve continues anteriorly in the incisive canal, providing sensory innervation to those teeth located anterior to the mental foramen. The nerve is always anesthetized when an inferior alveolar or mandibular nerve block is successful; therefore the incisive nerve block is not necessary when these blocks are administered.

The premolars, canine, lateral and central incisors, including their buccal soft tissues and bone, are anesthetized when the incisive nerve block is administered.

An important indication for the incisive nerve block is when the contemplated procedure will involve both the right and left sides of the mandible. It is my belief that bilateral inferior alveolar or mandibular nerve blocks are rarely needed (except in the case of bilateral surgical procedures in the mandible) because of the degree of discomfort and the inconvenience experienced by the patient both during and after the procedure. Where the dental treatment involves bilateral procedures on mandibular premolars and anterior teeth, bilateral incisive nerve blocks can be administered. Pulpal, buccal soft tissue, and bone anesthesia is readily obtained. Lingual soft tissues are *not* anesthetized with this block. If lingual soft tissues in very isolated areas require anesthesia, local infiltration can be accomplished readily by inserting a 27-gauge short needle through the interdental papilla on *both the mesial and distal aspect on the tooth* being treated. As the buccal soft tissues are already anesthetized (incisive nerve block), the penetration is atraumatic. Local anesthetic solution should be deposited as the needle is advanced through the tissue toward the lingual (Fig. 14-32). This technique will provide lingual soft tissue anesthesia adequate for deep curettage, root planing, and subgingival preparations. Where there is a significant requirement for lingual soft tissue anesthesia, an inferior alveolar or mandibular nerve block should be administered on that side, with the incisive nerve block administered on the contralateral side. In this manner the patient will not have to endure bilateral anesthesia of the tongue—a very disconcerting experience for many patients.

Another method of obtaining lingual anesthesia following the incisive nerve block is to administer a partial lingual nerve block (Fig. 14-33). Using a 25-gauge long needle, deposit 0.3 to 0.6 ml of local anesthetic under the posterior lingual mucosa just distal to the last tooth to be treated. This will provide lingual soft tissue anesthesia adequate for any dental procedure in this area.

It is not necessary for the needle to enter into the mental foramen for an incisive nerve block to be successful. The first edition of this book and other textbooks of local anesthesia for dentistry recommended insertion of the needle into the foramen.[11,14-15] There are at least two disadvantages to the needle entering into the mental foramen: (1) the administration of an incisive nerve block becomes technically more difficult and (2) the risk of traumatizing the mental and/or incisive nerves and their associated blood vessels is increased. As described below, for the incisive nerve block to be successful the anesthetic should be deposited just outside the mental foramen and, under pressure, directed into the foramen.

Indeed, the incisive nerve block may be considered the mandibular equivalent of the anterior superior alveolar nerve block, with the mental nerve block the equivalent of the infraorbital nerve block. Both of the disadvantages just mentioned are minimized by not entering into the mental foramen.

Other common name   Mental nerve block (inappropriate)

Nerves anesthetized   Mental and incisive

Areas anesthetized (Fig. 14-34)
1. Buccal mucous membrane anterior to the mental foramen, usually from the second premolar to the midline
2. Lower lip and skin of the chin
3. Pulpal nerve fibers to the premolars, canine, and incisors

Indications
1. Dental procedures requiring pulpal anesthesia on mandibular teeth anterior to the mental foramen
2. When inferior alveolar nerve block is not indicated
   a. When six or eight anterior teeth (e.g., canine to canine or premolar to premolar) are treated, the incisive nerve block is recommended in place of bilateral inferior alveolar nerve blocks.

Contraindication   Infection or acute inflammation in the area of injection

Advantages
1. Provides pulpal and hard tissue anesthesia *without* lingual anesthesia (which is uncomfortable and unnecessary for many patients); useful in place of bilateral inferior alveolar nerve blocks
2. High success rate

Disadvantages
1. Does not provide lingual anesthesia. The lingual tissues must be injected directly if anesthesia is desired.
2. Partial anesthesia may develop at the midline because of nerve fiber overlap with the opposite side (extremely rare). Local infiltration on the buccal of the mandibular central incisors may be necessary for complete pulpal anesthesia to be obtained.

Positive aspiration   5.7%

Alternatives
1. Local infiltration for buccal soft tissues and pulpal anesthesia of the central and lateral incisors
2. Inferior alveolar nerve block

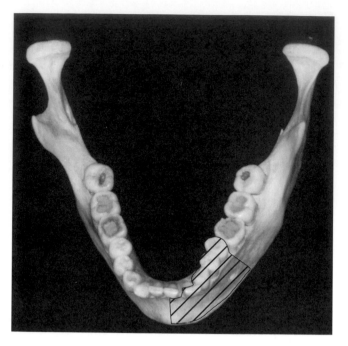

Fig. 14-34 Area anesthetized by an incisive nerve block.

3. Gow-Gates mandibular nerve block
4. Periodontal ligament injection

Technique
1. A 25-gauge short needle recommended (although a 27-gauge short is more commonly used and is perfectly acceptable)
2. Area of insertion: mucobuccal fold at or just anterior to the mental foramen
3. Target area: mental foramen, through which the mental nerve exits and inside of which the incisive nerve is located
4. Landmarks: mandibular premolars and mucobuccal fold
5. Orientation of the bevel: *toward* bone during the injection
6. Procedure
   a. Assume the correct position.
      (1) For a right or left incisive nerve block and a right-handed administrator, sit comfortably in front of the patient so that the syringe may be placed into the mouth below the patient's line of sight (Fig. 14-27).
      (2) The recommended position for this injection has been changed in this edition. I received many comments from doctors using this injection mentioning that the "old" position of choice—sitting behind the patient—was psychologically quite traumatic for the patient. The syringe was always in the patient's line of sight (Fig. 14-28).

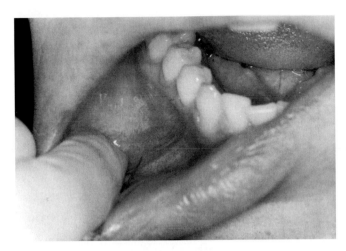

Fig. 14-35 Retract the lip to improve access and permit atraumatic needle insertion.

   b. Position the patient.
      (1) Supine is recommended, but semisupine is acceptable.
      (2) Request that the patient partially close; this will permit greater access to the injection site.
   c. Locate the mental foramen.
      (1) Place your thumb or index finger in the mucobuccal fold against the body of the mandible in the first molar area.
      (2) Move it slowly anteriorly until you feel the bone become irregular and somewhat concave.
        (a) The bone posterior and anterior to the mental foramen will feel smooth; however, the bone immediately around the foramen will feel rougher to the touch.
        (b) The mental foramen is usually found between the apices of the two premolars. However, it may be found either anterior or posterior to this site.
        (c) The patient will comment that finger pressure in this area produces soreness as the mental nerve is compressed against bone.
      (3) If radiographs are available, the mental foramen may easily be located (Fig. 14-30).
   d. Prepare tissues at the site of penetration.
      (1) Dry with sterile gauze.
      (2) Apply topical antiseptic (optional).
      (3) Apply topical anesthetic.
   e. With your left index finger pull the lower lip and buccal soft tissue laterally (Fig. 14-35).
      (1) Visibility will be improved.
      (2) Taut tissues permit atraumatic penetration.
   f. Orient the syringe with the bevel *toward* bone.

   g. Penetrate mucous membrane at the canine or first premolar, directing the needle toward the mental foramen.
   h. Advance the needle slowly until the mental foramen is reached. The depth of penetration will be 5 to 6 mm. There is no need to enter the mental foramen for the incisive nerve block to be successful.
   i. Aspirate.
   j. If negative, slowly deposit 0.6 ml (approximately one third of a cartridge) over 20 seconds.
      (1) During the injection, maintain gentle finger pressure directly over the injection site to increase the volume of solution entering into the mental foramen. This may be accomplished with either intraoral or extraoral pressure.
      (2) Tissues at the injection site should balloon, but very slightly.
   k. Withdraw the syringe and immediately make the needle safe.
   l. Continue to apply pressure at the injection site for 2 minutes.
   m. Wait approximately 3 minutes before commencing the dental procedure.
      (1) Anesthesia of the mental nerve (lower lip, buccal soft tissues) will be observed within seconds of the deposition.
      (2) Anesthesia of the incisive nerve will require additional time.

Signs and symptoms
1. Tingling or numbness of the lower lip
2. No pain during dental therapy

Safety feature   Anatomically "safe" region

Precaution   Usually an atraumatic injection unless the needle contacts periosteum or solution is deposited too rapidly

Failures of anesthesia
1. Inadequate volume of anesthetic solution in the mental foramen, with subsequent lack of pulpal anesthesia. To correct: Reinject into the proper region and apply pressure to the injection site.
2. Inadequate duration of pressure following injection. It is necessary to apply firm pressure over the injection site for a minimum of 2 minutes in order to force anesthetic solution into the mental foramen and to provide anesthesia of the second premolar, which lies *distal* to the foramen. Failure to achieve anesthesia of the second premolar is usually due to inadequate application of pressure following the injection.

TABLE 14-1 Mandibular Teeth and Available Local Anesthetic Techniques

Teeth	Pulpal	Soft tissue	
		Buccal	Lingual
Incisors	Incisive (Inc)	IANB	IANB
	Inferior alveolar (IANB)	GG	GG
	Gow-Gates (GG)	VA	VA
	Vazirani-Akinosi (VA)	Inc	PDL
	Periodontal ligament (PDL) injection	IS	IS
	Intraseptal (IS)	Mental	Inf
	Intraosseous (IO)	PDL	IO
	Infiltration (lateral incisor only)	Inf	
		IO	
Canine	Inferior alveolar	IANB	IANB
	Gow-Gates	GG	GG
	Vazirani-Akinosi	VA	VA
	Incisive	Inc	PDL
	Periodontal ligament injection	PDL	IS
	Intraseptal	IS	Inf
	Intraosseous	IO	IO
		Inf	
		Mental	
Premolars	Inferior alveolar	IANB	IANB
	Gow-Gates	GG	GG
	Vazirani-Akinosi	VA	VA
	Incisive	Inc	PDL
	Periodontal ligament injection	PDL	IS
	Intraseptal	IS	IO
	Intraosseous	IO	Inf
		Mental	
		Inf	
Molars	Inferior alveolar	IANB	IANB
	Gow-Gates	GG	GG
	Vazirani-Akinosi	VA	VA
	Periodontal ligament injection	PDL	PDL
	Intraseptal	IS	IS
	Intraosseous	IO	IO
		Inf	Inf

TABLE 14-2 Recommended Volumes of Local Anesthetic Solution for Mandibular Injection Techniques

Technique	Volume (ml)
Inferior alveolar	1.5
Buccal	0.3
Gow-Gates	1.8
Vazirani-Akinosi	1.5 to 1.8
Mental	0.6
Incisive	0.6 to 0.9

Complications

1. Few of any consequence
2. Hematoma (bluish discoloration and tissue swelling at injection site). Blood may exit the needle puncture site into the buccal fold. To treat: Apply pressure with gauze directly to the area for 2 minutes. This is rarely a problem, since proper incisive nerve block protocol includes the application of pressure at the injection site for 2 minutes.

• • •

Table 14-1 summarizes the various injection techniques applicable for mandibular teeth. Table 14-2 summarizes the recommended volumes for the various injection techniques.

REFERENCES

1. Kaufman E, Weinstein P, Milgrom P: Difficulties in achieving local anesthesia, *J Am Dent Assoc* 108:205-208, 1984.
2. Malamed SF: Unpublished clinical surveys at University of Southern California School of Dentistry, 1995.
3. Wilson S, Johns PI, Fuller PM: The inferior alveolar and mylohyoid nerves: an anatomic study and relationship to local anesthesia of the anterior mandibular teeth, *J Am Dent Assoc* 108:350-352, 1984.
4. Frommer J, Mele FA, Monroe CW: The possible role of the mylohyoid nerve in mandibular posterior tooth sensation, *J Am Dent Assoc* 85:113-117, 1972.
5. Roda RS, Blanton PL: The anatomy of local anesthesia, *Quint Intern* 25(1):27-38, 1994.
6. Gow-Gates GAE: Mandibular conduction anesthesia: a new technique using extraoral landmarks, *Oral Surg* 36:321-328, 1973.
7. Malamed SF: The Gow-Gates mandibular block: evaluation after 4275 cases, *Oral Surg* 51:463, 1981.
8. Fish LR, McIntire DN, Johnson L: Temporary paralysis of cranial nerves III, IV, and VI after a Gow-Gates injection, *J Am Dent Assoc* 119:127-130, 1989.
9. Akinosi JO: A new approach to the mandibular nerve block, *Br J Oral Surg* 15:83-87, 1977.
10. Murphy TM: *Somatic blockade.* In Cousins MJ, Bridenbaugh PO, editors: *Neural blockade in clinical anesthesia and management of pain,* Philadelphia, 1980, JB Lippincott.
11. Bennett CR: *Monheim's local anesthesia and pain control in dental practice,* ed 6, St Louis, 1978, Mosby–Year Book, pp115-116.
12. Vazirani SJ: Closed mouth mandibular nerve block: a new technique, *Dent Dig* 66:10-13, 1960.
13. Wolfe SH: The Wolfe nerve block: a modified high mandibular nerve block, *Dent Today* 11(5):34-37, 1992.
14. Malamed SF: *Handbook of local anesthesia,* St Louis, 1980, Mosby–Year Book.
15. Jastak JT, Yagiela JA, Donaldson D: *Local anesthesia of the oral cavity,* Philadelphia, 1995, WB Saunders.

fifteen

Supplemental Injection Techniques

In this chapter a group of injections are presented that are used in specialized clinical situations. Some of these injection techniques may be used as the sole technique for pain control for certain types of dental treatment. For example, the periodontal ligament (PDL) injection, intraseptal, and intraosseous techniques provide effective pulpal anesthesia without the need for other injections. On the other hand, use of the intrapulpal injection is almost always reserved for situations in which other injection techniques have failed or are contraindicated for use. The PDL, intraseptal, and intraosseous injections are also frequently used to supplement failed or only partially successful traditional injection techniques.

INTRAOSSEOUS ANESTHESIA

Intraosseous anesthesia involves the deposition of anesthetic solution into the bone that supports the teeth. Though not new—intraosseous anesthesia dates to the early 1900s—a resurgence of interest in this technique in dentistry has taken place over the past 15 years. Three techniques are discussed, two of which—the periodontal ligament injection and the intraseptal injection—are modifications of traditional intraosseous anesthesia.

Periodontal Ligament Injection

It is not possible to achieve adequate pulpal anesthesia of one solitary mandibular tooth in an adult patient with the techniques described in Chapter 14. On rare occasion, a supraperiosteal injection in the apical region of a mandibular lateral incisor will provide effective pulpal anesthesia. However, in other regions of the mandible a regional nerve block must be administered to provide pulpal anesthesia. In recent years an old technique has become repopularized. The technique, known as either the periodontal ligament (PDL) injection or the intraligamentary injection (ILI), was originally described as the peridental injection in local anesthesia textbooks dating from 1912 to 1923.[1,2]

The peridental injection was not well received in those early years, because it was claimed that the risk of producing blood-borne infection and septicemia was too great to warrant its use in patients. The technique never became popular but was used clinically by many doctors, though it was not referred to as the peridental technique. In clinical situations in which an inferior alveolar nerve block failed to provide adequate pulpal anesthesia to the first molar (usually its mesial root), the doctor would insert a needle along the long axis of the mesial root as far apically as possible and deposit, under pressure, a small volume of local anesthetic solution. This invariably provided effective pain control.

It was not until the early 1980s that the intraligamentary or PDL injection gained the popularity it still maintains today. Credit for its increased interest must go to the manufacturers of syringe devices designed to make the injection easier to administer. These original devices, the Peripress and Ligmaject (Fig. 15-1), provide a mechanical advantage that allows the administrator to deposit the anesthetic more easily (and sometimes too easily). They appear similar to the Wilcox-Jewett Obtunder (Fig. 15-2), which was widely advertised to the dental profession in

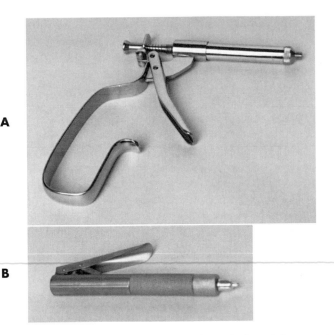

Fig. 15-1 A, Original pressure syringe designed for a periodontal ligament or intraligamentary injection. **B,** Second-generation syringe for a PDL injection.

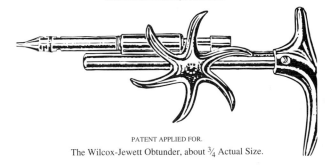

Fig. 15-2 Pressure syringe (1905) designed for a peridental injection.

a 1905 catalogue, *Dental Furniture, Instruments, and Materials,* perhaps reconfirming the adage that there is "nothing new under the sun."[3]

Why then has the PDL (née peridental) injection enjoyed renewed popularity? Because the primary thrust of the advertising for the new syringes has focused on being able to "avoid the mandibular block" injection with the PDL or intraligamentary technique—a concept to which the dental profession is quite receptive, given the fact that virtually all dentists have experienced periods when they have been unable to achieve adequate anesthesia with the inferior alveolar nerve technique.

The PDL injection may also be used quite successfully in the maxillary arch; however, with the ready availability of other highly effective and atraumatic techniques, such as the supraperiosteal (infiltration) injection to provide single-tooth pulpal anesthesia, there has been little compelling reason for use of the PDL in the upper jaw (although there is absolutely no other reason not to recommend it in this area). In my opinion the greatest potential benefit of the PDL injection lies in the fact that it provides pulpal and soft tissue anesthesia in a very localized area (one tooth) in the mandible without producing extensive soft tissue (i.e., tongue and lower lip) anesthesia as well. Virtually all dental patients prefer this technique to any of the "mandibular nerve blocks." In a clinical trial I reported that 74% of patients preferred the PDL injection primarily because of its lack of lingual and labial soft tissue anesthesia.[4] It is interesting that those preferring the inferior alveolar nerve block did so for a very important reason: with the inferior alveolar nerve

block, once patients' lips and tongues became "numb" they were able to relax because they knew that their dental treatment would not "hurt." Given the absence of lingual and labial soft tissue anesthesia in the PDL technique, they were unable to fully relax, for they were never certain that they had been adequately anesthetized.

Primary indications for the PDL injection include (1) the need for anesthesia of but one or two mandibular teeth in a quadrant, (2) treatment of isolated teeth in both mandibular quadrants (to avoid bilateral inferior alveolar nerve block), (3) treatment of children (because residual soft tissue anesthesia increases the risk of self-mutilation), (4) treatment in which nerve block anesthesia is contraindicated (e.g., in hemophiliacs), and (5) its use as a possible aid in the diagnosis of mandibular pain.

Contraindications to the PDL injection include infection or severe inflammation at the injection site, and primary teeth. Brannstrom et al reported the development of enamel hypoplasia or hypomineralization, or both, in 15 permanent teeth following the administration of the periodontal ligament injection.[5] Fortunately there is little need for this technique in the primary dentition—other techniques such as infiltration and nerve blocks being quite effective and easy to administer.

Several concerns have been expressed about this technique, most of which were addressed in a status report on the PDL injection in the *Journal of the American Dental Association.*[6] Two concerns were (1) the effect of the injection and deposition of the anesthetic solution under pressure into the confined space of the PDL and (2) the effect of the drug or vasoconstrictor on pulpal tissues. Walton and Garnick concluded that the PDL injection (administered with a conventional syringe) causes some slight damage to tissues in the region of needle penetration only.[7] Apical areas appeared normal; the epithelial and connective tissue attachment to enamel and cementum was not disturbed by the needle puncture; slight resorption of nonvital bone occurred in the crestal regions forming a wedge-shaped defect; soft tissue damage was minimal; the disruption of tissue that did occur showed repair in 25 days, with absence of inflammation, and formation of new bone in the regions of resorption; the injection of the solution was not in itself damaging. Damage produced by needle penetration alone (no drug administered) appeared similar to that seen when a drug had also been deposited. The authors concluded that the PDL injection is safe to the periodontium.[7] In addition, there is no evidence, to date, that the inclusion of a vasoconstrictor in the local anesthetic solution has any detrimental effect on pulpal microcirculation following the PDL injection.

It appears that the mechanism whereby the anesthetic solution reaches the periapical tissues with the PDL injection is diffusion apically and into the marrow spaces surrounding the teeth. The solution is not forced apically through the periodontal tissues, a procedure that might lead (as Nelson reported[8]) to avulsion of a tooth (premolar) because of the increased hydrostatic pressure being exerted in a confined space. The PDL injection therefore appears to produce anesthesia in much the same way as the intraosseous and intraseptal injections—by diffusion of anesthetic solution apically through marrow spaces in the intraseptal bone.

Another area of concern with the PDL injection is postinjection complications. Reported complications have included mild to severe postoperative discomfort, swelling and discoloration of soft tissues at the injection site, and prolonged ischemia of the interdental papilla followed by sloughing and exposure of crestal bone. Some of these complications are the direct result of poor operator technique, lack of familiarity with the pressure syringe, and injection of excessive volumes of anesthetic into the PDL. The most frequently voiced postinjection complications are mild discomfort and sensitivity to biting and to percussion for 2 or 3 days. The most common causes of postinjection discomfort are (1) too rapid injection (producing edema and slight extrusion of the tooth, thus sensitivity on biting) and (2) injection of excessive volumes into the site.

Prior to describing the PDL technique, it must be mentioned that although "special" PDL syringes can be used effectively and safely, there is usually no need for them. A conventional local anesthetic syringe is equally effective in providing PDL anesthesia. The use of a conventional syringe requires that the administrator apply significant force to deposit the solution into the periodontal tissues, but virtually all doctors and most hygienists are able to produce PDL anesthesia successfully without a special PDL syringe. Only when a doctor or hygienist is unable to achieve adequate PDL anesthesia with a conventional syringe is use of a PDL syringe recommended.

Arguments against using the conventional syringe for PDL injections (and my rebuttals) include the following:

1. It is too difficult to administer the solution with a conventional syringe

COMMENT: Slow administration of the anesthetic makes the PDL injection atraumatic. Improper use (read: "fast injection") of the PDL syringe produces both immediate and postinjection pain.

2. The extreme pressure applied to the glass may shatter the cartridge

The PDL syringes provide a metal or plastic covering for the glass cartridge, thereby protecting the patient from shards of glass should the cartridge shatter during injection.

COMMENT: Although I have read and heard of cartridges shattering during PDL injection, I have yet to experience this personally. There are, however, several ways to minimize the risk: since only small volumes of solution are injected (0.2 ml per root), a full, 1.8-ml cartridge is not required. Eliminate all but about 0.6 ml of solution before starting the PDL injection. This will minimize the area of glass being subjected to extreme pressures, decreasing the risk of breakage. In addition, glass cartridges have a thin Mylar plastic label that covers most or all of the glass. Should a cartridge break, the glass would not shatter but would be contained by the plastic covering. A piece of transparent adhesive tape might also be placed over the exposed glass portions of the metal or plastic syringe.

3. Many manufacturers of PDL syringes recommend use of 30-gauge short or 30-gauge ultrashort needles in this technique

COMMENT: In my early experience with the PDL technique I used the 30-gauge needle only to find that whenever pressure was applied to it (as in pushing it apically into the PDL) the 30-gauge needle bent quite easily. It was too fine a needle to withstand any pressure without bending. PDL injection failure rates were excessive. A 30-gauge ultrashort needle was manufactured specifically for use with this injection technique. Although somewhat more effective than the 30-gauge short, there was, in reality, absolutely no need to use a "special" needle for this injection. I have had great clinical success, with no increase in patient discomfort, using the more readily available 27-gauge short needle.

In summary, the PDL injection is an important addition to the armamentarium of local anesthetic techniques for providing mandibular and, to a lesser degree, maxillary pain control.

Other common names Peridental (original name) injection, intraligamentary injection, ILI

Nerves anesthetized Terminal nerve endings at the site of injection and at the apex of the tooth

Areas anesthetized Bone, soft tissue, and apical and pulpal tissues in the area of injection (Fig. 15-3)

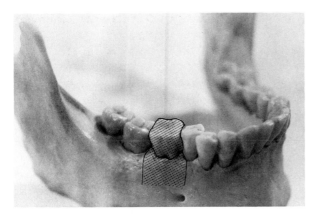

Fig. 15-3 Area anesthetized by a PDL injection.

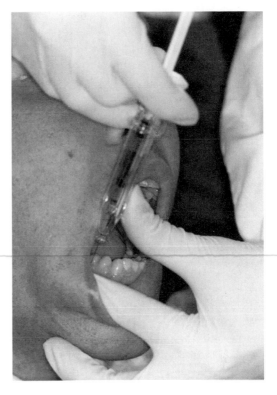

Fig. 15-4 Area of insertion for a PDL injection.

Indications
1. Pulpal anesthesia of one or two teeth in a quadrant
2. Treatment of isolated teeth in two mandibular quadrants (to avoid bilateral inferior alveolar nerve block)
3. Patients for whom residual soft tissue anesthesia is undesirable
4. Situations in which regional block anesthesia is contraindicated
5. As a possible aid in diagnosis of pulpal discomfort
6. As an adjunctive technique following nerve block anesthesia if partial anesthesia is present

Contraindications
1. Infection or inflammation at the site of injection
2. Primary teeth, when the permanent tooth bud is present[9]
   a. Enamel hypoplasia has been reported to occur in a developing permanent tooth when a PDL injection was administered to the primary tooth above it.
   b. As infiltration anesthesia and the incisive nerve block are quite effective in the primary dentition, there appears to be little reason for use of the PDL technique in primary teeth.
3. Patient who requires a "numb" sensation for psychological comfort

Advantages
1. Avoids anesthesia of the lip, tongue, and other soft tissues, thus facilitating treatment in multiple quadrants during a single appointment
2. Minimum dose of local anesthetic required to achieve anesthesia (0.2 ml per root)
3. An alternative to partially successful regional nerve block anesthesia
4. Rapid onset of profound pulpal and soft tissue anesthesia (30 seconds)
5. Less traumatic than conventional block injections
6. Well suited for procedures in children, for extractions, and for periodontal and endodontic, single-tooth, and multiple quadrant procedures

Disadvantages
1. Proper needle placement is difficult to achieve in some areas (i.e., distal of the second or third molar).
2. Leakage of anesthetic solution into the patient's mouth produces an unpleasant taste.
3. Excessive pressure or overly rapid injection may break the glass cartridge.
4. A special syringe may be required.
5. Excessive pressure can produce focal tissue damage.
6. Postinjection discomfort for several days may occur.
7. The potential for extrusion of a tooth exists if excessive pressure or volumes are used.

Positive aspiration   0%

Alternative   Supraperiosteal injection (entire maxilla and the mandibular lateral incisor region)

Technique
1. A 27-gauge short needle recommended
2. Area of insertion: long axis of the tooth to be treated on its mesial *or* distal of the root (one-rooted tooth) or on the mesial *and* distal roots (of multirooted tooth) interproximally (Fig. 15-4)
3. Target area: depth of the gingival sulcus

Fig. 15-5 If interproximal contacts are tight, the syringe should be directed in from the buccal, **A,** or lingual, **B,** side of the tooth.

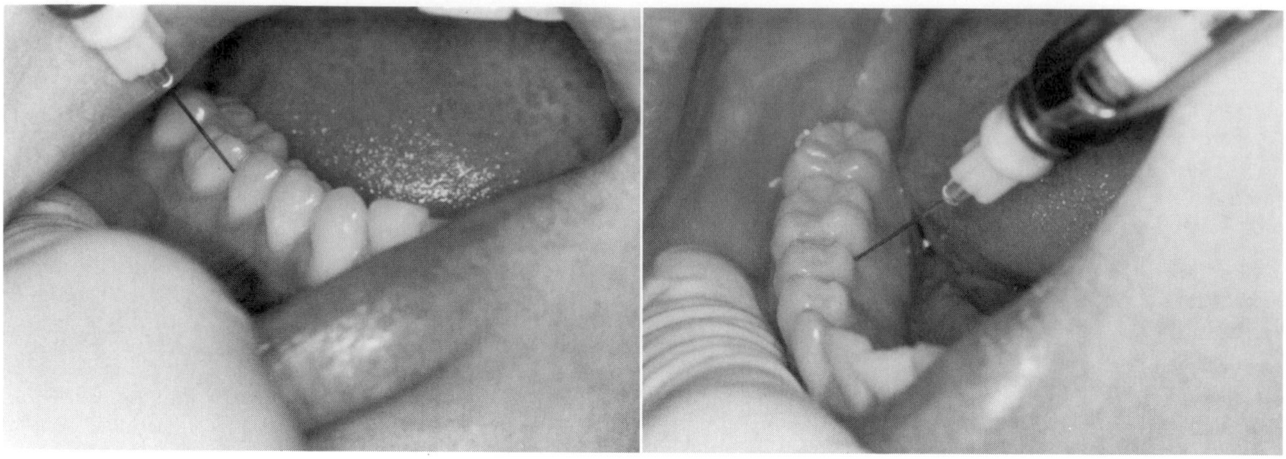

4. Landmarks
   a. Root(s) of the tooth
   b. Periodontal tissues
5. Orientation of the bevel: although not significant to success of the technique, I recommend that the bevel of the needle be facing *toward* the root to permit easy advancement of the needle in an apical direction.
6. Procedure
   a. Assume the correct position. (This will vary significantly with PDL injections on different teeth.) Sit comfortably, have adequate visibility of the injection site, and maintain control over the needle. It may be necessary to bend the needle to achieve proper angle, especially on the distal aspects of second and third molars.*
   b. Position the patient supine or semisupine, with the head turned to maximize access and visibility.
   c. Stabilize the syringe and direct it along the long axis of the root to be anesthetized.
      (1) The bevel faces the root of the tooth.
      (2) If interproximal contacts are tight, the syringe should be directed from either the lingual or the buccal surface of the tooth but maintained as close to the long axis as possible (Fig. 15-5).
      (3) Stabilize the syringe and your hand against the patient's teeth, lips, or face.
   d. With the bevel of the needle on the root, advance the needle apically until resistance is met.

e. Deposit 0.2 ml of local anesthetic solution in a minimum of 20 seconds.
   (1) When using the conventional syringe, notice that the thickness of the rubber stopper equals 0.2 ml on the syringe barrel. This may be used as a gauge for the volume of administration.
   (2) With the PDL syringe, each squeeze of the "trigger" provides a dose of 0.2 ml.
f. Two important items indicate the success of the injection
   (1) *Significant resistance to the deposition of solution*
      (a) This is especially noticeable when the conventional syringe is used; resistance is similar to that felt with the nasopalatine injection.
      (b) Anesthetic should not come back into the patient's mouth. If this occurs, repeat the injection at the same site, but from a different angle. Two tenths of a milliliter of solution must be deposited and must remain within the tissues for the PDL to be effective.
   (2) *Ischemia of the soft tissues adjacent to the injection site* (this is noted with all local anesthetic solutions but is more prominent with vasoconstrictor-containing solutions)
g. If the tooth has but one root, remove and cap the needle and start dental treatment within 30 seconds.
h. If the tooth is multirooted, remove the needle and repeat the procedure on the other root(s).

Signs and symptoms
1. There are no signs that absolutely assure adequate anesthesia; the anesthetized area is too circumscribed.

---

*Although I dislike bending needles for most injections, it may become necessary for the success of the PDL and intrapulpal injections to bend the needle so access can be gained to certain areas of the oral cavity. Because the needle does not enter into tissues more than a few millimeters, bending it is not as risk-prone as when the needle enters more completely into tissues.

When the following two signs are present, there is an excellent chance that profound anesthesia is present.
2. Ischemia of soft tissues at the injection site
3. Resistance to injection of solution

Safety feature Intravascular injection is extremely unlikely to occur

Precautions

1. Keep the needle against the tooth to prevent overinsertion into soft tissues on the lingual aspect.
2. Do not inject too rapidly (minimum 20 seconds for 0.2 ml).
3. Do not inject too much solution (0.2 ml per root retained within tissues).
4. Do not inject into infected or highly inflamed tissues.

Failures of anesthesia

1. Infected or inflamed tissues. The pH changes at the apex minimize the effectiveness of the local anesthetic.
2. Solution not retained. In this case, remove the needle and reenter at a different site(s) until 0.2 ml of solution is deposited and retained in the tissues.
3. Each root must be anesthetized with 0.2 ml of solution.

Complications

1. Pain during insertion of the needle
   Cause no. 1: The needle tip is in soft tissues. To correct: Keep the needle against tooth structure.
   Cause no. 2: The tissues are inflamed. To correct: Either avoid use of the PDL technique or apply a small amount of topical anesthetic for 1 minute prior to injection.
2. Pain during injection of solution
   Cause: Too rapid injection of local anesthetic solution. To correct: Slow down the rate of injection—minimum 20 seconds for 0.2 ml of solution, regardless of the syringe being used.
3. Postinjection pain
   Cause: Too rapid injection, excessive volume of solution, too many tissue penetrations (the patient usually complains of soreness and premature contact when occluding). To correct: Manage symptomatically with warm saline rinses and mild analgesics, if necessary (usually resolves within 2 to 3 days).

Duration of expected anesthesia The duration of pulpal anesthesia obtained with a successful PDL injection is extremely variable and not related to the drug administered. Administration of lidocaine with 1:100,000 epinephrine, for example, will provide pulpal anesthesia ranging in duration from 5 to 55 minutes. The PDL injection may be repeated if necessary to permit the completion of the dental procedure. It appears that the volume of anesthetic solution used with the PDL is too small to provide the usually expected duration of anesthesia of the drug.

• • •

Intraseptal Injection

The intraseptal injection is similar in technique and design to the PDL injection. It is included for discussion because of its usefulness in achieving osseous and soft tissue anesthesia and hemostasis for periodontal curettage and surgical flap procedures. In addition, it may be effective when the condition of the periodontal tissues in the gingival sulci precludes use of the PDL injection (infection, acute inflammation). Saadoun has shown that the path of diffusion of the anesthetic solution is through the medullary bone, as in the PDL injection.[10]

Other common names None

Nerves anesthetized Terminal nerve endings at the site of injection and in the adjacent soft and hard tissues

Areas anesthetized Bone, soft tissue, root structure in the area of injection (Fig. 15-6)

Indication When both pain control and hemostasis are desired for soft tissue and osseous periodontal treatment

Contraindication Infection or severe inflammation at the injection site

Advantages

1. Lack of lip and tongue anesthesia (appreciated by most patients)
2. Minimum volumes of anesthetic solution required
3. Minimized bleeding during the surgical procedure

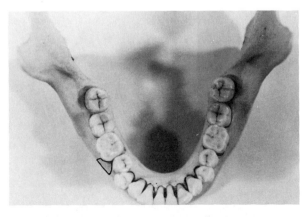

Fig. 15-6 Area anesthetized by an intraseptal injection.

4. Atraumatic
5. Immediate (< 30 seconds) onset of action
6. Very few postoperative complications
7. Useful on periodontally involved teeth (avoids infected pockets)

Disadvantages

1. Multiple tissue punctures may be required
2. Bitter taste of the anesthetic drug (if leakage occurs)
3. Short duration of pulpal anesthesia; limited area of soft tissue anesthesia (may necessitate reinjection)
4. Clinical experience necessary for success

Positive aspiration   0%

Alternatives

1. PDL injection, in the absence of infection or severe periodontal involvement
2. Regional nerve block with local infiltration for hemostasis

Technique

1. A 27-gauge short needle recommended
2. Area of insertion: center of the interdental papilla adjacent to the tooth to be treated (Fig. 15-7)
3. Target area: same
4. Landmarks: papillary triangle, about 2 mm below the tip, equidistant from adjacent teeth
5. Orientation of the bevel: not significant, although Saadoun recommends *toward* the apex[10]
6. Procedure
   a. Assume the correct position, which will vary significantly with different teeth. The administrator should be comfortable, have adequate visibility of the injection site, and maintain control over the needle.
   b. Position the patient supine or semisupine with the head turned to maximize access and visibility.

c. Prepare tissue at the site of penetration.
   (1) Dry with sterile gauze.
   (2) Apply topical antiseptic (optional).
   (3) Apply topical anesthetic.
d. Stabilize the syringe and orient the needle correctly (Fig. 15-8).
   (1) Frontal plane: 45 degrees to the long axis of the tooth
   (2) Sagittal plane: at right angle to the soft tissue
   (3) Bevel facing the *apex* of the tooth
e. Slowly inject a few drops of anesthetic as the needle enters soft tissue and advance the needle until contact with bone is made.
f. Applying pressure to the syringe, push the needle slightly deeper (1 to 2 mm) into the interdental septum.
g. Deposit 0.2 to 0.4 ml of local anesthetic in a minimum of 20 seconds.
   (1) With a conventional syringe, the thickness of the rubber plunger is equivalent to 0.2 ml.
h. Two important items indicate success of the intraseptal injection
   (1) *Significant resistance to the deposition of solution*
      (a) This is especially noticeable when a conventional syringe is used. Resistance is similar to that felt with the nasopalatine and PDL injections.
      (b) Anesthetic solution should not come back into the patient's mouth. If this occurs, repeat the injection with the needle slightly deeper.
   (2) *Ischemia of soft tissues adjacent to the injection site* (although noted with all local anesthetic solutions, more prominent with ones containing vasoconstrictor)
i. Repeat the injection as needed for the surgical procedure.

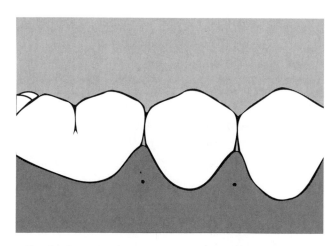

Fig. 15-7 Area of insertion for an intraseptal injection.

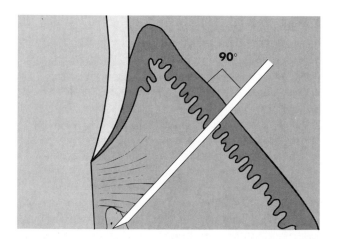

Fig. 15-8 Orientation of the needle for an intraseptal injection.

Signs and symptoms

1. As with the PDL injection, there are *no concrete symptoms* that ensure adequate anesthesia. The anesthetized area is too circumscribed.
2. Ischemia of soft tissues will be noted at the injection site.
3. Resistance to the injection of solution is felt.

Safety feature
Intravascular injection is extremely unlikely to occur.

Precautions

1. Do not inject into infected tissue.
2. Do not inject rapidly (minimum 20 seconds).
3. Do not inject too much solution (0.2 to 0.4 ml per site).

Failures of anesthesia

1. Infected or inflamed tissues. Changes in tissue pH minimize the effectiveness of the anesthetic.
2. Solution not retained in tissue. To correct: Advance the needle further into the septal bone and readminister 0.2 to 0.4 ml.

Complication
Postinjection pain is unlikely to develop because the injection site is within the area of surgical treatment. Saadoun demonstrated that postsurgical periodontal discomfort following the use of intraseptal anesthesia is no greater than that following a regional nerve block.[10]

Duration of expected anesthesia
The duration of osseous and soft tissue anesthesia is quite variable after an intraseptal injection. Using an epinephrine concentration of 1:50,000, Saadoun found pain control and hemostasis adequate for completion of the planned procedure without reinjecting in most patients.[10] However, there may be some patients who require a second intraseptal injection.

• • •

Intraosseous Injection

Deposition of local anesthetic solution into the interproximal bone between two teeth has been practiced in dentistry since the start of the twentieth century.[11] Originally intraosseous anesthesia required the use of a half-round bur to provide entry into interseptal bone that had been surgically exposed. Once the hole had been made, a needle would be inserted into this hole and local anesthetic solution deposited.

The periodontal ligament and intraseptal injections, previously described, are modifications of intraosseous anesthesia. In the PDL injection the anesthetic solution enters the interproximal bone through the periodontal tissues surrounding a tooth, while in the intraseptal tech-

nique the needle is gently embedded into the interproximal bone without the use of a bur.

In recent years the intraosseous technique has been modified with the introduction of a new device* that simplifies the procedure. The system consists of two parts: a perforator, a solid needle that perforates the cortical plate of bone with a conventional slow-speed contraangle handpiece, and an 8 mm long, 27-gauge needle that is inserted into this predrilled hole for anesthetic administration.

Experience with the intraosseous technique has shown that the perforation of the interproximal bone is usually entirely atraumatic. However, some persons have some difficulty placing the needle of the local anesthetic syringe back into the previously drilled hole in the interproximal bone. I have been able to overcome this problem by not taking my eyes off the perforation at any time during the entire procedure. In this way I am able to locate the hole with the anesthetic needle with little or no difficulty.

The intraosseous injection technique can provide anesthesia of a single tooth or of multiple teeth in a quadrant. To a significant degree the area of anesthesia will be dependent upon both the site of injection and the volume of anesthetic solution deposited. It is recommended that 0.45 to 0.6 ml of anesthetic be administered when treatment is to be confined to not more than one or two teeth. Greater volumes, up to 1.8 ml, may be administered when treatment of multiple teeth in one quadrant is contemplated. The intraosseous injection may be used when managing six or eight mandibular anterior teeth (first premolar to first premolar bilaterally, for example). Bilateral intraosseous injections are necessary, the perforation being made between the canine and first premolar on both sides. This will provide pulpal anesthesia of eight teeth.

As the injection site is relatively vascular, it is suggested that the volume of local anesthetic delivered be kept to the recommended minimum to avoid possible overdose.[12] In addition, because of the high incidence of palpitations noted when vasopressor-containing anesthetics are used, I recommend use of a "plain" local anesthetic in the intraosseous injection.

Other common names
None

Nerves anesthetized
Terminal nerve endings at the site of injection and in the adjacent soft and hard tissues

Areas anesthetized
Bone, soft tissue, root structure in the area of injection

*Stabident Local Anesthesia System, Fairfax Dental, Miami, Fla.

Indication Pain control for dental treatment on single or multiple teeth in a quadrant.

Contraindication Infection or severe inflammation at the injection site

Advantages
1. Lack of lip and tongue anesthesia (appreciated by most patients)
2. Atraumatic
3. Immediate (< 30 seconds) onset of action
4. Very few postoperative complications

Disadvantages
1. Requires a special syringe (e.g., Stabident System)
2. Bitter taste of the anesthetic drug (if leakage occurs)
3. Occasional difficulty in placing anesthetic needle into predrilled hole
4. High occurence of palpitations when vasopressor-containing local anesthetic is used

Positive aspiration 0%

Alternatives
1. PDL injection, in the absence of infection or severe periodontal involvement
2. Intraseptal injection
3. Supraperiosteal injections
4. Regional nerve blocks

Technique*
1. Selection of site for injection
    a. Lateral perforation
       (1) At a point 2 mm apical to the intersection of lines drawn horizontally along the gingival margins of the teeth and a vertical line through the interdental papilla
       (2) The site should be located *distal* to the tooth to be treated.
       (3) *Avoid* injecting in the mental foramen area.
    b. Vertical perforation (for edentulous areas)
       (1) Perforate at a point on the alveolar crest either mesial or distal to the treatment area.
2. Technique
    a. *Preparation of soft tissues at perforation site*
       (1) Prepare tissue at the injection site with 2 × 2 inch sterile gauze
       (2) Apply topical anesthetic to the injection site
       (3) Place bevel of needle against gingiva, injecting a small volume of local anesthetic until blanching occurs (optional)
    b. *Perforation of the cortical plate*
       (1) Place perforator in handpiece and remove cap
       (2) Holding the perforator perpendicular to the cortical plate, gently push the perforator through the attached gingiva until its tip rests against bone
       (3) Activate the handpiece in short spurts, applying light pressure on the perforator until a sudden loss of resistance is felt. Cortical bone will be perforated within 2 seconds.
       (4) Withdraw the perforator and dispose of it safely (sharps)
    c. *Injection into cancellous bone*
       (1) Compress a cotton roll against the mucosa to absorb any bleeding
       (2) Hold syringe in a "pen grip" and insert needle into perforation
       (3) *Slowly* and *gently* inject the local anesthetic solution
    d. *Stabident mandibular doses**

To anesthetize	Injection site	Dose (ml)
1 tooth	Immediately distal or immediately mesial	0.45 to 0.6
2 adjacent teeth	Between the 2 teeth or immediately distal to most distal tooth	0.6 to 0.9
3 adjacent teeth	Immediately distal to the middle tooth	0.9
6 anterior teeth + premolars	Give 2 injections, 1 on each side, between canine and 1st premolar	0.9 per side

e. *Stabident maxillary doses**

To anesthetize	Injection site	Dose (ml)
1 tooth	Immediately distal or mesial	0.45
2 adjacent teeth	Between the 2 teeth	0.45
4 adjacent teeth	Midway between teeth	0.9
Up to 8 teeth on one side	Midway between teeth	1.8

Signs and symptoms
1. As with the PDL injection, there are *no concrete symptoms* that ensure adequate anesthesia. The anesthetized area is too circumscribed.
2. Ischemia of soft tissues will be noted at the injection site.

Safety feature Intravascular injection is extremely unlikely, although the area injected into is quite vascular. Slow injection of the recommended volume of solution is important in making intraosseous anesthesia safe.

Precautions
1. Do not inject into infected tissue.
2. Do not inject rapidly.

*From the instruction manual, Stabident Local Anesthesia System, Fairfax Dental, Miami, Fla.

3. Do not inject too much solution. (See the recommendations on p. 228).
4. Do not use a vasopressor-containing local anesthetic.

Failures of anesthesia

1. Infected or inflamed tissues. Changes in tissue pH minimize the effectiveness of the anesthetic.
2. Inability to perforate cortical bone. If cortical bone is not perforated within 2 seconds, it is recommended that drilling be stopped and an alternative site be used.

Complications

1. Palpitation: frequent when a vasopressor-containing local anesthetic is used. To minimize the risk, use a "plain" local anesthetic.
2. Postinjection pain is unlikely following intraosseous anesthesia. The use of mild analgesics (nonsteroidal antiinflammatory drugs) is recommended if discomfort occurs in the postinjection period.

Duration of expected anesthesia   Pulpal anesthesia of between 15 and 30 minutes can be expected. If a vasopressor-containing solution is used, the duration will approach 30 minutes; if a plain solution is used, a 15 minute duration is usual.

• • •

INTRAPULPAL INJECTION

Obtaining profound pulpal anesthesia in the pulpally involved tooth is a potential problem. Specifically the problem usually occurs with mandibular molars since there are few alternative anesthetic techniques available with which the doctor may obtain profound anesthesia. Maxillary teeth are usually anesthetized with either a supraperiosteal injection or a nerve block such as the posterior superior alveolar (PSA), anterior superior alveolar (ASA), or (rarely) a maxillary nerve block. Mandibular teeth anterior to the molars are anesthetized with the incisive nerve block. Anesthesia of mandibular molars, however, is limited to nerve block anesthesia, which may prove to be ineffective in the presence of infection and inflammation. Methods of obtaining anesthesia for endodontics will be described in Chapter 16.

Deposition of local anesthetic directly into the pulp chamber of a pulpally involved tooth provides effective anesthesia for pulpal extirpation and instrumentation. The intrapulpal injection may be used on any tooth when difficulty in providing profound pain control exists, but from a practical view it is required most commonly on mandibular molars.

The intrapulpal injection provides pain control both by the pharmacological action of the local anesthetic and by applied pressure. This technique may be used once the pulp chamber is exposed, either surgically or pathologically.

Other common names   None

Nerves anesthetized   Terminal nerve endings at the site of injection in the pulp chamber and canals of the involved tooth

Areas anesthetized   Tissues within the injected tooth

Indication   When pain control is required for pulpal extirpation or other endodontic treatment in the absence of adequate anesthesia from other techniques

Contraindication   None. The intrapulpal injection may be the only local anesthetic technique available in some clinical situations.

Advantages

1. Lack of lip and tongue anesthesia (appreciated by most patients)
2. Minimum volumes of anesthetic solution required
3. Immediate onset of action
4. Very few postoperative complications

Disadvantages

1. Traumatic
   a. The intrapulpal injection is associated with a brief period of pain as anesthetic is deposited.
2. Bitter taste of the anesthetic drug (if leakage occurs)
3. May be difficult to enter certain root canals
   a. Bending of the needle may be required
4. Need a small opening into the pulp chamber for optimum effectiveness
   a. Large areas of decay make it more difficult to achieve profound anesthesia with the intrapulpal injection.

Positive aspiration   0%

Alternatives   None, as intrapulpal injection is always used as a supplement to other, more traditional, injection techniques.

Technique

1. Insert a 25- or 27-gauge short or long needle into the pulp chamber or the root canal as needed (Fig. 15-9).
2. Ideally, wedge the needle firmly into the pulp chamber or root canal.
   a. Occasionally the needle will not fit snugly into the canal. In this situation the anesthetic can be deposited in the chamber or canal. Anesthesia

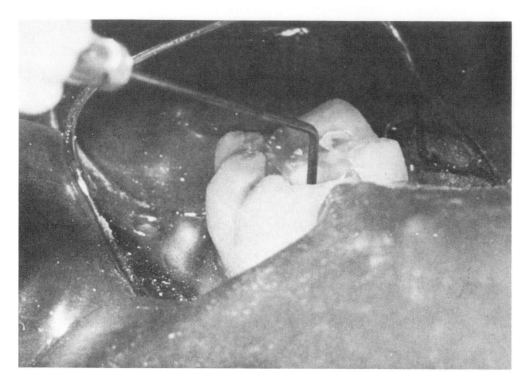

Fig. 15-9 For the intrapulpal injection a 25-gauge 1 or 1⁵/₈ inch needle is inserted into the pulp chamber or specific root canal. Bending the needle may be necessary to gain access. *(From Cohen S, Burns RC: Pathways of the pulp, ed 6, St Louis, 1994, Mosby-Year Book.)*

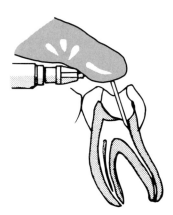

Fig. 15-10 The needle may have to be bent to gain access to a canal. *(Modified from Cohen S, Burns RC: Pathways of the pulp, ed 6, 1994, Mosby-Year Book.)*

will in this case be produced only by the pharmacological action of the local; there will not be any pressure anesthesia.

3. Deposit anesthetic solution under pressure.
   a. A very small volume of anesthetic (0.2 to 0.3 ml) is required for successful intrapulpal anesthesia—if the anesthetic stays within the tooth. In many situations the anesthetic simply flows back out of the tooth into the aspirator tip.
4. Resistance to the injection of the drug should be felt.
5. Bend the needle, if necessary, to gain access to the canal (Fig. 15-10).

   a. Although there is a greater risk of breakage with a bent needle, this is not a problem during intrapulpal anesthesia since the needle is inserted into the tooth itself, not into soft tissues; if the needle should break, retrieval is relatively simple.
6. When the intrapulpal injection is performed properly, a brief period of sensitivity (ranging from mild to very painful) usually accompanies the injection. Pain relief usually occurs immediately thereafter, permitting instrumentation to proceed atraumatically.
7. Instrumentation may begin approximately 30 seconds after the injection.

Signs and symptoms
1. As with the PDL, intraseptal, and intraosseous injections, there are *no concrete symptoms* that ensure adequate anesthesia. The area is too circumscribed.
2. The endodontically involved tooth is able to be treated painlessly

Safety features
1. Intravascular injection is extremely unlikely to occur.
2. Small volumes of anesthetic are administered.

Precautions
1. Do not inject into infected tissue.
2. Do not inject rapidly (minimum 20 seconds).
3. Do not inject too much solution (0.2 to 0.3 ml).

Failures of anesthesia
1. Infected or inflamed tissues. Changes in tissue pH

minimize the effectiveness of the anesthetic. However, intrapulpal anesthesia invariably works to provide effective pain control.

2. Solution not retained in tissue. To correct: Try to advance the needle further into the pulp chamber or root canal and readminister 0.2 to 0.3 ml of anesthetic drug.

Complication   Discomfort during the injection of anesthetic. The patient may experience a very brief period of intense discomfort as the injection of the anesthetic drug is started. Within a second (literally) the tissue is anesthetized and the discomfort ceases. The use of inhalation sedation (nitrous oxide/oxygen) can help to minimize or to alter the feeling experienced.

Duration of expected anesthesia   The duration of anesthesia is quite variable after intrapulpal injection. In most instances the duration is adequate to permit atraumatic extirpation of the pulpal tissues.

REFERENCES

1. Bethel LP, editor: *Dental summary,* vol 32, Toledo, Ohio, 1912, Ranson & Randolph, p 167.

2. Fischer G: *Local anesthesia in dentistry,* ed 3, Philadelphia, 1923, Lea & Febiger, p 197.

3. *Illustrated catalogue of dental furniture, instruments, and materials,* ed 4, Pittsburgh, 1905, Lee S Smith & Son.

4. Malamed SF: The periodontal ligament (PDL) injection: an alternative to inferior alveolar nerve block, *Oral Surg* 53:117-121, 1982.

5. Brannstrom M, Lindskog S, Nordenvall KJ: Enamel hypoplasia in permanent teeth induced by periodontal ligament anesthesia of primary teeth, *J Am Dent Assoc* 109(5):735-736, 1984.

6. Council on Dental Materials, Instruments, and Equipment: Status report: the periodontal ligament injection, *J Am Dent Assoc* 106:222-224, 1983.

7. Walton RE, Garnick JJ: The periodontal ligament injection: histologic effects on the periodontium in monkeys, *J Endodod* 8:22-26, 1982.

8. Nelson PW: Injection system, *J Am Dent Assoc* 103.692, 1981 (letter).

9. Brannstrom N, Nordenvall KJ, Hedstrom KG: Periodontal tissue changes after intraligamentary anesthesia, *ADSC J Dent Child* 49:417, 1982.

10. Saadoun A, Malamed SF: Intraseptal anesthesia in periodontal surgery, *J Am Dent Assoc* 111:249-256, 1985.

11. Fischer G: *Local anesthesia in dentistry,* ed 3, Philadelphia, 1923, Lea & Febiger, pp 244- 248.

12. Leonard M: The efficacy of an intraosseous injection system of delivering local anesthetic, *J Am Dent Assoc* 126(1):81-86, 1995.

CHAPTER
sixteen

Local Anesthetic Considerations in Dental Specialties

The techniques of local anesthesia described previously in this section are of value to doctors in virtually all areas of dental practice. There are, however, very specific needs and problems associated with pain control in particular areas of dental practice. This chapter discusses the dental specialties listed below and their peculiar needs in the area of pain control:

Endodontics
Pediatric dentistry
Periodontics
Oral surgery
Fixed prosthodontics
Long-duration anesthesia
Dental hygiene

ENDODONTICS

Effects of Inflammation on Local Anesthesia

Inflammation and infection lower tissue pH, altering the ability of a local anesthetic to provide clinically adequate pain control. As a review, most local anesthetics are weak bases (pK_a, 7.5 to 9.5). Local anesthetics are injected in their acid-salt form (through combination with hydrochloric acid), improving both their water solubility and stability. When a local anesthetic is injected into tissue, it is rapidly neutralized by tissue fluid buffers, and a part of the cationic form (RNH^+) is converted to the nonionized base (RN), according to the Henderson-Hasselbalch equation. (See Chapter 1.) The nonionized base is able to diffuse into the nerve. Pulpal and periapical inflammation or infection can cause tissue pH in the affected region to be lowered (e.g., pus has a pH of 5.5 to 5.6). Increased acidity does several things. (1) It limits the formation of nonionized base (RN), favoring formation of the cationic form (RNH^+). The RN that does penetrate the nerve once again encounters a normal tissue pH (7.3) inside the nerve and reequilibrates to both the RN and RNH^+ forms. This RNH^+ is available to block sodium channels—but with fewer cations available inside the nerve sheath, there is a greater likelihood of incomplete anesthesia developing. The overall effect of ion entrapment is to delay the onset of anesthesia and possibly interfere with nerve blockade. (2) It changes the products of inflammation so they inhibit anesthesia by directly affecting the nerve. Brown demonstrated that inflammatory exudates enhance nerve conduction by lowering the response threshold of the nerve, which may inhibit local anesthesia.[1] (3) It causes blood vessels in the region of inflammation to become unusually dilated, allowing for a more rapid uptake of anesthetic from the site of injection. Thus there is an increased possibility that local anesthetic blood levels may be elevated (from those seen in normal tissue).

There are two primary methods of obtaining adequate nerve block anesthesia in the presence of tissue inflammation. First, administer the local anesthetic away from the area of inflammation. It is undesirable to inject anesthetic solutions into areas of infection because of the possibility of spreading the infection to uninvolved regions.[2,3] The administration of local anesthetic solution into a site distant from the involved tooth is more likely to provide adequate pain control because of the presence of more normal tissue conditions. *Regional nerve block anesthesia is a major factor in pain control for pulpally involved teeth.* Second, deposit a larger volume of anesthetic into the region. This will provide a greater number of uncharged base molecules able to diffuse through the nerve sheath, with the increased likelihood of a satisfactory anesthetic block.

Methods of Achieving Anesthesia

The following techniques are recommended for providing pain control in pulpally involved teeth: local infiltration (supraperiosteal injection), regional nerve block, intrapulpal injection, periodontal ligament injection, intraseptal injection, and intraosseous injection. The order in which these techniques is discussed is the typical sequence in which they are normally used to achieve pain control.

Local Infiltration (Supraperiosteal Injection)

Local infiltration is commonly used to provide pulpal anesthesia in maxillary teeth. It is usually effective in endodontic procedures when severe inflammation or infection is not present. Local infiltration should *not* be attempted in a region where infection is obviously (clinically or radiographically) present because of the possible spread of infection to other regions and a greatly decreased rate of success. When infection is present, other techniques of pain control should be relied upon. Infiltration anesthesia is often effective at subsequent endodontic visits, if adequate debridement and shaping of the canals have previously been accomplis. '

Regional Nerve Block

Regional nerve block anesthesia is recommended where infiltration anesthesia may be ineffective or contraindicated. These techniques are discussed in detail in Chapters 13 and 14. Regional nerve block is likely to be effective because the anesthetic solution is deposited at a distance from the inflammation, where tissue pH and other factors are more normal.

Intrapulpal Injection

The intrapulpal injection achieves pain control both by the pharmacological action of the local anesthetic and by applied pressure. This technique may be used once the pulp chamber is exposed, either surgically or pathologically. The technique is described in Chapter 15.

When intrapulpal injections are administered properly, a brief period of sensitivity, ranging from mild to quite severe, may accompany the injection. Clinical pain relief follows almost immediately, permitting instrumentation to proceed atraumatically.

Occasionally the anesthetic needle does not fit snugly into the canal, preventing the increased pressure normally found in the intrapulpal injection. In this situation the anesthetic can be deposited in the chamber or canal. Anesthesia will be produced only by the pharmacological action of the local; there will not be any pressure anesthesia. Instrumentation may begin approximately 30 seconds after the injection.

Periodontal Ligament Injection

The periodontal ligament (PDL) injection may be an effective method of providing anesthesia in pulpally involved teeth if infection and severe inflammation are not present. This technique is discussed in Chapter 15. By way of review, a 27-gauge short needle is firmly placed between the interproximal bone and the tooth to be anesthetized. The bevel of the needle should face the tooth (though bevel orientation is not critical to success). It is appropriate to bend the needle if necessary to gain access. A small volume (0.2 ml) of local anesthetic is deposited under pressure. It may be necessary to repeat the PDL injection on all four sides of the tooth.

Intraseptal Injection

This is a variation of the intraosseous and PDL injections. It is easier and used more often than the intraosseous injection, but it does not enjoy as high a success rate. It is more successful in young patients because of the decreased density of bone. Intraseptal anesthesia is discussed more fully in Chapter 15 and proceeds as follows:[4]

1. Anesthetize the soft tissues at the injection site via local infiltration.
2. Insert a 27-gauge short needle into the intraseptal bone distal to the tooth to be anesthetized (Fig. 16-1).
3. Advance the needle firmly into the cortical plate of bone.

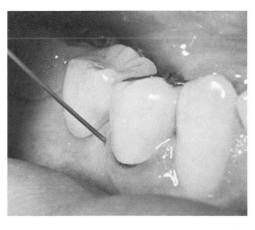

Fig. 16-1 For the intraseptal injection a 27-gauge 1-inch needle is inserted into the intraseptal bone distal to the tooth to be anesthetized.

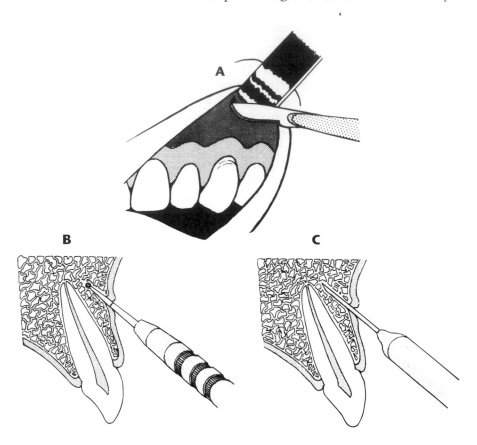

Fig. 16-2 Intraosseous anesthesia is often used to obtain adequate pulpal anesthesia when other techniques have failed. The soft tissue over the site has previously been anesthetized through local infiltration. **A,** An incision is made down to the periosteum. **B,** By means of a small ($\frac{1}{2}$ or 1) round bur, a hole is opened in the cortical plate. **C,** A 25-gauge needle is placed in the opening, and anesthetic solution is deposited. *(From Cohen S, Burns RC: Pathways of the pulp, ed 6, St Louis, 1994, Mosby-Year Book.)*

4. Inject about 0.2 ml of anesthetic. Considerable resistance must be encountered as the anesthetic is being deposited. If the administration is easy, the needle tip is most likely in soft tissue, not bone.

Intraosseous Injection

The intraosseous injection has experienced a resurgence of enthusiasm in recent years.[5] It can produce anesthesia deep enough to permit access into the pulp chamber, at which time intrapulpal anesthesia can be administered (if necessary). The technique for the intraosseous injection is described in Chapter 15 and is reviewed here (Fig. 16-2):

1. Apply topical anesthetic at the site of the injection to anesthetize the soft tissue.
2. Holding the perforator perpendicular to the cortical plate, gently push it through the attached gingiva until its tip rests against bone.
3. Activate the handpiece in short spurts, applying light pressure on the perforator until a sudden loss of resistance is felt.
4. Withdraw the perforator and dispose of it safely.
5. Insert a 30-gauge short needle on the syringe into the hole and deposit 0.45 to 0.6 ml of local anesthetic.

Cardiovascular absorption of local anesthetic following intraosseous injection is more rapid than after the other techniques described.[6] Therefore the volume of local anesthetic should not exceed recommended values, and a non–vasopressor-containing local anesthetic should be used to minimize palpitations.

• • •

There are occasions, happily rare, when all the previously discussed techniques fail to provide clinically acceptable pain control, and intrapulpal anesthesia cannot be attempted until the pulp is exposed. The following sequence of treatment may then be of value:

1. Use slow-speed high-torque instrumentation (which is usually less traumatic than the high-speed low-torque option).
2. Use conscious sedation (which helps to moderate the patient's response to painful stimuli). Nitrous oxide–oxygen inhalation sedation is a readily available, safe, and highly effective method of elevating a patient's pain reaction threshold.
3. If available, consider the use of electronic dental anesthesia. (See the discussion in Chapter 19.)
4. If, following Steps 1 and 2, the pulp chamber is opened, administer direct intrapulpal anesthesia. This will usually be effective despite the brief period of pain associated with its administration.
5. If a high level of pain persists and it is still not possible to enter the pulp chamber, then the following sequence should be considered:

a. Place a cotton pellet saturated with local anesthetic loosely on the pulpal floor of the tooth.

b. Wait 30 seconds, after which press the pellet more firmly into the dentinal tubules or the area of pulpal exposure. This area may be initially sensitive but should become insensitive within 2 to 3 minutes.

c. Remove the pellet and continue use of the slow-speed drill until pulpal access is gained, at which time direct injection into the pulp can be performed.

In most endodontic procedures it is only at the first appointment that there may be difficulty in providing adequate anesthesia. Once the pulp tissue has been extirpated, the need for pulpal anesthesia disappears. Soft tissue anesthesia may be necessary at ensuing appointments for comfortable placement of the rubber dam clamp; but if there is adequate tooth structure remaining, even that may not be necessary. Some patients respond unfavorably to instrumentation of their root canals, even when the canals have been thoroughly debrided. If this occurs, infiltration (in the maxilla) or intrapulpal anesthesia, or topical anesthetic, may be used. Apply a small amount of topical anesthetic ointment onto the file or reamer prior to inserting it into the canal. This helps to desensitize the periapical tissues during instrumentation of canals. Patients may also react to filling the canals. Local anesthesia should be considered before this stage of treatment is started.

PEDIATRIC DENTISTRY

Pain control is one of the most important aspects of behavioral control in children undergoing dental treatment. Unpleasant childhood experiences have made many adults acutely phobic with regard to dental treatment. Today, however, many local anesthetic drugs are available to make pain management relatively easy. Special concerns in pediatric dentistry relevant to local anesthesia include anesthetic overdose, complications related to the long duration of soft tissue anesthesia, and technique variations related to the smaller skulls and differing anatomy of young patients.

Local Anesthetic Overdose

Overdose from a drug develops when its blood level in a target organ (e.g., brain) becomes excessive. (See Chapter 18.) Undesirable (toxic) effects may be caused by intravascular injection or the administration of large volumes of the drug. Local anesthetic toxicity develops when the blood level of the drug in the brain or heart becomes too high. Local anesthetic toxicity, therefore, relates to the volume of drug reaching the cerebrovascular and cardiovascular systems and to the volume of blood in the patient. Once a drug has reached toxic levels, it exerts unwanted and possibly deleterious systemic actions. Local anesthetic toxicity produces central nervous system (CNS) and cardiovascular system (CVS) depression, with reactions ranging from mild tremor to tonic-clonic convulsions (CNS), from a slight decrease in blood pressure and cardiac output to cardiac arrest (CVS).

Uncommonly high numbers of deaths and serious morbidity caused by local anesthetic overdose have occurred in children, leading to the assumption that local anesthetics are more toxic in children than in adults.[7,8] This is untrue; it is the safety margin of local anesthetics in small children that is low. Given an equal dose of local anesthetic, a healthy patient with a greater blood volume will have a lower blood level of anesthetic than a patient with a lesser blood volume. Blood volume, to a large degree, relates to body weight: the greater the body weight, the greater the blood volume (except when the patient is obese).

Maximum recommended doses (MRDs) of all drugs administered by injection should be calculated by body weight and should not be exceeded, unless it is absolutely essential to do so.[8] For example, two cartridges of 3% mepivacaine (54 mg per cartridge) will exceed the maximum recommended dose for a 15 kg (33 lb) child of 66 mg. Unfortunately, the lack of awareness of maximum doses has led to fatalities in children.[9] The ease with which a child may be overdosed with local anesthetics is compounded by the practice of multiple quadrant dentistry and the concomitant use of sedative drugs (especially narcotics).[7] When treating a child, the dentist should maintain strict adherence to maximum doses (Table 16-1) and anesthetize only that quadrant currently being treated.

Primosch et al surveyed 117 dentists who regularly treated children regarding their local anesthetic usage.[13] They found that the lighter the weight of the patient, the more likely the doctor was to administer an overly large dose of the local anesthetic, based upon milligrams per kilogram of body weight. For example, a 13 kg patient should receive no more than 91 mg of lidocaine (based on a high maximum recommended dose of 7.0 mg/kg). The range of doses administered by dentists treating children was from 0.9 to 19.3 mg/kg. As the patient's weight increased, the number of milligrams per pound or kilogram reached lower and safer levels, the maximum mg/kg range falling to 12.6 mg/kg in the 20 kg patient and to 7.2 mg/kg in the 35 kg patient. The mean dose of local anesthetic also fell when the patient's weight increased, from 5.4 mg/kg in the 13 kg patient to 4.8 mg/kg in the 20 kg patient to 3.8 mg/kg in the 35 kg patient (Table 16-2).

TABLE 16-1 Maximum Recommended Doses of Local Anesthetics

Drug	Formulation	Adult MRD*	mg/lb (mg/kg)*		Author's MRD	mg/kg[11,12]
Lidocaine	Plain	300	2.0	(4.4)	300	4.4
	With epinephrine	500	3.3	(7.0)	300	4.4
Mepivacaine	Plain	400	2.6	(5.7)	300	4.4
	With levonordefrin	400	2.6	(5.7)	300	4.4
Prilocaine	Plain	600	4.0	(8.8)	400	6.0
	With epinephrine	600	4.0	(8.8)	400	6.0

*Manufacturer's recommendations.[10]

TABLE 16-2 Local Anesthetic Administration by Dentists Who Treat Children (n = 117)

Patient			
Age (yrs)	2	5	10
Weight (kg)	13	20	35
Dose (mg)	69.9	96.5	135
Mean (mg/kg)	5.4	4.8	3.8
(mg)	12 to 252	18 to 252	36 to 252
Range (mg/kg)	0.9 to 19.3	0.9 to 12.6	1.0 to 7.2
Recommended	Lidocaine 4.4 to 7.0 mg/kg		
	Mepivacaine 4.4 to 6.0 mg/kg		

Modified from Cheatham BD, Primosch RE, Courts FJ: A survey of local anesthetic usage in pediatric patients by Florida dentists, *J Dent Child* 59:401-407, 1992.

The administration of large volumes of local anesthetic is not necessary when seeking pain control in younger patients. Because of differences in anatomy (see "techniques" below), smaller volumes of local anesthetics provide the depth and duration of pain control usually required to successfully complete the planned dental treatment in younger patients.

Because injectable local anesthetics possess vasodilating properties, leading to more rapid vascular uptake and to a shorter duration of adequate anesthesia, it is strongly recommended that a vasopressor be included in the local anesthetic solution unless there is a compelling reason for it to be excluded.[14] Many treatment appointments in pediatric dentistry do not exceed 30 minutes in duration; therefore the use of a local anesthetic containing a vasopressor is considered to be unnecessary and unwarranted. It is thought that the increased duration of soft tissue anesthesia, especially following inferior alveolar nerve block, will increase the risk of the patient suffering self-inflicted injury to the soft tissues. A non–vasopressor-containing local anesthetic is frequently used—most often mepivacaine 3%. Providing 20 to 40 minutes of pulpal anesthesia, mepivacaine 3% is considered the appropriate drug for this group of patients—and it is, provided that treatment is limited to one quadrant per visit. However, when multiple quadrants are to be treated (and anesthetized) in one visit on a smaller patient,

> *When treating more than one quadrant in a younger, smaller patient, a local anesthetic containing a vasopressor should be used.*
>
> *A local anesthetic without a vasopressor may be used in the younger, smaller patient when dental treatment is of short duration and is confined to one quadrant.*

the administration of a "plain" drug into multiple injection sites increases the potential risk of overdose. The use of a local anesthetic containing a vasopressor is strongly recommended whenever multiple quadrants are anesthetized in the smaller pediatric patient. Sixty-nine percent of doctors treating children administered lidocaine with epinephrine as their primary anesthetic (Table 16-3).[13]

Complications of Local Anesthesia

Accidental biting or chewing of the lip, tongue, or cheek is a complication of residual soft tissue anesthesia (Fig. 16-3). Soft tissue anesthesia always lasts longer than pulpal anesthesia and may be present for 4 to 5 hours or more after local anesthetic administration. Fortunately, most patients do not encounter problems related to pro-

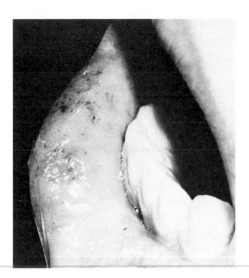

Fig. 16-3 Lip trauma caused by biting while the area was anesthetized.

TABLE 16-3 Local Anesthetic Choice by Dentists Who Treat Children (n = 117)

Anesthetic formulation	Percent employing
2% lidocaine + 1:100,000 epinephrine	69
3% mepivacaine	11
2% lidocaine	8
2% mepivacaine + 1:20,000 levonordefrin	8
Other anesthetics	4

Adapted from Cheatham BD, Primosch RE, Courts FJ: A survey of local anesthetic usage in pediatric patients by Florida dentists, *J Dent Child* 59:401-407, 1992.

TABLE 16-4 Relative Durations of Pulpal and Soft Tissue Anesthesia

Drug	Approximate pulpal anesthesia (min)	Approximate soft tissue anesthesia (hr)
Mepivacaine plain	20 to 40	3 to 4
Prilocaine plain	(infiltration) 10	1½ to 2
Lidocaine plain	5 to 10	1 to 1½

longed soft tissue anesthesia; but the majority of those who do are young or mentally or physically disabled. Problems related to soft tissue anesthesia most often involve the lower lip. Much less frequently is the tongue injured and quite rarely is the upper lip involved.

Several preventive measures can be implemented:

1. Select a local anesthetic with a duration of action that is appropriate for the length of the planned procedure. There are drugs that provide pulpal anesthesia of adequate duration (20 to 40 minutes) for restorative procedures, with a relatively shorter duration of soft tissue anesthesia (1 to 3 hours instead of 4 or 5) (Table 16-4). It should be kept in mind, however, that there is no research to demonstrate a relationship between reduced soft tissue trauma and the use of plain local anesthetics. The clinician must also consider the advisability of using a local anesthetic with vasopressor in view of the decreased margin of safety of local anesthetics in smaller children.
2. Advise both the patient and the accompanying adult about the possibility of injury if the patient bites, sucks, or chews on the lips, tongue, or cheeks or ingests hot substances while anesthesia persists.
3. Some doctors reinforce the verbal warning to the patient and adult by placing a cotton roll in the mucobuccal fold (held in position by dental floss through the teeth) if soft tissue anesthesia is still present at the time of the patient's discharge. Warning stickers are also available to help prevent soft tissue trauma.

The management of soft tissue trauma involves reassuring the patient, allowing time for the anesthetic effects to diminish, and coating the involved area with a lubricant (petroleum jelly) to help prevent drying, cracking, and pain.

Techniques of Local Anesthesia in Pediatric Dentistry

Local anesthetic techniques in children do not differ greatly from those used in adults. Skulls of children do have some anatomical differences from those of adults, however. For instance, maxillary and mandibular bone in children is generally less dense, which works to the dentist's advantage. Decreased density permits a more rapid and complete diffusion of the anesthetic solution. Children are also smaller, thus the standard injection techniques can usually be completed with a decreased depth of needle penetration.

Maxillary Anesthesia

All primary teeth, as well as permanent molars, can be anesthetized by supraperiosteal infiltration in the mucobuccal fold. The *posterior superior alveolar nerve block* is often not necessary because of the effectiveness of infiltration in children. However, in some individuals the morphology of the bone surrounding the apex of the permanent first molar does not permit effective infiltration of local anesthetic. This is because the zygomatic process lies closer to the alveolar bone in children. A posterior superior alveolar (PSA) nerve block may be warranted in this clinical situation. A short dental needle should be used and the depth of needle penetration modified to meet the smaller dimensions of the pediatric patient in order to minimize the risk of hematoma. As an alternative to the PSA, Rood[15] has suggested using buccal infiltrations on both the mesial and distal of the maxillary first molar to avoid a prominent zygomatic process. The *anterior superior alveolar nerve block* can also be used in children, as long as it is realized that the depth of penetration is probably just slightly greater than with a supraperiosteal injection (due to the lower height of the maxillae in children). Generally there are few indications for either the posterior superior alveolar or anterior superior alveolar nerve block in children because of the lack of need for multiple restorations in one quadrant.

Occasionally a maxillary tooth will remain sensitive after a supraperiosteal injection because of accessory innervation from the palatal nerves[16] or because of widely flared palatal roots. Palatal anesthesia can be obtained in children through the nasopalatine and greater (anterior) palatine nerve blocks. The technique for a *nasopalatine nerve block* proceeds exactly as described in Chapter 13. That for a *greater palatine nerve block* is as follows: the administrator visualizes a line from the gingival border of the most posterior molar that has erupted to the midline. The needle is inserted from the opposite side of the mouth, distal to the last molar, bisecting this line. If the child has only primary dentition, the needle is inserted approximately 10 mm posterior to the distal surface of the second primary molar, bisecting the line drawn toward the midline.

An intrapapillary injection can also be used to achieve palatal anesthesia in young children. Once buccal anesthesia is effective, the needle (27-gauge short) is inserted horizontally into the buccal papilla just above the interdental septum. Local anesthetic is injected as the needle is advanced toward the palatal side. This should cause ischemia of the soft tissue.[17]

Mandibular Anesthesia

Supraperiosteal infiltration is usually effective in providing pain control of mandibular primary teeth. This is due to the decreased density of bone in the mandible in younger children. The rate of success of mandibular infiltration anesthesia decreases somewhat for primary mandibular molars as the child increases in age. The technique of supraperiosteal infiltration in the mandible is the same as in the maxilla. The tip of the needle is directed toward the apex of the tooth, in the mucobuccal fold, and approximately one fourth to one third (0.45 ml to 0.6 ml) cartridge is slowly deposited.

The *inferior alveolar nerve block* has a greater success rate in children than in adults because of the location of the mandibular foramen. The mandibular foramen in children lies distal and more inferior to the occlusal plane. Benham[18] demonstrated that the mandibular foramen lies at the height of the occlusal plane in children and rises an average 7.4 mm above the occlusal plane in

adults. He also found that there is no age-related difference as to the anteroposterior position of the foramen on the ramus.

The technique for an inferior alveolar nerve block is essentially identical for adults and children. Differences include placing the syringe barrel over the primary molars on the opposite side of the mouth and using an average penetration depth of 15 mm (though this varies with the size of the mandible and the age of the patient). Bone should be contacted before any solution is deposited. In general, the more inferior location of the mandibular foramen in children provides a greater opportunity for successful anesthesia. "Low" injections are more likely to be successful. In clinical situations the success rate for well-behaved children usually exceeds 90% to 95%.

Because of the decreased thickness of soft tissue overlying the inferior alveolar nerve (about 15 mm) a 25- or 27-gauge short needle may be recommended in the inferior alveolar nerve block in younger patients. Once the patient is of sufficient size that a short needle does not reach the injection site without entering tissue almost to its hub, a long needle should be used.

The *buccal nerve* may be anesthetized if anesthesia of the buccal tissues in the permanent molar region is necessary. The needle tip is placed distal and buccal to the most posterior tooth in the arch. Deposit approximately 0.3 ml of solution.

The *Vazirani-Akinosi* and *Gow-Gates mandibular nerve blocks* can also be used in children. Akinosi[19] advocates the use of short needles with this technique. He also states that the technique appears less reliable in children, which he relates to the difficulty of judging the depth of penetration necessary in a growing child. The Gow-Gates mandibular block can be used successfully in children.[20] However, rarely are either of these injections required in pediatric dentistry because of the relative ease with which one can achieve inferior alveolar and incisive nerve block anesthesia.

The *incisive nerve block* provides pulpal anesthesia of the five primary mandibular teeth in a quadrant. Deposition of anesthetic solution outside the mental foramen and the application of finger pressure for 2 minutes provide a very high degree of success. The mental foramen is usually located between the two primary mandibular molars.

The *PDL injection* has been well accepted in pediatric dentistry. It provides the doctor with the means to achieve anesthesia of proper depth and duration on one tooth, without unwanted residual soft tissue anesthesia. The PDL is also useful when a child has discrete carious lesions in multiple quadrants. See Chapter 15 for a complete discussion of technique for the PDL injection. It is recommended that the described technique be scrupulously adhered to in order to avoid both physiological (pain) and psychological (fear) trauma to the patient. The PDL injection is not recommended for use on primary teeth because of the possibility of the development of enamel hypoplasia in the developing permanent tooth.[21]

PERIODONTICS

The special requirements for local anesthesia in periodontal procedures center on the use of vasopressors to provide hemostasis and the use of long-duration local anesthetics for postoperative pain control. Long-duration anesthesia is discussed as a separate subject later in this chapter.

Soft tissue manipulation and surgical procedures are associated with hemorrhage, especially when the tissues involved are not healthy. Administration of local anesthetics without vasopressors proves to be counterproductive because the vasodilating properties of the local anesthetic increase bleeding in the region of the injection. Vasopressors are added to counteract this unwanted action.

The pharmacology of vasopressors is more completely discussed in Chapter 3. As a review, vasopressors produce arterial smooth muscle contraction by direct stimulation of α receptors located in the wall of the blood vessel. So it follows that local anesthetics with vasopressors used for hemostasis must be injected directly into the region where the bleeding is to occur.

Pain control for periodontal procedures should be achieved through nerve block techniques, such as the posterior superior alveolar, inferior alveolar, and infraorbital nerve blocks. Saadoun[22] has shown that the *intraseptal technique* is very effective for periodontal flap surgical procedures. It decreases the total volume of administered anesthetic and volume of blood lost during the procedure. Local anesthetic solutions used for nerve blocks should include a vasopressor in a concentration not greater than 1:100,000 epinephrine or 1:20,000 levonordefrin. An epinephrine concentration of 1:50,000 is not recommended for pain control since depth, duration, and success rates are no greater than those seen with anesthetics containing 1:100,000 epinephrine.

Epinephrine is the drug of choice for local hemostasis. Norepinephrine can produce marked tissue ischemia, which can lead to necrosis and sloughing and is not recommended for use in hemostasis.[23,24] Epinephrine is most commonly used for hemostasis in a

concentration of 1:50,000 (0.2 mg/ml). Generally small volumes are deposited (not exceeding 0.1 ml) when it is used for hemostasis. Epinephrine also provides excellent hemostasis in a concentration of 1:100,000. Surgical bleeding is inversely proportional to the concentration of vasopressor administered. When a plain anesthetic is infiltrated (e.g., 3% mepivacaine) during periodontal surgery, blood loss is two to three times that noted when 2% lidocaine with 1:100,000 epinephrine is administered.[25] Buckley et al demonstrated that the use of a 1:50,000 epinephrine concentration produced a 50% decrease in bleeding during periodontal surgery from that seen with a 1:100,000 concentration (with 2% lidocaine).[26] However, epinephrine is not a drug without systemic effects and some undesirable local effects. Studies have shown that even the small volumes of epinephrine used in dentistry can significantly increase the concentrations of plasma catecholamine and alter cardiac function.[27] It is therefore prudent to administer the smallest volume of the least concentrated form of epinephrine that provides clinically effective hemostasis.

As tissue levels of epinephrine decrease following its injection for hemostasis, a rebound vasodilation develops. Sveen demonstrated that postsurgical bleeding (at 6 hours) occurred in 13 of 16 (81.25%) patients receiving 2% lidocaine with epinephrine for surgical removal of a third molar, while 0 of 16 patients who underwent surgery with 3% mepivacaine bled at 6 hours postsurgery.[25] Bleeding interfered with postoperative healing in 9 of 16 (56.25%) patients receiving lidocaine with epinephrine, compared with 25% of patients receiving no epinephrine. There is also evidence that the use of epinephrine in local anesthetics during surgery may produce an increase in postoperative pain.[28]

Many doctors use a 30-gauge short needle to deposit anesthetics for hemostasis—their rationale being that the thinner needle produces a smaller defect (puncture) in the tissue. If a small puncture is important, then the 30-gauge needle should be used, but only for this purpose. The 30-gauge short needle should not be used if there is the possibility of positive aspiration of blood or if any depth of soft tissue must be penetrated. The aspiration of blood through a 30-gauge needle (though possible) is difficult. A 27-gauge needle can be used for local infiltration to achieve hemostasis when vascularity is a problem, or in any other area of the oral cavity without any increase in patient discomfort.

ORAL AND MAXILLOFACIAL SURGERY

Pain control during surgical procedures is achieved through the administration of local anesthetics, either alone or in combination with inhalation sedation, intra-

> *Local anesthetics with vasopressors used for hemostasis must be injected directly into the region where the bleeding is to occur.*

venous sedation, or general anesthesia. As is the case with periodontal surgery, the long-duration local anesthetics play an important role in postoperative pain control and will be discussed separately.

Local anesthesia techniques used in oral surgery do not differ from those employed in nonsurgical procedures. It should therefore be expected that instances of either partial or incomplete anesthesia will develop. Oral surgeons frequently treat patients who have received intravenous sedation or general anesthesia prior to the start of the surgery. These techniques act to modify the patient's reaction to pain, tending to decrease the number of reported instances of inadequate local anesthesia.

Local anesthesia is administered almost routinely to patients for third molar extractions under general anesthesia. The reasons for this are as follows:

1. Pain control during the surgery permits a lessened exposure to general anesthetic agents, allowing for a faster postanesthetic recovery period and a minimization of drug-related complications.
2. Hemostasis is possible if a vasopressor is included.
3. Residual local anesthesia in the postoperative period minimizes the requirement for opioid oral analgesics.

The rate at which local anesthetics are administered is important in all areas of dental practice, but it is probably most important during the extraction of teeth from multiple quadrants. When four third molars are extracted, effective pain control must be obtained in all four quadrants. This requires multiple injections of local anesthetics, which usually occur within a relatively short period of time. Four cartridges or more of local anesthetic are frequently used.* The rate at which these local anesthetics are administered must be closely monitored to lessen the occurrence of complications. Complications arising from the rapid administration of local anesthetic include any of the following:

1. Pain during the injection
2. Greater possibility of a serious overdose reaction, if the local anesthetic is administered intravascularly (speed of injection significantly affects the clinical manifestations of toxicity)
3. Postanesthetic pain caused by tissue trauma during the injection

---

*Typical local anesthetic injections for four third molar extractions include the following:

1. Right and left inferior alveolar and buccal nerve blocks, 1.8 ml each (3.6 ml)
2. Right and left posterior superior alveolar nerve blocks or supraperiosteal infiltration over the third molar, 1.3 to 1.8 ml each (2.6 to 3.6 ml)
3. Right and left palatal infiltration over the third molar, 0.45 ml each, or right and left greater palatine nerve block, 0.45 ml each (0.9 ml)

Total volume of solution: 8.1 ml or 162 mg of a 2% solution, 243 mg of a 3% solution, or 324 mg of a 4% solution.

These complications and their prevention, recognition, and management are discussed in greater depth in Chapters 17 and 18.

It should be noted that in some persons the inferoposterior border of the mandible is not innervated by the trigeminal nerve. Any of the mandibular nerve blocks described in Chapter 14 will provide only partial anesthesia in this situation. The PDL injection usually corrects the lack of pain control in this situation.

FIXED PROSTHODONTICS

When preparing a tooth for full coverage (crown or bridge), it is necessary to place a temporary restoration over the prepared tooth. Although achieving pain control might not be difficult at the initial visit, there may be subsequent visits during which it is difficult to adequately anesthetize the prepared tooth. The reason for this is probably the temporary restoration. Overly high restorations produce traumatic occlusion, which after about a day can lead to considerable sensitivity. Poorly adapted gingival margins develop microleakage, which also causes sensitivity. The procedure itself can also cause tooth sensitivity, through desiccation of tooth structure, possible pulpal involvement, and periodontal irritation. The longer these sources of irritation are present, the greater the trauma to the tooth is likely to be and the more difficult it is to achieve adequate anesthesia. Usually a regional nerve block is effective. Supraperiosteal injections generally do not provide adequate pain control in these situations (depth may be adequate but duration is considerably shorter than that usually expected from the drug).

LONG-DURATION LOCAL ANESTHESIA
Prolonged Dental/Surgical Procedures

Several specialty areas of dental practice have a need for longer than usual pulpal and/or soft tissue anesthesia. They are fixed prosthodontics, oral surgery, and periodontics. During longer procedures (2 or more hours) an adequate duration of pulpal anesthesia may be difficult to achieve with the more commonly used anesthetics: lidocaine, mepivacaine, and prilocaine. Bupivacaine (Marcaine) and etidocaine (Duranest) are two long-acting drugs currently available that can then be used. They are discussed more completely in Chapter 4.

Bupivacaine, a homologue of mepivacaine, has a long duration of clinical effectiveness when used for regional nerve block. Its duration of action when administered by supraperiosteal injection, though still long, is somewhat shorter (shorter even than that of lidocaine with epinephrine).[29] Its postoperative analgesic period lasts an average of 8 hours in the mandible and 5 hours in the maxilla. Etidocaine, similar in structure to lidocaine, is less toxic and less potent than bupivacaine.[30] Although it is clinically similar to bupivacaine, it has a considerably shorter duration of postoperative analgesia when administered via infiltration.[31] Etidocaine administered via nerve block provides the same long duration as bupivacaine.

Both bupivacaine and etidocaine are available with vasopressor (1:200,000 epinephrine). It is interesting to note that the addition of vasopressor to bupivacaine does not prolong its duration of action. This is in contrast to etidocaine, whose effect is prolonged by the addition of vasopressor.[32]

Postprocedural Pain Control

Often, after extensive surgical procedures, the patient may experience considerable pain when the anesthetic effect dissipates. It was, and still is in many cases, common practice to treat postoperative pain through the use of narcotic (opioid) analgesics. However, opioids have a high incidence of undesirable side effects such as nausea, vomiting, constipation, respiratory depression, and postural hypotension, especially in ambulatory patients.[33]

Long-acting local anesthetics administered to surgical patients offer a means of providing successful postoperative pain control with a minimal risk of development of adverse reactions. An advantage of using long-duration local anesthetics is their longer postoperative analgesia, which leads to a reduced need for the administration of postoperative opioid analgesic drugs.[34] Dentists often use an intermediate-acting local anesthetic, such as lidocaine, mepivacaine, or prilocaine with a vasopressor, during the surgical period and administer the long-acting local anesthetic just before the termination of the surgery. Danielsson et al compared bupivacaine, etidocaine, and lidocaine with regard to their effect on postoperative pain, and found that both bupivacaine and etidocaine were more effective in controlling postoperative

pain when compared with lidocaine.[29] They also reported that bupivacaine was more effective than etidocaine in providing postoperative analgesia and that patients receiving bupivacaine used significantly fewer analgesics.

It is pertinent to note that there appears to be a difference between etidocaine and bupivacaine with respect to their ability to provide adequate hemostasis, even though they contain the same concentration of vasopressor (1:200,000). Danielsson et al noted that bupivacaine and lidocaine provided adequate hemostasis in 90%, and etidocaine in only 75%, of the procedures.[32] It is possible that a higher concentration of local anesthetic may require a higher concentration of vasopressor to provide comparable hemostasis. Also keep in mind the different vasodilating properties of the solutions.[35]

Protocol for Perioperative and Postoperative Pain Control in Surgical Patients

Postoperative pain associated with most uncomplicated dental surgical procedures is mild and well managed by oral administration of nonsteroidal antiinflammatory drugs (NSAIDs) such as aspirin and ibuprofen. The preoperative administration of the NSAID appears to delay the onset of postoperative pain and to lessen its severity.[34,36] When a patient is unable to tolerate aspirin or other NSAIDs, acetaminophen can provide acceptable analgesia.

Other dental surgical procedures, such as removal of bony impactions and osseous periodontal or endodontic surgery, are more traumatic and typically are associated with more intense and prolonged postoperative pain. The onset of such pain can be delayed by the presurgical administration of an NSAID followed by the administration of a long-acting local anesthetic (bupivacaine or etidocaine) at the completion of the surgery.[36]

When postoperative pain does emerge, it may require the addition of an opioid to the nonsteroidal regimen. Codeine, at a dosage level of 30 to 60 mg every 4 to 6 hours, is frequently prescribed and often very effective.

TABLE 16-5 Pain Control Regimen for Surgical Procedures

Preoperative:	Administer 1 or 2 oral doses of NSAID, minimally 1 hour prior to the scheduled surgical procedure
Perioperative:	Administer local anesthetic of adequate duration for procedure (lidocaine, mepivacaine, prilocaine with or without vasopressor)
	If surgery is planned at < 30 min duration: *immediately* follow initial local anesthetic injection with long-acting local anesthetic (bupivacaine, etidocaine [via block only])
	If surgery is planned at > 30 min duration: at the *conclusion* of the surgical procedure reinject the patient with long-acting local anesthetic (bupivacaine, etidocaine)
Postoperative:	Have patient continue to take oral NSAID on a timed basis (e.g., bid, tid, qid) for the number of days considered necessary by the surgeon
	Contact patient via telephone the evening of the surgery to determine level of comfort. *If considerable pain is present*, add opioid to NSAID: codeine, oxycodone, propoxyphene

From Malamed SF: Local anesthetics: dentistry's most important drugs, *J Am Dent Assoc* 125:1571-1576, 1994.

TABLE 16-6 Nonsteroidal Antiinflammatory Drugs

Generic	Proprietary	Availability	Dosage regimen
Diclofenac	Voltaren	25, 50, and 75 mg tablets	50 mg bid or tid or 75 mg bid
Etodolac	Lodine	200 and 300 mg capsules and tablets	200 to 400 mg q 6 to 8 hr
Fenoprofen	Nalfon	200 and 300 mg tablets	200 mg q 4 to 6 hr
Flurbiprofen	Ansaid	50 and 100 mg tablets	200 to 300 mg total dose divided tid or qid
Ibuprofen	Motrin	300, 400, 600, and 800 mg tablets	300, 400, 600, 800 mg tid or qid
	Nuprin	200 mg tablets	200 mg q 4 to 6 hr
Indomethacin	Indocin	25 and 50 mg capsules	25 to 50 mg bid or tid
Ketoprofen	Orudis	25, 50, and 75 mg capsules	150 to 300 mg tid
Ketorolac	Toradol	10 mg tablets	10 mg q 4 to 6 hr
Meclofenamate	Meclomen	50 and 100 mg capsules	50 mg q 4 to 6 hr
Mefenamic acid	Ponstel	250 mg capsules	500 mg initially then 250 mg qid
Naproxen	Anaprox	75 mg tablets	50 mg followed by 275 q 6 to 8 hr
	Naprosyn	250, 375, and 500 mg tablets	250 to 500 mg bid
Nabumetone	Relafen	500 and 750 mg tablets	1 to 2 g/day—single or bid
Piroxicam	Feldene	10 and 20 mg capsules	20 mg once a day
Sulindac	Clinoril	150 and 200 mg tablets	150 to 300 mg bid
Tolmetin	Tolectin	200, 400, and 600 mg tablets	400 mg tid

Data from *Drug Handbook*, Springhouse, Pa, 1994, Springhouse; Olin BR, editor: *Drug Facts and Comparisons*, St Louis, 1992, Facts and Comparisons.

Alternative opioids include propoxyphene or oxycodone administered in doses that are equianalgesic to 30 to 60 mg of codeine.[36]

Table 16-5 outlines a recommended protocol for the management of intraoperative and postoperative pain associated with dental surgical procedures.[37] Common NSAIDs and their recommended doses are listed in Table 16-6.

DENTAL HYGIENE

Registered dental hygienists in 20 states in the United States and several provinces in Canada are permitted to administer local anesthesia to dental patients (Table 16-7).[38] The inclusion of this expanded function in the Dental Practice Act in these areas has proved of great benefit to the hygienist, the doctor, and the dental patient.[39]

Not all patients require local anesthesia for scaling, root planing, and subgingival curettage, but many do. The periodontal tissues being treated are normally sensitive to stimuli and are even more so when inflammation is present. Such is frequently the case when a patient is being treated by the dental hygienist.

The hygienist who is permitted to administer local anesthetics to dental patients requires the same technique armamentarium as the doctor. Regional block anesthesia, especially in the maxilla (posterior superior or anterior superior alveolar nerve block), is an integral part of the hygienist's anesthetic armamentarium since hygienists usually treat whole quadrants in one appointment. The hygiene patient requires the same depth of

TABLE 16-7 States Permitting Administration of Local Anesthetics by Dental Hygienists

Alaska	1981
Arizona	1976
Arkansas	1995
California	1984
Colorado	1982
Hawaii	1986
Idaho	1975
Kansas	1993
Missouri	1973
Montana	1985
Nevada	1982
New Mexico	1972
Oklahoma	1980
Oregon	1975
South Dakota	1992
Utah	1983
Vermont	1993
Washington	1971

Data from American Dental Hygienists Association, Chicago, 1995.

anesthesia as that obtained by the doctor doing restorative dentistry or surgery. Root planing without discomfort requires pulpal, along with soft tissue and osseous, anesthesia.[40]

Before dental hygienists were permitted to administer local anesthetics, pain control required that the doctor administer local anesthesia or inhalation sedation (nitrous oxide and oxygen) for the hygienist's patients, or the hygienist applied topical anesthetic to the buccal and linguopalatal soft tissue in all four quadrants. Although these alternatives are workable, they do not compare with permitting a well-trained dental hygienist to administer local anesthetics to patients. Over 70% of respondents to a survey on dental hygiene patients' need for pain control reported that their patients needed anesthesia but did not receive it.[40]

Feedback from dentists whose hygienists administer local anesthesia has been uniformly positive, with negative comments extremely rare.[39] Dental patients themselves are aware of the difference in local anesthesia administered by the dental hygienist and that administered by the dentist. They frequently comment on the lack of discomfort when the hygienist injects the local anesthetic. Be it a slower rate of administration, more attention to the details of atraumatic injection technique, or greater empathy, it works.

REFERENCES

1. Brown RD: The failure of local anaesthesia in acute inflammation, *Br Dent J* 151:47-51, 1981.
2. Kitay D, Ferraro N, Sonis ST: Lateral pharyngeal space abscess as a consequence of regional anesthesia, *J Am Dent Assoc* 122(7):56-59, 1991.
3. Connor JP, Edelson JG: Needle tract infection: a case report, *Oral Surg* 65(4):401-403, 1988.
4. Saadoun AP, Malamed SF: Intraseptal anesthesia in periodontal surgery, *J Am Dent Assoc* 111:249, 1985.
5. Leonard M: The efficacy of an intraosscous injection system of delivering local anesthetic, *J Am Dent Assoc* 126(1):81-86, 1995.
6. Berg RA: Emergency infusion of catecholamines into bone marrow, *Am J Dis Child* 138:810-811, 1984.
7. Goodsen JM, Moore PA: Life-threatening reactions after pedodontic sedation: an assessment of narcotic, local anesthetic, and antiemetic drug interaction, *J Am Dent Assoc* 107:239-245, 1983.
8. Moore PA: Preventing local anesthesia toxicity, *J Am Dent Assoc* 123:60-64, 1992.
9. Berquist HC: The danger of mepivacaine 3% toxicity in children, *Can Dent Assoc J* 3:13, 1975.
10. *Prescribing information: dental*, Westborough, Mass, 1990, Astra Pharmaceutical Products.
11. Council on Dental Therapeutics of the American Dental Association: *Accepted dental therapeutics*, ed 40, Chicago, 1984, American Dental Association.
12. *USP dispensing information*, ed 13, Rockville, Md, 1993, United States Pharmacopeial Convention.
13. Cheatham BD, Primosch RE, Courts FJ: A survey of local anesthetic usage in pediatric patients by Florida dentists, *J Dent Child* 59:401-407, 1992.
14. Yagiela JA: Regional anesthesia for dental procedures, *Int Anesthesiol Clin* 27(2):68-82, 1989.
15. Rood JP: Notes on local analgesia for the child patient, *Dent Update* 8:377-381, 1981.
16. Kaufman L, Sowray JH, Rood JP: *General anaesthesia, local analgesia, and sedation in dentistry*, Oxford, 1982, Blackwell Scientific.
17. O'Sullivan VR, Holland T, O'Mullane DM, Whelton H: A review of current local anaesthetic techniques in dentistry for children, *J Irish Dent Assoc* 32(3):17-27, 1986.
18. Benham NR: The cephalometric position of the mandibular foramen with age, *J Dent Child* 43:233-237, 1976.
19. Akinosi JO: A new approach to the mandibular nerve block, *Br J Oral Surg* 15:83-87, 1977.
20. Yamada A, Jastak JT: Clinical evaluation of the Gow-Gates block in children, *Anesth Prog* 28:106-109, 1981.
21. Brannstrom M, Lindskog S, Nordenvall KJ: Enamel hypoplasia in permanent teeth induced by periodontal ligament anesthesia of primary teeth, *J Am Dent Assoc* 109(5):735-736, 1984.
22. Saadoun AP, Malamed SF: Intraseptal anesthesia in periodontal surgery, *J Am Dent Assoc* 111:249-256, 1985.
23. van der Bijl P, Victor AM: Adverse reactions associated with norepinephrine in dental local anesthesia, *Anesth Prog* 39(3):87-89, 1992.
24. Jakob W: Local anaesthesia and vasoconstrictive additional components, *Newslett Int Fed Dent Anesthesiol Soc* 2(1):3, 1989.
25. Sveen K: Effect of the addition of a vasoconstrictor to local anesthetic solution on operative and postoperative bleeding, analgesia and wound healing, *Int J Oral Surg* 8:301-306, 1979.
26. Buckley JA, Ciancio SG, McMullen JA: Efficacy of epinephrine concentration in local anesthesia during periodontal surgery, *J Periodontol* 55:653-657, 1984.
27. Jastak JT, Yagiela JA: Vasoconstrictors and local anesthesia; a review and rationale for use, *J Am Dent Assoc* 107:623-630, 1983.
28. Skoglund LA, Jorkjend L: Postoperative pain experience after gingivectomies using different combinations of local anaesthetic agents and periodontal dressings, *J Clin Periodontol* 18:204-209, 1991.
29. Danielsson K, Evers H, Nordenram A: Long-acting local anesthetics in oral surgery: an experimental evaluation of bupivacaine and etidocaine for oral infiltration anesthesia, *Anesth Prog* 32:65-68, 1985.
30. Sisk AL, Dionne RA, Wirdzek PR: Evaluation of etidocaine hydrochloride for local anesthesia and postoperative pain control in oral surgery, *J Oral Maxillofac Surg* 42:84-88, 1984.
31. Yagiela JA: Local anesthetics. In Neidle EA, Yagiela JA, editors: *Pharmacology and therapeutics for dentistry*, cd 3, St Louis, 1989, Mosby-Year Book.
32. Danielsson K, Evers H, Holmlund A, et al: Long-acting local anaesthetics in oral surgery, *Int J Oral Maxillofac Surg* 15:119-126, 1986.
33. Gilman AG, Goodman LS, Gilman A, editors: *The pharmacological basis of therapeutics*, ed 6, New York, 1980, Macmillan, pp 494-509.
34. Jackson DL, Moore PA, Haegreaves KM: Pre-operative nonsteroidal antiinflammatory medication for the prevention of postoperative dental pain, *J Am Dent Assoc* 119:641-647, 1989.
35. Linden ET, Abrams H, Matheny J, et al: A comparison of postoperative pain experience following periodontal surgery using two local anesthetic agents, *J Periodontol* 57(10):637-642, 1986.
36. Acute Pain Management Guideline Panel: *Acute pain management: operative or medical procedures and trauma. Clinical practice guideline*, AHCPR Pub No 92-0032, Rockville, Md, 1992, Agency for Health Care Policy and Research, Public Health Service, US Department of Health and Human Services.
37. Malamed SF: Local anesthetics: dentistry's most important drugs, *J Am Dent Assoc* 125:1571-1576, 1994.
38. American Dental Hygienists Association, Chicago, 1995.
39. Sisty-LePeau N, Boyer EM, Lutjen D: Dental hygiene licensure specifications on pain control procedures, *J Dent Hygiene* 64(4):179-185, 1990.
40. Sisty-LePeau N, Nielson-Thompson N, Lutjen D: Use, need and desire for pain control procedures by Iowa hygienists, *J Dent Hygiene* 66(3):137-146, 1992.

in this part

four

Complications, questions, and future trends

Despite careful patient evaluation, proper tissue preparation, and meticulous administration technique, local and systemic complications associated with dental anesthesia occasionally develop. These problems are addressed in Chapters 17 and 18. Emphasis is placed on prevention, recognition, and management of the complications.

Chapter 19, Future Trends in Pain Control, first appeared in the third edition and is updated here. There has been considerable interest demonstrated in recent years in improving local anesthesia as "the" technique of pain control. Additionally, alternative techniques for providing clinically pain-free dental and medical care are continually being sought. In the past decade the electronic dental anesthesia (EDA) technique has been shown to be a viable alternative to injectable local anesthetics in certain areas of dental care. EDA is described and the current literature reviewed.

In Chapter 20 I present a series of questions related to local anesthesia and pain control in dentistry. These are questions commonly asked of me by doctors who have had peculiar situations arise in connection with this technique of pain control. They are presented here as a matter of interest and in the hope that the answer to one of your questions or problems might be included.

seventeen

Local Complications

There are a number of potential complications associated with the administration of local anesthetics:

Needle breakage
Pain on injection
Burning on injection
Persistent anesthesia or paresthesia
Trismus
Hematoma
Infection
Edema
Sloughing of tissues
Soft tissue injury
Facial nerve paralysis
Postanesthetic intraoral lesions

For purposes of convenience these complications may be separated into those that occur *locally* in the region of the injection and those that are *systemic*. Systemic complications associated with local anesthesia are discussed in Chapter 18; local complications are described in this chapter.

It must be emphasized that whenever a complication associated with local anesthetic administration occurs, a written note should be entered on the patient's dental chart. For complications that become chronic, a note should appear whenever the patient is reevaluated.

NEEDLE BREAKAGE

Since the introduction of disposable needles, breakage and loss of needles within tissues have become extremely rare. However, reports of needle breakage still appear, despite the fact that virtually all such instances are preventable (Fig. 17-1).[1-4]

Causes

The primary cause of needle breakage is *sudden unexpected movement* by the patient as the needle penetrates muscle or contacts periosteum. If the patient's movement is opposite that of the needle, the force of contact may prove adequate to break the needle.

1. *Smaller* needles (i.e., 30-gauge) are more likely to break than larger needles (25-gauge).
2. Needles that have previously been *bent* (in an attempt to direct them more accurately into the tissue) are weakened and more likely to break than unbent needles are.
3. Needles may prove to be defective in manufacture (an exceedingly rare cause of needle breakage).

Problem

Needle breakage per se is not a significant problem. If a broken needle can be retrieved without surgical intervention, no emergency exists. A Magill intubation forceps or hemostat can be used to grasp the visible proximal end of the needle fragment and remove it from the soft tissue.

Needles that break off within tissues and cannot readily be retrieved do not usually migrate more than a few millimeters. They become encased in scar tissue within a few weeks. Localized or systemic infection produced by such needles is extremely rare. Electing to leave a needle frag-

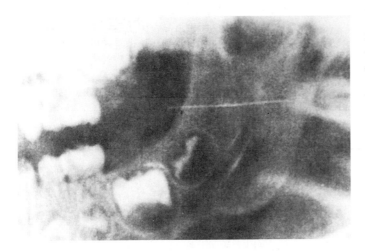

Fig. 17-1 Radiograph of a broken dental needle in the ptery-gomandibular space. *(From Marks RB, Carlton DM, McDonald S: Management of a broken needle in the ptery-gomandibular space: report of a case,* J Am Dent Assoc *109:263-264, 1984. Copyright the American Dental Association. Reprinted by permission.)*

ment in the tissue instead of attempting its removal usually leads to fewer problems than the extensive, involved, and often traumatic surgical procedure required for its removal.

Prevention

Use larger-gauge needles for injections requiring penetration of significant depths of soft tissue; 25-gauge needles are appropriate for an inferior alveolar, mandibular, posterior superior alveolar, anterior superior alveolar, and maxillary nerve block.

Use long needles for injections requiring penetration of significant (>18 mm) depths of soft tissues.

Do not insert a needle into tissues to its hub, unless it is absolutely essential for the success of the technique; the point at which the needle shaft meets the hub is the weakest part of the needle and the site at which needle breakage usually occurs. Select a needle of adequate length for the contemplated procedure.

Do not redirect a needle once it is inserted into tissues. Excessive lateral force on the needle is a factor in breakage. Withdraw the needle *almost completely* before redirecting it.

Management

Shira has presented a description of the management of broken needles.[5] A summary of his prudent suggestions follows:

1. When a needle breaks
   a. Remain calm; do not panic.
   b. Instruct the patient not to move. Do not remove your hand from the patient's mouth; keep the patient's mouth open. If available, place a bite block in the patient's mouth.
   c. If the fragment is visible, try to remove it with a small hemostat or a Magill intubation forceps. (See Chapter 8.)
2. *If the needle is lost (not visible) and cannot be readily retrieved*

   a. Do *not* proceed with an incision or probing.
   b. Calmly inform the patient; attempt to allay fears and apprehension.
   c. Note the incident on the patient's chart. Keep the remaining needle fragment. Inform your insurance carrier immediately.
   d. Refer the patient to an oral and maxillofacial surgeon for *consultation*, not for removal of the needle.
3. *When a needle breaks, consideration should be given to its immediate removal*
   a. If it is superficial *and* easily located through radiological and clinical examination, then removal by a competent dental surgeon is possible.
   b. If, despite its superficial location, attempted retrieval is unsuccessful in a reasonable length of time, it is prudent to abandon the attempt and allow the needle fragment to remain.
   c. If it is located in deeper tissues or is hard to locate, permit it to remain *without* an attempt at removal.

There is considerable precedent to justify the retention of a broken needle if removal appears difficult.

Unfortunately, the chance of litigation ensuing following a broken needle incident is high.

PAIN ON INJECTION

Pain on deposition of a local anesthetic can best be prevented through careful adherence to the basic protocol of atraumatic injection. (See Chapter 11.)

Causes

1. Careless injection technique and callous attitude ("Palatal injections always hurt" or "This will hurt a little") all too often become self-fulfilling prophesies.
2. A needle can become dull from multiple injections.

3. Rapid deposition of the anesthetic solution may cause tissue damage.
4. Needles with barbs (from impaling on bone) may produce pain as they are withdrawn from tissue.

Problem

Pain on injection increases patient anxiety and may lead to sudden unexpected movement, increasing the risk of needle breakage.

Prevention

1. Adhere to proper techniques of injection, both anatomical and psychological.
2. Use sharp needles.
3. Use topical anesthetic prior to injection.
4. Use sterile local anesthetic solutions.
5. Inject local anesthetics slowly.
6. Be certain that the temperature of the solution is correct. A solution that is too hot or too cold will be more uncomfortable than one that is at room temperature.

Management

No management is required. However, steps should be taken to prevent the recurrence of pain associated with the injection of local anesthetics.

BURNING ON INJECTION

Causes

A burning sensation occurring during injection of a local anesthetic is not uncommon. There are several potential causes.

The primary cause of a mild burning sensation is the pH of the solution being deposited into the soft tissues. The pH of local anesthetic solutions as prepared for injection is approximately 5 whereas that of solutions containing a vasopressor is even more acidic (around 3).

Rapid injection of local anesthetic, especially in the denser more adherent tissues of the palate, produces a burning sensation.

Contamination of the local anesthetic cartridges can result when they are stored in alcohol or other sterilizing solutions, leading to diffusion of these solutions into the cartridge.

Solutions warmed to normal body temperature are usually considered "too hot" by the patient.

Problem

Although usually transient, the sensation of burning on injection of a local anesthetic indicates that tissue irritation is occurring. If this is caused by the pH of the solution, it rapidly disappears as the anesthetic action develops. There is usually no residual sensitivity noted when the anesthetic action terminates.

When a burning sensation occurs as a result of rapid injection, contaminated solution, or overly warm solution, there is a greater likelihood that tissue may be damaged, with subsequent development of other complications such as postanesthetic trismus, edema, or possible paresthesia.

Prevention

It is difficult, if not impossible, to eliminate the mild burning sensation that some patients experience during injection of a local anesthetic solution. However, the duration of this sensation is but a few seconds, its intensity is quite low, and many patients are not even aware of it.

Slowing the injection should help. The *ideal* rate is 1 ml/min. Do not exceed the *recommended* rate of 1.8 ml in 1 minute.

The cartridge of anesthetic should be stored at room temperature either in the container in which it was shipped or in a suitable container *without* alcohol or other sterilizing agents. (See Chapter 7 for proper care and handling of dental cartridges.)

Management

Since most instances of burning on injection are transient and do not lead to prolonged tissue involvement, formal treatment is not usually indicated. In those few situations in which postinjection discomfort, edema, or paresthesia becomes evident, management of the specific problem is indicated.

PERSISTENT ANESTHESIA OR PARESTHESIA

On occasion a patient will report feeling numb ("frozen") many hours or days after a local anesthetic injection. Normal distribution of patient response to drugs allows for the rare individual (hyperreactor) who may experience prolonged soft tissue anesthesia following local anesthetic administration persisting for many hours longer than that which is expected. This is not a problem. When anesthesia persists for days, weeks, or months there is an increased potential for the development of problems. Paresthesia or persistent anesthesia is a disturbing yet sometimes unpreventable complication of local anesthetic administration. Paresthesia is also one of the most frequent causes of dental malpractice litigation.

Causes

Trauma to any nerve may lead to persistent anesthesia. Injection of a local anesthetic solution contaminated by alcohol or sterilizing solution near a nerve produces irritation, resulting in edema and increased pressure in the region of the nerve, leading to paresthesia. These contaminants, especially alcohol, are neurolytic and can produce long-term trauma to the nerve (paresthesia lasting for months to years).

Trauma to the nerve sheath can be produced by the needle during injection. The patient reports the sensation of an "electric shock" throughout the distribution of the involved nerve. Though it is difficult to actually sever a nerve trunk or even its fibers with the small needles used in dentistry, trauma to a nerve produced by contact with the needle is all that may be needed to produce paresthesia. Insertion of a needle into a foramen, as in the second division (maxillary) nerve block via the greater palatine foramen, also increases the likelihood of nerve injury.

Hemorrhage into or around the neural sheath is another cause. Bleeding increases pressure on the nerve, leading to paresthesia.

Problem

Persistent anesthesia, rarely total, in most cases partial, can lead to self-inflicted injury. Biting or thermal or chemical insult can occur without a patient's awareness, until the process has progressed to a serious degree. When the lingual nerve is involved, the sense of taste (via the chorda tympani nerve) may also be impaired.

In some instances a loss of sensation (paresthesia) is not the clinical manifestation of nerve injury. *Hyperesthesia* (an increased sensitivity to noxious stimuli) and *dysesthesia* (a painful sensation occurring to usually nonnoxious stimuli) may also be noted. Haas and Lennon reported that pain was present in 22% of the 143 cases of paresthesia they reviewed.[6] Paresthesia appears to occur more commonly with prilocaine than with other injectable local anesthetics.[6]

Prevention

Strict adherence to injection protocol and proper care and handling of dental cartridges help minimize the risk of paresthesia. Nevertheless, cases of paresthesia will still occur despite our care in injection.

Management

Most paresthesias resolve within approximately 8 weeks without treatment.[7] Only if damage to the nerve is severe will the paresthesia be permanent, and then only rarely. In most situations paresthesia is minimal, with the patient retaining most sensory function to the affected area. The risk of self-inflicted tissue injury is therefore minimal. Haas and Lennon, in a 21 year retrospective study of Canadian dentists, have reported that most paresthesias involved the tongue, with the lower lip the next most common site of involvement.[6]

McCarthy has recommended the following sequence in managing the patient with a persistent sensory deficit following local anesthesia:[8]

1. *Be reassuring.* The patient usually telephones the office the day following the dental procedure complaining of still being a little numb.
   a. *Speak with the patient personally!* Do not relegate the duty to an auxiliary.
   b. Explain that paresthesia is not uncommon following local anesthetic administration. Sisk et al have reported that paresthesia may develop in up to 22% of patients in very selected circumstances.[9]
   c. *Arrange an appointment to examine the patient.*
   d. *Record the incident on the dental chart.*
2. *Examine the patient.*
   a. *Determine the degree and extent of paresthesia.*
   b. *Explain to the patient that paresthesia normally persists for at least 2 months* before resolution begins and that it may last up to a year or longer.
   c. "Tincture of time" is the recommended medicine.
   d. *Record all findings on the patient's chart.*
3. Reschedule the patient for examination every 2 months for as long as the sensory deficit persists.
4. If sensory deficit is still evident 1 year after the incident, consultation with an oral surgeon or neurologist is recommended. Consultation should be considered earlier if the patient and/or doctor consider it prudent.
5. Dental treatment may continue, but avoid readministering local anesthetic into the region of the previously traumatized nerve. Use alternate local anesthetic techniques if possible.

TRISMUS

Trismus, from the Greek *trismos,* is defined as a prolonged, tetanic spasm of the jaw muscles by which the normal opening of the mouth is restricted (locked jaw). The designation was originally used only in tetanus, but as an inability to open the mouth may be seen in a variety of conditions, the term is currently used in restricted jaw movement regardless of etiology.[10] Although postinjection pain is the most common local complication of local anesthesia, trismus can become one of the more chronic and complicated problems to manage.

Causes

Trauma to muscles or blood vessels in the infratemporal fossa is the most common etiological factor in trismus associated with dental injections of local anesthetics.

Local anesthetic solutions into which alcohol or cold sterilizing solutions have diffused will produce irritation of tissues (e.g., muscle), leading potentially to trismus.

Local anesthetics have been demonstrated to have slight myotoxic properties on skeletal muscles. The injection of local anesthetic solution either intramuscularly or supramuscularly leads to a rapidly progressive necrosis of the exposed muscle fibers.[11-13]

Hemorrhage is another cause of trismus. Large volumes of extravascular blood can produce tissue irritation, leading to muscle dysfunction as the blood is slowly resorbed.

A low-grade infection following injection can also cause trismus.[14]

Every needle insertion produces some insult to the tissue through which it passes. It stands to reason, then, that multiple needle penetrations would correlate with a greater incidence of postinjection trismus. In addition, Stacy and Hajjar found that of 100 needles used for the administration of the inferior alveolar nerve block, 60% were barbed on removal from the tissues. The barb occurred when the needle came into contact with the medial aspect of the mandibular ramus. Withdrawal of the needle from tissue increased the likelihood of involvement of the lingual or inferior alveolar nerve and the development of trismus.[15]

Excessive volumes of local anesthetic solution deposited into a restricted area produce distention of tissues, which may lead to postinjection trismus. This is more common following multiple missed inferior alveolar nerve blocks.

Problem

Though the limitation of movement associated with postinjection trismus is usually minor, it is possible for much more severe limitation to develop. The average interincisal opening in cases of trismus is 13.7 mm (range 5 to 23 mm).[12] Stone and Kaban reported four cases of severe trismus following multiple inferior alveolar or posterior superior alveolar nerve blocks, three of which required surgical intervention.[16] Before this treatment the patients had limited mandibular openings of approximately 2 mm, despite usual treatment regimens.

In the acute phase of trismus, pain produced by hemorrhage leads to muscle spasm and limitation of movement.[17,18] The second, or chronic, phase usually develops if treatment is not begun. Chronic hypomobility is secondary to organization of the hematoma, with subsequent fibrosis and scar contracture.[19] Infection may also produce hypomobility through increased pain, increased tissue reaction (irritation), and scarring.[14]

Prevention

1. Use a sharp, sterile, disposable needle.
2. Properly care for and handle dental local anesthetic cartridges.
3. Use aseptic technique. Contaminated needles should be changed immediately.
4. Practice atraumatic insertion and injection technique.

> **Trismus is not always preventable.**

5. Avoid repeat injections and multiple insertions into the same area through knowledge of anatomy and proper technique. Use regional nerve blocks instead of local infiltration (supraperiosteal injection) wherever possible and rational.
6. Use minimum effective volumes of local anesthetic. Refer to specific protocols for recommendations.

Management

In most cases a patient will report pain and some difficulty opening the mouth on the day following dental treatment in which a posterior superior alveolar or inferior alveolar nerve block was administered. Hinton et al reported that the onset of trismus occurred between 1 to 6 days posttreatment (average 2.9 days).[12] The degree of discomfort and dysfunction varies but is usually mild.

With mild pain and dysfunction the patient reports minimum difficulty opening the mouth. Arrange an appointment for examination. In the interim, prescribe heat therapy, warm saline rinses, analgesics, and, if necessary, muscle relaxants to manage the initial phase of muscle spasm.[20,21] *Heat therapy* consists of applying hot, moist towels to the affected area for approximately 20 minutes every hour. For a *warm saline rinse,* a teaspoon of salt is added to a 12 ounce glass of warm water and held in the mouth on the involved side (and spit out) to help relieve the discomfort of trismus. Aspirin is usually adequate as an *analgesic* in managing the pain associated with trismus. Its antiinflammatory properties are also beneficial. Codeine may be required (30 to 60 mg q6h) if the discomfort is more intense (extremely rare). Diazepam (approximately 10 mg bid) or other benzodiazepine is used for *muscle relaxation* if deemed necessary.

The patient should be advised to initiate physiotherapy consisting of opening and closing the mouth, as well as lateral excursions of the mandible for 5 minutes every 3 to 4 hours. Chewing gum (sugarless, of course!) is yet another means of providing lateral movement of the temporomandibular joint.

Record the incident, findings, and treatment on the patient's dental chart. Avoid further dental treatment in the involved region until symptoms resolve and the patient is more comfortable.

If continued dental care in the area is urgent, as with an infected painful tooth, it may prove difficult to achieve effective pain control when trismus is present. The Vazirani-Akinosi mandibular nerve block will usually provide relief of the motor dysfunction, permitting the patient to open the mouth and allow the administration of the appropriate injection for clinical pain control, if needed.

In virtually all cases of trismus related to intraoral injections that are managed as described, patients report improvement within 48 to 72 hours. Therapy should be continued until the patient is free of symptoms. If pain and dysfunction continue unabated beyond 48 hours, consider the possibility of infection. Antibiotics should be added to the treatment regimen described and continued 7 full days. Complete recovery from injection-related trismus takes about 6 weeks, with a range of from 4 to 20 weeks.[12]

For severe pain or dysfunction, if no improvement is noted within 2 or 3 days without antibiotics or within 5 to 7 days with antibiotics, or if the ability to open the mouth has become quite limited, the patient should be referred to an oral and maxillofacial surgeon for evaluation. Other therapies, including the use of ultrasound or appliances, are available for use in these situations.[22,23]

Temporomandibular joint involvement is quite rare in the first 4 to 6 weeks following injection. Surgical intervention to correct chronic dysfunction may be indicated in some instances.[12,16]

HEMATOMA

The effusion of blood into extravascular spaces can result from inadvertently nicking a blood vessel (artery or vein) during the injection of a local anesthetic. A hematoma developing subsequent to the nicking of an artery will usually increase rapidly in size until treatment is instituted, due to the significantly greater blood pressure within the artery. Nicking a vein may or may not result in the formation of a hematoma. Tissue density surrounding the injured vessel will be a determining factor.

Cause

Because of the density of tissue in the hard palate and its firm adherence to bone, hematoma rarely develops after a palatal injection. A rather large hematoma may result from either arterial or venous puncture following posterior superior alveolar or inferior alveolar nerve block. The tissues surrounding these vessels more readily accommodate significant volumes of blood. The blood effuses from vessels until extravascular exceeds intravascular pressure or until clotting occurs. Hematomas following the inferior alveolar nerve block are usually only visible intraorally, while posterior superior alveolar hematomas are visible extraorally.

Problem

A hematoma rarely produces significant problems, aside from the resulting "bruise," which may or may not be visible extraorally. Possible complications of hematoma include trismus and pain. The swelling and discoloration of the region usually subside within 7 to 14 days.

A hematoma constitutes an inconvenience to the patient and an embarrassment to the person administering the drug (Fig. 17-2).

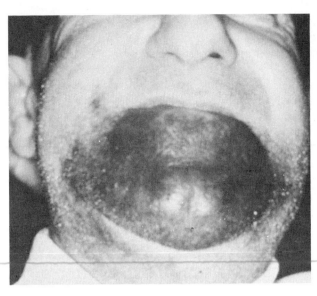

Fig. 17-2 Hematoma that developed after bilateral mental nerve blocks.

Hematoma is not always preventable.

Prevention

1. Knowledge of the normal anatomy involved in the proposed injection is important. Certain techniques have a greater risk of hematoma. The posterior superior alveolar nerve block is the most common, followed by the inferior alveolar nerve block (a distant second) and the mental/incisive nerve block (a close third when the foramen is entered, a distant third if the technique described in Chapter 14 is adhered to).
2. Modify the injection technique as dictated by the patient's anatomy. For example, the depth of penetration for a posterior superior alveolar nerve block may be decreased in a patient with smaller facial characteristics.
3. Use a short needle for the posterior superior alveolar nerve block to decrease the risk of hematoma.
4. Minimize the number of needle penetrations into tissue.
5. Never use a needle as a probe in tissues.

Management

Immediate

When swelling becomes evident during or immediately following a local anesthetic injection, direct pressure should be applied to the site of bleeding. For most injections the blood vessel lies between the skin and bone, on which pressure should be applied for not less than 2 minutes. This will effectively stop the bleeding.

Inferior alveolar nerve block Pressure is applied to the medial aspect of the mandibular ramus. Clinical manifestations of the hematoma are intraoral: possible tissue discoloration and probable tissue swelling on the medial (lingual) aspect of the mandibular ramus.

Infraorbital nerve block Pressure is applied to the skin directly over the infraorbital foramen. Clinical manifestation is discoloration of the skin below the lower eyelid. Hematoma is unlikely to arise with infraorbital nerve block because the technique described requires application of pressure to the injection site throughout drug administration and for a period of 2 to 3 minutes after.

Mental or incisive nerve block Pressure is placed directly over the mental foramen, on the skin or mucous membrane. Clinical manifestations are discoloration of skin over the mental foramen and/or swelling in the mucobuccal fold in the region of the mental foramen (Fig. 17-2). As with the infraorbital nerve block, pressure applied during the administration of the drug effectively minimizes the risk of hematoma formation during incisive (not mental) nerve block.

Buccal nerve block or any palatal injection Place pressure at the site of bleeding. In these injections the clinical manifestations of hematoma are usually visible only within the mouth.

Posterior superior alveolar nerve block The posterior superior alveolar nerve block usually produces the largest and most esthetically unappealing hematoma. The infratemporal fossa, into which bleeding occurs, can accommodate a large volume of blood. The hematoma is usually not recognized until swelling appears on the side of the face (usually a few minutes after the injection is completed), progressing inferiorly and anteriorly toward the lower anterior region of the cheek. It is difficult to apply pressure to the site of bleeding in this situation because of the location of the involved blood vessels. It is also relatively difficult to apply pressure directly to the posterior superior alveolar artery (the primary source of bleeding), the facial artery, and the pterygoid plexus of veins. They are located posterior, superior, and medial to the maxillary tuberosity. Bleeding normally halts when external pressure on the vessels exceeds the internal pressure or when clotting occurs. Digital pressure can be applied to the soft tissues in the mucobuccal fold as far distally as can be tolerated by the patient (without eliciting a gag reflex). Apply pressure in a medial and superior direction. If available, ice should be used (extraorally) to exert pressure on the site and help constrict the vessel.

Subsequent

Once bleeding stops the patient may be discharged. Make a note of the hematoma on the patient's dental chart.

Advise the patient about possible soreness and limitation of movement. If either of these develops, begin treatment as described previously for trismus. There will probably be discoloration as a result of extravascular blood elements, which will gradually be resorbed over 7 to 14 days.

If soreness develops, advise the patient to take an analgesic such as aspirin. *Do not apply heat* to the area for at least 4 to 6 hours after the incident. Heat produces vasodilation, which may further increase the size of the hematoma. Heat may be applied to the region beginning the next day. It will serve as an analgesic, and its vasodilating properties may increase the rate at which blood elements are resorbed, although its benefits are debatable. The patient should apply warm moist towels to the affected area for 20 minutes every hour.

Ice *may* be applied to the region immediately on recognition of a developing hematoma. It acts as both an analgesic and a vasoconstrictor and it may aid in minimizing the size of the hematoma.

Time (tincture of time) is the most important element in managing a hematoma. With or without treatment, a hematoma will be present for 7 to 14 days. Avoid additional dental therapy in the region until symptoms and signs resolve.

INFECTION

Infection following the administration of a local anesthetic solution in dentistry has become an extremely rare occurrence since the introduction of sterile disposable needles and glass cartridges.

Causes

The major cause of postinjection infection is contamination of the needle prior to administration of the anesthetic. Contamination of a needle always occurs when the needle touches mucous membrane in the oral cavity. This cannot be prevented, nor is it a significant problem since the normal flora of the oral cavity does not lead to tissue infection.

Improper technique in the handling of the local anesthetic equipment and improper tissue preparation for injection are other possible causes of infection.

Injecting local anesthetic solution into an area of infection As already discussed, local anesthetics are less effective when deposited into infected tissues. However, if deposited under pressure, as in the periodontal ligament injection, the force of their administration might transport bacteria into adjacent, healthy tissues, spreading infection.

Problem

Contamination of needles or solutions may cause a low-grade infection when the needle or solution is placed in deeper tissue. This may lead to trismus if it is not recognized and proper treatment is not initiated.[14]

Prevention

1. Use disposable needles.
2. Properly care for and handle needles. Take precautions to avoid contamination of the needle through contact with nonsterile surfaces; avoid multiple injections with the same needle, if possible.
3. Properly care for and handle dental cartridges of local anesthetic.
   a. Use a cartridge only once (one patient).
   b. Store cartridges aseptically in their original container, covered at all times.
   c. Cleanse the diaphragm with a sterile disposable alcohol wipe immediately prior to use.
4. Properly prepare the tissues prior to penetration. Dry them and apply topical antiseptic (optional).

Management

Low-grade infection, which is quite rare, will seldom be recognized immediately. The patient will report postinjection pain and dysfunction 1 or more days following dental care. There rarely will be any overt signs and symptoms of infection. Immediate treatment should consist of the procedures used to manage trismus: heat and analgesic if needed, muscle relaxant if needed, and physiotherapy. Trismus produced by factors other than infection normally responds with resolution or improvement within several days. If signs and symptoms of trismus do not begin to respond to conservative therapy within 3 days, the possibility of a low-grade infection should be entertained and the patient started on a 7-day course of antibiotics. Prescribe 29 tablets of penicillin V (250 mg tablets). The patient takes 500 mg immediately and then 250 mg four times a day until all tablets have been taken. Erythromycin may be substituted if the patient is allergic to penicillin.

Record the progress and management of the patient on the dental chart.

EDEMA

Swelling of tissues is not a syndrome but a clinical sign of the presence of some disorder.

Causes

1. Trauma during injection
2. Infection
3. Allergy (angioedema is a common response to topical anesthetics in an allergic patient; localized tissue swelling occurs as a result of vasodilation secondary to histamine release)
4. Hemorrhage (effusion of blood into soft tissues produces swelling)

5. Injection of irritating solutions (alcohol or cold sterilizing solution–containing cartridges)

Problem

Edema related to local anesthetic administration is seldom intense enough to produce significant problems such as airway obstruction. Most instances of local anesthetic-related edema result in pain and dysfunction of the region and embarrassment for the patient.

Angioneurotic edema produced by topical anesthetic in an allergic individual can compromise the airway. Edema of the tongue, pharynx, or larynx may develop and represents a potentially life-threatening situation that requires vigorous management.[24]

Prevention

1. Properly care for and handle the local anesthetic armamentarium.
2. Use atraumatic injection technique.
3. Complete an adequate medical evaluation of the patient prior to drug administration.

Management

The management of edema is predicated on reduction of the swelling as quickly as possible and on the cause of the edema. When produced by traumatic injection or introduction of irritating solutions, edema is usually of minimal degree and resolves in several days without formal therapy. In this and all situations in which edema is present, it may be necessary to prescribe analgesics for pain.

After hemorrhage, edema resolves more slowly (over 7 to 14 days) as extravasated blood elements are resorbed into the vascular system. If signs of hemorrhage are evident (e.g., bluish discoloration progressing to green and other colors), management follows that discussed previously for hematoma.

Edema produced by infection will not resolve spontaneously but may, in fact, become progressively more intense if untreated. If signs and symptoms of infection (pain, mandibular dysfunction, edema, warmth) do not appear to resolve within 3 days, institute antibiotic therapy as just outlined.

Allergy-induced edema is potentially life-threatening. Its degree and location are highly significant. If swelling develops in buccal soft tissues and there is absolutely no airway involvement, treatment consists of intramuscular and oral antihistamine administration and consultation with an allergist to determine the precise cause of the edema.

If edema occurs in any area where it compromises breathing, treatment consists of the following:

1. If unconscious, the patient is placed supine.
2. Basic life support (airway, breathing, circulation) is administered, as needed.
3. Emergency medical service (e.g., 911) is summoned.

4. Epinephrine is administered: 0.3 mg (adult), 0.15 mg (child), IM or IV, every 5 minutes until respiratory distress resolves.
5. Antihistamine is administered IM or IV.
6. Corticosteroid is administered IM or IV.
7. Preparation is made for cricothyrotomy if total airway obstruction appears to be developing. This is extremely rare, but is the reason for summoning emergency medical services early.
8. The patient's condition is thoroughly evaluated prior to the next appointment to determine the cause of the reaction.

SLOUGHING OF TISSUES

Prolonged irritation of gingival soft tissues may lead to a number of unpleasant complications, including epithelial desquamation and sterile abscess.

Causes

Epithelial Desquamation

1. Application of a topical anesthetic to the gingival tissues for a prolonged period
2. Heightened sensitivity of the tissues to a local anesthetic
3. Reaction in an area where a topical has been applied

Sterile Abscess

1. Secondary to prolonged ischemia resulting from the use of a local anesthetic with vasoconstrictor (usually norepinephrine)
2. Almost always in the tissues of the hard palate

Problem

Pain, at times quite severe, may be a consequence of epithelial desquamation or a sterile abscess. There is a remote possibility that infection may develop in these areas.

Prevention

Use topical anesthetics as recommended. Allow the solution to contact the mucous membranes for 1 to 2 minutes to maximize its effectiveness and to minimize toxicity.

When using vasoconstrictors for hemostasis, do not use overly concentrated solutions. Norepinephrine (Levophed) 1:30,000 is the agent most likely to produce ischemia of sufficient duration to cause tissue damage and a sterile abscess (Fig. 17-3). Epinephrine (1:50,000) may also produce this problem, if reinjection of the solution occurs whenever ischemia resolves, over a long period of time. The palatal tissues are virtually the only place in the oral cavity where this phenomenon occurs.

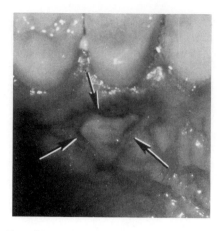

Fig. 17-3 Sloughing of tissue (*arrows*) on the palate caused by prolonged ischemia secondary to the use of local anesthetic with vasoconstrictor.

Management

Usually no formal management is required for either epithelial desquamation or sterile abscess. Be certain to reassure the patient of this fact.

Management may be symptomatic. For pain, analgesics such as aspirin or codeine and a topically applied ointment (Orabase) to minimize irritation to the area are recommended.

Epithelial desquamation will resolve within a few days; the course of a sterile abscess may run 7 to 10 days. Record data on the patient's chart.

SOFT TISSUE INJURY

Self-inflicted trauma to the lips and tongue is frequently caused by the patient inadvertently biting or chewing these tissues while still anesthetized (Fig. 17-4).

Cause

Trauma occurs most frequently in children and in mentally or physically disabled children or adults, but it can, and does, occur in patients of all ages. The primary cause is the fact that soft tissue anesthesia lasts significantly longer than does pulpal anesthesia. The patient will usually be dismissed from the dental office with residual soft tissue numbness.

Problem

Trauma to anesthetized tissues can lead to swelling and significant pain when the anesthetic actions of the drug resolve. A young child or handicapped individual may have difficulty coping with the situation, and this may lead to behavioral problems. The possibility that infection will develop is quite remote in most instances.

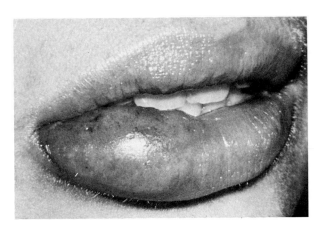

Fig. 17-4 Traumatized lip caused by inadvertent biting while it was still anesthetized.

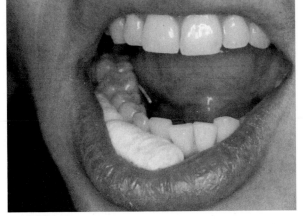

Fig. 17-5 Cotton roll placed between lips and teeth secured with dental floss.

Prevention

If dental appointments are brief, a local anesthetic of appropriate duration should be selected. (Refer to the discussion of lip chewing and duration of anesthesia for specific drugs, p. 236.)

A cotton roll can be placed between the lips and teeth if they are still anesthetized at the time of discharge. Secure the roll with dental floss wrapped around the teeth (this will also prevent inadvertent aspiration of the roll) (Fig. 17-5).

Warn the patient and guardian against eating, drinking hot fluids, and biting on the lips or tongue to test for anesthesia.

A self-adherent warning sticker may be used on children. It states: "Watch me, my lips and cheeks are numb." The sticker is placed on the patient's forehead (Fig. 17-6).

Management

Management of the patient with self-inflicted soft tissue injury secondary to lip or tongue biting or chewing is symptomatic:

1. Analgesics for pain
2. Antibiotics, in the unlikely situation that infection results
3. Lukewarm saline rinses to aid in decreasing any swelling that may be present
4. Petroleum jelly or other lubricant to cover a lip lesion and minimize irritation

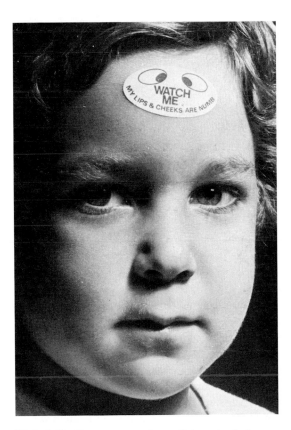

Fig. 17-6 Self-adherent warning sticker to help prevent accidental trauma to anesthetized tissues in children.

FACIAL NERVE PARALYSIS

The seventh cranial nerve carries motor impulses to the muscles of facial expression, of the scalp and external ear, and of other structures. Paralysis of some of its terminal branches occurs whenever an infraorbital nerve block is administered or when maxillary canines are infiltrated. Muscle droop is also observed when, occasionally, the motor fibers are anesthetized by inadvertent deposition of local anesthetic into their vicinity. This may occur when anesthetic is introduced into the deep lobe of the parotid gland, through which terminal portions of the facial nerve extend.

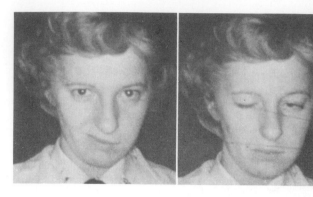

Fig. 17-7 A, Transient facial nerve paralysis following an inferior alveolar nerve block on the left side. **B,** The patient was unable to close the eyelid.

The facial nerve branches and the muscles they innervate are listed below:

1. Temporal branches
   a. Frontalis
   b. Orbicularis oculi
   c. Corrugator supercilii
2. Zygomatic branches
   a. Orbicularis oculi
3. Buccal branches: supplying the region inferior to the eye and around the mouth
   a. Procerus
   b. Zygomaticus
   c. Levator labii superioris
   d. Buccinator
   e. Orbicularis oris
4. Mandibular branch: supplying muscles of the lower lip and chin
   a. Depressor anguli oris
   b. Depressor labii inferioris
   c. Mentalis

Cause

Transient facial nerve paralysis is commonly caused by the introduction of local anesthetic into the capsule of the parotid gland, which is located at the posterior border of the mandibular ramus, clothed by the medial pterygoid and masseter muscles.[25] Directing the needle posteriorly or inadvertently deflecting it in a posterior direction during an inferior alveolar nerve block, or overinserting it during a Vazirani-Akinosi nerve block, may place the tip of the needle within the substance of the parotid gland. If local anesthetic is deposited, transient paralysis can result.

Problem

Loss of motor function to the muscles of facial expression produced by local anesthetic deposition is *transitory*. It will last no more than several hours depending on the agent used, the volume injected, and the proximity to the facial nerve. There is usually minimal or no sensory loss involved.

During this time the patient will have unilateral paralysis and be unable to use these muscles (Fig. 17-7). The primary problem associated with transient facial nerve paralysis therefore is cosmetic: the person's face appears lopsided. There is no treatment other than waiting until the action of the drug resolves.

A secondary problem is that the patient is unable to voluntarily close one eye. The protective lid reflex of the eye is abolished. Winking and blinking become impossible. The cornea, however, does retain its innervation; thus, if it is irritated, the corneal reflex is intact and tears will lubricate the eye.

Prevention

Transient facial nerve paralysis is almost always preventable by adhering to protocol with the inferior alveolar and Vazirani-Akinosi nerve blocks (as described in Chapter 14).

A needle tip in contact with bone (medial aspect of the ramus) prior to deposition of solution virtually precludes the possibility that local anesthetic solution will be deposited into the parotid gland with the inferior alveolar nerve block. If the needle deflects posteriorly during this block and bone is not contacted, the needle should be withdrawn *almost entirely* from the soft tissues, the barrel of the syringe brought posteriorly (the needle tip therefore being directed more anteriorly), and the needle readvanced until it contacts bone. Since there is no contact with bone during the Vazirani-Akinosi nerve block, overinsertion of the needle, either absolute (>25 mm) or relative (25 mm in a smaller patient), should be avoided.

Management

Within seconds to minutes following the deposition of local anesthetic into the parotid gland, the patient will sense a weakening of the muscles on the affected side of the face. Anesthesia will *not* be present in this situation. Management includes the following:

1. Reassure the patient. Explain that the situation is transient, will last for a few hours, and will resolve without residual effect. Mention that it is produced

by anesthetic drug actions on the facial nerve, which is the motor nerve to the muscles of facial expression.

2. An eyepatch should be applied to the affected eye until muscle tone returns. If resistance is offered by the patient, advise the patient to manually close the lower eyelid periodically to keep the cornea lubricated.

3. Contact lenses should be removed until muscular movement returns.

4. Record the incident on the patient's chart.

5. Although there is no contraindication to reanesthetizing the patient to achieve mandibular anesthesia, it may be prudent to forego further dental care at this appointment.

POSTANESTHETIC INTRAORAL LESIONS

Patients will occasionally report that approximately 2 days after an intraoral injection of local anesthetic, ulcerations developed in their mouth, primarily around the site(s) of the injection(s). The primary initial symptom is pain, usually of a relatively intense nature.

Cause

Recurrent aphthous stomatitis and/or herpes simplex can occur intraorally after a local anesthetic injection or after any trauma to the intraoral tissues.

Recurrent aphthous stomatitis is the more frequently observed manifestation, developing on gingival tissues that are *not* attached to underlying bone (i.e., movable tissue), such as the buccal vestibule. It is definitely not viral but thought to be either an autoimmune process (most widely held theory) or an L-form bacterial infection.

Herpes simplex can also develop intraorally, although it more commonly is observed extraorally. It is viral and becomes manifest as small bumps on tissues that are attached to underlying bone (i.e., fixed) such as the soft tissue of the hard palate (Fig. 17-8).

Trauma to tissues by a needle, local anesthetic solution, cotton swab, or any other instrument (e.g., rubber dam clamp or handpiece) may activate the latent form of the disease process that has been present in the tissues prior to injection.

Problem

The patient will complain of acute sensitivity in the ulcerated area. Many will consider that the tissue has become infected as a result of the local anesthetic injection they received. However, the risk of a secondary infection developing in this situation is small.

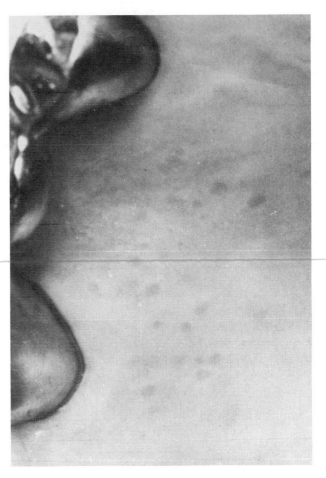

Fig. 17-8 Intraoral lesion (herpes simplex) on the palate following a local anesthetic injection.

Prevention

Unfortunately, there is no means of preventing these intraoral lesions from developing in susceptible patients. Extraoral herpes simplex may, on occasion, be prevented or its clinical manifestations minimized if treated in its prodromal phase. The prodrome consists of a mild burning or itching sensation at the site where the virus is present (e.g., lip). Antiviral agents, such as *acyclovir*, applied qid to the affected area effectively minimize the acute phase of this process.

Management

Primary management is symptomatic. Pain is the major initial symptom, developing approximately 2 days after injection. Reassure the patient that the situation is *not* due to a bacterial infection secondary to the local anesthetic injection but in fact is an exacerbation of a process that has been present, in latent form, in the tissues prior to injection. Indeed, most of these patients will have experienced this response before and will be resigned to its happening again.

If the pain is not severe, no management is required. However, if it causes the patient to complain, treatment can be instituted, usually with varying degrees of success. The objective is to keep the ulcerated areas covered and/or anesthetized.

Topical anesthetic solutions (e.g., viscous lidocaine) may be applied as needed to the painful areas. A mixture of equal amounts of diphenhydramine (Benadryl) and milk of magnesia rinsed in the mouth will effectively coat the ulcerations and provide relief from pain. Orabase, a protective paste, *without* Kenalog can provide a degree of pain relief. Kenalog, a corticosteroid, is not recommended because its antiinflammatory actions increase the risk of either viral or bacterial involvement. A tannic acid preparation (Zilactin) can be applied topically to the lesions either extraorally or intraorally (dry the tissues first). Studies from the University of Alabama have demonstrated that most patients achieve substantial pain relief with a duration of up to 6 hours.[26,27]

The ulcerations usually last 7 to 10 days with or without treatment. Negatol, a chemical cauterizing agent, will often provide dramatic relief from pain. Because of its permanent effect on tissues, however, its use in the management of herpetic or aphthous lesions cannot be recommended.

Maintain records on the patient's chart.

REFERENCES

1. Orr DL II: The broken needle: report of a case, *J Am Dent Assoc* 107(4):603-604, 1983.
2. Burgess JO: The broken dental needle: a hazard, *Spec Care Dentist* 8(2):71-73, 1988.
3. Fox LJ, Belfiglio EK: Report of a broken needle, *Gen Dent* 34:102-106, 1986.
4. Marks RB, Carlton DM, McDonald S: Management of a broken needle in the pterygomandibular space: report of a case, *Am Dent Assoc* 109:263-264, 1984.
5. Shira RB: *Surgical emergencies.* In McCarthy FM, editor: *Emergencies in dental practice*, ed 3, Philadelphia, 1979, WB Saunders.
6. Haas DA, Lennon D: A 21 year retrospective study of reports of paresthesia following local anesthetic administration, *J Can Dent Assoc* 61(4):319-320, 323-326, 329-330, 1995.
7. Nickel AA Jr: A retrospective study of paresthesia of the dental alveolar nerves, *Anesth Prog* 37(1):42-45, 1990.
8. McCarthy FM: Personal communication, 1979.
9. Sisk AL, Hammer WB, Shelton DW, Joy ED: Complications following removal of impacted third molars, *J Oral Maxillofac Surg* 44:855-859, 1986.
10. Tveter-as K, Kristensen S: The aetiology and pathogenesis of trismus, *Clin Otolaryngol* 11(5):383-387, 1986.
11. Benoit PW, Yagiela JA, Fort NF: Pharmacologic correlation between local anesthetic-induced myotoxicity and disturbances of intracellular calcium distribution, *Toxic Appl Pharmacol* 52:187-198, 1980.
12. Hinton RJ, Dechow PC, Carlson DS: Recovery of jaw muscle function following injection of a myotonic agent (lidocaine-epinephrine), *Oral Surg Oral Med Oral Pathol* 59:247-251, 1986.
13. Jastak JT, Yagiela JA, Donaldson D: *Complications and side effects.* In Jastak JT, Yagiela JA, Donaldson D, editors: *Local anesthesia of the oral cavity*, Philadelphia, 1995, WB Saunders.
14. Kitay D, Ferraro N, Sonis ST: Lateral pharyngeal space abcess as a consequence of regional anesthesia, *J Am Dent Assoc* 122(7):56-59, 1991.
15. Stacy GC, Hajjar G: Barbed needle and inexplicable paresthesias and trismus after dental regional anesthesia, *Oral Surg Oral Med Oral Pathol* 77(6):585-588, 1994.
16. Stone J, Kaban LB: Trismus after injection of local anesthetic, *Oral Surg*, 48:29-32, 1979. .
17. Eanes WC: A review of the considerations in the diagnosis of limited mandibular opening, *Cranio* 9(2):137-144, 1991.
18. Luyk NH, Steinberg B: Aetiology and diagnosis of clinically evident jaw trismus, *Aust Dent J* 35(6):523-529, 1990.
19. Brooke RI: Postinjection trismus due to formation of fibrous band, *Oral Surg Oral Med Oral Pathol* 47:424-426, 1979.
20. Himel VT, Mohamed S, Luebke RG: Case report: relief of limited jaw opening due to muscle spasm, *LDA J* 47:6-7, 1988.
21. Kouyoumdjian JH, Chalian VA, Nimmo A: Limited mandibular movement: causes and treatment, *J Prosthet Dent* 59(3):330-333, 1988.
22. Carter EF: Therapeutic ultrasound for the relief of restricted mandibular movement, *Dent Update* 13(10):503, 504, 506, 508-509, 1986.
23. Lund TW, Cohen JI: Trismus appliances and indications for use, *Quintessence Int* 24(4):275-279, 1993.
24. Hayes SM: Allergic reaction to local anesthetic: report of a case, *Gen Dent* 28(1):30-31, 1980.
25. Cooley RL, Coon DE: Transient Bell's palsy following mandibular block: a case report, *Quintessence Int* 9:9, 1978.
26. Raborn GW, McGaw WT, Grace M, et al: Herpes labialis treatment with acyclovir 5% modified aqueous cream: a double-blind randomized trial, *Oral Surg Oral Med Oral Pathol* 67(6):676-679, 1989.
27. Raborn GW, McGaw WT, Grace M, Percy J: Treatment of herpes labialis with acyclovir. Review of three clinical trials, *Am J Med* 85(2A):39-42, 1988.

CHAPTER
eighteen

Systemic Complications

The use of medications is commonplace in the practice of dentistry, and the administration of local anesthetics is considered essential whenever potentially painful procedures are contemplated. It is estimated (conservatively) that dental professionals in the United States administer in excess of 6 million dental cartridges per week, or more than 300,000,000 per year.

Local anesthetics are relatively safe drugs when used as recommended. However, when any drug, including local anesthetics, is used there exists the potential for development of unwanted responses. In this chapter systemic adverse reactions to drugs in general, and local anesthetics in particular, are reviewed.

Several general principles of toxicology (the study of the harmful effects of chemicals or drugs on biological systems) will be presented to further an understanding of the material in this chapter.

Harmful effects of drugs range from those that are inconsequential to the patient and entirely reversible once the chemical is withdrawn, to those that are uncomfortable but not seriously harmful, to those that can seriously incapacitate or prove fatal to the patient.

Whenever any drug is administered, two types of actions may be observed: (1) desired actions, which are clinically sought and usually beneficial, and (2) undesired actions, which are additional and not sought.

Principle 1: No drug ever exerts a single action

All drugs exert many actions, desirable and undesirable. In ideal circumstances the right drug in the right dose is administered via the right route to the right patient at the right time for the right reason and will not produce any unwanted effects.[1] This clinical situation is rarely if ever attained, since no drug is so specific that it produces only the desired actions in all patients.

Principle 2: No clinically useful drug is entirely devoid of toxicity

The aim of rational treatment is to maximize the therapeutic and minimize the toxic effects of a given drug. No drug is completely safe or completely harmful. All drugs are capable of producing harm if handled improperly; conversely, any drug may be handled safely if proper precautions are observed.

Principle 3: The potential toxicity of a drug rests in the hands of the user

A second factor in the safe use of drugs (after the drug itself) is the person to whom the drug is being administered. Individuals react differently to the same stimulus. Patients therefore vary in their reactions to a drug. Before administering any drug, the doctor must ask specific questions of the patient concerning his or her medical and drug history. Physical evaluation related to local anesthetic administration is discussed in Chapters 4 and 10.

CLASSIFICATION OF ADVERSE DRUG REACTIONS

Classifying adverse drug reactions has, in the past, been the object of much confusion; reactions were labeled as side effects, adverse experience, drug-induced disease, diseases of medical progress, secondary effects, and intolerance. The term *adverse drug reaction* (ADR) is preferred at this time.

The box at right outlines the three major methods by which drugs produce adverse reactions.

Overdose reactions, allergy, and idiosyncrasy are very important topics in relation to local anesthetics and pain control in dentistry. A brief overview of each will be presented, followed by an in-depth look at overdose and allergy.

Overdose reactions are those clinical signs and symptoms that manifest as a result of an absolute or relative overadministration of a drug, which produces elevated levels in the blood. Clinical manifestations of overdose are related to a direct extension of the normal pharmacological effects of the agent in the various tissues and organs of the body. Local anesthetics are drugs that act to depress excitable membranes (i.e., the central nervous system [CNS] and heart). When administered properly and in therapeutic dosages, they cause little or no clinical evidence of CNS or CVS (cardiovascular system) depression. However, with increased levels in the cerebral circulation or myocardium, signs and symptoms of selective CNS and CVS depression are observed.

Allergy is a hypersensitive state acquired through exposure to a particular allergen (a substance capable of inducing altered bodily reactivity), reexposure to which brings about a heightened capacity to react. Clinical manifestations of allergy vary and include the following:

Fever
Angioedema
Urticaria
Dermatitis
Depression of blood-forming organs
Photosensitivity
Anaphylaxis

In contrast to the overdose reaction, in which clinical manifestations are related directly to the pharmacological properties of the causative agent, in allergy the clinically observed reaction is always produced by an exaggerated response of the immune system. Allergic responses to a local anesthetic, antibiotic, latex, or to shellfish, a bee sting, or strawberries are produced by the same mechanism and may appear clinically similar. All require the same basic management. Overdose reactions to these substances are clinically quite different, necessitating entirely different modes of management.

Another point of contrast between overdose and allergic responses relates to the amount of drug required to produce or provoke a reaction. For an overdose reaction to develop, a large enough amount of the drug must have been administered so that excessive blood levels occur in the target organ or tissues. *Overdose reactions are dose related.* In addition, the degree of intensity (severity) of the clinical signs and symptoms relates to the blood level of the administered drug. The greater the dose administered, the higher will be the blood level and the more severe the reaction. By contrast, *allergic reac-*

CAUSES OF ADVERSE DRUG REACTIONS

Toxicity caused by *direct extension of the usual pharmacological effects* of the drug:

1. Side effects
2. Overdose reactions
3. Local toxic effects

Toxicity caused by *alteration in the recipient* of the drug:

1. A disease process (hepatic dysfunction, congestive heart failure, renal dysfunction)
2. Emotional disturbances
3. Genetic aberrations (atypical plasma cholinesterase, malignant hyperthermia)
4. Idiosyncrasy

Toxicity caused by *allergic responses* to the drug

---

tions are not dose related. A large dose of a medication (i.e., "overdose") administered to a nonallergic patient will not provoke an allergic response, whereas a minuscule amount (say, 0.1 ml) of a drug to which the patient is allergic can provoke life-threatening anaphylaxis.

Idiosyncrasy, the third category of true adverse drug reactions, is a response that cannot be explained by any known pharmacological or biochemical mechanism. A second definition considers an idiosyncratic reaction to be any adverse response that is neither an overdose nor an allergic reaction. An example would be stimulation or excitation that develops in some patients following administration of a CNS-depressant drug (e.g., an antihistamine). Unfortunately, it is virtually impossible to predict which persons will have such reactions or the nature of the resulting idiosyncrasy.

It is thought that virtually all instances of idiosyncratic reaction have an underlying genetic mechanism. These aberrations remain undetected until the individual receives a specific drug, which then produces its bizarre (nonpharmacological) clinical expression.

Specific management of idiosyncratic reactions is difficult to discuss because of the unpredictable nature of the response. Treatment is necessarily symptomatic: positioning, airway, breathing, circulation, and definitive care.

Table 18-1 compares allergy and overdose.

OVERDOSE

A drug overdose reaction has previously been defined as those clinical signs and symptoms that result from an overly high blood level of a drug in various target organs and tissues. Overdose reactions are the most common of

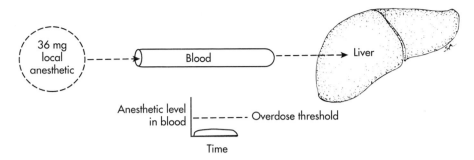

Fig. 18-1 Under normal conditions there is both a constant absorption of local anesthetic from the site of deposition into the CVS and a constant removal of the agent from the blood by the liver. Local anesthetic levels in the blood remain low and below the threshold for overdose.

TABLE 18-1 Comparison of Allergy and Overdose

	Allergy	Overdose
Clinical response		
Dose	Non–dose related	Dose related
S&S	Similar, regardless of allergen	Relate to pharmacology of drug administered
Management	Similar (epinephrine, histamine blockers)	Differ: specific for drug administered

S&S, Signs and symptoms.

all true adverse drug reactions, accounting for up to 99% in some estimates.[2]

For an overdose reaction to occur the drug must first gain access to the circulatory system in quantities sufficient to produce adverse effects on various tissues of the body. Normally there is both a constant absorption of the drug from its site of administration into the circulatory system and a steady removal of the drug from the blood as it undergoes redistribution (e.g., to skeletal muscle and fat) and biotransformation in other parts of the body (e.g., liver). In this situation overly high drug levels in the blood and target organs rarely develop (Fig. 18-1).

There are, however, a number of ways in which this "steady state" can be altered, leading to either a rapid or a more gradual elevation of the drug's blood level. In either case a drug overdose reaction is caused by a sufficiently high level of a drug in the blood adequate to produce adverse effects in various organs and tissues of the body. The reaction continues only as long as the blood level of the agent in those tissues remains above the threshold for overdose.

Predisposing Factors

Overdose reaction to local anesthetics is related to the blood level of the agent occurring in certain tissues after the agent is administered. Many factors have a profound effect on the rate at which this level is elevated and the length of time it remains elevated. The presence of one or more of these factors predisposes the patient to the development of overdose. The first group of factors concerns

the patient; the second group concerns the agent and the area into which it is administered (see box, p. 263).

Patient Factors

Age Although adverse drug reactions, including overdose, can occur in persons of any age, individuals at either end of the age spectrum experience a higher incidence of such reaction. The functions of absorption, metabolism, and excretion may be imperfectly developed in young persons and may be diminished in old persons, thereby increasing the half-life of the drug, elevating circulating blood levels, and increasing the risk of overdose.[3]

Weight The greater the (lean) body weight of a patient (within certain limits), the larger will be the dose of a drug that can be tolerated before overdose reactions occur. Most drugs are distributed evenly throughout the body. Larger individuals have a greater blood volume and consequently a lower level of the drug per milliliter of blood. Maximum recommended doses (MRDs) of local anesthetics are normally calculated on the basis of milligram of drug per kilogram or pound of body weight. One of the major factors involved in producing local anesthetic overdose in the past was a lack of consideration of this extremely important factor. Determination of maximum doses according to milligram per pound or kilogram of body weight is based on the responses of the "normal-responding" patient, which are calculated from the responses of thousands of patients. Individual patient response to drug administration, however, may demon-

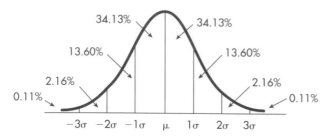

Fig. 18-2 Normal distribution curve (bell curve). *(From Freilich JD, Bennett CR: Conscious-sedation in a patient on combined tranylcypromine and lithium therapy: a case report,* Anesth Prog *30:86-88, 1983.)*

strate significant variation. The normal distribution curve (Fig. 18-2) illustrates this fact. The usual blood level of lidocaine required to induce seizure activity is approximately 7.5 µg/ml in the brain. However, patients on the hypo-responding side of this curve may not demonstrate seizure until a significantly higher brain-blood level is reached, whereas others (hyperresponders) may have seizures at a brain-blood level considerably below 7.5 µg/ml.

Other medications Administration of concomitant medications may influence local anesthetic drug levels. Patients taking *meperidine* (Demerol), *phenytoin* (Dilantin), *quinidine* (an antidysrhythmic), and *desipramine* (a tricyclic antidepressant) have increased free local anesthetic blood levels and thus may experience toxic effects at lower administered doses because of protein binding competition. The H_2 histamine blocker *cimetidine* slows the biotransformation of lidocaine by competing for hepatic oxidative enzymes with the local anesthetic, leading to somewhat elevated lidocaine blood levels.[4-6]

Sex Studies in animals have shown that sex is a factor in drug distribution, response, and metabolism; but it is not of major importance in humans. In humans, the only instance of sexual difference affecting a drug response is pregnancy. During pregnancy, renal function may be disturbed, leading to impaired excretion of certain drugs, their accumulation in the blood, and increased risk of overdose. However, local anesthetic seizure thresholds for the fetus, newborn, and mother are significantly different.[5-9] In the adult female the seizure threshold was reported to be 5.8 mg/kg, in the newborn 18.4, and in the fetus 41.9 mg/kg. This was thought to be a result of the efficient placental clearance of lidocaine into the mother's plasma.

Presence of disease Disease may affect the ability of the body to transform a drug into an inactive product. *Hepatic* and *renal dysfunction* impair the body's ability to break down and excrete local anesthetic, leading to an increased anesthetic level in the blood, whereas *congestive heart failure* decreases liver perfusion (the volume of blood flowing through the liver during a specific period), thereby increasing the half-lives of amide local anesthetics and increasing the risk of overdose.[10,11]

Genetics Genetic deficiencies may alter a patient's response to certain drugs. A genetic deficiency in the enzyme serum pseudocholinesterase (serum cholinesterase, plasma pseudocholinesterase, plasma cholinesterase) is an important example. This enzyme, produced in the liver, circulates in the blood and is responsible for the biotransformation of the ester local anesthetics. A deficiency in this enzyme either quantitatively or qualitatively can prolong the half-life of an ester local anesthetic as well as increase its blood level. Approximately 1 in 2820 persons or 6% to 7% of patients in most surgical populations possess atypical serum pseudocholinesterase.[12]

Mental attitude and environment A patient's psychological attitude influences the ultimate effect of a drug. Although of greater importance with regard to antianxiety or analgesic drugs, it is also of importance with regard to local anesthetics. Psychological attitude affects the patient's response to various stimuli. The apprehensive patient who overreacts to stimulation (experiencing pain when gentle pressure is applied) is more likely to require a larger dose of local anesthetic. It has also been demonstrated that the local anesthetic seizure threshold is lower in patients who are fearful and apprehensive than in nonfearful patients.[13] Both of these factors—larger dose requirement and the lower seizure threshold—increase the likelihood of local anesthetic overdose. The concomitant judicious use of psychosedation can minimize this risk.

Drug Factors

Vasoactivity All local anesthetics currently used in dental practice have vasodilating properties. Injection of these drugs into soft tissues increases the vascularity of the area, leading to an increased rate of absorption from the site of injection into the cardiovascular system. This causes two undesirable effects: a shorter duration of clinical anesthesia and an increased blood level of the local anesthetic.

Concentration The greater the concentration (% solution injected) of the local anesthetic administered, the greater will be the number of milligrams per milliliter of solution and the greater the circulating blood volume of the drug in the patient. For example, 1.8 ml of a 4% solution is 72 mg of the drug, but 1.8 ml of a 2% solution represents only 36 mg. If the drug is clinically effective as a 2% concentration, higher concentrations should not be used. *The lowest concentration of a given drug that is clinically effective should be selected for use.* For the commonly used local anesthetics in dentistry these ideal concentrations have been determined and are represented in the commercially available forms of these agents.

Dose The larger the dose of a local anesthetic agent used, the greater the number of milligrams injected and the higher the circulating blood level. *The smallest dose of a given drug that is clinically effective should be*

LOCAL ANESTHETIC OVERDOSE: PREDISPOSING FACTORS

Patient factors
Age

Weight

Other drugs

Sex

Presence of disease

Genetics

Mental attitude and environment

Drug factors
Vasoactivity

Concentration

Dose

Route of administration

Rate of injection

Vascularity of the injection site

Presence of vasoconstrictors

Many local anesthetic overdose reactions occur as a result of the combination of inadvertent intravascular injection and too rapid rate of injection, both of which are virtually 100% preventable.

---

administered. For each of the injection techniques discussed in this book a recommended dose has bu presented. Whenever possible, this dose should not be exceeded. Although "dental" doses of local anesthetics are relatively small compared to those used in many nondental nerve blocks, significantly high blood levels of anesthetic can be achieved in dental situations because of the vascularity of the injection site or inadvertent intravascular injection.

Route of administration Local anesthetics used for pain control produce their clinical effect in the area of injection. The drug need not enter into the cardiovascular system and reach a minimum therapeutic blood level, as most other drugs do. Local anesthetics administered for antidysrhythmic purposes must reach a therapeutic blood level to be effective. Indeed, one factor involved in terminating pain control by a local anesthetic is diffusion of the drug out of the nerve tissue, and its absorption into the CVS and removal from the area of injection.

An important factor in local anesthetic overdose in dentistry is inadvertent *intravascular injection.* Extremely high drug levels can be reached in minimal time, leading to serious overdose reactions.

Absorption of local anesthetics through oral mucous membranes is also potentially dangerous because of the rate at which some topically applied anesthetics enter the circulatory system. Lidocaine and tetracaine are absorbed well following topical application to mucous membranes. Benzocaine, on the other hand, is poorly absorbed, if at all.

Rate of injection The rate at which a drug is injected is a very important factor in the causation or prevention of overdose reactions. (In my view, rate of injection is *the* singlemost important factor.) Whereas intravascular injection may or may not produce signs and symptoms of overdose (indeed, lidocaine is frequently administered intravenously in doses of 75 to 100 mg to manage cardiac dysrhythmias), the rate at which the drug is injected is a major factor in determining whether drug administration will prove clinically safe or hazardous. Malagodi et al demonstrated that the incidence of seizures with etidocaine went up when the rate of intravenous infusion was increased.[14]

Rapid intravenous administration (≤15 seconds) of 36 mg of lidocaine produces greatly elevated levels and virtually ensures an overdose reaction. Slow (≥60 seconds) IV administration produces significantly lower levels in the blood, with a lesser risk that a severe overdose reaction will develop.

Vascularity of the injection site The greater the vascularity of an injection site, the more rapid the absorption of the drug will be from that area into the circulation. Unfortunately (in this regard) for dentistry, the oral cavity is one of the most highly vascularized areas of the entire body. However, there are some areas within the oral cavity that are less well perfused (e.g., the site for a Gow-Gates injection), and these are usually more highly recommended than other, better-perfused, sites (i.e., those for the inferior alveolar or posterior superior alveolar nerve block).

Presence of vasoconstrictors The addition of vasoconstrictor to a local anesthetic produces a decrease in the perfusion of an area and a decreased rate of systemic absorption of the drug. This greatly reduces the clinical toxicity of the local anesthetic. (See Table 3-1.)

Causes

Elevated blood levels of local anesthetics may result from one or more of the following:

1. Biotransformation of the drug is unusually slow.
2. The drug is too slowly eliminated from the body through the kidneys.
3. Too large a total dose is administered.

4. Absorption from the injection site is unusually rapid.
5. Inadvertent intravascular administration.

Biotransformation and Elimination

Ester local anesthetics, as a group, undergo more rapid biotransformation in the liver and blood than the amides. Plasma pseudocholinesterase is primarily responsible for their hydrolysis to para-aminobenzoic acid.

Atypical pseudocholinesterase occurs in approximately 1 out of every 2820 individuals or 6% to 7% of patients in a surgical population.[12] Patients with a familial history of this disorder may be unable to biotransform ester agents at the usual rate, and subsequently higher levels of ester anesthetics may develop in their blood.

Atypical pseudocholinesterase represents a relative contraindication to the administration of ester local anesthetics. Amide local anesthetics may be used without increased risk of overdose in patients with pseudocholinesterase deficiency.

Amide local anesthetics are biotransformed in the liver by hepatic microsomal enzymes. A history of liver disease does not, however, absolutely contraindicate their use. In an ambulatory patient with a history of liver disease (ASA II or III), amide local anesthetics may be used, but judiciously (*relative contraindication*) (Fig. 18-3).

Minimum effective volumes of anesthetic should be used. Average, even low-average, doses may be capable of producing an overdose if liver function is compromised to a great enough degree (ASA IV, V); however, this situation is unlikely to be seen in an ambulatory patient.[11]

Renal dysfunction can also delay elimination of active local anesthetic from the blood. A percentage of all anesthetics is eliminated unchanged through the kidneys: 2% procaine, 10% lidocaine, 1% to 15% mepivacaine and prilocaine. Renal dysfunction may lead to a gradual increase in the level of active local anesthetic in the blood.[10]

Excessive Total Dose

Given in excess, *all* drugs are capable of producing signs and symptoms of overdose (Fig. 18-4). Precise milligram dosages or the blood levels at which clinical effects are noted are impossible to predict. Biological variability has a great influence on the manner in which persons respond to drugs.

The maximum recommended dose (MRD) of parenterally administered (injected) drugs is commonly calculated after consideration of a number of factors, including:

1. Patient's age. Individuals at either end of the age spectrum may be unable to tolerate normal doses, which should be decreased accordingly.
2. Patient's physical status. For medically compromised individuals (ASA III, IV, and V) the calculated MRD should be decreased.
3. Patient's weight. The larger the person (within limits), the greater the distribution of the drug will be. With a normal dose the blood level of the drug is lower in the larger patient, and a larger milligram dose can be administered safely. Although this rule is generally valid, there are always exceptions; care must be exercised when any drug is administered.

Maximum recommended doses of local anesthetics should be determined following consideration of the patient's age, physical status, and body weight. Table 18-2 provides maximum recommended doses based on

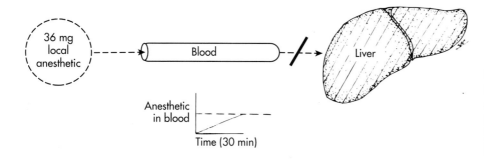

Fig. 18-3 In patients with significant liver dysfunction, removal of a local anesthetic agent from the blood may be slower than its absorption into the blood, leading to a slow but steady rise in the blood anesthetic level.

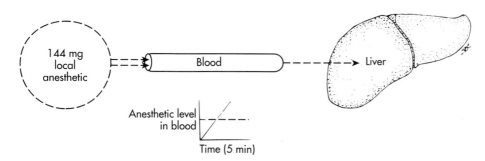

Fig. 18-4 Even in a patient with normal liver function, a large dose of local anesthetic may still be absorbed into the CVS more rapidly than the liver can remove it. This produces a relatively rapid elevation of the blood anesthetic level.

body weight for lidocaine, mepivacaine, prilocaine, and articaine.

It is highly unlikely that the maximum figures indicated in Table 18-2 will be reached in the typical dental practice. Rarely is there occasion to administer more than three or four cartridges during a dental appointment. Regional block anesthesia is capable of obtunding the full mouth in an adult with six cartridges. Yet despite this ability to achieve widespread anesthesia with minimum volumes of anesthetic, the administration of excessive volumes is the most frequently seen cause of local anesthetic overdose.[19,20]

Rapid Absorption into the Circulation

Vasoconstricting drugs are considered an integral component of all local anesthetics whenever depth and duration of anesthesia are important. There are few indications in dentistry for the use of local anesthetics without a vasoconstrictor. Vasoconstrictors increase the duration of anesthesia and reduce the systemic toxicity of most local anesthetics by delaying their absorption into the CVS. Vasoconstrictors should be included in local anesthetic solutions unless specifically contraindicated by the medical status of the patient or by the duration of the planned treatment.[21]

Rapid absorption of local anesthetics may also occur following their application to oral mucous membranes. Absorption of some topically applied local anesthetics into the circulation is quite rapid, exceeded in rate only by direct intravascular injection.[22] Local anesthetics designed for topical application are used in a greater

> *Vasoconstrictors should be included in local anesthetic solutions unless specifically contraindicated by the medical status of the patient or by the duration of the planned treatment.*

concentration than formulations suitable for parenteral administration.

From the perspective of overdose, amide topical anesthetics, when applied to wide areas of mucous membrane, increase the risk of serious reactions. Benzocaine, an ester anesthetic, which is poorly, if at all, absorbed into the cardiovascular system, is less likely to produce an overdose reaction than amides. The risk of allergy (more likely with esters than amides) must be addressed prior to using any drug.

Serious overdose reactions have been reported following topical application of amide local anesthetics.[23-26]

The area of application of a topical anesthetic should be limited. There are few indications for applying a topical to more than a full quadrant (buccal and lingual/palatal) at one time. Application of an amide topical to a wide area would require a large quantity of the agent and increase the likelihood of overdose.

I recommend the use of metered dosage forms of topical anesthetics whenever and wherever possible. Disposable nozzles are now available for metered sprays that make maintenance of sterility more simple (Fig. 18-5). Ointments or gels, if used in small amounts (as on the tip of a cotton applicator stick), may be applied with minimal risk of overdose.

Intravascular Injection

An intravascular injection may occur with any type of intraoral nerve block but is more likely with the following[27]:

Nerve block	Percent positive aspiration
Inferior alveolar	11.7
Mental/incisive	5.7
Posterior superior alveolar	3.1
Anterior superior alveolar	0.7
(Long) buccal	0.5

Both intravenous (IV) and intraarterial (IA) injections are capable of producing overdose (Fig. 18-6). A rapid IA

T A B L E   1 8 - 2   Maximum Recommended Doses of Local Anesthetics

Drug	Formulation	MRD	mg/lb	(mg/kg)	Author's MRD	mg/kg[17,18]
Articaine	With epinephrine	500†	3.2 (adult)†	(7.0)	3.2 (adult)	7.0
			2.3 (child)†	(7.6)	2.3 (child)	7.6
Lidocaine	Plain	300*	2.0	(4.4)*	300	4.4
	With epinephrine	500*	3.3	(7.0)*	300	4.4
Mepivacaine	Plain	400*	2.6	(5.7)*	300	4.4
	With levonordefrin	400*	2.6	(5.7)*	300	4.4
Prilocaine	Plain	600*	4.0	(8.8)*	400	6.0
	With epinephrine	600*	4.0	(8.8)*	400	6.0

*Manufacturer's recommendation.[15]
†Manufacturer's recommendation.[16]

injection can cause retrograde blood flow in the artery as the anesthetic drug is deposited (Fig. 18-7).[28] Intravascular injections within the usual practice of dentistry should not occur. With care and knowledge of the anatomy of the area to be anesthetized, and proper technique of aspiration prior to injecting the anesthetic solution, overdose as a result of inadvertent intravascular injection is minimized.

Prevention   To prevent intravascular injection, *use an aspirating syringe.* In an unpublished survey I conducted, 23% of dentists questioned stated that they routinely use nonaspirating syringes to administer local anesthetics. Indeed, even today, I am often asked by doctors if use of an aspirating syringe is necessary! There is no justification for the use of nonaspirating syringes for any intraoral injection technique, since it is impossible to determine the precise location of the needle tip without aspirating.

> *There is no justification for the use of nonaspirating syringes for any intraoral injection technique, since it is impossible to determine the precise location of the needle tip without aspirating.*

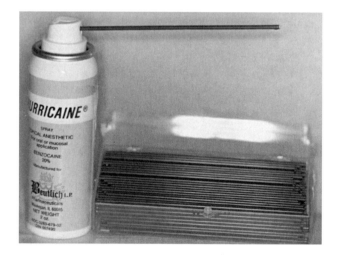

Fig. 18-5 Metered spray with disposable nozzle.

Use a needle no smaller than 25 gauge   when the risk of aspiration is high. Though aspiration of blood is possible through smaller-gauge needles, more force needs to be applied to the plunger in order to aspirate blood reliably, with an increased likelihood of an inadequate aspiration test. Injection techniques with a greater likelihood of positive aspiration therefore dictate the use of a 25-gauge needle.

Aspirate in at least two planes before injection
Figure 18-8 illustrates how an aspiration test may be negative even though the needle tip lies within the lumen of a blood vessel. Multiple aspiration tests prior to injecting solution, with the needle bevel in different planes, overcome this potential problem. After aspiration, rotate the syringe about 45 degrees to reorient the needle bevel relative to the wall of the blood vessel and reaspirate.

Slowly inject the anesthetic   Rapid intravascular injection of 1.8 ml of a 2% local anesthetic solution produces a level in the blood greatly in excess of that required for overdose. "Rapid injection" is defined (by me) as the administration of the entire volume of a dental cartridge in 30 seconds or less. The same volume of anesthetic deposited intravascularly slowly (minimum 60 seconds) produces blood levels below the minimum for serious overdose (seizure). In the event that the level does exceed this minimum, the onset of the reaction will be slower, with signs and symptoms less severe than those observed following a more rapid injection. Slow injection is the most important factor in preventing adverse drug reactions, even more so than aspiration. The ideal rate of local anesthetic administration is 1 ml/min. *Under no circumstances should the rate of drug deposition be less than 60 seconds for a 1.8 ml cartridge.* However, because the recommended volumes of local anesthetic for most intraoral injection techniques are considerably less than 1.8 ml, most injections can be safely administered in less than 1 minute.

Clinical Manifestations

Clinical signs and symptoms of local anesthetic overdose appear whenever the anesthetic blood level in an organ becomes overly high for that individual. The rate of onset of signs and symptoms and, to an extent, their severity correspond to this level. Table 18-3 compares the various forms of local anesthetic overdose.

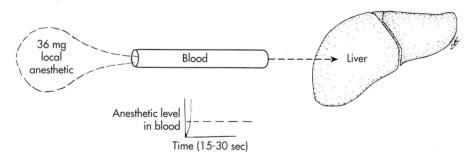

Fig. 18-6 Direct intravascular administration of one cartridge of local anesthetic produces marked elevation of the blood anesthetic level in a very short time.

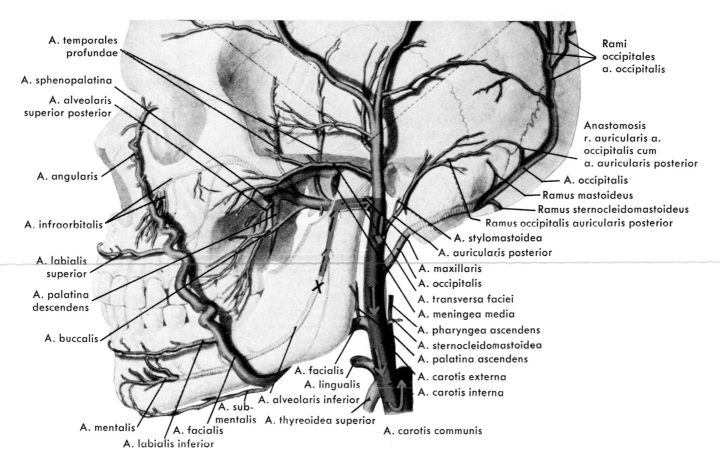

Fig. 18-7 Reverse carotid blood flow. Rapid intraarterial deposition of local anesthetic into the inferior alveolar artery (X) produces an overdose reaction. Blood flow in the arteries is reversed because of the high pressure produced by the rate of injection. *Arrows* indicate the path of the solution into the cerebral circulation.

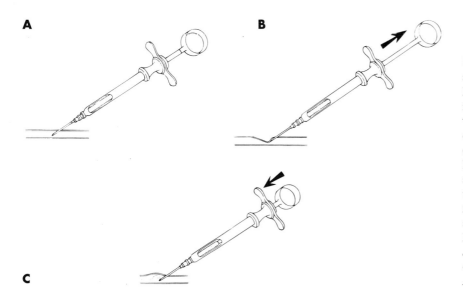

Fig. 18-8 Intravascular injection of local anesthetic. **A,** Needle is inserted in the lumen of the blood vessel. **B,** Aspiration test is performed. Negative pressure pulls the vessel wall against the bevel of the needle—therefore no blood enters the syringe (negative aspiration). **C,** Drug is injected. Positive pressure on the plunger of the syringe forces local anesthetic solution out through the needle. Wall of the vessel is forced away from the bevel, and anesthetic solution is deposited directly into the lumen of the blood vessel. *(From Malamed SF: Medical emergencies in the dental office, ed 4, St Louis, 1993, Mosby–Year Book.)*

TABLE 18-3 Comparison of Forms of Local Anesthetic Overdose

	Rapid intravascular	Too large a total dose	Rapid absorption	Slow bio-transformation	Slow elimination
Likelihood of occurrence	Common	Most common	Likely with "high normal" doses if no vasoconstrictors are used	Uncommon	Least common
Onset of signs and symptoms	Most rapid (seconds); intraarterial faster than intravenous	3 to 5 min	3 to 5 min	10 to 30 min	10 min to several hr
Intensity of signs and symptoms	Usually most intense	Gradual onset with increased intensity; may prove quite severe		Gradual onset with slow increase in intensity of symptoms	
Duration of signs and symptoms	2 to 3 min	Usually 5 to 30 min; depends on dose and ability to metabolize or excrete		Potentially longest duration because of inability to metabolize or excrete agents	
Primary prevention	Aspirate, slow injection	Administer minimal doses	Use vasoconstrictor; limit topical anesthetic use or use nonabsorbed type (base)	Adequate pretreatment physical evaluation of patient	
Drug groups	Amides and esters	Amides; esters only rarely	Amides; esters only rarely	Amides and esters	Amides and esters

From Malamed SF: *Medical emergencies in the dental office*, ed 4, St Louis, 1993, Mosby–Year Book.

Minimal to Moderate Overdose Levels

Signs
Talkativeness
Apprehension
Excitability
Slurred speech
Generalized stutter, leading to muscular twitching and tremor in the face and distal extremities
Euphoria
Dysarthria
Nystagmus
Sweating
Vomiting
Failure to follow commands or be reasoned with
Disorientation
Loss of response to painful stimuli
Elevated blood pressure
Elevated heart rate
Elevated respiratory rate

Symptoms (progressive with increasing blood levels)
Light-headedness and dizziness
Restlessness
Nervousness
Numbness
Sensation of twitching before actual twitching is observed (see "Generalized stutter" under "Signs")
Metallic taste
Visual disturbances (inability to focus)
Auditory disturbances (tinnitus)
Drowsiness and disorientation
Loss of consciousness

Moderate to High Overdose Levels
Tonic-clonic seizure activity followed by
Generalized CNS depression
Depressed blood pressure, heart rate, and respiratory rate

Note: It is also possible that the excitatory phase of the overdose reaction may be extremely brief or may not occur at all, in which case the first clinical manifestation of overdose may be drowsiness progressing to unconsciousness and respiratory arrest. This appears to be more common with lidocaine than with other local anesthetics.[29]

The clinical manifestations of local anesthetic overdose will continue until anesthetic blood levels in the affected organs (brain, heart) fall below the minimum value or until clinical signs and symptoms are terminated through the use of appropriate drug therapy.

Pathophysiology

The blood or plasma level of a drug is the amount absorbed into the circulatory system and transported in plasma throughout the body. Levels are measured in micrograms per milliliter (µg/ml). Recall that 1000 µg = 1 mg. Figure 18-9 illustrates clinical manifestations observed with increasing blood levels of lidocaine in the CNS and heart. Blood levels are approximate, as significant individual variation can occur.

Local anesthetics exert a depressant effect on all excitable membranes. In the clinical practice of anesthesia a local anesthetic is applied to a specific region of the body, where it produces its primary effect: a reversible depression of peripheral nerve conduction; other effects are related to its absorption into the circulation and its subsequent actions on excitable membranes, including smooth muscle, the myocardium, and the CNS.

Following the intraoral administration of 40 to 160 mg of a local anesthetic (lidocaine) the blood level rises to a maximum of approximately 1 µg/ml. (The usual range is between 0.5 and 2 µg/ml, but remember that response to drugs varies according to the individual.) Adverse reactions to the anesthetic are extremely uncommon in most individuals at these normal blood levels.

Central Nervous System Actions

The CNS is extremely sensitive to the actions of local anesthetics. As the cerebral blood level of anesthetic increases, clinical signs and symptoms are noted.

Local anesthetics cross the blood-brain barrier, producing CNS depression. At nonoverdose levels of lidocaine (<5 µg/ml) there are no clinical signs of adverse CNS effects. Indeed, therapeutic advantage may be taken of lidocaine at blood levels between 0.5 and 4 µg/ml, for then lidocaine possesses anticonvulsant properties.[30-32] The mechanism of this action is depression of hyperexcitable neurons found in the amygdala of seizing patients.

Signs of CNS toxicity appear at a cerebral blood level greater than 4.5 µg/ml. There is generalized cortical sensitivity: agitation, talkativeness, and irritability. Tonic-clonic seizures generally occur at levels greater than 7.5 µg/ml. With further increases in the anesthetic blood level, seizure activity terminates and a state of generalized CNS depression develops. Respiratory depression and arrest are manifestations of this. Chapter 2 describes the method through which a CNS-depressant drug, such as a local anesthetic, produces clinical signs and symptoms of CNS stimulation.

Cardiovascular System Actions

The CVS is much less sensitive to the actions of local anesthetic drugs. Adverse reactions do not usually develop until long after adverse CNS actions have occurred.

Local anesthetics, primarily lidocaine, have been increasingly used in the management of cardiac dysrhythmias, especially ventricular extrasystoles and ventricular tachycardias. The minimum effective level of

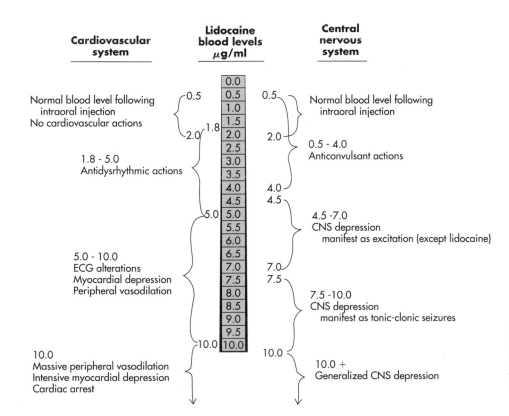

Fig. 18-9 Local anesthetic blood levels and actions on cardiovascular and central nervous sytems. *(From Malamed SF: Medical emergencies in the dental office, ed 4, St Louis, 1993, Mosby–Year Book.)*

lidocaine for this action is 1.8 µg/ml, and the maximum is 5 µg/ml, the level at which undesirable actions become more common.[33]

Increased levels (5 to 10 µg/ml) lead to minor alterations on the electrocardiogram, myocardial depression, decreased cardiac output, and peripheral vasodilation. Above 10 µg/ml there is an intensification of these effects—primarily massive peripheral vasodilation, marked reduction in myocardial contractility, severe bradycardia, and possible cardiac arrest.[34,35]

Management

The management of a local anesthetic overdose is based on the severity of the reaction. In most cases the reaction will be mild and transitory, requiring little or no specific treatment. In other instances, however, it may be more severe and longer lasting, in which case prompt therapy is required.

Most local anesthetic overdose reactions are self-limiting, since the blood level in tissues (e.g., brain and heart) continually decreases as the reaction progresses and redistribution and biotransformation take place (*if* the heart is still beating effectively). Only rarely are drugs other than oxygen required to terminate a local anesthetic overdose. When any of the signs and symptoms of overdose develop, do *not* simply label the patient "allergic" to local anesthetics, for this will further complicate future treatment. (See p. 279.)

Mild Overdose Reaction

Signs and symptoms of a mild overdose are retention of consciousness, talkativeness, and agitation, along with increased heart rate, blood pressure, and respiratory rate usually developing between 5 and 10 minutes after completion of the anesthetic injection(s).

Slow onset (≥5 minutes following administration) The possible causes of reactions with a slow onset are unusually rapid absorption, and too large a total dose. Use the following protocol to deal with a slow onset of symptoms.

Step 1 Reassure the patient that everything will be all right.

Step 2 Administer oxygen via nasal cannula or nasal hood. This is indicated as a means of preventing acidosis, a situation in which the cerebral blood level of local anesthetic required for seizure activity is decreased. The greater the arterial carbon dioxide tension, the lower the anesthetic blood level required to induce or perpetuate tonic-clonic activity.[36]

Step 3 Monitor and record vital signs. Postexcitation depression is usually mild, with little or no therapy required.

Step 4 (optional) If trained, establish an IV infusion. Use of anticonvulsants (e.g., diazepam or midazolam) is usually not indicated at this time, although

diazepam may be administered *slowly intravenously* and titrated at a rate of 5 mg/minute (midazolam at 1 mg/min) if CNS stimulation appears to be intensifying toward a more severe reaction.

Step 5 Permit the patient to recover for as long as necessary. Dental care may or may not be continued following an evaluation of the patient's physical and emotional status. The patient may leave the dental office unescorted only if you believe that full recovery has occurred. Vital signs should be recorded and compared with baseline values, and the patient evaluated thoroughly before discharge. If any anticonvulsant drug was administered or if doubt exists as to the level of recovery, do not allow the patient to leave and seek emergency medical assistance.

Slower onset (≥15 minutes following administration) Possible causes of reactions of a slower onset are abnormal biotransformation and renal dysfunction. Follow this protocol for dealing with the slower onset of signs and symptoms in a conscious patient.

Step 1 Reassure the patient.

Step 2 Administer oxygen.

Step 3 Monitor vital signs.

Step 4 Administer an anticonvulsant. Overdose reactions caused by abnormal biotransformation or renal dysfunction usually progress somewhat in intensity and last longer (because the drug cannot be eliminated rapidly). If venipuncture can be performed, titrate 5 mg of diazepam/minute (or midazolam 1 mg/min) until the clinical signs and symptoms of overdose subside.

Step 5 Summon medical assistance. When venipuncture is not practical or if an anticonvulsant drug has been administered, seek emergency medical assistance as soon as possible. Postexcitement depression is usually moderate following a mild excitement phase. Administration of diazepam, midazolam, or any other anticonvulsant will intensify this depression slightly. Monitoring the patient's condition and adhering to the steps of basic life support are normally more than adequate for this situation.

Step 6 After termination of the reaction, be sure that the patient is examined by a physician or hospital staff member to determine possible causes of this reaction. The examination should include blood tests and hepatic and renal function tests.

Step 7 Do not let the patient leave the dental office alone. Arrangements should be made for an adult companion if hospitalization is not deemed necessary.

Step 8 Determine the cause of the reaction before proceeding with therapy requiring additional local anesthetics.

Severe Overdose Reaction

Rapid onset (within 1 minute) Signs and symptoms are unconsciousness with or without convulsions. The probable cause is intravascular injection. A treatment protocol follows:

> *An adequate airway and oxygenation are of utmost importance during management of local anesthetic–induced seizures.*

Step 1 Remove the syringe from the mouth (if still present) and place the patient supine with their feet elevated slightly. Subsequent management is based on the presence or absence of convulsions.

Step 2 If convulsions are present, protect the patient's arms, legs, and head. Loosen tight clothing, such as ties, collars, and belts, and remove the pillow (or "doughnut") from the headrest.

Step 3 Immediately summon emergency medical assistance.

Step 4 Basic life support. Maintenance of an adequate airway and oxygenation are of utmost importance during management of local anesthetic–induced tonic-clonic seizures. Increased oxygen utilization and hypermetabolism, with increased production of carbon dioxide and lactic acid, occur during the seizure and lead to acidosis; this, in turn, lowers the seizure threshold (the blood level at which local anesthetic–induced seizures begin), prolonging the reaction.[37] Cerebral blood flow during such a seizure is also increased, elevating still further the anesthetic blood levels within the CNS.

Step 5 Administer an anticonvulsant. The blood level of the anesthetic will decline as the drug undergoes redistribution and, if acidosis is not present, within 2 or 3 minutes seizures will cease. Anticonvulsant therapy is usually *not* indicated. If a seizure is protracted (4 to 5 minutes with no indication of terminating), consider administering an anticonvulsant. IV diazepam, titrated at a rate of 5 mg/minute or midazolam (1 mg/min) until seizures cease is the preferred treatment.[38,39] If venipuncture is not feasible, 5 mg of midazolam may be given IM.[40,41] Maintain basic life support and obtain the assistance of emergency medical personnel.

Step 6 Postseizure CNS depression is usually present at an intensity equal that of the excitation phase (Fig. 18-10). The patient may be drowsy or unconscious; breathing may be shallow or absent; the airway may be partially or totally obstructed; blood pressure and heart rate may be depressed or absent. Implementation of the steps of basic life support is crucial: airway, breathing, and circulation must be provided as needed. In all postseizure situations, maintenance of an adequate airway will be required; in some other cases assisted or controlled ventilation may be indicated; for a small percentage of the most severe reactions, artificial circulation must be added to the first two steps of basic life support.

Step 7 Additional management such as use of a vasopressor (phenylephrine or methoxamine) IM is indicated if hypotension persists for extended periods (≥30

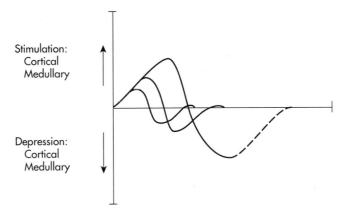

Fig. 18-10 Effects of local anesthetics on the CNS. Notice that the intensity of depression is equal to the intensity of the preceding stimulation. *(From Bennett CR: Monheim's local anesthesia and pain control in dental practice, ed 7, St Louis, 1984, Mosby-Year Book.)*

minutes). Preferred initial management for hypotension in this situation is positioning of the patient and the administration of intravenous fluids.

Step 8 Allow the patient to rest until recovery is sufficient to permit discharge. This means a return of vital signs to approximate baseline levels. Do not permit the patient to leave unescorted. In all situations in which local anesthetic induced seizures develop and emergency medical services are required, evaluation of the patient in an emergency department of a hospital will usually be required.

Slow onset (5 to 15 minutes) Possible causes of severe reactions of slow onset are too large a total dose, rapid absorption, abnormal biotransformation, and renal dysfunction. *Note*: Overdose reactions that develop very slowly (15 to 30 min) are unlikely to progress to severe clinical manifestations if the patient is continually observed and management is started promptly.

Step 1 Terminate dental treatment as soon as the signs of toxicity first appear.

Step 2 Provide basic life support as necessary. As in the preceding protocol, the prevention of acidosis and hypoxia through airway management and adequate pulmonary ventilation is of primary importance to a successful outcome.

Step 3 Administer an anticonvulsant. If symptoms are mild at the onset but progress in severity, and if an intravenous line can be established, definitive treatment with IV anticonvulsants and continued oxygen administration is indicated. IM midazolam may be considered when the IV route is not available.

Step 4 Summon emergency medical assistance immediately if seizures develop.

Step 5 Postseizure management includes basic life support and the IM or IV administration of a vasopressor for hypotension, as needed. The administration of IV fluids is recommended for management of hypotension.

Step 6 Permit the patient to recover for as long as necessary before discharge to hospital or home (in the custody of an adult). Completely evaluate the patient's condition before readministering a local anesthetic. The patient should be examined by a physician before discharge.

• • •

Overdose reactions are the most common "true" adverse drug reactions associated with the administration of amide local anesthetics. Most overdose reactions are preventable through adequate pretreatment evaluation of the patient and the rational use of these drugs. In the few instances in which clinical manifestations of overly high local anesthetic blood levels become evident, a successful outcome will be noted if the condition is promptly recognized and the patient effectively treated. Primary among the steps of management are maintenance of a patent airway and adequate oxygenation. Data indicate that if local anesthetic–induced seizures are brief and well managed no permanent neurological or behavioral sequelae remain postictally.[42] In other words, ischemic CNS damage is *not* inevitable with well-managed, brief, local anesthetic–induced seizures.

Epinephrine Overdose

Precipitating Factors and Prevention

A number of vasoconstrictors are currently used in dental practice, with epinephrine the most effective and most widely used. Overdose reactions, though possible, are uncommon with vasoconstrictors other than epinephrine. Table 18-4 outlines the milligram per milliliter concentrations of several vasoconstrictors currently in use.

The optimum concentration of epinephrine for prolongation of pain control (with lidocaine) appears to be 1:250,000.[43] Use of 1:50,000 epinephrine for pain control cannot be recommended. Epinephrine 1:50,000 or 1:100,000 is useful via local infiltration in the control of bleeding when applied directly to the surgical area.

Epinephrine or local anesthetic overdose reactions occurring under these conditions are quite rare.

Epinephrine overdose is more common following its use in gingival retraction cord before impressions are taken for a crown and bridge procedure. Currently available cords contain approximately 225.5 μg of racemic epinephrine per inch of cord.[44] Epinephrine is readily absorbed through gingival epithelium that has been disturbed (abraded) by the dental procedure. About 64% to 94% of applied epinephrine is absorbed into the CVS.[44] There is extreme variability in absorption according to the degree and duration of vascular exposure (bleeding). With regard to vasoconstrictors used for gingival retraction purposes, the American Dental Association states in *Accepted Dental Therapeutics*: "Since effective agents which are devoid of systemic effects are available, it is not advisable to use epinephrine for gingival retraction, and its use is contraindicated in individuals with a history of cardiovascular disease."[45]

Clinical Manifestations

Clinical symptoms of epinephrine or other vasopressor overdose include:

Fear, anxiety
Tenseness
Restlessness
Throbbing headache
Tremor
Perspiration
Weakness
Dizziness
Pallor
Respiratory difficulty
Palpitations

Signs of the epinephrine overdose reaction include:

Sharp elevation in blood pressure, primarily systolic
Elevated heart rate
Possible cardiac dysrhythmias (premature ventricular contractions, ventricular tachycardia, ventricular fibrillation)

TABLE 18-4 Dilutions of Vasoconstrictors Used in Dentistry

Dilution	Drug available	mg/ml	mg per cartridge (1.8 ml)	Maximum no. of cartridges used for healthy patient and cardiac-impaired patient
1:1000	Epinephrine (emergency kit)	1.0	Not applicable	Not available in local anesthetic cartridge
1:10,000	Epinephrine (emergency kit)	0.1	Not applicable	Not available in local anesthetic cartridge
1:20,000	Levonordefrin	0.5	0.09	10 (H), 2 (C)
1:30,000	Levarterenol	0.034	0.06	5 (H), 2 (C)
1:50,000	Epinephrine	0.02	0.036	5 (H), 1 (C)
1:100,000	Epinephrine	0.01	0.018	10 (H), 2 (C)
1:200,000	Epinephrine	0.005	0.009	20 (H), 4 (C)

From Malamed SF: *Medical emergencies in the dental office*, ed 4, St Louis, 1993, Mosby–Year Book.
H, Healthy patient; *C*, cardiac-impaired patient.

Management

Most instances of epinephrine overdose are of such short duration that little or no formal management is required. On occasion, however, the reaction may be prolonged and some management is desirable.

Step 1 Terminate the dental procedure. If possible, remove the source of epinephrine. Stopping the injection of local anesthetic does not remove epinephrine that has been deposited; however, endogenous epinephrine and norepinephrine release from the adrenal medulla and nerve endings will be lessened once the anxiety-inducing stimulus is eliminated. Epinephrine-impregnated gingival retraction cord, if present, should be removed.

Step 2 Position the patient. A conscious patient should be comfortable. The supine position is not recommended, because it accentuates the CVS effects. A semisitting or erect position minimizes any further elevation in cerebral blood pressure.

Step 3 Reassure the patient that the signs and symptoms will subside momentarily. Anxiety and restlessness are common clinical manifestations of epinephrine overdose.

Step 4 Monitor blood pressure and administer oxygen. The blood pressure and heart rate should be checked every 5 minutes during the episode. Striking elevations in both parameters are noted but gradually return toward baseline. Oxygen may be administered if deemed necessary. The patient may complain of difficulty breathing. An apprehensive patient may hyperventilate (increased rate and depth of breathing). Oxygen is not indicated in the management of hyperventilation, for it might exacerbate symptoms and possibly lead to carpopedal tetany.

Step 5 Recovery. Permit the patient to remain in the dental chair as long as necessary to recover. The degree of postexcitation fatigue and depression noted will vary but will usually be prolonged. Do not discharge the patient if any doubt remains about ability for self-care.

ALLERGY

Allergy is a hypersensitive state, acquired through exposure to a particular allergen, reexposure to which produces a heightened capacity to react. Allergic reactions cover a broad spectrum of clinical manifestations ranging from mild and delayed responses occurring as long as 48 hours after exposure to the allergen, to immediate and life-threatening reactions developing within seconds of exposure (Table 18-5).

TABLE 18-5 Classification of Allergic Diseases (after Gell and Coombs)

Type	Mechanism	Principal antibody or cell	Time of reactions	Clinical examples
I	Anaphylactic (immediate, homocytotropic, antigen-induced, antibody-mediated)	IgE	Seconds to minutes	Anaphylaxis (drugs, insect venom, antisera) Atopic bronchial asthma Allergic rhinitis Urticaria Angioedema Hay fever
II	Cytotoxic (antimembrane)	IgG IgM (activate complement)	—	Transfusion reactions Goodpasture's syndrome Autoimmune hemolysis Hemolytic anemia Certain drug reactions Membranous glomerulonephrosis
III	Immune complex (serum sickness–like)	IgG (form complexes with complement)	6 to 8 hr	Serum sickness Lupus nephritis Occupational allergic alveolitis Acute viral hepatitis
IV	Cell-mediated (delayed) or tuberculin-type response	—	48 hr	Allergic contact dermatitis Infectious granulomas (tuberculosis, mycoses) Tissue graft rejection Chronic hepatitis

Adapted from Krupp MA, Chatton MJ: *Current medical diagnosis and treatment*, Los Altos, Calif, 1994, Lange Medical.

Predisposing Factors

The incidence of allergy in the population is not low: about 15% of patients with allergy have conditions severe enough to require medical management, and some 33% of all chronic disease in children is allergic in nature.[46]

Allergy to local anesthetics does occur, but its incidence has decreased dramatically since the introduction of amide anesthetics in the 1940s. Brown et al stated: "The advent of the amino-amide local anesthetics which are not derivatives of para-aminobenzoic acid markedly changed the incidence of allergic type reactions to local anesthetic drugs. Toxic reactions of an allergic type to the amino amides are extremely rare, although several cases have been reported in the literature in recent years which suggest that this class of agents can on rare occasions produce an allergic type of phenomenon."[47]

Allergic responses to local anesthetics include dermatitis (common in dental office personnel), bronchospasm (asthmatic attack), and systemic anaphylaxis. The most frequently encountered are localized dermatological reactions. Life-threatening allergic responses related to local anesthetics are indeed rare.[48]

Hypersensitivity to ester local anesthetics is much more frequent: procaine, propoxycaine, benzocaine, tetracaine, and related compounds such as procaine penicillin G and procainamide.

Amide local anesthetics are essentially free of this propensity. However, reports from the literature and from medical history questionnaires indicate that *alleged* allergy to amide drugs appears to be increasing, despite the fact that subsequent evaluation of these reports usually finds them describing cases of overdose, idiosyncrasy, or psychogenic reactions.[49,50]

Allergic reactions have been documented for the various contents of the dental cartridge. Table 18-6 lists the functions of these components. Of special interest with regard to allergy is the preservative *methylparaben*. The parabens (methyl, ethyl, and propyl) are included, as bacteriostatic agents, in many multiuse drugs, cosmetics, and on some foods. Their increasing use has led to more frequent sensitization to them. In evaluating local anesthetic allergy, Aldrete and Johnson demonstrated positive reactions to methylparaben but negative reactions to the amide anesthetic without the preservative.[2] Table 18-7 presents Aldrete and Johnson's dermal reaction findings in patients exposed to various ester and amide local anesthetic solutions. The authors reported no signs of systemic anaphylaxis occurring in any of the subjects. Allergy to *sodium bisulfite* or *metabisulfite* is being reported today with increasing frequency.[51-53] Bisulfites are antioxidants, commonly sprayed onto fruits and vegetables to keep them appearing "fresh" for long periods of time. For example, apple slices sprayed with bisulfite do not turn brown (become oxidized). Persons allergic to bisulfites (most often steroid-dependent asthmatics) may develop a severe response (bronchospasm).[53,54] The U.S. Food and Drug Administration has enacted regulations that limit the use of bisulfites on foods. A history of allergy to bisulfites should alert the dentist to the possibility of this same type of response if sodium bisulfite or metabisulfite is included in the local anesthetic solution. Sodium bisulfite or metabisulfite is found in all dental local anesthetic cartridges that contain a vasoconstrictor, but is not found in "plain" local anesthetic solutions.

Topical anesthetics possess a potential to induce allergy. Most of the commonly used topicals in dentistry are esters, such as benzocaine and tetracaine. The incidence of allergy to this classification of local anesthetics far

---

TABLE 18-6 Contents of Local Anesthetic Cartridge

Ingredient	Function
Local anesthetic agent	Conduction blockade
Vasoconstrictor	Decrease absorption of local anesthetic into blood, thus increasing duration of anesthesia and decreasing toxicity of anesthetic
Sodium metabisulfite	Antioxidant for vasoconstrictor
Methylparaben*	Preservative to increase shelf life; bacteriostatic
Sodium chloride	Isotonicity of solution
Sterile water	Diluent

From Malamed SF: *Medical emergencies in the dental office,* ed 4, St Louis, 1993, Mosby–Year Book.
*Methylparaben has been excluded from all local anesthetic cartridges manufactured in the United States since January 1984, although it is still found in multidose vials of medication.

TABLE 18-7 Frequency of Dermal Reactions in Patients Exposed to Various Local Anesthetic Agents

Agent	Nonallergic patients (n = 60)	Allergic patients (n = 11)
NaCl	0	0
Procaine	20	8
Chloroprocaine	11	8
Tetracaine	25	8
Lidocaine	0	0
Mepivacaine	0	0
Prilocaine	0	0
Methylparaben	8	NA

From Aldrete JA, Johnson DA: Evaluation of intracutaneous testing for investigation of allergy to local anesthetic agents, *Anesth Analg* 49:173-183, 1970.
NA, Not available.

exceeds that of the amide local anesthetics. However, as benzocaine (an ester topical anesthetic) is not absorbed systemically, allergic responses that might develop in response to its application are limited to the site of application.[55] When other topical formulations, ester or amide, that are absorbed systemically are applied to mucous membranes, allergic responses may be either localized or systemic. Many also contain preservatives such as methylparaben, ethylparaben, or propylparaben.

Prevention

Medical History Questionnaire

The medical history questionnaire contains several questions related to allergy:

Question: *Are you allergic to (i.e., have itching, rash, swelling of hands, feet, or eyes) or made sick by penicillin, aspirin, codeine, or any other medications?*

Question: *Have you ever had asthma, hay fever, sinus trouble, or allergies or hives?*

COMMENT: These questions seek to determine if the patient has experienced any adverse drug reactions. Adverse drug reactions are not uncommon; those most frequently reported are labeled as "allergy." If the patient mentions any reaction to local anesthetics, the following protocol should be observed before use of the questionable drug is considered. If the patient relates a history of alleged local anesthetic allergy, it is imperative that the dentist consider the following factors:

1. Assume that the patient is truly allergic to the drug in question and take whatever steps are necessary to determine whether the alleged "allergy" is indeed an allergy.
2. Any drug or closely related agent to which a patient claims to be allergic *must not* be used until the alleged allergy can be absolutely disproved.
3. For almost all drugs commonly implicated in allergic reactions, equally effective alternate drugs exist (i.e., antibiotics and analgesics).
4. The only drug group in which alternatives are not equally effective is the local anesthetics.

• • •

Two major components are useful for determining the veracity of a claim of allergy: (1) *dialogue history*, whereby additional information is sought directly from the patient, and (2) *consultation* for a more complete evaluation if doubt still persists.

Dialogue History

The following questions are included in the dialogue history between the dentist and a patient with an alleged allergy to local anesthetics. The first two questions are the most critical, for they immediately establish in the

evaluator's mind a feeling that allergy either does or does not exist.[56]

Question: *Describe exactly what happened.*

Question: *What treatment was given?*

After these two questions the evaluator may consider others that will help elucidate the actual reaction:

Question: *What position were you in during the injection of the local anesthetic?*

Question: *What was the time sequence of events?*

Question: *Were the services of emergency personnel required?*

Question: *What drug was used?*

Question: *What volume of the drug was administered?*

Question: *Did the local anesthetic solution contain a vasoconstrictor?*

Question: *Were you taking any other drugs or medications at the time of the incident?*

Question: *Can you provide the name, address, and telephone number of the doctor (dentist or physician) who was treating you when the incident occurred?*

The answers to these questions will provide enough information to permit a doctor to make an informed determination as to whether or not a true allergic reaction to a drug occurred. This is the initial step in managing alleged local anesthetic allergy. The dialogue history follows.

Question: *Describe exactly what happened.*

COMMENT: This is probably the most important question, as it allows the patient to describe the actual sequence of events. The "allergy" will, in most instances, be explained by the answer to this question. The symptoms described by the patient should be recorded and evaluated to help in formulating a tentative diagnosis of the adverse reaction. Did the patient lose consciousness? Did convulsions occur? Was there skin involvement or respiratory distress? The manifestations of allergic reactions are discussed below. Knowing them can aid the evaluator in rapidly determining the nature of the reaction that occurred.

Allergic reactions involve one or more of the following: skin (itching, hives, rash, edema), gastrointestinal system (cramping, diarrhea, nausea, vomiting), exocrine glands (runny nose, watery eyes), respiratory system (wheezing, laryngeal edema), and cardiovascular system (angioedema, vasodilation, hypotension). Most patients describe their local anesthetic "allergic" reaction as one in which they experienced palpitations, severe headache, sweating, and mild shaking (tremor). Such reactions are almost always of psychogenic origin or are related to the administration of overly large doses of vasoconstrictor (i.e., epinephrine). They are not allergic in nature. Hyperventilation, an anxiety-induced reaction in which the patient loses control over breathing (exhaling and inhaling rapidly and deeply), is accompanied by dizziness, light-headedness, and peripheral paresthesias (fingers, toes, and lips). Complaints of itching, hives, rash, or edema lead to the conclusion that an allergic reaction may actually have occurred.

Question: *What treatment was given?*

COMMENT: When the patient is able to describe the management of the reaction, the evaluator can usually determine its cause. *Were drugs injected?* If so, *what drugs? Epinephrine, histamine blockers, or anticonvulsants? Was aromatic ammonia used? Oxygen?* Knowledge of the specific management of these situations can lead to an accurate diagnosis.

Drugs used in the management of allergic reactions include three categories: *vasopressors* (epinephrine [Adrenalin]), *histamine blockers* (diphenhydramine [Benadryl] or chlorpheniramine [Chlor-Trimeton]), and *corticosteroids* (hydrocortisone sodium succinate [Solu-Cortef]).

Mention of the use of one or more of these drugs increases the likelihood that an allergic response did occur. *Anticonvulsants*, such as diazepam (Valium), midazolam (Versed), and pentobarbital (Nembutal), are administered intravenously to terminate seizures induced by overdose of local anesthetic. *Aromatic ammonia* is frequently used in the treatment of syncopal episodes. *Oxygen* may be administered in any or all of these reactions.

Question: *What position were you in when the reaction took place?*

COMMENT: Injection of a local anesthetic into an upright patient is most likely to produce a psychogenic reaction (vasodepressor syncope). This does not exclude the possibility that another type of reaction may occur; but with the patient supine during the injection, vasodepressor syncope is a less likely etiology, even though the transient loss of conciousness may (on very rare occasion) develop in these circumstances.[57] In some of the evaluations of allergy to local anesthetics that I have carried out, the patient had been given an intracapsular injection of corticosteroid in the knee. Seated upright on a table in the physician's treatment room, the patient was able to watch the entire procedure—and it was profoundly disturbing. In an effort to make such injections more tolerable, lidocaine or another local anesthetic is added to the steroid mixture. In spite of this, however, the intracapsular injection of corticosteroid/lidocaine is extremely uncomfortable. Many patients experience their "allergic reaction" at this time. The supine position is therefore recommended as being physiologically best tolerated for the administration of all local anesthetic injections.

Question: *What was the time sequence of events?*

COMMENT: When, in relation to the administration of the local anesthetic, did the reaction occur? Most adverse drug reactions associated with local anesthetic administration occur during or immediately (within seconds) after the injection. Syncope, hyperventilation, overdose, and (sometimes) anaphylaxis are most likely to develop immediately during the injection or within minutes thereafter, although they all may occur later, during dental therapy. Also, seek to determine the amount of time that elapsed during the entire episode. *How long was it before the patient was discharged from the office? Did dental treatment continue after the episode?* The fact that dental treatment continued following this episode indicates that the response was probably minor and of a nonallergic nature.

Question: *Were the services of a physician, paramedic, or hospital required?*

COMMENT: A positive response to this usually indicates the occurrence of a more serious reaction. Most psychogenic reactions are ruled out by a positive answer, although an overdose or allergic reaction may indeed have occurred.

Question: *What local anesthetic was administered?*

COMMENT: A patient who is truly allergic to a drug should be told the exact (generic) name of the substance. Many persons with documented allergic histories wear a medical-alert tag or bracelet that lists specific items to which they are sensitive. However, some patients respond to this question with: "I'm allergic to local anesthetics" or "I'm allergic to Novocain" or "I'm allergic to all 'caine' drugs." Of 59 patients reporting allergy to local anesthetics, 54 could name one or more local anesthetics they believed were responsible. Five referred to only caine drugs.[58] Novocain (procaine), and other esters, are rarely used today as injectable local anesthetics in dentistry (though the esters are still popular in medicine), the amides having virtually replaced the esters in clinical practice. Yet patients throughout the world frequently call the local anesthetics they receive "shots of Novocain." Two reasons exist for this. First, many older patients at one time received Novocain as a dental local anesthetic, and its name has become synonymous with intraoral dental injections. Second, despite the fact that most dentists do not inject procaine or procaine-propoxycaine, many still describe local anesthetics as Novocain when talking with their patients. Thus the usual response of a patient to this question remains "I'm allergic to Novocain." This response, received from a patient who has been managed properly in the past fol-

> *A response of "I'm allergic to Novocain" is too general an answer and requires more in-depth evaluation before labeling the patient allergic to local anesthetics.*

lowing an adverse reaction, indicates that the patient was sensitive to ester local anesthetics but not necessarily to amide local anesthetics. However, the answers usually are too general and too vague for any conclusions to be drawn.

Question: *What amount of drug was administered?*

COMMENT: This question seeks to determine whether there was a definite dose-response relationship, as might occur with an overdose reaction. The problem is that patients rarely know these details and can provide little or no assistance. The doctor who was involved in the prior episode(s) may be of greater assistance.

Question: *Did the anesthetic solution contain a vasoconstrictor or preservative?*

COMMENT: The presence of vasoconstrictor might lead to the thought of an overdose reaction (relative or absolute) to this component of the solution. A preservative, such as methylparaben or sodium bisulfite, in the solution might lead to the belief that an allergic reaction did occur to the preservative, not to the local anesthetic. Unfortunately, however, most patients are unable to furnish this information. Methylparaben is found only in multiple-dose vials of local anesthetics (and most other drugs). Bisulfites are found in all dental local anesthetic cartridges containing a vasopressor.

Question: *Were you taking any other drugs or medications at the time of the reaction?*

COMMENT: This question seeks to determine the possibility of a drug/drug interaction or a side effect of other drugs as being responsible for the reported adverse response. Reidenburg and Lowenthal, reporting in 1968 on adverse *nondrug* reactions, demonstrated that "adverse" effects and side effects, which are so often blamed on medications, occur with considerable regularity in persons who have received no drugs or medications for weeks.[59] In other words, many so-called adverse drug reactions may be nothing more than a coincidental event: the person's becoming overly tired, irritable, nauseated, or dizzy for reasons unrelated to drugs. Unfortunately, however, it seems that whenever such symptoms develop in a patient taking a medication the drug is immediately thought to be responsible, with the label "allergy" often applied.

Question: *Can you provide the name and address of the doctor (dentist, physician, or hospital) who was treating you at the time of the incident?*

COMMENT: If possible, it is usually valuable to speak to the person who managed the previous episode. In most instances this person will be able to locate patient records and describe in detail what transpired. If it is not possible to locate or contact the doctor, the patient's primary care physician should be consulted. Direct discussion with the patient and doctor can provide a wealth of information that the knowledgeable dentist can use to determine more precisely the nature of the previous reaction.

Consultation and Allergy Testing

Consultation should be considered if any doubt remains as to the cause of the reaction following the dialogue history. Referral to a doctor who will test for allergy to local anesthetics is recommended.

Though no form of allergy testing is 100% reliable, skin testing is the primary mode of assessing a patient for local anesthetic allergy. Intracutaneous injections are among the most reliable means available, being 100 times more sensitive than cutaneous testing, and involve depositing 0.1 ml of test solution into the patient's forearm.[2,58,60-63] In all such instances, anesthetic solutions should contain neither vasoconstrictor nor preservative. Methylparaben, if evaluated, should be tested separately.[64]

The protocol for intracutaneous testing for local anesthetic allergy used at the University of Southern California School of Dentistry for the past 20 years involves the administration of 0.1 ml of each of the following: 0.9% sodium chloride, 1% or 2% lidocaine, 3% mepivacaine, and 4% prilocaine, without methylparaben, bisulfites, or vasopressors. After successful completion of this phase of testing, 0.9 ml of one of the above-noted local anesthetic solutions that produced no reaction is injected intraorally via supraperiosteal infiltration atraumatically (but without topical anesthesia) above a maxillary right or left premolar or anterior tooth. This is termed an *intraoral challenge test*, and it frequently provokes the "allergic" reaction: fainting, sweating, and palpitations.

After more than 200 local anesthetic allergy testing procedures, I have encountered four allergic responses to the paraben preservative (before 1984 the protocol included testing for parabens) and none to the amide local anesthetic agent itself. Numerous psychogenic responses have been observed during either the intracutaneous or the intraoral testing phases (syncope, hyperventilation, palpitations).

Such testing may be carried out by any person who is knowledgeable in the procedure and is also fully prepared to manage whatever adverse reactions may develop. It must be remembered that skin testing is not without risk. Severe immediate allergic reactions may be precipitated by as little as 0.1 ml of drug in a sensitized patient. Emergency drugs, equipment, and trained per-

> *Emergency drugs, equipment, and trained personnel must always be available whenever allergy testing is performed.*

sonnel must always be available whenever allergy testing is performed.

Intracutaneous allergy testing should be carried out only following an intensive dialogue history in which the evaluator has become convinced that the prior reaction to the local anesthetic was not allergy. The testing procedure is used to confirm this fact to the patient. The intraoral challenge test was added to the protocol when several patients with negative responses to intracutaneous testing stated, "But the dentist will give me a larger amount in the mouth." It was intended to provide the patient with the psychological support needed to receive intraoral local anesthetic injections safely.

Informed consent is obtained prior to allergy testing. The consent includes, among other possible complications, acute allergy (anaphylaxis), cardiac arrest, and death.

A continuous intravenous infusion is started prior to all allergy testing procedures, and emergency drugs and equipment are readily available throughout the testing.

Dental Management in the Presence of Alleged Local Anesthetic Allergy

When doubt persists concerning a history of allergy to local anesthetics, do not administer these drugs to the patient. *Assume that allergy exists. Do not use local anesthetics unless and until allergy has been absolutely disproved.*

Elective Dental Care

Dental treatment requiring local anesthesia (topical or injectable) should be postponed until a thorough evaluation of the patient's "allergy" is completed. Dental care not requiring local anesthesia may be completed during this time.

Emergency Dental Care

Pain or oral infection presents a more difficult situation in the "local anesthesia allergic" patient. Commonly the patient is new to the office, requiring tooth extraction, pulpal extirpation, or incision and drainage (I & D) of an abscess, with a normal medical history except for their "allergy to Novocain." If, after dialogue history, the "allergy" appears to have been a psychogenic reaction but some doubt remains, consider one of several courses of action.

Emergency protocol no. 1 The most practical approach to this patient is *no treatment of an invasive nature*. Arrange an appointment for immediate consultation and allergy testing. Do *not* carry out any dental care requiring the use of either injectable or topical local anesthetics. For incision and drainage of an abscess, inhalation sedation with nitrous oxide and oxygen may be an acceptable alternative.

Pain may be managed with oral analgesics; infection with oral antibiotics. These constitute temporary measures only. After evaluation of the allergy, definitive dental care may proceed.

Emergency protocol no. 2 Use *general anesthesia* in place of local anesthesia for management of a dental emergency. When properly used, general anesthesia is a highly effective and relatively safe alternative. Its lack of availability is a major problem in most dental practices.

When general anesthesia is used, be careful to avoid local anesthetics in these procedures:

1. Topical application (via spray) to the pharynx and tracheal mucosa immediately prior to intubation
2. Infiltration of the skin with local anesthetic prior to venipuncture to decrease discomfort

General anesthesia, within either the dental office or a hospital operating room, is a viable alternative to local anesthetic administration in managing the "allergic" patient, provided adequate facilities and well-trained personnel are available.

Emergency protocol no. 3 *Histamine blockers as local anesthetics* should be considered if general anesthesia is not available and if it is deemed necessary to intervene physically in the dental emergency. Most injectable histamine blockers have local anesthetic properties. Diphenhydramine hydrochloride in a 1% solution with 1:100,000 epinephrine provides pulpal anesthesia for up to 30 minutes.[65] Although the quality of soft and hard tissue anesthesia obtained with diphenhydramine and lidocaine are equivalent, an unwanted side effect frequently noted during injection of diphenhydramine is a burning or stinging sensation, which limits the use of this agent for most patients to emergency procedures only.[66] Nitrous oxide and oxygen used along with diphenhydramine minimize patient discomfort while increasing their pain reaction threshold. Another side effect of diphenhydramine and many histamine blockers is sedation (drowsiness), which may prove somewhat beneficial during treatment but forces an adult guardian to be available in order to take the patient home following treatment.

Emergency protocol no. 4 *Electronic dental anesthesia* (EDA) or other nondrug techniques of pain control, such as hypnosis, may provide effective pain control in some situations in which local anesthetics are contraindicated. The adjunctive use of nitrous oxide–oxygen inhalation sedation will increase the effectiveness of EDA and might permit the successful completion of painful procedures without the need for local anesthetic administration.[67,68]

Management of the Patient with Confirmed Allergy

Management of the dental patient with a confirmed allergy to local anesthetics will vary according to the nature of the allergy. If the allergy is limited to ester anesthetics, an amide anesthetic may be used (provided it does not contain a paraben preservative, which is closely related to the esters). No dental cartridges manufactured in the United States since January 1984 contain methylparaben.

If allergy does truly exist to amide and ester local anesthetics, dental treatment may be safely completed via one of the following:

1. Use of histamine blockers as local anesthetics
2. General anesthesia
3. Alternative techniques of pain control
   a. Electronic dental anesthesia
   b. Hypnosis

On occasion it is reported that a patient is "allergic to all 'caine' drugs." Such a report should provoke close scrutiny by the dentist, and the method by which this conclusion was reached should be reexamined.

All too often patients are mislabeled "allergic to local anesthetics." Such patients ultimately must have dental treatment carried out in a hospital setting, usually under general anesthesia, when a proper evaluation might have saved the patient time and money and decreased the risk of dental care.[50]

Clinical Manifestations

Table 18-5 lists the various forms of allergic reactions. It is also possible to classify allergic reactions by the time that elapses between contact with the antigen and the onset of clinical manifestations of allergy. *Immediate reactions* develop within seconds to hours of exposure. (They include Types I, II, and III in Table 18-5.) With *delayed reactions*, clinical manifestations develop hours to days following antigenic exposure (Type IV).

Immediate reactions, particularly Type I, anaphylaxis, are significant. Organs and tissues involved in immediate allergic reactions include the skin, cardiovascular system, respiratory system, and gastrointestinal system. Generalized (systemic) anaphylaxis involves all these systems. Type I reactions may also involve only one system, in which case they are termed *localized allergy*. Examples of localized anaphylaxis and their "targets" are bronchospasm (respiratory system) and urticaria (skin).

Time of Onset of Symptoms

The time elapsing between a patient's exposure to the antigen and the development of clinical signs and symptoms is important. In general, the more rapidly signs and symptoms develop following antigenic exposure, the more intense the reaction is likely to be. Conversely, the more time between exposure and onset, the less intense the reaction. Cases have been reported of systemic anaphylaxis arising many hours after exposure.[69]

The rate of progression of signs and symptoms once they appear is also significant. Situations in which signs and symptoms rapidly increase in intensity are likely to be more life threatening than those progressing slowly or not at all once they appear.

Signs and Symptoms

Dermatological Reactions

The most common allergic drug reaction associated with local anesthetic administration is urticaria and angioedema.

Urticaria is associated with *wheals*, which are smooth, elevated patches of skin. Intense itching (pruritus) is frequently present.

Angioedema is localized swelling in response to an allergen. Skin color and temperature are usually normal (unless urticaria or erythema is present.) Pain and itching are uncommon.

Angioedema most frequently involves the face, hands, feet, and genitalia, but it can also involve the lips, tongue, pharynx, and larynx. It is more common following the application of topical anesthetics to oral mucous membranes. Within 30 to 60 minutes the tissue in contact with the allergen appears swollen.

Allergic skin reactions, if the sole manifestation of an allergic response, are normally not life threatening; however, those occurring rapidly following drug administration may be the first indication of a more generalized reaction to follow.

Respiratory Reactions

Clinical signs and symptoms of allergy may be solely related to the respiratory tract, *or* respiratory tract involvement may occur along with other systemic responses.

Bronchospasm is the classic respiratory allergic response. Following are its signs and symptoms:

Respiratory distress
Dyspnea
Wheezing
Flushing
Cyanosis
Perspiration
Tachycardia
Increased anxiety
Use of accessory muscles of respiration

Laryngeal edema, an extension of angioneurotic edema to the larynx, is a swelling of the soft tissues surrounding the vocal apparatus with subsequent obstruction of the airway. Little or no exchange of air from the lungs is possible. Laryngeal edema represents the effects of allergy on the upper airway, whereas bronchospasm represents the effects on the lower airway (smaller bronchioles). Laryngeal edema is a life-threatening emergency.

Generalized Anaphylaxis

The most dramatic and acutely life-threatening allergic reaction is generalized anaphylaxis. Clinical death can occur within a few minutes. Generalized anaphylaxis can develop after the administration of an antigen by any route but is more common following parenteral administration (injection). Time of response is variable, but the reaction typically develops rapidly, reaching maximum intensity within 5 to 30 minutes. It is unlikely that this reaction will ever be noted following the administration of amide local anesthetics.

Signs and symptoms of generalized anaphylaxis, listed according to their typical progression, follow:

1. Skin reactions
2. Smooth muscle spasm of the gastrointestinal and genitourinary tracts and respiratory smooth muscle (bronchospasm)
3. Respiratory distress
4. Cardiovascular collapse

In fatal anaphylaxis, respiratory and cardiovascular disturbances predominate and are evident early in the reaction. The typical reaction progression follows:

1. Early phase: *skin reactions*
   a. Patient complains of feeling sick
   b. Intense itching (pruritus)
   c. Flushing (erythema)
   d. Giant hives (urticaria) over the face and upper chest
   e. Nausea and possibly vomiting
   f. Conjunctivitis
   g. Vasomotor rhinitis (inflammation of mucous membranes in the nose, marked by increased mucus secretion)
   h. Pilomotor erection (feeling of hair standing on end)
2. Associated with skin responses are various *gastrointestinal and/or genitourinary* disturbances related to smooth muscle spasm
   a. Severe abdominal cramps
   b. Nausea and vomiting
   c. Diarrhea
   d. Fecal and urinary incontinence
3. *Respiratory symptoms* usually develop next
   a. Substernal tightness or pain in chest
   b. Cough may develop
   c. Wheezing (bronchospasm)
   d. Dyspnea
   e. If the condition is severe, cyanosis of the mucous membranes and nail beds
   f. Possible laryngeal edema
4. The *cardiovascular system* is next to be involved
   a. Pallor
   b. Light-headedness
   c. Palpitations
   d. Tachycardia
   e. Hypotension
   f. Cardiac dysrhythmias
   g. Unconsciousness
   h. Cardiac arrest

In rapidly developing reactions *all signs and symptoms may occur within a very short time with considerable overlap.* In particularly severe reactions respiratory and cardiovascular signs and symptoms may be the only ones present. The reaction or any part of it can last from minutes to a day or more.[70]

With prompt and appropriate treatment the entire reaction may be terminated rapidly. However, hypotension and laryngeal edema may persist for hours to days despite intensive therapy. Death, which may occur at any time during the reaction, is usually secondary to upper airway obstruction produced by laryngeal edema.[71]

Management

Skin Reactions

Management is predicated on the rate at which the reaction appears following antigenic challenge.

Delayed skin reactions Signs and symptoms developing 60 minutes or more after exposure usually do not progress and are not considered life threatening. Examples are a localized mild skin and mucous membrane reaction following application of topical anesthetic.

Step 1 Oral histamine blocker: 50 mg diphenhydramine or 10 mg chlorpheniramine; a prescription for diphenhydramine, 50 mg capsules, one q6h for 3 to 4 days should be given to the patient.

Step 2 Obtain medical consultation to determine the cause of the reaction. A complete list of all drugs and chemicals administered to or taken by the patient should be compiled for use by the allergy consultant.

Immediate skin reactions Signs and symptoms of allergy developing within 60 minutes require more vigorous management. Examples are conjunctivitis, rhinitis, urticaria, pruritus, and erythema.

Step 1 Administer 0.3 mg (0.15 mg for a child) epinephrine IM or subcutaneously (SC).

Step 2 Administer IM histamine blocker: 50 mg diphenhydramine (25 mg for a child) or 10 mg chlorpheniramine (5 mg for a child).

Step 3 Obtain medical consultation with a physician, allergist, or hospital emergency room *before discharge* from the dental office, if epinephrine has been administered. It may be necessary to transfer the patient to the physician or hospital for observation before discharge. This should be done via emergency medical services (911).

Step 4 Observe the patient a minimum of 60 minutes for evidence of recurrence. Discharge in the custody of an adult if any parenteral drugs have been given.

Step 5 Prescribe an oral histamine blocker for 3 days.

Step 6 Fully evaluate the patient's reaction before further dental care.

Respiratory Reactions

Bronchial constriction (bronchospasm)

Step 1 Terminate dental therapy.

Step 2 Place the patient in a comfortable (semi-erect) position.

Step 3 Administer oxygen via full face mask, nasal hood, or nasal cannula at a flow of 5 to 6 liters/min.

Step 4 Administer epinephrine or other appropriate bronchodilator via aerosol inhaler (Medihaler Epi, albuterol) *or* IM/SC injection (0.3 mg [adult] or 0.15 mg [child]) of epinephrine (Fig. 18-11). Dose may be repeated every 5 minutes, if needed.

Step 5 Observe the patient for 60 minutes before considering discharge. If relapse occurs, readminister 0.3 mg epinephrine via IM injection or aerosol. Summon outside medical assistance (911), if there is no response to treatment.

Step 6 Administer a histamine blocker to minimize relapse possibility (50 mg IM diphenhydramine [25 mg child] or 10 mg IM chlorpheniramine [5 mg child]).

Step 7 After medical consultation and observation the patient may be discharged or transferred to a hospital via ambulance with paramedical personnel.

Step 8 Prescribe an oral histamine blocker and complete a thorough allergy evaluation before subsequent dental therapy.

Laryngeal edema Laryngeal edema may be present when movement of air through the patient's nose and mouth cannot be heard or felt in the presence of spontaneous respiratory movements *or* when it is impossible to carry out artificial ventilation in the presence of a patent airway (tongue *not* causing obstruction). Partial obstruction of the larynx produces stridor (a characteristic highpitched crowing sound), in contrast to the wheezing associated with bronchospasm. A partial obstruction may gradually or rapidly progress to total obstruction: accompanied by the ominous "sound" of silence. The patient rapidly loses consciousness from lack of oxygen.

Step 1 Place the patient supine with the feet elevated slightly.

Step 2 Summon medical assistance and administer oxygen.

Step 3 Administer 0.3 mg (0.15 mg for a child) epinephrine IM or SC. Epinephrine may be administered every 5 minutes, as needed.

Step 4 Maintain the airway. If it is partially obstructed, epinephrine may halt or reverse the progress of edema.

Step 5 Provide additional drug management: histamine blocker IM or IV (50 mg diphenhydramine or 10 mg chlorpheniramine), corticosteroid IM or IV (100 mg hydrocortisone sodium succinate to inhibit and decrease edema and capillary dilation).

Step 6 Perform cricothyrotomy. If the preceding steps have failed to secure a patent airway, an emergency procedure to create an airway is essential for survival. Figures 18-12 and 18-13 illustrate the anatomy of the region and the technique. Once established, the airway

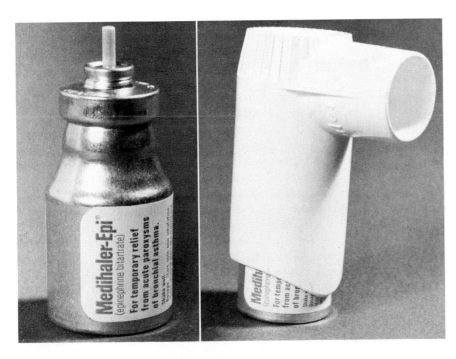

A **B**

Fig. 18-11 A, Bronchodilator. **B,** Epinephrine aerosol inhaler.

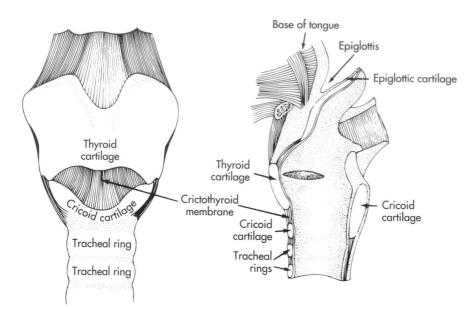

Fig. 18-12 Anatomical relationships of importance for cricothyrotomy. *(From Malamed SF: Medical emergencies in the dental office, ed 4, St Louis, 1993, Mosby–Year Book.)*

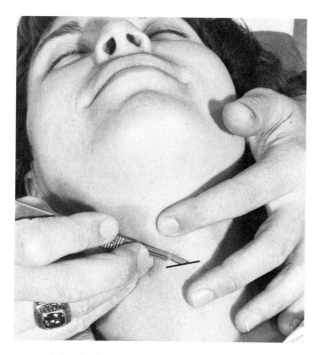

Fig. 18-13 With fingers placed on the thyroid and cricoid cartilages, make a horizontal incision into the trachea.

must be maintained, oxygen administered, and artificial ventilation used as needed. Monitor the patient's vital signs. The patient definitely requires hospitalization following transfer from the dental office by paramedical personnel.

Generalized Anaphylaxis

Generalized anaphylaxis is highly unlikely to develop in response to local anesthetic administration. Its manage-

ment is included here, however, for completeness. The most common causes of death from anaphylaxis are parenterally administered penicillin and stinging insects (the *Hymenoptera*: wasps, hornets, yellow jackets, and bees).

Signs of allergy present   When signs and symptoms of allergy are present (e.g., urticaria, erythema, pruritus, and wheezing), they should signal an immediate diagnosis of allergy. The patient will usually be unconscious.

Step 1   Position patient. The unconscious patient is placed into the supine position with the legs elevated slightly.

Step 2   Basic life support, as indicated. The airway is opened (head tilt), and the steps of basic life support are carried out as needed (Fig. 18-14).

Step 3   Summon medical assistance. As soon as a severe allergic reaction is considered a possibility, emergency medical care should be summoned.

Step 4   Administer epinephrine. The doctor should have previously called for the office emergency team. Epinephrine from the emergency kit (0.3 ml of 1:1000 for adults, 0.15 ml for children, and 0.075 ml for infants) is administered IM as quickly as possible, or IV. Because of the immediate need for epinephrine in this situation, a preloaded syringe of epinephrine is recommended for the emergency kit (Fig. 18-15). Epinephrine is the only injectable agent that need be kept in a preloaded form so as to prevent confusion when looking for the drug in this near-panic situation.

Should the clinical picture fail to improve or continue to deteriorate (increased severity of symptoms) within 5 minutes of the initial epinephrine dose, a second dose is administered. Subsequent doses may be administered as needed every 5 to 10 minutes, if the potential

Fig. 18-14 Summary of basic life support. (*From Malamed SF:* Medical emergencies in the dental office, *ed 4, St Louis, 1993, Mosby–Year Book.*)

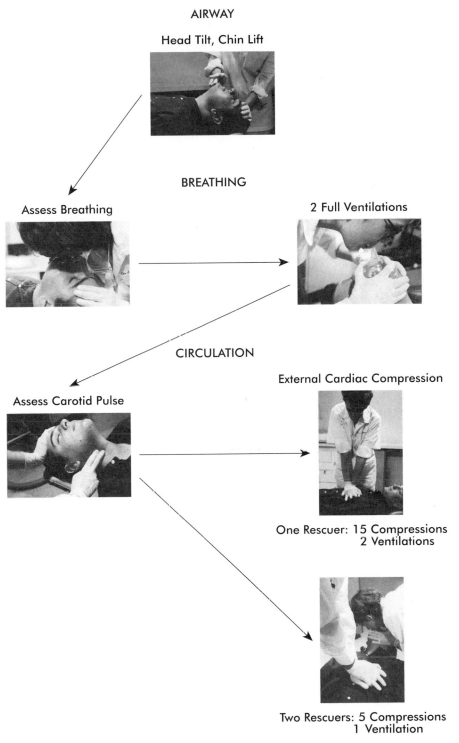

AIRWAY

Head Tilt, Chin Lift

BREATHING

Assess Breathing

2 Full Ventilations

CIRCULATION

Assess Carotid Pulse

External Cardiac Compression

One Rescuer: 15 Compressions
2 Ventilations

Two Rescuers: 5 Compressions
1 Ventilation

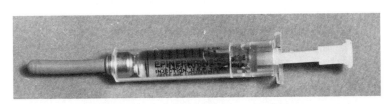

Fig. 18-15 Syringe preloaded with 1:1000 epinephrine.

risk of epinephrine administration (excessive cardiovascular stimulation) is kept in mind and the patient is adequately monitored.

Step 5 Administer oxygen.

Step 6 Monitor vital signs. The patient's cardiovascular and respiratory status must be monitored continuously. Blood pressure and heart rate (at the carotid artery) should be recorded at least every 5 minutes, and closed chest compression should be started if cardiac arrest occurs.

During this acute, life-threatening phase of what is obviously an anaphylactic reaction, management consists of basic life support; the administration of oxygen and epinephrine; and continual monitoring of vital signs. Until an improvement in the patient's status is noted, no additional therapy is indicated.

Step 7 Additional drug therapy. Once clinical improvement is noted (increased blood pressure, decreased bronchospasm), additional drug therapy may be started. This includes the administration of a histamine blocker and a corticosteroid (both drugs IM or IV, if possible). Their function is to prevent a possible recurrence of symptoms and to obviate the need for the continued administration of epinephrine. They are not administered during the acute phase of the reaction because they are too slow in onset and they do not do enough immediate good to justify their use at this time. Epinephrine and oxygen are the only drugs to administer during the acute phase of the anaphylactic reaction.

No signs of allergy present If a patient receiving a local anesthetic injection loses consciousness and no signs of allergy are present, the differential diagnosis includes psychogenic reaction (vasodepressor syncope), overdose reaction, and allergic reaction involving only the cardiovascular system, among other possibilities.

Step 1 Terminate dental treatment.

Step 2 Position patient. Management of this situation, which might prove to result from any of a number of causes, will require immediately placing the patient in the supine position with the legs elevated slightly.

Step 3 Basic life support, as indicated. Victims of vasodepressor syncope or postural hypotension rapidly recover consciousness once they are properly positioned with an ensured airway. Patients who do not recover at this point should continue to have the elements of basic life support applied (breathing, circulation).

Step 4 Summon medical assistance. If consciousness does not return rapidly following the institution of the steps of basic life support, emergency medical assistance should be sought immediately.

Step 5 Administer oxygen.

Step 6 Monitor vital signs. Blood pressure, heart rate and rhythm, and respirations should be monitored at least every 5 minutes, with the elements of basic life support started at any time they are required.

Step 7 Definitive management. On arrival, the emergency medical personnel will seek to make a diagnosis of the cause of the loss of consciousness. If this is possible, appropriate drug therapy will be instituted, and the patient stabilized and then transferred to a local hospital emergency department.

In the absence of any definitive signs and symptoms of allergy, such as edema, urticaria, or bronchospasm, epinephrine and other drug therapy are not indicated. Any of a number of other situations may be the cause of the unconsciousness—for example, drug overdose, hypoglycemia, cerebrovascular accident, acute adrenal insufficiency, or cardiopulmonary arrest may be causative factors. Continuation of the steps of basic life support until medical assistance arrives is the most rational mode of management in this situation.

SUMMARY

Systemic complications of local anesthetic drug administration and techniques are frequently preventable. Following is a summary of those procedures recommended to minimize their occurrence:

1. Preliminary medical evaluation should be completed prior to local anesthetic administration.
2. Anxiety, fear, and apprehension should be recognized and managed before administration of a local anesthetic.
3. All dental injections should be administered with the patient supine or semisupine. Patients should not receive local anesthetic injections in the upright position unless special conditions dictate (e.g., severe cardiorespiratory disease).
4. Topical anesthetic should be applied before all injections for a minimum of 1 minute.
5. The weakest effective concentration of local anesthetic solution should be injected in the *minimum volume* compatible with successful anesthesia.
6. The anesthetic solution selected should be appropriate for the dental treatment contemplated (*duration of action*).
7. Vasoconstrictors should be included in all local anesthetics unless specifically contraindicated by the desired duration of effect or the patient's physical status.
8. Needles should be disposable, sharp, rigid, capable of reliable aspiration, and of adequate length for the contemplated injection techniques.
9. Aspirating syringes must *always* be used for all injections.
10. Aspiration should be carried out in at least two planes prior to injection.

11. Injection should be made slowly, a *minimum* of 60 seconds for deposition of 1.8 ml of anesthetic.
12. Observe the patient both during and after the administration for signs of undesirable reaction. *Never* give the injection and leave the patient alone while doing other procedures.

REFERENCES

1. Pallasch TJ: *Pharmacology for dental students and practitioners*, Philadelphia, 1980, Lea & Febiger.
2. Aldrete JA, Johnson DA: Evaluation of intracutaneous testing for investigation of allergy to local anesthetic agents, *Anesth Analg* 49:173-183, 1970.
3. Prince BS, Goetz CM, Rihn TL, Olsky M: Drug-related emergency department visits and hospital admissions, *Am J Hosp Pharm* 49 (7):1696-1700, 1992
4. Kishikawa K, Namiki A, Miyashita K, Saitoh K: Effects of famotidine and cimetidine on plasma levels of epidurally administered lignocaine, *Anaesthesia* 45(9):719-721, 1990.
5. Shibasaki S, Kawamata Y, Ueno F, et al: Effects of cimetidine on lidocaine distribution in rats, *J Pharmacobio-dynam* 11(12):785-793, 1988.
6. Dailey PA, Hughes SC, Rosen MA, et al: Effect of cimetidine and ranitidine on lidocaine concentrations during epidural anesthesia for cesarian section, *Anesthesiology* 69(6):1013-1017, 1988.
7. de Jong RH: Bupivacaine preserves newborns' muscle tone, *JAMA* 237:53-54, 1977.
8. Steen PA, Michenfelder JD: Neurotoxicity of anesthetics, *Anesthesiology* 50:437-453, 1979.
9. Hazma J: Effect of epidural anesthesia on the fetus and the neonate, *Cah Anesthesiol* 42(2):265-273, 1994.
10. Shammas FV, Dickstein K: Clinical pharmacokinetics in heart failure: an updated review, *Clin Pharmacokinet* 15(2):94-113, 1988.
11. Hammermeister KE: Adverse hemodynamic effects of antiarrhythmic drugs in congestive heart failure, *Circulation* 81(3):1151-1153, 1990.
12. Pedersen NA, Jensen FS: Clinical importance of plasma cholinesterase for the anesthetist, *Ann Acad Med Singapore* 23(suppl 6):120-124, 1994.
13. Englesson S: The influence of acid-base changes on central nervous system toxicity of local anaesthetic agents, *Acta Anaesth Scand* 18:88-103, 1974.
14. Malagodi MH, Munson ES, Embro MJ: Relation of etidocaine and bupivacaine toxicity to rate of infusion in rhesus monkeys, *Br J Anaesth* 49:121-125, 1977.
15. *Prescribing information: dental*, Westborough, Mass, 1990, Astra Pharmaceutical Products.
16. *Prescribing information*, Montreal, 1993, Hoechst AG.
17. Council on Dental Therapeutics of the American Dental Association: *Accepted dental therapeutics*, ed 40, Chicago, 1984, American Dental Association.
18. *USP dispensing information*, ed 13, Rockville, Md, 1993, United States Pharmacopeial Convention.
19. Hersh EV, Helpin ML, Evans OB: Local anesthetic mortality: report of a case, *ASDC J Dent Child* 58(6):489-491, 1991.
20. Moore PA: Preventing local anesthetic toxicity, *J Am Dent Assoc* 123(3):60-64, 1992.
21. Yagiela JA: Local anesthetics, *Anesth Prog* 38(4-5):128-141, 1991.
22. Adriani J, Campbell D: Fatalities following topical application of local anesthetics to mucous membrane. *J Am Med Assoc* 162:1527, 1956.
23. Smith M, Wolfram W, Rose R: Toxicity: seizures in an infant caused by (or related to) oral viscous lidocaine use, *J Emerg Med* 10:587-590, 1992.
24. Hess GP, Walson PD: Seizures secondary to oral viscous lidocaine, *Ann Emerg Med* 17:725-727, 1988.
25. Garrettson LK, McGee EB: Rapid onset of seizures following aspiration of viscous lidocaine, *J Pediatr* 30:413-422, 1992.
26. Rothstein P, Dornbusch J, Shaywitz BA: Prolonged seizures associated with the use of viscous lidocaine, *J Pediatr* 101:461-463, 1982.
27. Bartlett SZ: Clinical observations on the effects of injections of local anesthetics preceded by aspiration, *Oral Surg Oral Med Oral Pathol* 33:520, 1972.
28. Aldrete JA, Narang R, Sada T, et al: Reverse carotid blood flow: a possible explanation for some reactions to local anesthetics, *J Am Dent Assoc* 94:1142-1145, 1977.
29. Munson ES, Tucker WK, Ausinsch B, Malagodi H: Etidocaine, bupivacaine, and lidocaine seizure thresholds in monkeys, *Anesthesiology* 42:471-478, 1975.
30. Rey E, Radvanyi-Bouvet MF, Bodiou C, et al: Intravenous lidocaine in the treatment of convulsions in the neonatal period: monitoring plasma levels, *Ther Drug Monit* 12(4):316-320, 1990.
31. Aggarwal P, Wali JP: Lidocaine in refractory status epilepticus: a forgotten drug in the emergency department, *Am J Emerg Med* 11(3):243-244, 1993.
32. Pascual J, Ciudad J, Berciano J: Role of lidocaine (lignocaine) in managing status epilepticus, *J Neurol Neurosurg Psychiatry* 55(1):49-51, 1992.
33. Jaffe AS: The use of antiarrhythmics in advanced cardiac life support, *Ann Emerg Med* 22:307-316, 1993.
34. Bruelle P, de La Coussaye JE, Eledjam JJ: Convulsions and cardiac arrest after epidural anesthesia: prevention and treatment, *Cah Anesthesiol* 42(2):241-246, 1994.
35. de La Coussaye JE, Eledjam JJ, Brugada J, Sassine A: Cardiotoxicity of local anesthetics, *Cah Anesthesiol* 41(6):589-598, 1993.
36. Bachmann MB, Biscoping J, Schurg R, Hempelmann G: Pharmacokinetics and pharmacodynamics of local anesthetics, *Anaesthesiol Reanim* 16(6):359-373, 1991.
37. Ryan CA, Robertson M, Coe JY: Seizures due to lidocaine toxicity in a child during cardiac catheterization, *Pediatr Cardiol* 14(2):116-118, 1993.
38. Rivera R, Segnini M, Baltodano A, Perez V: Midazolam in the treatment of status epilepticus in children, *Crit Care Med* 21(7):991-994, 1993.
39. Bertz RJ, Howrie DL: Diazepam by continuous intravenous infusion for status epilepticus in anticonvulsant hypersensitivity syndrome, *Ann Pharmacother* 27(3):298-301, 1993.
40. Lahat E, Aladjem M, Eshel G, et al: Midazolam in treatment of epileptic seizures, *Pediatr Neurol* 8(3):215-216, 1992.
41. Wroblewski BA, Joseph AB: Intramuscular midazolam for treatment of acute seizures or behavioral episodes in patients with brain injuries, *J Neurol Neurosurg Psychiatr* 55(4):328-329, 1992.
42. Feldman HS, Arthur GR, Pitkanen M, et al: Treatment of acute systemic toxicity after the rapid intravenous injection of ropivacaine and bupivacaine in the conscious dog, *Anaesth Analg* 73(4):373-384, 1991.
43. de Jong RH: *Vasoconstrictor*. In de Jong RH, editor: *Local anesthetics*, St Louis, 1994, Mosby–Year Book, pp 158-160.
44. Kellam SA, Smith JR, Scheffel SJ: Epinephrine absorption from commercial gingival retraction cords in clinical patients, *J Prosth Dent* 68(5):761-765, 1992.
45. American Dental Association: *Accepted dental therapeutics, 1984-1985*, Chicago, 1984, The Association.
46. Burr ML: Epidemiology of clinical allergy: introduction, *Monogr Allergy* 31:1-8, 1993.
47. Brown DT, Beamish D, Wildsmith JA: Allergic reaction to an amide local anaesthetic, *Br J Anaesth* 53:435-437, 1981.
48. Aldrete JA, O'Higgins JW: Evaluation of patients with history of allergy to local anesthetic drugs, *South Med J* 64:1118-1121, 1971.

49. Jackson D, Chen AH, Bennett CR: Identifying true lidocaine allergy, *J Am Dent Assoc* 125(10):1362-1366, 1994.

50. Doyle KA, Goepferd SJ: An allergy to local anesthetics? The consequences of a misdiagnosis, *ASDC J Dent Child* 56(2):103-106, 1989.

51. Schwartz HJ, Sher TH: Bisulfite sensitivity manifesting as allergy to local dental anesthesia, *J Allergy Clin Immunol* 75(4):525-527, 1985.

52. Seng GF, Gay BJ: Dangers of sulfites in dental local anesthetic solutions: warnings and recommendations, *J Am Dent Assoc* 113(5):769-770, 1986.

53. Perusse R, Goulet JP, Turcotte JY: Sulfites, asthma and vasoconstrictors, *Can Dent Assoc J* 55:55-56, 1989.

54. Perusse R, Goulet JP, Turcotte JY: Contraindications to vasoconstrictors in dentistry: Part II. Hyperthyroidism, diabetes, sulfite sensitivity, cortico-dependent asthma, and pheochromocytoma, *Oral Surg Oral Med Oral Pathol* 74:687-691, 1992.

55. Bruze M, Gruvberger B, Thulin I: PABA, benzocaine, and other PABA esters in sunscreens and after-sun products, *Photodermatol Photoimmunol Photomed* 7(3):106-108, 1990.

56. Malamed SF: *Medical emergencies in the dental office*, ed 4, St Louis, 1993, Mosby–Year Book.

57. Peter R: Sudden unconsciousness during local anesthesia, *Anesth Pain Control Dent* 2(3):140-142, 1993.

58. Chandler MJ, Grammer LC, Patterson R: Provocative challenge with local anesthetics in patients with a prior history of reaction, *J Allergy Clin Immunol* 79(6):883-886, 1987.

59. Riedenburg MM, Lowenthal DT: Adverse nondrug reaction, *N Engl J Med* 279:678-679, 1968.

60. Hodgson TA, Shirlaw PJ, Challacombe SJ: Skin testing after anaphylactoid reactions to dental local anesthetics. A comparison with controls, *Oral Surg Oral Med Oral Pathol* 75(6):706-711, 1993.

61. Rozicka T, Gerstmeier M, Przybilla B, Ring J: Allergy to local anesthetics: comparison of patch test with prick and intradermal test results, *J Am Acad Dermatol* 16(6):1202-1208, 1987.

62. Escolano F, Aliaga L, Alvarez J, et al: Allergic reactions to local anesthetics, *Rev Esp Anestesiol Reanim* 37(3):172-175, 1990.

63. Canfield DW, Gage TW: A guideline to local anesthetic allergy testing, *Anesth Prog* 34(5):157-163, 1987.

64. Swanson JG: An answer for a questionable allergy to local anesthetics, *Ann Emerg Med* 17(5):554, 1988.

65. Malamed SF: The use of diphenhydramine HCl as a local anesthetic in dentistry, *Anesth Prog* 20:76-82, 1973.

66. Ernst AA, Anand P, Nick T, Wassmuth S: Lidocaine versus diphenhydramine for anesthesia in the repair of minor lacerations, *J Trauma* 34(3):354-357, 1993.

67. Quarnstrom F, Milgrom P: Clinical experience with TENS and TENS combined with nitrous oxide–oxygen, *Anesth Prog* 36:66-69, 1989.

68. Donaldson D, Quarnstrom F, Jastak T: The combined effect of nitrous oxide and oxygen and electrical stimulation during restorative dental treatment, *J Am Dent Assoc* 118:733-736, 1989.

69. Oh VM: Treatment of allergic adverse drug reactions, *Singapore Med J* 30(3):290-293, 1989.

70. Orange RP, Donsky GJ: *Anaphylaxis*. In Middleton E, Ellis FF, Reed CE, editors: *Allergy: principles and practice*, ed 2, St Louis, 1983, Mosby–Year Book

71. Stafford CT: Life-threatening allergic reactions. Anticipating and preparing are the best defenses, *Postgrad Med* 86(1):235-242, 245, 1989.

CHAPTER

nineteen

Future Trends in Pain Control

Though local anesthesia remains the backbone of pain control in dentistry, research has continued, in both medicine and dentistry, to seek new and better means of managing pain associated with many surgical treatments. Much of this research has focused on improvements in the area of local anesthesia—safer needles and syringes, more successful techniques of regional nerve block (especially important in the mandible), and newer drugs. Several of these advances have been discussed at some depth in the preceding chapters: the Gow-Gates and Vazirani-Akinosi mandibular nerve blocks (Chapter 14), the periodontal ligament injection and intraosseous anesthesia (Chapter 15), the nondeflecting needle (Chapter 6), and the self-aspirating, pressure, and safety syringes (Chapter 5).

Considerable interest has focused on improvements in drugs that are injected to block pain impulses from reaching the brain. Several have been mentioned previously: *centbucridine* (Chapter 2) and *articaine* (Chapter 4). They are but two of the newly developed local anesthetics that possess potentially useful characteristics; another is *ropivacaine*, an amide local anesthetic receiving considerable scrutiny at this time in the area of epidural anesthesia.

Also in the realm of local anesthetic improvements, initially in medicine but of potential interest as well in dentistry, have been efforts to increase the ability of the anesthetic to cross (diffuse through) a relatively impervious barrier, such as intact skin. *EMLA* (eutectic mixture of local anesthetics) is one agent that has been used, with considerable success, in many areas of medicine requiring the insertion of needles into skin. Additionally,

the desire to speed the onset of anesthesia as well as make the administration of local anesthetics (into the skin or any tissue) more comfortable for the patient has given rise to altering the *pH* of the anesthetic solution. *Hyaluronidase* has been added to local anesthetic solutions because it permits injected solutions to spread and penetrate tissues more effectively than plain solutions.

Tetrodotoxin and *saxitoxin* (Chapter 1) and the vasoconstrictor *felypressin* (Chapter 3) are also reviewed.

Most of the drugs mentioned above are attempts at making the injection of local anesthetics into tissue more comfortable for the patient—important because most adverse reactions to local anesthetics arise *not as a reaction to the drug being administered, but as a response to the act of administering the drug*. The use of a needle to deliver local anesthetics (and other) drugs into tissues increases the likelihood of development of psychogenic reactions. This is true not only in dentistry but also in medical specialties that frequently require local anesthetic administration (e.g., dermatology, ophthalmology).

With this in mind, a second area of research into pain control that we should consider is techniques that do not involve the injection of drugs—that is, *electronic dental anesthesia* (the modification of TENS for dentistry) and *ultrasonics*. TENS is currently used in medicine for managing chronic pain, most often in orthopedic and sports medicine but increasingly in other areas as well. Ultrasonics involves the application of high-frequency sound waves to drive drugs, such as local anesthetics, through intact skin without the requirement of a needle.

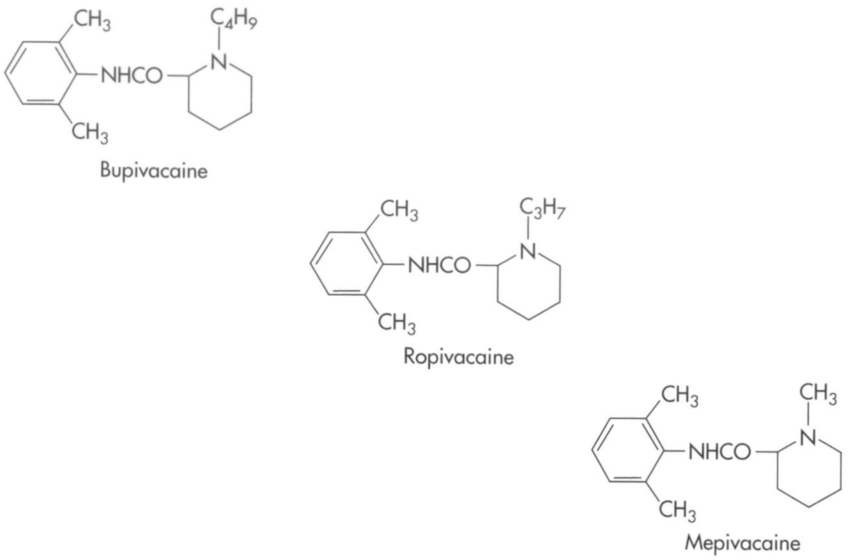

Fig. 19-1 Chemical structures of bupivacaine, ropivacaine, and mepivacaine.

LOCAL ANESTHETICS

Centbucridine

Centbucridine, a quinoline derivative, was first discussed in the second edition of this book as a drug with five to eight times the potency of lidocaine and with an equally rapid onset and an equivalent duration of action. Significantly, it does not affect the central nervous system (CNS) or cardiovascular system (CVS) adversely except when administered in very large doses.[1] Most of the research on this drug has been conducted in India.

Centbucridine has been used in subarachnoid and extradural anesthesia,[2] and in intravenous regional[3] anesthesia. In the only reported dental trial with centbucridine, Vacharajani et al compared the efficacy of a 0.5% centbucridine concentration with that of 2% lidocaine for dental extractions in 120 patients.[4] They reported a degree of analgesia attained with centbucridine that compared well to that obtained with lidocaine. Centbucridine was well tolerated, with no significant changes in cardiovascular parameters and no serious side effects. When administered to overdose, centbucridine functions, unlike lidocaine, as a true stimulant of the central nervous system.[5]

Developments Since the Third Edition of This Book

Since the third edition of this textbook, in 1990, little research has been published relative to centbucridine. The only trial of centbucridine in dentistry showed it to be as effective, in a 0.5% concentration, as lidocaine 2%.[4] More research into centbucridine is required before its ultimate place in the dental local anesthetic armamentarium can be determined.

Ropivacaine

Ropivacaine is a long-acting amide anesthetic, similar to bupivacaine and etidocaine in duration of activity. It is similar structurally to mepivacaine and bupivacaine (Fig. 19-1) but is unique in that ropivacaine is prepared as an isomer rather than as a racemic mixture. Data indicate that it has a greater margin of safety between convulsive and lethal doses than does bupivacaine[6] and also a lower arrhythmogenic potential than bupivacaine.[7] The elimination half-life of ropivacaine is 25.9 minutes, which is considerably shorter than that of other amides.[8] Ropivacaine has demonstrated decreased cardiotoxicity relative to bupivacaine, but its clinical duration of action is approximately 20% shorter.[9,10] The primary use of ropivacaine in anesthesiology has been for regional nerve block, primarily epidural. Its potential for use in dentistry as another long-acting local anesthetic appears great, but awaits clinical evaluation.[11]

Developments Since the Third Edition of This Book

Much has been learned about the clinical properties of ropivacaine since the last edition of this book. To date, no clinical trial has been published using ropivacaine as a dental local anesthetic. Such work is eagerly awaited.

EMLA

Intact skin is an impervious barrier to the penetration of drugs, including topical anesthetics. Yet once skin is damaged, as occurs in sunburn or injury, anesthetic drugs such as Solarcaine could be applied topically for the relief of pain. For years a drug or a technique was sought that would permit needles to be inserted painlessly through intact skin. The development of an oil-in-water emulsion containing high concentrations of lidocaine and prilocaine in base form resulted in *EMLA (eutectic mixture of local anesthetics)*, which has been shown to provide anesthesia of intact skin profound enough to permit venipuncture to be performed painlessly.[12-14]

EMLA consists of a 5% cream containing 25 mg/g lidocaine and 25 mg/g prilocaine. It is applied to the skin for at least 1 hour before the anticipated procedure. The cream is covered with an occlusive dressing. Since its introduction in the United States, research has demonstrated the effectiveness of EMLA in many aspects of pediatrics, including venipuncture; vaccination;[15] suture removal; lumbar puncture; minor otological surgery; minor gynecological and urological procedures; and dermatological surgery, including split thickness skin graft harvesting, argon laser treatments, postherpetic neuralgia, debridement of infected ulcers, and inhibition of itching and burning in adults.[16]

The potential for toxic local anesthetic blood levels developing with EMLA is minimal. Peak plasma anesthetic concentrations occurring 180 minutes after application have been quite low.[17] The use of EMLA in infants under the age of 6 months is contraindicated because of the possibility of a metabolite of prilocaine inducing methemoglobinemia.[12] Adverse responses noted included transient and mild skin blanching and erythema. There is one report of an allergic contact dermatitis developing in response to EMLA application to the skin.[18]

Several studies have reported on the intraoral use of EMLA cream. EMLA decreased patient reports of pain to needle insertion and anesthetic administration significantly in both the greater palatine and nasopalatine injection compared to placebo application.[19] However, the use of EMLA in an attempt to obtain pulpal anesthesia has provided conflicting reports. Vickers and Punnia-Moorthy reported that 92% (12 of 13) of subjects reported no pain to the maximum setting of a pulp tester (300 V) following a 15 to 30 minute application of EMLA,[20] whereas Meechan and Donaldson reported that EMLA did not differ significantly from placebo in the changes in pulpal responses of maxillary primary teeth to electrical stimulation before and after application in a double-blind split mouth study in 20 children.[21]

Developments Since the Third Edition of This Book

EMLA is now available in North America (Canada, 1991; United States, 1993). It has gained acceptance as an effective means of minimizing or eliminating the pain associated with percutaneous needle insertion. Though useful in all age groups, EMLA has been most readily accepted in pediatric populations. The intraoral application of EMLA, as a topical anesthetic, appears to provide anesthesia as effective as traditional topical formulations, but

it does require an extended period of application—a significant drawback.[22] Whether EMLA is capable of providing clinically effective pulpal anesthesia, in either primary or permanent teeth, is questionable and in need of considerably more research.

pH Alterations

The administration of local anesthetics into skin and, to a lesser degree, oral mucous membranes is frequently uncomfortable. Though many factors are involved in this, including the speed of injection, volume of solution, density of the tissues, and a lot of psychology, the acidic pH of the anesthetic solution plays a significant role in provoking discomfort during local anesthetic injections. The pH of a "plain" local anesthetic solution is approximately 5.5, whereas that of a vasopressor-containing solution is about 4.5. The addition of substances to the anesthetic that alkalinize the solution should make the drug's administration more comfortable. In addition, the anesthetic drug, at a higher pH, should have a more rapid onset of action and greater potency.

Two strategies have been used to achieve this effect: the addition of sodium bicarbonate to the anesthetic solution, and the addition of carbon dioxide. Carbonation of local anesthetics is not really new, their use being described as early as 1965.[23]

The addition of *sodium bicarbonate* to a local anesthetic solution immediately prior to injection alkalinizes the solution, increasing the number of uncharged base molecules (RN). As it is this uncharged ionic form of the drug that is lipid soluble and able to diffuse through the nerve membrane, a formulation of lidocaine with epinephrine plus sodium bicarbonate (pH 7.2) provides a more rapid onset of anesthetic block (onset = 2 minutes) than commercially prepared (pH 4.55) lidocaine plus epinephrine (onset = 5 minutes).[24-26] However, if the pH of the solution is too high, local anesthetic will precipitate out as the drug base. The stability of the local anesthetic decreases as pH increases, leading to considerably shorter shelf lives. Stewart et al demonstrated that a solution of lidocaine 1% with epinephrine 1:100,000 and sodium bicarbonate (80 mEq/L) provided the same depth and area of anesthesia after 1 week of storage as that provided by a freshly prepared solution.[27] However, the preparation of such solutions into dental cartridges with a 2- to 3-year shelf life seems impractical at this point. Alkalinization of epinephrine-free anesthetic solutions proffers no benefit.[25] Clinical trials in blepharoplasty and rhinoplasty found a more rapid onset of clinical action and increased patient comfort along with no discernible difference in hemostasis or duration of action.[26,28] Recommendations for preparation of the local anesthetic with bicarbonate appear divided between 1 part 4.2% bicarbonate with 10 parts local anesthetic,[25,29] and 1 part 8.4% bicarbonate in 5 parts local anesthetic.[26,28]

Carbon dioxide enhances diffusion of local anesthetic through nerve membranes, providing a more rapid onset of nerve block. As CO_2 diffuses through the nerve membrane, intracellular pH is decreased, raising the intracellular concentration of charged cations (RNH^+), the form of the anesthetic that attaches to receptor sites in sodium channels. Since the cationic form of the drug does not readily diffuse out of the nerve, the anesthetic becomes concentrated within the nerve trunk (termed "ion trapping"), providing a longer duration of anesthesia.[30] The problem clinically has been that if the carbonated local anesthetic agent is not injected almost immediately after opening of the vial the CO_2 will diffuse out of solution, significantly diminishing the solution's effectiveness. The anesthetic drug must be administered within a short time after preparing the syringe.

Developments Since the Third Edition of This Book

The use of alkalinized local anesthetics has received considerable attention in areas of medicine where skin surgery is performed. Sodium bicarbonate has received most of the attention, since it is easier to work with than CO_2. Most studies have concluded that pain on injection is diminished and speed of onset increased, with no deleterious effect upon either duration of action or area of anesthesia. The only published dental study reported no clinical difference between lidocaine hydrochloride and lidocaine hydrocarbonate solutions with 1:100,000 epinephrine when administered via inferior alveolar nerve block.[31]

Hyaluronidase

Hyaluronidase is an enzyme that breaks down intracellular cement. It has been advocated as an additive to local anesthetics because it permits injected solutions to spread and penetrate tissues.[32]

The primary use of hyaluronidase has been in plastic surgery, dermatology, and ophthalmologic procedures, primarily in retrobulbar nerve blocks, where it has been demonstrated to speed both the onset of anesthesia and the area of anesthesia significantly when compared with non–hyaluronidase-containing anesthetic solutions.[33-35] The duration of anesthesia is slightly decreased when hyaluronidase is added, but the benefits associated with its addition more than outweigh this minor inconvenience.[35]

The use of hyaluronidase in dental local anesthetic solutions has been discussed for many years. The first paper in dental literature discussing the use of hyaluronidase in local anesthetics appeared in 1949,[36] but there is little mention of hyaluronidase in dental literature in the ensuing years. However, a considerable number of dentists in the United States and elsewhere do add hyaluronidase to their anesthetic solutions and report, anecdotally, a considerably more rapid onset of nerve block anesthesia and an increase in success rate, especially in the inferior alveolar nerve block. The negative factor of a decreased duration of anesthesia is considered a minor inconvenience since the duration provided when a vasopressor-containing solution is used is more than adequate to permit completion of the procedure painlessly.

Hyaluronidase is available as Wydase (Wyeth-Ayerst) in a lyophilized powder, as well as in a stabilized solution. It is added to the anesthetic cartridge just before administration by removing approximately one third of the anesthetic solution and refilling the cartridge with hyaluronidase.

Allergic reactions have been reported following hyaluronidase administration.[37]

Developments Since the Third Edition of This Book

Hyaluronidase was not included in previous editions. It has been added to this fourth edition because of a seeming resurgence of interest in its use in dentistry among dentists communicating on the Internet. Caution is advised before considering the use of hyaluronidase in dental local anesthetics. Clinical research trials to demonstrate the efficacy, safety, and proper dosage of this combination should be completed before its widespread use.

Ultra–long-acting Local Anesthetics

Tetrodotoxin (TTX) and *saxitoxin* (STX) are classified as biotoxins. Found in the puffer fish (TTX) and in certain species of dinoflagellates (STX), they specifically block sodium channels on nerve membranes when applied to the outer membranous surface and thus produce conduction blockade. Though these agents are about 250,000 times as potent as procaine in providing conduction blockade of isolated nerve preparations,[38] they both are highly toxic and will not pass readily through the epineurium surrounding peripheral nerves; they therefore provide little or no conduction blockade of the sciatic nerve.[39] However, when administered via subarachnoid block in sheep, they have induced spinal anesthesia of almost 24 hours' duration.[40] Unfortunately, both TTX and SSX are extremely difficult to synthesize and are not very stable in aqueous solutions, thereby significantly limiting their usefulness. There is little likelihood that they will be of any clinical value in anesthesiology or dentistry in the near future.

Developments Since the Third Edition of This Book

None of significance in the areas of anesthesiology or dentistry

Felypressin

Felypressin, an analogue of vasopressin (the antidiuretic hormone), has been available in dental local anesthetic cartridges in many European countries for a number of years, most often in combination with prilocaine. It is a direct stimulator of vascular smooth muscle (primarily venous), having little direct effect on the heart or on adrenergic nerve transmission. It may be used safely in patients in whom a medical problem (e.g., hyperthyroidism, high blood pressure) contraindicates the administration of epinephrine.[41] Because it acts primarily on the venous circulation, felypressin is not as effective as conventional vasoconstrictors in providing hemostasis during surgical procedures.[42] It is marketed under the trade name Octapressin and is used in a concentration of 0.03 IU/ml. When felypressin with prilocaine was compared to lidocaine with epinephrine for the removal of third molars, both agents produced similar effects on blood pressure and heart rate.[43]

Developments Since the Third Edition of This Book

Felypressin is not presently available in the United States; however, it is available in Canada and Mexico. Because of its lack of significant action on the myocardium, it seems reasonable that it should be made available in dental local anesthetic cartridges, especially with the continuing increase in the number of older adults in the population and patients with compromised cardiovascular systems.[44]

ELECTRONIC DENTAL ANESTHESIA

The use of electricity as a therapeutic modality in medicine and dentistry is not new. The first recorded report of electrotherapy dates from 46 A.D., when Scribonius Largus, physician to the emperor Claudius, used the torpedo fish to relieve the pains of gout.[45] Electricity continued to be used into the eighteenth century, when interest in its therapeutic potential reached new heights. With the ability to produce electricity, devices were designed to treat a wide range of disorders in the human body. Textbooks in the late eighteenth and early nineteenth centuries illustrated the technique of electrotherapy for managing ulcers and toothache (Fig. 19-2).[46,47] It must be remembered that local anesthetics were not available at this time. Unfortunately, "electroquackery" also became popular during the late 1700s. Elisha Perkins, a Connecticut physician, created "Perkins Patent Tractors"—two brass and iron rods about 3 inches long, rounded at one end and pointed at the other. He claimed that by moving these devices downward from the site of pain to the patient's extremities he could draw disease out of the body.[48] Sales of the tractors netted enormous wealth for Perkins, but feeling was so strong against him and his tractors that the Connecticut Medical Society expelled him from membership in 1796.

In 1883 Erb wrote "At the present time we possess in the electrical current one of the most certain and brilliant remedies for neuralgia, although we must admit that much progress has not been made in our knowledge concerning its mode of action in these forms of disease."[49]

References to electroanalgesia continued into the early 1900s, but after this time there was scarce mention of the use of electrical stimulation for pain relief in either the medical or the dental literature.[50] This gap extended into the mid-1960s, when interest in the field of electronic anesthesia was renewed. One example (circa 1970) of "new" electroanesthesia equipment was the Desensor handpiece (Fig. 19-3), a high-speed device that carried low-voltage electrical current through a bur directly onto the tooth being treated. Its lack of consistent reliability led to its rapid demise.

The use of transcutaneous electrical nerve stimulation (TENS) and, more recently, its dental progeny, electronic dental anesthesia (EDA), has developed since the mid-1960s into techniques that appear to have utility in the battle against pain. Only time will tell whether EDA rep-

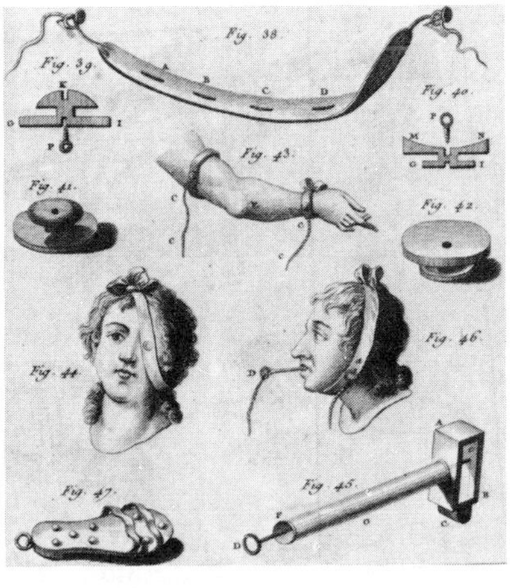

Fig. 19-2 Electrodes available in 1786.

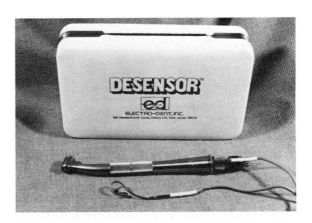

Fig. 19-3 Electroanesthesia handpiece, circa 1970.

resents just another fad that will once again die out, only to reappear at some other time in the future, or will prove valuable enough to gain a strong foothold in the dental armamentarium for pain control.

Mechanism of Action

At the low-frequency setting of 2 Hz (hertz or cycles per second), which is most often used in the *management of chronic pain*, TENS produces measurable changes in the blood levels of L-tryptophan, serotonin, and beta-endorphins. L-Tryptophan, a precursor of serotonin, is present in the blood in decreasing amounts as the duration of TENS increases. By contrast, serotonin levels in the blood increase with time.[51] Serotonin possesses analgesic actions, elevating the pain reaction threshold. At the same time, levels of beta-endorphins and enkephalins in the cerebral circulation also increase. Beta-endorphins and enkephalins are potent analgesics produced by the body in response to certain types of stimulation.[52] It appears that elevated blood levels of these chemicals are not achieved for a period of about 10 minutes after the start of TENS or EDA stimulation—findings that provide a clearer understanding of the mechanism whereby TENS may aid in the management of chronic pain. Because blood levels of serotonin and beta-endorphins remain elevated for several hours following the termination of TENS therapy, patients benefit from this residual analgesic action in the immediate posttreatment period. Opioid-agonist analgesics prescribed for posttreatment pain are rarely required when TENS or EDA has been used during or after treatment.

The mechanism by which EDA operates to prevent *acute pain* during surgery or dentistry is somewhat different. It is felt that the Melzack and Wall gate control theory of pain provides an adequate explanation for the prevention of acute pain provided by EDA.[53] Used at a higher frequency (120 Hz or greater), EDA causes the patient to experience a sensation most often described as "vibrating," "throbbing," "pulsing," or "twitching." This involves the stimulation of larger-diameter nerves (A fibers), which transmit the sensations of touch, pressure, and temperature. If the patient can maintain a minimum "threshold" intensity of A fiber stimulation, the pain impulse produced by the high-speed drill, scalpel, or curette, which is transmitted to the central nervous system more slowly along the smaller A-delta and C fibers, will come upon a "closed" gate and be unable to reach the brain, where it is translated into physical pain. Thus, large-fiber input is said to inhibit central transmission of the overall effects of small-fiber input. When the pain impulse fails to reach the brain, the sensation of pain does not occur.

Blood levels of serotonin and endorphins are likewise elevated during high-frequency stimulation and probably play a secondary, albeit important, role in providing acute pain control during most dental treatment.

Electrotherapy in Medicine

During the 1960s neurosurgeons began the use of implanted electrodes in the spinal cord as an alternative to cordotomy in patients with chronic debilitating back pain. Neurosurgical procedures, though effective, did not possess an exceptionally high success rate in eliminating the chronic pain being experienced.

In 1967 Shealy et al reported that through direct stimulation of the dorsal column of the spinal cord intractable pain could be suppressed without the need for an irreversible surgical procedure.[54] The success rate of this technique was quite satisfactory, and the use of direct electrical stimulation became a more accepted mode of therapy for patients with chronic debilitating pain.

In the early 1970s Shealy[55] and Long,[56] working with electrode pads placed on the patient's skin over the spinal cord, were able to eliminate pain without the need for implanting electrodes into the cord. The technique of transcutaneous electrical nerve stimulation (TENS) was thus founded.

Today TENS is an accepted treatment modality in the management of an ever-growing variety of chronic pain disorders. (See the box below.) However, it is in the realm of sports medicine that TENS has had its greatest acceptance.[57] The application of a low-frequency electrical current to an area that has recently been injured can be of benefit to the patient in two ways:

1. First, it acts to increase tissue perfusion produced by capillary and arteriolar dilation while stimulating the contraction of skeletal muscles. The net effect of these two processes is to provide a pumping action in the area of application of the current.

MEDICAL USES OF TENS

Causalgia
Phantom limb pain
Postherpetic neuralgia
Intractable cancer pain
Lower back pain
Spinal cord injury
Ileus
Peripheral nerve injury
Bursitis
Parturition
Polycythemia vera
Cervical back pain
Postoperative pain
Diabetic ulceration

Therapeutically, a 1-hour treatment at a low frequency (2.5 Hz) helps to decrease edema (skeletal muscle–stimulating effect) and the increased perfusion and skeletal muscle stimulation act to "cleanse" the area of tissue-injury breakdown products. The use of TENS in this manner speeds the recovery process, enabling the athlete to return to the field of play sooner.

2. A second benefit in the recovery from injury is the analgesic action it possesses. Low-frequency stimulation for longer than 10 minutes produces elevated blood levels of serotonin and endorphins. These increased levels persist for several hours after the termination of TENS, helping to block the pain "cycle" that has been partially responsible for the chronicity of the pain experienced by the patient. Once this pain cycle is broken, it becomes considerably easier to keep the patient comfortable.

TENS in Dentistry

TMJ/MPD

TENS has been used with great success in dentally related chronic pain in the management of temporomandibular joint (TMJ) problems for many years. Until recently the management of TMJ pain and dysfunction with TENS was almost exclusively limited to physical therapists. In recent years dentistry has begun to incorporate TENS into its armamentarium for the treatment of these patients. Meizels,[58] Clark et al,[59] and Geissler and McPhee[60] have all demonstrated the efficacy and ease of using this technique for TMJ and myofascial pain dysfunction (MPD) syndrome. For the management of limited mandibular opening secondary to TMJ problems, EDA has been used in a manner similar to that described above in medicine—that is, low-frequency extraoral stimulation of the area. Clark et al,[59] Christensen,[61] and others who have been working with EDA for TMJ/MPD patients have had significant success rates (increased range of motion and decreased discomfort) compared with those achieved with placebo.

Acute Dental Pain

The next step in the development of EDA in dentistry was to determine whether the technique could provide pain relief during procedures in which acute, not chronic, pain was being encountered. To do this, it became apparent that a higher frequency of electronic stimulation would be required. The most often used frequency for acute pain management has been 120 Hz, although one EDA unit provided 16,000 Hz.

To date, the areas that have received greatest interest have been restorative dentistry, periodontal procedures, fixed prosthodontics, and endodontics, although clinical trials have been pursued in other areas (removable prosthodontics, oral surgery, and orthodontics).

Using EDA alone (no local anesthesia or sedation) in *restorative dentistry*, Clark et al demonstrated a statistically significant success rate when EDA was used (13 of 14) versus a placebo EDA unit (4 of 7).[59] Hochman, using a much larger patient sample, had a success rate of 76% in 473 restorative dentistry procedures.[62] Patients, using a visual analogue scale, evaluated the degree of pain control achieved, from 0% (painful) to 100% (no pain). Those indicating pain relief of better than 90% were considered successes. My colleagues and I have demonstrated a success rate of 80% in 109 restorative procedures in both arches.[63] Success rates for restorative dentistry utilizing EDA approach those seen with local anesthesia. Mellor, comparing local anesthesia with EDA for restorative dentistry, found that 60% of patients (n = 25) preferred EDA to local anesthesia, whereas 28% had no preference.[64] The degree of pain control obtained by both techniques was evaluated as equal.

EDA has had its greatest success to date in periodontal procedures. The procedures being considered are *nonsurgical periodontics* (i.e., root planing, curettage, and subgingival scaling). Periodontal and other surgical procedures are discussed below. Success rates in excess of 90% for EDA alone have been found by Clark (100%) and myself (97%). Hochman reported an 83% success rate in 71 patients undergoing "scaling and prophylaxis."[62] The use of EDA as an alternative to local anesthesia in nonsurgical periodontics appears quite well founded. This may be of special interest in those countries, states, and provinces where dental hygienists are not permitted to inject local anesthetics.

In *fixed prosthodontics*, results to date for EDA have not been as impressive as in restorative and periodontal procedures, a success rate of 53% in 29 procedures being reported by Hochman.[62] More recently I have reported a success rate in crown-and-bridge of about 75%.[65] Fixed prosthodontics is an area in which EDA can usually provide adequate pain control for the preparation of the tooth. Most failures in the past have occurred when gingival retraction cord was being placed, or following that, when the impression was being taken (because of the need to remove the intraoral electrode pads from the patient's mouth during the period of impression taking). Modifications in EDA technique, using more adhesive and less obtrusive electrodes or extraoral electrodes, have provided a satisfying increase in its success rate and patient acceptance in fixed prosthodontics.

In *endodontics*, Clark et al reported a 0% success rate (n = 4).[59] Until recently I too had met with little success using EDA alone for pain control in the pulpally involved tooth. However, when EDA is employed as an adjunctive technique to local anesthesia and/or sedation (preferably inhalation sedation with N_2O/O_2), I have achieved considerable success in extirpating the pulps of some very difficult to anesthetize teeth (mandibular molars). Though much more work needs to be done in the area of EDA and endodontics, EDA can provide the doctor with one more technique of pain control when seeking to open up the pulp chamber of the infected tooth.

Clark et al were able to remove comfortably 50% (2 of 4) of nonimpacted teeth with EDA versus 0% with a placebo EDA unit.[59] EDA can be used effectively in *simple exodontia* and other surgical (periodontal, endodontic) procedures, but the immediate cessation of anesthesia when the unit is turned off after the procedure may leave the patient with little postsurgical pain control if the surgical procedure is of short duration. Fortunately, a degree of pain relief is present following surgery as the blood levels of serotonin and beta-endorphins remain elevated (for several hours) after the unit has been turned off. If the procedure was very short (<10 minutes), there will be little or no increased blood level of these chemicals and the patient may experience immediate posttreatment pain.

The elevated serotonin and beta-endorphin levels following EDA greatly benefit the patient undergoing restorative, crown-and-bridge, or periodontal procedures—in which there may normally be a slight degree of soreness in the immediate posttreatment period. Following lengthy surgical procedures in which EDA was used, I have been quite impressed with the general lack of discomfort experienced by the patient. Considerable work is presently being undertaken to determine the efficacy of EDA as a postsurgical pain prevention modality in dentistry.

Two other areas in which EDA has been used with success in dentistry include the following:

1. Providing pain control for the administration of local anesthetics. EDA produces excellent soft tissue anesthesia. It may be used when local anesthetic injections must be given, as in multiple palatal infiltrations to achieve hemostasis.

   In a recently completed, randomized, double-blind clinical trial comparing EDA and topical anesthesia for the control of pain during the administration of the inferior alveolar nerve block and long buccal and palatal infiltration, EDA was significantly superior to both placebo and topical anesthesia in permitting comfortable injections to be administered in all three areas.[66]

2. Reversing local anesthesia. Following successful inferior alveolar nerve block with lidocaine/epinephrine, soft tissue anesthesia of approximately 5 hours is to be expected but perhaps not welcomed by the patient. EDA (applied unilaterally [see below]) at its low-frequency setting (thereby maximizing vasodilation and muscle contraction) for a period of 10 to 15 minutes can successfully remove a large volume of residual anesthetic solution and thereby partially or totally reverse the anesthetic effect.

EDA Plus Sedation

The studies reported above have involved the use of EDA as an alternative to local anesthesia. No other technique of pain control or sedation was used. Quarnstrom has demonstrated significantly higher success rates when EDA was used in combination with nitrous oxide–oxygen inhalation sedation (N_2O/O_2) than when either technique was used alone.[67,68] He reported success rates of 32% for EDA alone and 39% for N_2O/O_2 alone whereas an overall success rate of 86% was achieved with a combination of the two techniques. EDA and N_2O/O_2 complement each other quite well (as does the combination of local anesthesia and N_2O/O_2).

Where local anesthesia is less than 100% successful in blocking transmission of pain impulses to the brain, N_2O/O_2 may increase the pain reaction threshold to a point that no pain is interpreted by the patient. Yet when local anesthesia fails entirely, merely adding N_2O/O_2 will not provide adequate pain relief.

This same interaction occurs with EDA and N_2O/O_2. These three techniques are extremely complementary and may be used with impunity in combination. Always consider potential contraindications, however, to each procedure before using it clinically.

Technique of EDA

Temporomandibular Joint Pain and Limitation of Motion

When using electronic dental anesthesia (EDA) for treatment of chronic pain, as in TMJ/MPD, a low-frequency setting is used. For most units this is in the range of 2.5 Hz.

Electrodes are placed bilaterally, extraorally, over the TMJ region (Fig. 19-4) and the intensity is slowly increased until visible muscle contraction is noted. A cotton roll may be placed between the maxillary and mandibular central incisors to prevent the teeth from continually coming into contact as the skeletal muscles contract.

The patient receives treatment for a period of from 40 to 60 minutes depending on the degree of limitation of mandibular movement. If pain is not a component of the patient's condition, treatment is terminated at the end of this time.

Where pain is a component, at the end of approximately 40 minutes of low-frequency treatment the patient (or doctor) turns the frequency control to as high a level as is tolerable yet still comfortable (maximum = 120 Hz). The patient remains at this level for the balance of the 1-hour session.

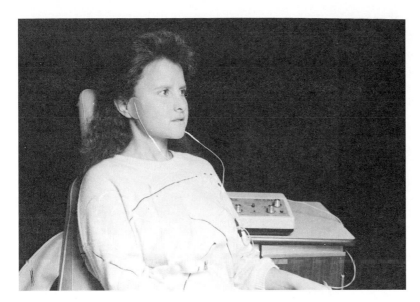

Fig. 19-4 EDA being used for TMJ/MPD treatment. The electrodes are placed bilaterally over the TMJs.

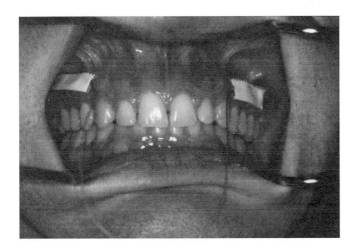

Fig. 19-5 Intraoral bilateral placement.

Low-frequency treatment usually leads to an immediately noticeable increase in the patient's range of motion. Additionally, there are increased blood levels of serotonin and beta-endorphins following this 1-hour treatment session. Higher-frequency stimulation produces muscle fatigue and increased blood levels of these pain threshold–elevating chemicals.

At the onset of treatment patients are often seen for two 1-hour appointments per week. As symptoms and signs subside, visits may be limited to once a week for 1 hour. Other modalities of TMJ/MPD therapy are frequently used concurrently.

Acute Pain (i.e., Restorative and Nonsurgical Periodontics)

For management of acute pain (operative, periodontics, endodontics, crown-and-bridge), the conductive electrode pads are placed into the buccal folds bilaterally in

the arch being treated (Fig. 19-5) or extraorally bilaterally (Fig. 19-6). Other placements are possible (unilateral buccal and lingual, unilateral maxillary and mandibular), but the bilateral placement has proved quite effective and easy to stabilize.

The frequency control on the EDA unit is set at maximum (120 Hz) setting and the intensity control to the 12:00 position (Fig. 19-7). This will limit the maximum output to no more than 17.5 volts. The patient-managed controller (Fig. 19-8) limits the output to the electrodes in the mouth. The controller should *not yet* be attached to the wires leading to the electrode pads in the patient's mouth. Before doing so, recheck that the controller knob is turned to the minimum position. When the EDA unit is initially turned on, the patient should not feel any sensation. Instruct the patient to turn the control dial clockwise as quickly as possible while remaining comfortable. Initial movements of the dial will provide little change in sensation, perhaps a slight feeling of "tingling," "vibrating," or "pulsing." The patient continues to turn the dial until the *threshold* position is reached. The threshold position is one in which an intense but nonpainful sensation is experienced by the patient (if they were to increase the intensity any further, it would be uncomfortable). This is usually at approximately the 2:00 position.

Most patients are not able to turn the control dial continuously to the 2:00 position. As stimulation increases, they may state that the feeling is "getting intense." Have them stop moving the dial for 20 to 30 seconds, after which time the "sensation" will no longer be present. They have "accommodated" to that level of sensation. As they continue to turn the dial, patients will find that they are now able to go beyond this level comfortably. Though it may take three or four accommodation "stops," most

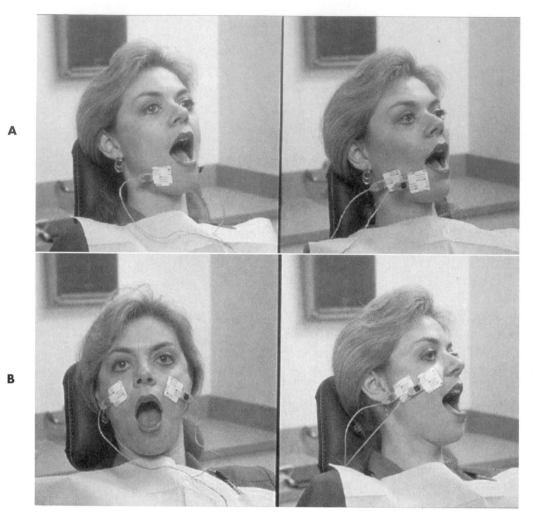

Fig. 19-6 A, Pad placement for mandibular procedures, 3M Patient Comfort System. *Left,* Anterior and premolar teeth; *right,* posterior teeth. **B,** Pad placement for maxillary procedures, 3M Patient Comfort System. *Left,* Anterior and premolar teeth; *right,* posterior teeth.

patients are able to achieve the threshold level within about 4 minutes.

Once threshold is reached, the dental procedure may start. The patient has been told that during treatment the level of nonpainful stimulation can be increased (or decreased). If pain is felt during treatment, it is necessary merely to turn up the dial on the controller. By increasing the level of nonpainful stimulation, it is possible for the patient to "dial" away their pain.

A clinically more efficient means of accomplishing this is for the doctor or hygienist to anticipate the possibility of pain and tell the patient to increase the controller slightly. As the drill cuts through enamel, the threshold level may be comfortable, but the dentinoenamel junction (DEJ) will be the first real test of anesthesia. Have the patient turn the controller up slightly just prior to entering this area. In periodontal procedures, if one area of soft tissue is considerably more inflamed than surrounding regions, the controller may remain at

threshold until this area is approached, at which time it is increased slightly.

In this manner, for both restorative and periodontal procedures, the patient may remain comfortable throughout the planned treatment.

At the completion of dental treatment, turn off the EDA unit before removing the electrode pads from the patient's mouth. The pads, cotton rolls, and wires to the patient controller are all disposable single-use items.

As soon as the EDA unit is turned off, the nonpainful proprioceptive sensation that was present earlier will terminate and the patient's mouth feel "back to normal."

Because of the release of beta-endorphins and serotonin in response to prolonged stimulation (>10 min) with EDA, the patient will remain comfortable into the immediate posttreatment period even though there may have been some trauma to the local soft tissues secondary to the dental intervention.

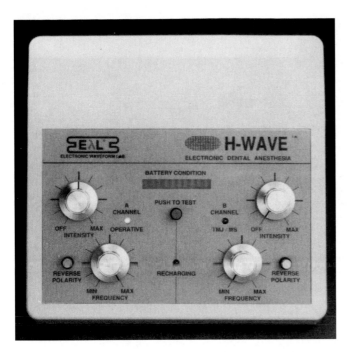

Fig. 19-7 EDA unit for acute pain management. The channel A intensity is set at 12:00, and the channel A frequency at maximum. *(Courtesy Electronic Waveform Laboratories, Huntington Beach, Calif.)*

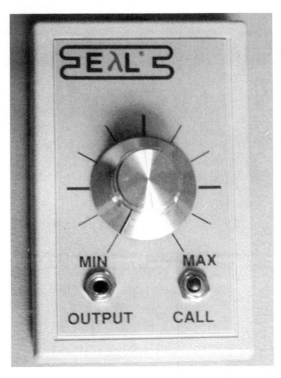

Fig. 19-8 Patient controller for EDA unit.

Acute Pain (i.e., Fixed Prosthodontics)

When using EDA during the preparation of crowns on vital teeth, follow the same technique as described in the preceding section (acute pain: operative and periodontal procedures). Little difficulty will be encountered in preparation of the tooth or in placing the gingival retraction cord (the latter being a very uncomfortable procedure for many patients when local anesthetics are used).

The lower success rates that were encountered in prosthodontics occurred when the EDA unit using intraoral electrodes had to be turned off and the electrode pads removed to permit the use of impression materials. Sensitivity frequently develops at this time. The problem can be diminished or eliminated if the time required for tooth preparation is not too short. (Elevated blood levels of beta-endorphins and serotonin are noted in 10 minutes and increase thereafter.) In this situation, therefore, "slower is better." When more time is needed, the concurrent use of N_2O/O_2 will raise the pain reaction threshold to an acceptable level in most patients, permitting the successful and comfortable taking of impressions. The availability of electronic dental anesthesia units with extraoral electrodes has added to the success rate observed in fixed prosthodontics.

When intraoral electrodes are used, the EDA unit should remain on, with the electrode pads in place, until the last possible moment. Then turn off the machine and remove the pads as the impression tray is placed.

When the impression tray is removed, replace the electrode pads and reattain threshold level. The threshold level for treatment can almost always be reattained in less than a minute at this time.

Administering Local Anesthesia

EDA may be used effectively for the intraoral administration of local anesthetics. A hand-held electrode is placed at the needle penetration site, providing a very localized area of intense anesthesia, permitting both the painless penetration of intraoral soft tissues with dental needles and administration of local anesthetics (Fig. 19-9). In a recently completed clinical trial, local anesthetics administered via the inferior alveolar nerve block and long buccal and palatal infiltration were rated as more comfortable when EDA was used during the injection than with either placebo or topical anesthetic.[66]

EDA in Pediatric Dentistry

Electronic dental anesthesia requires a considerable degree of patient cooperation and participation in order to be successful. Patients are responsible for determining when "threshold" has been achieved and are to understand that they must increase their level of stimulation should they experience any pain during the dental pro-

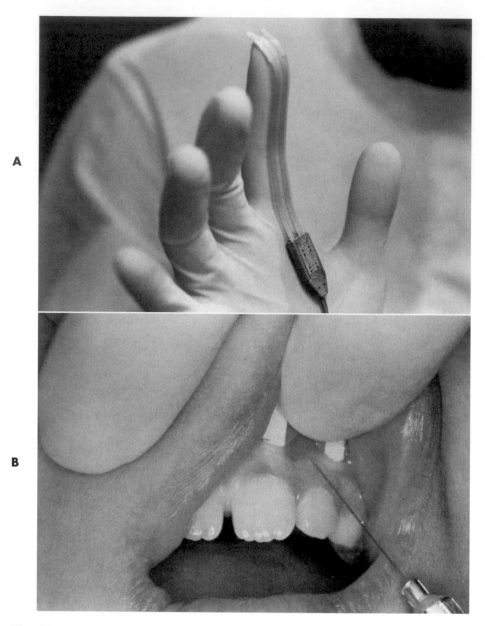

Fig. 19-9 A, Injection Assist electrode adheres to glove, 3M Patient Comfort System. **B,** Injection Assist is placed at site of needle penetration. Needle is inserted between electrodes, 3M Patient Comfort System.

cedure. With this in mind, the use of EDA in younger populations, though not contraindicated, requires a more intensive evaluation of patients' abilities to both understand the concept of EDA and their ability to perform their tasks properly.

teDuits et al used EDA on 27 children between the ages of 6 and 12 years for restorative dentistry.[69] Two opposing teeth were treated, one with local anesthesia, the other with EDA. There was no overall significant difference in pain perception between the two modalities of treatment, regarding dentin sensitivity and rubber dam

clamp placement. When asked for a preference of techniques, 78% chose EDA over local anesthesia.

EDA Indications

The most significant indication for the utilization of EDA as a major technique in pain control is *needle phobia* (fear of injections). Patients who state that they "hate shots" but once numb are "okay" are ideal candidates for EDA. The combination of the technique's success rate and a positive placebo response in this patient group (they want it to work) provides a unique situation for a successful procedure—in stark contrast to the situation in the dental phobic who is fearful of all aspects of dentistry, including EDA.

Other indications for EDA, either alone or in combination with local anesthetics and N_2O/O_2, include:

1. Ineffective local anesthesia
2. Where local anesthetics cannot be administered (i.e., with a history of true, documented reproducible allergy)

The most likely dental procedures to prove successful with EDA are (in descending order of anticipated success):

1. TMJ/MPD (chronic pain)
2. Administration of local anesthesia
3. Nonsurgical periodontal procedures (acute pain)
4. Restorative dentistry (acute pain)
5. Fixed prosthodontic procedures (acute pain)
6. Endodontics (recommended in conjunction with local anesthesia and/or N_2O/O_2)

EDA Contraindications

Specific medical contraindications to the use of EDA are those stated for TENS (ASA IVs remain contraindications for all modes of dental care, including EDA):

1. Cardiac pacemakers
2. Neurological disorders
   a. Status post–cerebrovascular accident (stroke)
   b. History of transient ischemic attacks
   c. History of epilepsy
3. Pregnancy
4. Immaturity (inability to understand the concept of patient control of pain)
   a. Very young pediatric patient
   b. Older patients with senile dementia
   c. Language communication difficulties

Perhaps the most significant nonmedical contraindication to the use of EDA is patients who are *dental phobics*—that is, fearful of everything dental: the smells, the sounds, and the sensations involved with therapeutic interventions in the mouth. To them everything a dentist does represents a threat. EDA is looked upon by them as just one more thing to be afraid of. The likelihood of success in such circumstances is negligible. In Hochman's study of 600 patients, in which the level of "concern" toward this new technique (EDA) was evaluated, patients who considered themselves as "trusting," "ambivalent," or "slightly anxious" had an EDA success rate of 73%, whereas those rating themselves as "extremely apprehensive" had a success rate of 53%.[62] With EDA (as with most dental therapies) patient selection becomes an important component of success.

Another factor, which is somewhat confusing to the doctor, is the few patients who undergo a very successful EDA treatment (i.e., no pain experienced), but when asked which pain control technique, EDA or local anesthesia, they would prefer if required to undergo the same type of dental care at the next visit, state that they would choose local anesthesia. When questioned, these patients often mention that although they did not experience any pain, they disliked EDA for one of two reasons:

1. The "feeling" involved in the EDA was too intense, bordering on uncomfortable.
2. They were unable to "relax" with EDA. Following a local anesthetic injection (which they disliked intensely) they were at least able to relax because they knew that they would not experience any further pain during their treatment. With EDA, however, they had to remain alert throughout the entire procedure, ready to increase the level of stimulation if they became uncomfortable.

EDA Advantages

The advantages of using electronic dental anesthesia over injectable local anesthetics include the following:

1. No need for needle
2. No need for injection of drugs
3. Patient is in control of the anesthesia
4. No residual anesthetic effect at the end of the procedure
5. Residual analgesic effect remains for several hours

EDA Disadvantages

1. Cost of the unit
2. Training
3. "Learning curve"—initial success may be low but will increase with experience
4. Intraoral electrodes—weak link in the entire system
   a. The availability of extraoral electrodes on some units has lessened this disadvantage; however, clinical experience with extraoral electrodes has demonstrated that the depth of anesthesia obtained may not always be as great as that with intraoral electrodes.

EDA Units

Several EDA units are currently marketed in the United States and have received FDA approval for use in intraoral pain control. These include the following units:

- Cedeta*
- H-Wave†
- 3M Patient Comfort System‡

*Cedeta Mk2 Targeted Electronic Anesthesia System: Cedeta Dental International, Trumbull, Conn.
†H-Wave Machine: Electronic Waveform Laboratory, Huntington Beach, Calif.
‡3M Patient Comfort System: 3M Dental Products, St. Paul, Minn.

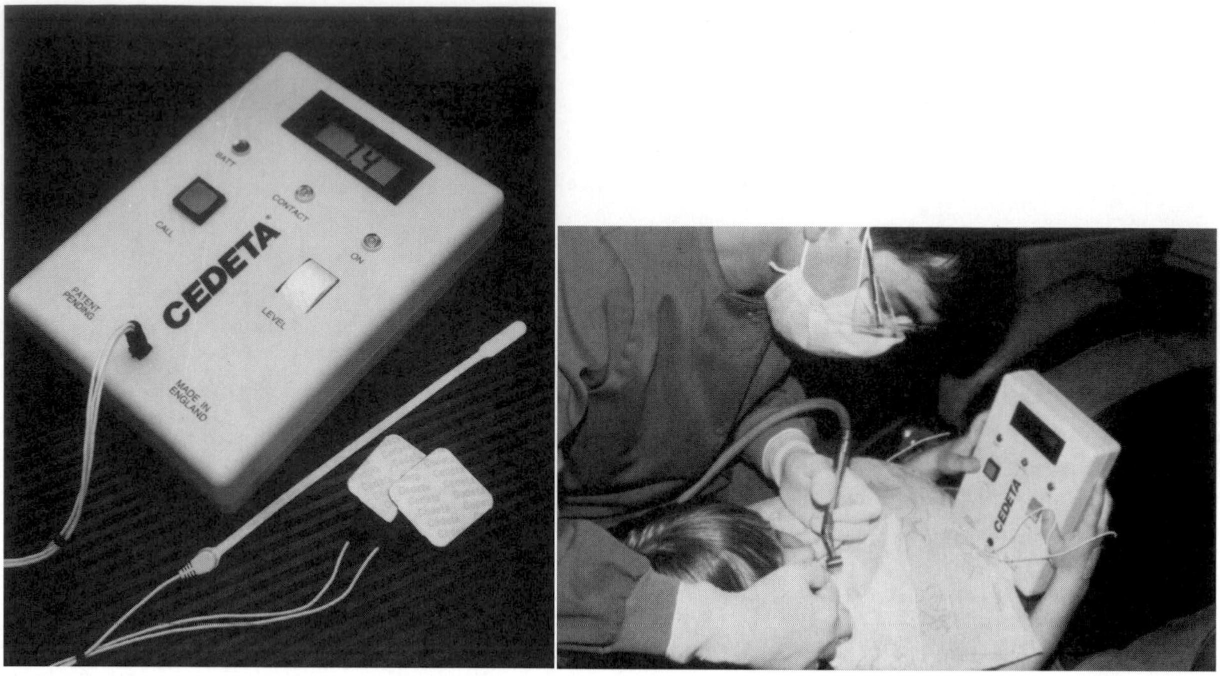

Fig. 19-10 **A,** Cedeta machine and electrodes. **B,** Cedeta machine in clinical setting.

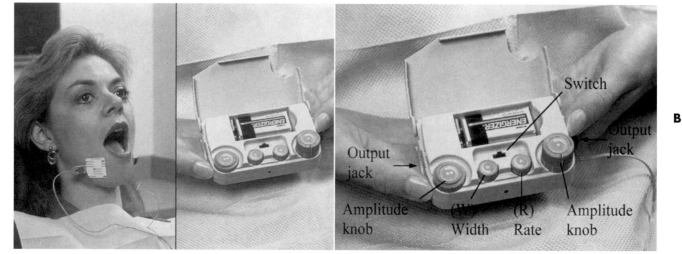

Fig. 19-11 **A,** 3M Patient Comfort System. **B,** Components of the 3M Patient Comfort System.

The H-Wave has two channels, each with a control for intensity and one for frequency (Fig. 19-7). This unit may be used at either a low- or a high-frequency setting to manage chronic or acute pain.

The Cedeta unit uses one extraoral electrode placed on the web of the thumb, with another electrode placed intraorally at the site of treatment (Fig. 19-10).

The 3M Patient Comfort System is a smaller hand-held device, which operates in a manner similar to the H-Wave, except that the electrodes are placed extraorally (Fig. 19-11). Table 19-1 compares these units.

Other EDA units have become available and then faded into obscurity over the past several years—the UltraCalm Machine, Comfort Machine, Pain Suppressor, and Dentron 4000. However, the units mentioned above have thus far withstood the test of time.

Developments Since the Third Edition of This Book
The introduction of electrodes that are more firmly adherent, even when wet, has improved the utility of systems using intraoral electrodes. Additionally, the entry of a major international corporation (3M) into the field of

TABLE 19-1 **Comparison of Electronic Dental Anesthesia Units**

	Cedeta	H-Wave	3M
Frequency range (output)	Two frequencies in the rf range*	2.5 to 120 Hz	2.5 to 120 Hz
Battery	Four 1.5V AA batteries	One 12V battery	One 9V battery
Chronic pain (TMJ)	Yes (medical version of device)	Yes	No
Acute pain	Yes	Yes	Yes
Local anesthesia administration	Yes	Yes	Yes (injection assist)

*Two radio frequencies mix at treatment site to create a specific low-frequency waveform that interrupts the sodium/potassium ion exchange.

electronic dental anesthesia with a relatively inexpensive EDA unit has opened up this area of therapy to many doctors who had previously been unwilling or unable to invest a much larger sum of money to try this new technology.

It is obvious that dentists throughout the world are unwilling to abandon local anesthesia as their primary technique of pain control. However, EDA has been demonstrated to be a highly effective and easy to use method of pain control *during* the injection of local anesthetics. It appears that this may prove to be one of the most important uses of this technique in dentistry.

Postsurgical pain and swelling can be minimized through the use of EDA *following* surgical procedures. The use of EDA at a low-frequency setting for 30 to 60 minutes at the completion of surgery provides a more comfortable postoperative recovery for many patients.

The administration of nitrous oxide–oxygen in conjuction with EDA adds to the success of EDA.

REFERENCES

1. Gupta PP, Tangri AN, Saxena RC, Dhawan BN: Clinical pharmacology studies on 4-N-butylamino-1,2,3,4,-tetrahydroacridine hydrochloride (centbucridine), a new local anaesthetic agent, *Indian J Exp Biol* 20:344-346, 1982.
2. Suri YV, Singhal AP, Phadke VK, et al: Double blind study on centbucridine for subarachnoid and extradural anaesthesia, *Indian J Med Res* 76:875-881, 1982.
3. Suri YV, Patnaik GK, Nayak BC, et al: Evaluation of centbucridine for intravenous regional anaesthesia, *Indian J Med Res* 77:722-727, 1983.
4. Vacharajani GN, Parikh N, Paul T, Satoskar RS: A comparative study of centbucridine and lidocaine in dental extraction, *Int J Clin Pharmacol Res* 3:251-255, 1983.
5. Samsi AB, Bhalerao RA, Shah SC, et al: Evaluation of centbucridine as a local anesthetic, *Anesth Analg* 62:109-111, 1983.
6. Reiz S, Haggmark S, Johansson G, Nath S: Cardiotoxicity of ropivacaine: a new amide local anesthetic, *Acta Anaesthesiol Scand* 33:93-98, 1989.
7. Arthur GR, Feldman HS, Covino BG: Comparative pharmacokinetics of bupivacaine and ropivacaine, a new amide local anesthetic, *Anesth Analg* 67:1053-1058, 1988.
8. Arthur GR, Covino BG: What's new in local anesthetics? *Anesthesiol Clin North Am* 6:357-370, 1988.
9. Brown DL, Carpenter RL, Thompson GE: Comparison of 0.5% ropivacaine and 0.5% bupivacaine for epidural anesthesia in patients undergoing lower-extremity surgery, *Anesthesiology* 72:633-636, 1990.
10. Moller RA, Covino BG: Effect of progesterone on the cardiac electrophysiologic alterations produced by ropivacaine and bupivacaine, *Anesthesiology* 77:735-741, 1992.
11. Sisk AL: Long-acting local anesthetics in dentistry, *Anesth Prog* 39(3):53-60, 1992 .
12. Buckley MM, Benfield P: Eutectic lidocaine/prilocaine cream. A review of the topical anaesthetic/analgesic efficacy of a eutectic mixture of local anaesthetics (EMLA), *Drugs* 46(1):126-151, 1993.
13. Brodin A, Nyqvist-Mayer A, Wadsten T, et al: Phase diagram and aqueous solubility of the lidocaine-prilocaine binary system, *J Pharm Sci* 73:481-484, 1984.
14. Evers H, von Dardel O, Juhlin L, et al: Dermal effects of compositions based on the eutectic mixture of lignocaine and prilocaine (EMLA): Studies in volunteers, *Br J Anaesth* 57:997-1005, 1985.
15. Taddio A, Nulman I, Goldbach M, et al: Use of lidocaine-prilocaine cream for vaccination pain in infants, *J Pediatr* 124(4):643-648, 1994.
16. Lycka BA: EMLA: a new and effective topical anesthetic, *J Dermatol Surg Oncol* 18(10):859-862, 1992.
17. Buckley MM, Benfield P: Eutectic lidocaine/prilocaine cream: a review of the topical anaesthetic/analgesic efficacy of an eutectic mixture of local anaesthetics (EMLA), *Drugs* 46(1):126-151, 1993.
18. van den Hove J, Decroix J, Tennstedt D, Lachapelle JM: Allergic contact dermatitis from prilocaine, one of the local anaesthetics in EMLA cream, *Contact Dermatitis* 30(4):239, 1994.
19. Svennson P, Petersen JK: Anesthetic effect of EMLA occluded with Orahesive oral bandages on oral mucosa, *Anesth Prog* 39:79-82, 1992.
20. Vickers ER, Punnia-Moorthy A: Pulpal anesthesia from an application of a eutectic topical anesthetic, *Quintess Intern* 24(8):547-551, 1993.
21. Meechan JG, Donaldson D: The intraoral use of EMLA cream in children: a clinical investigation, *ASDC J Dent Child* 61(4):260-262, 1994.
22. Vickers ER, Punnia-Moorthy A: A clinical evaluation of three topical anaesthetic agents, *Austral Dent J* 37(4):267-270, 1992.
23. Bromage PR: A comparison of the hydrochloride and carbon dioxide salts of lidocaine and prilocaine in epidural analgesia, *Acta Anaesthesiol Scand* Suppl 16:55-69, 1965.
24. DiFazio CA, Carron H, Grosslight KR, et al: Comparison of pH-adjusted lidocaine solutions for epidural anaesthesia, *Anaesth Analg* 65:760-764, 1986.
25. Berrada R, Chassard D, Bryssine S, et al: In vitro effects of alkalinization of 0.25% bupivacaine and 2% lidocaine, *Ann Fr Anesth Reanim* 13(2):165-168, 1994.
26. Metzinger SE, Rigby PL, Bailey DJ, Brousse RG: Local anesthesia in blepharoplasty: a new look? *South Med J* 87(2):225-227, 1994.
27. Stewart JH, Chinn SE, Cole GW, Klein JA: Neutralized lidocaine with epinephrine for local anesthesia—II, *J Derm Surg Oncol* 16(9):842-845, 1990.

28. Metzinger SE, Bailey DJ, Boyce RG, Lyons GD: Local anesthesia in rhinoplasty: a new twist? *Ear Nose Throat J* 71(9):405-406, 1992.

29. Redd DA, Boudreaux AM, Kent RB III: Towards less painful local anesthesia, *Ala Med* 60(4):18-19, 1990.

30. Bokesch PM, Raymond SA, Strichartz GR: Dependence of lidocaine potency on pH and PCO_2, *Anesth Analg* 66:9-17, 1987.

31. Chaney MA, Kerby R, Reader A, et al: An evaluation of lidocaine hydrocarbonate compared with lidocaine hydrochloride for inferior alveolar nerve block, *Anesth Prog* 38:212-216, 1991.

32. Courtiss EH, Ransil BJ, Russo J: The effects of hyaluronidase on local anesthesia: a prospective, randomized, controlled, double-blind study, *Plast Reconstr Surg* 95(5):876-883, 1995.

33. Johansen J, Kjeldgård M, Corydon L: Retrobulbar anaesthesia: a clinical evaluation of four different anaesthetic mixtures, *Acta Ophthalm* 71(6):787-790, 1993.

34. Watson D: Hyaluronidase, *Br J Anaesth* 71(3):422-425, 1993.

35. Clark LE, Mellette JR Jr: The use of hyaluronidase as an adjunct to surgical procedures, *J Dermatol Surg Oncol* 20(12):842-844, 1994.

36. Looby JP, Kirby CK: Use of hyaluronidase with local anesthetic agents in dentistry, *J Am Dent Assoc* 38:1-4, 1949.

37. Kempeneers A, Dralands L, Ceuppens L: Hyaluronidase induced orbital pseudotumor as complication of retrobulbal anesthesia, *Bull Soc Belge Ophthalmol* 243:159-166, 1992.

38. Covino BG, Vassallo HG: *Local anesthetics: mechanisms of action and clinical use*, New York, 1976, Grune & Stratton.

39. Adams HJ, Blair MR Jr, Takman VH: The local anaesthetic activity of tetrodotoxin alone and in combination with vasoconstrictors and local anaesthetics, *Anaesth Analg* 55:568-573, 1976.

40. Akerman GR, Feldman HS, Norway SB: Acute IV toxicity of LEA-103, a new local anesthetic, compared to lidocaine and bupivacaine in the awake dog, *Anesthesiology* 65:182, 1986.

41. Anderson LD, Reagan SE: Local anesthetics and vasoconstrictors in patients with compromised cardiovascular systems, *Gen Dent* 41(2):161-164, 1993.

42. McClymont LG, Crowther JA: Local anaesthetic with vasoconstrictor combinations in septal surgery, *J Laryngol Otol* 102:793-795, 1988.

43. Meechan JG, Rawlins MD: The effects of two different dental local anesthetic solutions on plasma potassium levels during third molar surgery, *Oral Surg* 66:650-653, 1988.

44. Nordenram A, Danielsson K: Local anaesthesia in elderly patients. An experimental study of oral infiltration anaesthesia, *Swed Dent J* 14(1):19-24, 1990.

45. Scribonius Largus: *De compositione medicamentorum*, Liber CLXII, Paris, 1528, C Wechel.

46. Wesley J: *The desideratum: or electricity made plain and useful*, London, W Flexney, 1760.

47. Ferguson J: *An introduction to electricity*, London, 1770.

48. Malamed SF, Joseph C: Electricity in dentistry, *J Calif Dent Assoc* 15:12-14, 1987.

49. Erb W: *Handbook of electrotherapeutics*, New York, 1883, W Wood, p. 234.

50. Sturridge E: *Dental electro-therapeutics*, ed 2, Philadelphia, 1918, Lea & Febiger.

51. Silverstone L: Electronic dental anesthesia, *Dent Pract* 27:4-6, 1989.

52. Hughes J, Smith TW, Kosterlitz HW: Identification of two related pentapeptides from the brain with potent opiate agonist activity, *Nature* 258:577-580, 1975.

53. Melzack R, Wall PD: Pain mechanisms: a new theory, *Science* 150:971-979, 1965.

54. Shealy CN, Mortimer JT, Reswick JB: Electrical inhibition of pain by stimulation of the dorsal column: preliminary clinical report, *Anesth Analg* 45:489-491, 1967.

55. Shealy CN: Transcutaneous electrical stimulation for control of pain, *Clin Neurosurg* 21:269-277, 1974.

56. Long DM: External electrical stimulation as a treatment of chronic pain, *Minn Med* 57:195-198, 1974.

57. Smith MJ, Hutchins RC, Hehenberger D: Transcutaneous neural stimulation use in postoperative knee rehabilitation, *Am J Sport Med* 11:75-82, 1983.

58. Meizels P: H-wave and TMJ treatment, *J Calif Dent Assoc* 15:42-44, 1987.

59. Clark MS, Silverstone LM, Lindemuth J, et al: An evaluation of the clinical analgesia/anesthesia efficacy on acute pain using the high frequency neural modulator in various dental settings, *Oral Surg* 63:501-505, 1987.

60. Geissler PR, McPhee PM: Electrostimulation in the treatment of pain in the mandibular dysfunction syndrome, *J Dent* 14:62-64, 1986.

61. Christensen GJ: Electronic anesthesia: research and thoughts, *J Calif Dent Assoc* 15:46-48, 1987.

62. Hochman R: Neurotransmitter modulator (TENS) for control of dental operative pain, *J Am Dent Assoc* 116:208-212, 1988.

63. Malamed SF, Quinn CL, Torgerson RT, Thompson W: Electronic dental anesthesia for restorative dentistry, *Anesth Prog* 36:195-198, 1989.

64. Mellor AC: A comparison of injectable local anesthesia and electronic dental anesthesia in restorative dentistry, *Anesth Pain Control Dent* 2(3):177-179, 1993.

65. Malamed SF: Unpublished data, 1989.

66. Malamed SF: The effectiveness of electronic anesthesia for pain control during intraoral injections, Unpublished data, 1995.

67. Quarnstrom FC: Electrical anesthesia, *J Calif Dent Assoc* 16:35-40, 1988.

68. Quarnstrom FC: Clinical experience with TENS and TENS combined with nitrous oxide–oxygen, *Anesth Prog* 36:66-69, 1989.

69. teDuits E, Goepferd S, Donly K, et al: The effectiveness of electronic dental anesthesia in children, *Pediatr Dent* 15(3):191-196, 1993.

CHAPTER
t w e n t y

Questions

LOCAL ANESTHETICS

Question: Why is it said that intravascular administration of local anesthetics is dangerous when physicians frequently administer intravenous (IV) lidocaine to correct serious cardiac dysrhythmias?

The intravenous administration of local anesthetics is potentially hazardous at all times and in all patients. However, IV local anesthetics, such as lidocaine and procainamide, do have an important place in the management of various ventricular dysrhythmias, such as premature ventricular contractions and ventricular tachycardia. Several factors, including weighing the risk versus the benefit, must be considered whenever local anesthetics are to be administered "safely" intravenously.

1. *The patient's physical status.* Patients receiving IV lidocaine or other antiarrhythmic drugs have potentially life-threatening cardiac dysrhythmias. The myocardium is highly irritable (usually secondary to ischemia), one of the reasons for the dysrhythmia's presence. Local anesthetics are myocardial depressants. By depressing myocardial activity they decrease the incidence of dysrhythmias. Patients with normal cardiac rhythms receiving IV local anesthetics also have their myocardium depressed; in this circumstance their cardiac function may be impaired by the local anesthetic.

2. *The form of lidocaine used.* Lidocaine for IV use in the management of ventricular dysrhythmias, so-called "cardiac lidocaine," is prepared in single-use ampules. These ampules contain only lidocaine and sodium chloride. The typical dental cartridge of lidocaine contains lidocaine, distilled water, vasopressor, sodium bisulfite, and sodium chloride. IV injection of these ingredients, in and of itself, might precipitate unwanted cardiovascular responses rather than terminate them.

3. *The rate of injection.* Lidocaine for antiarrhythmic use is titrated slowly into the cardiovascular system to achieve a therapeutic blood level in the myocardium. Typically, a 75 to 100 mg bolus (1 mg/kg) is administered slowly under electrocardiographic monitoring, titrating to clinical effect. In the typical dental practice a 1.8-ml cartridge of lidocaine (36 mg) is deposited in 15 seconds or less. The rate at which the drug is administered intravenously has a significant bearing upon the peak blood level of the drug. Overly rapid intravenous administration results in lidocaine blood levels that quickly enter into the overdose range, whereas a more slowly administered dose results in blood levels well within the therapeutic range for terminating dysrhythmias.

4. *Risk versus benefit.* An overdose reaction is always a possibility whenever IV lidocaine is administered. Even under controlled conditions in a hospital, adverse reactions related to overly high blood levels do develop. The risk of administering local anesthetics intravenously must always be weighed against the potential benefit to be gained from their use. For high-risk patients with a specific life-threatening dysrhythmia, the benefit clearly outweighs the risk. For

dental patients seeking relief from intraoral pain, IV local anesthetic administration confers no benefit yet adds many risks.

Question: What shall I do when a patient claims to be allergic to a local anesthetic?

Believe the patient! Do not use any form of local anesthetic (including topical preparations) on this patient. Seek to determine what actually happened to the patient to prompt such a claim. (A detailed discussion of this problem is found in Chapter 18.)

Question: Are any local anesthetics safer than others? Some appear to be implicated more than others in adverse reactions.

No. When used properly, all currently available local anesthetics are highly effective and safe. "Used properly" is the key phrase. Aspiration before injection, to minimize the risk of intravascular administration, and slow administration of the drug are vital. A medical history and physical evaluation, to determine potential contraindications to specific local anesthetics or additives, must be completed prior to their use. Maximum dosage of a drug should be determined for a given patient and not exceeded. Charts for the most commonly used local anesthetics are found in Chapters 4 and 18. The figures cited are maximum recommended doses. They should be decreased in patients with certain medical complications and in older individuals. Most systemic reactions to local anesthetics are entirely avoidable. Overdose reactions that have led to death are frequently the result of the administration of too large a dose or following accidental IV administration. Psychogenic reactions, by far the most common adverse response to local anesthetic administration, may be virtually eliminated through increased rapport with the patient, use of an atraumatic injection technique (Chapter 11), placement of the patient in a supine position during injection, and ample doses of empathy.

Question: How do I select the proper local anesthetic for a given patient and a given procedure?

Two factors are particularly important:

1. The patient's physical status (i.e., ASA classification), hypersensitivity, methemoglobinemia, or sulfur allergy, which may preclude the use of some drugs
2. The duration of pain control required to complete the procedure (Table 4-2 lists currently available local anesthetics by their approximate duration of action.)

For most patients the duration of desired pain control is the ultimate deciding factor in local anesthetic selection, since there is usually no contraindication to the administration of any particular agent.

Question: What local anesthetics should be available in my office?

It is suggested that a number of local anesthetics be available at all times. The nature of the dental practice will dictate the number and types of local anesthetics needed. In a typical dental practice the selection of a drug will be based on the desired duration of anesthesia—for example, less than 30 minutes, approximately 60 minutes, in excess of 90 minutes. One local anesthetic preparation from each group necessitated by the nature of the doctor's practice should be available. For example, the pediatric dentist may have little need or desire for long-acting local anesthetics, such as bupivacaine and etidocaine, whereas the oral and maxillofacial surgeon may have little need for shorter-acting drugs like mepivacaine plain, but a greater need for bupivacaine and etidocaine. Remember that not all patients have similar local anesthetic requirements and the same patient may require a different local anesthetic for a dental procedure of a different duration. In general, amide local anesthetics are preferred to the esters because of their decreased incidence of allergy.

Question: Do topical anesthetics really work?

Yes, if the topical anesthetic preparation is applied to mucous membrane for an adequate length of time. The American Dental Association recommends a 1 minute application.[1] The Food and Drug Administration recommends application for a minimum of 1 minute. Gill and Orr recommend application for 2 to 3 minutes.[2] Topical anesthetics containing benzocaine are not absorbed from their site of application into the cardiovascular system. Risk of overdose is therefore minimal when benzocaine-containing topical anesthetic preparations are used. Because of the rapid absorption of some topically applied local anesthetics, such as lidocaine, it is recommended that their use be restricted to the following situations:

1. Locally, at the site of needle puncture prior to injection
2. For scaling or curettage, over no more than three or four teeth at a time

Pressurized sprays of topical anesthetics cannot be recommended unless they release a metered dose of the drug, not a steady uncontrolled dose. Sterilization of the spray nozzle must be possible if a spray is used. Many pressurized topical anesthetic sprays are available in metered form with disposable spray nozzles.

VASOCONSTRICTORS

Question: Are there any contraindications to the use of vasopressors in dental patients?

Yes. Use of local anesthetics with vasopressors should be avoided or kept to an absolute minimum in the following cases:[3]

1. Patients with blood pressure in excess of 200 mm Hg systolic or 115 mm Hg diastolic
2. Patients with uncontrolled hyperthyroidism
3. Patients with severe cardiovascular disease
   a. Less than 6 months after myocardial infarction
   b. Less than 6 months after cerebrovascular accident
   c. Daily episodes of angina pectoris or unstable (preinfarction) angina
   d. Cardiac dysrhythmias despite appropriate therapy
   e. Post–coronary artery bypass surgery, less than 6 months
4. Patients who are undergoing general anesthesia with halogenated agents
5. Patients receiving nonspecific beta blockers, monoamine oxidase inhibitors, or tricyclic antidepressants

Patients in categories 1 to 3a through 3d above are classified as ASA IV risk and are *not* candidates for elective or emergency dental treatment in the office. (Refer to Chapter 3 for a more detailed discussion; also see the next question.)

Question: Very often medical consultants recommend against inclusion of a vasopressor in a local anesthetic for a cardiovascular risk patient. Why? And what can I do to achieve effective pain control?

As indicated previously, there are several instances in which it is prudent to avoid the use of vasopressors in local anesthetics. Most of these situations (high blood pressure, severe cardiovascular disease) also represent absolute contraindications to elective dental care because of the greater potential risk to the patient. If a dental patient with cardiovascular disease is deemed treatable (ASA II or III), then local anesthetics for pain control are indicated. The patient's physician often will state that, although local anesthetics can be used, epinephrine should be avoided.

Question: When should epinephrine be avoided?

One of the few valid reasons for avoiding epinephrine is the patient with cardiac rhythm abnormalities that are unresponsive to medical therapy. The presence of dysrhythmias (especially ventricular) usually indicates an irritable or ischemic myocardium. Epinephrine, either exogenous or endogenous, pharmacologically increases the sensitivity of the myocardium even more, predisposing this patient to a greater frequency of dysrhythmias or to more significant types of dysrhythmias, such as ventricular tachycardia or ventricular fibrillation. In these patients epinephrine-containing local anesthetics should be avoided, if at all possible. However, many cardiologists today do not even consider the ischemic myocardium a valid reason for excluding vasoconstrictors from local anesthetics, provided the dose of epinephrine administered is minimal and intravascular administration is avoided.

It is my recommendation that with a patient able to tolerate the stresses of dental therapy a vasoconstrictor should be included in the local anesthetic if it is needed. As Bennett has stated, the greater the medical risk of a patient, the more important effective control of pain and anxiety becomes.[4]

Question: Why do many physicians still recommend against the use of epinephrine (and other vasopressors) in cardiovascular risk patients?

Most physicians never, or at best rarely, use epinephrine in their practice. The only physicians doing so on a regular basis are anesthesiologists, emergency medicine specialists, and surgeons. As used in medicine, epinephrine is almost always used in emergency situations. At those times the dose is considerably higher than that used in dentistry. The average emergency dose of intramuscular (IM) or IV epinephrine (used in a 1:1000 or 1:10,000 concentration) for anaphylaxis or cardiac arrest is 0.3 to 1 mg, whereas one dental cartridge with 1:100,000 epinephrine contains but 0.018 mg.

It is therefore understandable that physicians, lacking an intimate knowledge of the practice of dentistry, would think of epinephrine in terms of the doses used in emergency medicine and not in the much more dilute forms used for anesthesia in dentistry.

An example follows. In a hospital situation a patient with a serious cardiovascular problem (ASA IV) who requires a surgical procedure (e.g., appendectomy) may be considered too great a risk for general anesthesia. Many anesthesiologists would opt to use a regional local anesthetic (spinal) block with an IV antianxiety agent (diazepam or midazolam) for sedation in place of general anesthesia. The local anesthetic would usually contain a vasopressor such as epinephrine in a 1:100,000 or 1:200,000 concentration, added primarily to decrease the rate at which the local anesthetic was absorbed into the cardiovascular system but also to minimize bleeding and prolong the duration of clinical action.

Question: Why is the use of vasopressors in local anesthetics recommended for cardiac risk patients?

Pain is stressful to the body. During stress endogenous catecholamines (epinephrine, norepinephrine) are released from their storage sites into the cardiovascular system at a level approximately 40 times greater than at the resting level (Table 20-1). (Refer to Chapter 3 for a review of the pharmacology of this group of drugs.)

Release of epinephrine and norepinephrine into the blood increases the cardiovascular workload, and thus the myocardial oxygen requirement increases. In patients with compromised (partially occluded) coronary arteries, this greater myocardial oxygen require-

TABLE 20-1 Catecholamine Blood Levels		
	Epinephrine (µg/min)	Norepinephrine (µg/min)
Resting adrenal medullary secretion	7	1.5
Stress	280	56
Local anesthesia (1:50,000 epinephrine in 1.8 ml)	< 1	—

From Malamed SF: *Medical emergencies in the dental office,* ed 4, St Louis, 1993, Mosby–Year Book.

ment may not be met—with the subsequent development of ischemia, leading to dysrhythmias, anginal pain (if transient), or myocardial infarction (if prolonged). Increased cardiac workload may also lead to acute exacerbation of congestive heart failure. Elevated catecholamine levels can produce a dramatic increase in blood pressure, which can precipitate another life-threatening situation (cerebrovascular accident [CVA]).

The goal, therefore, is to minimize endogenous catecholamine release during dental therapy. The stress reduction protocol is designed to accomplish this. A local anesthetic without vasopressor produces pulpal anesthesia of shorter duration than the same drug with a vasopressor. Profound pain control of adequate duration is less likely to be achieved when a vasopressor is excluded from a local anesthetic solution. If the patient experiences pain during treatment, an exaggerated stress response is observed.

With the proper use (aspiration and slow injection) of a local anesthetic with minimum concentration of exogenous vasopressor (e.g., 1:100,000 or 1:200,000), pain control of longer duration is virtually guaranteed and the exaggerated stress response is avoided. Levels of catecholamine in the blood are elevated when exogenous epinephrine is administered, but these levels are not of clinical significance.

An oft-repeated, and essentially true, statement is that the cardiovascularly impaired patient is more at risk from endogenously released catecholamines than from exogenous epinephrine administered in a proper manner.

Question: Can I administer a local anesthetic with a vasopressor even if a physician has advised against it?

Yes. A medical consultation is simply a request for advice, usually from a person with more knowledge of the matter being discussed. You need not always heed this advice if you feel it may be inaccurate. When doubt persists in your mind concerning proper treatment protocol, additional opinions should be sought, preferably from specialists in the "area" of concern, such as a cardiologist, anesthesiologist, or dental expert in local anesthesia. There will, of course, be patients for whom exogenous catecholamines may prove too great a risk, in which case "plain" local anesthetic solutions will be administered. It should always be remembered that the primary responsibility for the care and well-being of a patient rests solely in the hands of the person who performs the treatment, not the one who gives advice.

A recent incident concerning a medical consultation is worth relating here. A periodontal graduate student was planning four quadrants of osseous surgery on a patient whose medical history was within normal limits except for a torticollis for which she was receiving imipramine, a tricyclic antidepressant. A written consultation was sent to the patient's physician requesting that the patient be taken off of the imipramine prior to the surgical procedure. The response, not surprisingly, was that the patient could not be taken off of the drug, as it had taken over a year to get her medical condition stabilized. Moreover, it was recommended that epinephrine be avoided during this patient's surgery. It was decided to contact the physician directly to discuss the matter and attempt to explain the importance of epinephrine during the surgical procedure. In the ensuing conversation it was agreed that epinephrine could be used, but in a limited dose, and that the patient was to be monitored (vital signs) throughout the procedure. The surgery was carried off without incident. The lesson to be learned from this episode is that the wording of the original consult was too constricting, or indeed might have been construed as threatening, to the physician. Whenever possible, direct contact and discussion, with both parties explaining their needs, should be obtained, as this is more likely to lead to a satisfactory compromise and to better and safer patient management.

Question: If epinephrine is used in cardiac risk patients, is there a maximum dose?

Yes. Bennett recommends, and I concur, that the maximum dose of epinephrine in a cardiac risk patient should be 0.04 mg.[4] This equates to approximately

- One cartridge of 1:50,000 epinephrine
- Two cartridges of 1:100,000 epinephrine
- Four cartridges of 1:200,000 epinephrine

I do *not* recommend the use of 1:50,000 epinephrine for pain control purposes. (Further information on dental management of the cardiovascular risk patient is available.[4,5])

Question: What about epinephrine-containing gingival retraction cord?

Racemic epinephrine gingival retraction cord should *never* be used in cardiovascular risk patients, and it is my opinion that it should not be used for any patient. Gingival retraction cord contains 8% racemic epinephrine. Half of this is the levorotatory form, which provides a concentration of active epinephrine of 4% (or 40 mg/ml). This is *40 times* the concentration used in the management of anaphylaxis or cardiac arrest. Absorption of epinephrine through mucous membrane into the cardiovascular system is normally rapid but is even more so with active bleeding such as that occurring after subgingival tooth preparation. Levels of epinephrine in the blood rise rapidly, leading to cardiovascular manifestations of epinephrine overdose (p. 272). In patients with preexisting clinically evident or subclinical cardiovascular disease, this increase in cardiovascular activity may prove to be life-threatening.

Question: If I elect not to use a vasopressor for a patient, which local anesthetics are clinically useful?

The clinically available local anesthetics are listed by their duration of action in Table 4-2. Mepivacaine 3% can provide up to 40 minutes of pulpal anesthesia (via nerve block) for the average patient, while prilocaine 4% can provide up to 60 minutes with nerve blocks.

SYRINGES

Question: What kind of syringe is recommended?

Although a wide variety are available, there are two factors of primary importance in their selection.

1. A syringe must be capable of aspiration. *Never* use a syringe that does not permit aspiration.
2. A syringe must be sterilizable, unless it is disposable.

In addition, with the introduction of so-called safety syringes, it is my recommendation that every consideration be given to the use of a syringe that is designed to minimize the risk of accidental needle stick after injection is completed. Though the unit cost of the disposable safety syringe will increase office expenses, the decreased liability faced by the doctor in needle-stick injuries should more than cover this consideration.

NEEDLES

Question: What gauge and length of needles are recommended for injection?

Selection of a needle depends on several factors, foremost among which are the aspiration potential of the injection and the estimated depth of soft tissue penetration.

1. A long needle is recommended for the inferior alveolar, Gow-Gates mandibular, Vazirani-Akinosi mandibu-

lar, infraorbital, buccal, and maxillary nerve blocks in adults.
2. A short needle is recommended for the posterior superior alveolar, mental, and incisive nerve blocks; maxillary infiltration (supraperiosteal injection); palatal nerve blocks and infiltration; and periodontal ligament and intraseptal injections.

In previous editions I had specified the gauge of the needle for each injection. A 25-gauge needle was recommended for no. 1 above, a 27-gauge needle for no. 2. This remains my recommendation today.

If but two needles were to be available in my dental office, I would opt for a 25-gauge long and a 27-gauge short. I have absolutely no need, nor any desire, to ever use a 30-gauge needle for an intraoral injection. However, this is not the case in dentistry in the United States. Information received from needle manufacturers indicates that the most commonly used needles in dentistry are the 27-gauge long and the 30-gauge short.

I do not recommend a 30 gauge short, but it may be used for local infiltration to produce hemostasis.

CARTRIDGES

Question: Why do you (the author) call this a "cartridge" when everyone else calls it a "carpule"?

Carpule is a proprietary name for the glass cartridge. The name is trademarked by the Cook-Waite Corporation.

Question: Can glass cartridges be autoclaved?

No. Autoclaving of glass cartridges destroys the seals on them. The heat of autoclaving will also degrade the heat-labile vasopressor.

Question: Should local anesthetic cartridges be stored in alcohol or cold sterilizing solution?

No. Alcohol or cold sterilizing solution will diffuse into the cartridge. Injection of these into tissues may produce burning, irritation, or paresthesia. (The care and handling of local anesthetic cartridges are discussed in Chapter 8.)

Question: Are cartridge warmers effective in making local anesthetic solutions more comfortable on injection?

No. Most cartridge warmers make the local anesthetic solution too warm, leading to increased discomfort on injection as well as possible destruction of the heat-sensitive vasopressor. Cartridges stored at room temperature produce no discomfort to patients and are greatly preferred.

Question: Why do some patients complain of a burning sensation when a local anesthetic is injected?

Because of its pH, any local anesthetic may cause a slight burning sensation during the initial injection. The pH of a plain solution is in the 5.5 range, that of a vaso-pressor-containing solution in the mid 4s. Other causes include an overly warm solution, the presence of alcohol or cold sterilizing solution within the cartridge, or solution with a vasopressor at or near its expiration date.

Question: What causes local anesthetic solution to run down the outside of the needle into a patient's mouth?

Improper preparation of the armamentarium is to blame here. (See Chapter 9.) The recommended sequence for preparation is as follows (using a metal syringe and disposable needle):

1. Place the cartridge in the syringe.
2. Embed the aspirating harpoon.
3. Place the needle on the syringe.

This sequence provides a perfectly centric perforation of the rubber diaphragm by the needle, with a tight seal formed around the needle. No leakage of anesthetic occurs.

When the needle is placed onto the syringe first, followed by the cartridge, it is possible for the perforation of the diaphragm to be ovoid, not round. The ovoid perforation does not seal itself as well around the metal needle, leading to leakage of anesthetic around this area as the anesthetic drug is injected.

Question: What causes cartridges to break during injection?

1. Damage during shipping
   Visually check cartridges before use.
2. Using excessive force to engage the aspirating harpoon in the rubber stopper
   Proper preparation of the needle, cartridge, and syringe (see previous question) precludes breakage due to excessive force. When the needle is placed onto the syringe before the cartridge it is necessary to "hit" the plunger in order to embed the harpoon into the rubber stopper. This may cause a cartridge to shatter.
3. Attempting to force a cartridge with an extruded plunger into the syringe
4. Using a syringe with a bent aspirating harpoon
5. Bent needle with an occluded lumen
   Always expel a small volume of anesthetic from the syringe prior to inserting the needle into the patient's mouth to ensure patency of the needle.

TECHNIQUES OF REGIONAL ANESTHESIA IN DENTISTRY

Question: What should always be done prior to local anesthetic administration in a patient?

Review of the patient's medical history questionnaire (visually and/or verbally) and a physical examination, including vital signs and visual inspection, are recommended when a patient is seen for the first time or following a long absence from the office. This will identify possible contraindications to the use of local anesthetics or vasopressors and in general determine a patient's ability to tolerate physically and psychologically the stresses of dental care without undue risk.

Question: What are the medical contraindications to use of local anesthetics and vasopressors?

These are discussed in Chapter 4 and in an excellent review article by Perusse, Goulet, and Turcotte.[3]

Question: Should a patient be advised that a local anesthetic injection will hurt, before the injection is started?

No. Local anesthetic injections need not hurt. Careful adherence to the atraumatic injection protocol described in Chapter 11 can make virtually all injections, including palatal, painless.

Question: Is there any chair position that is best for administration of local anesthetics?

Yes. Since the most commonly observed adverse reactions to local anesthetics are psychogenic, the position of choice during intraoral injections is one in which the patient's chest and head are parallel to the floor with the feet slightly elevated. Presyncopal episodes may still occur (pallor, light-headedness), but actual loss of consciousness is extremely unlikely to develop with the patient in this position.

Following completion of several mandibular injections (inferior alveolar, Gow-Gates mandibular, and Vazirani-Akinosi mandibular nerve blocks) it is suggested that the patient be returned to a comfortable, more upright position during the ensuing 5 to 10 minutes. This change in patient position appears to help speed the onset of mandibular block anesthesia.

Question: Why do you recommend regional block anesthesia in the maxilla instead of infiltration (supraperiosteal) anesthesia?

Regional block anesthesia in the maxilla is preferred over infiltration whenever more than two teeth are to be treated. Its advantages include the following:

1. Fewer penetrations of tissue, thus less likelihood of postinjection problems
2. Smaller volume of local anesthetic (e.g., than for infiltration of the same area), thereby decreasing the risk of systemic reactions such as overdose
3. Clinically adequate anesthesia more likely when infiltration is ineffective because of the presence of infection

Question: Do palatal injections always hurt?

No. Careful adherence to the protocol for atraumatic injections can do much to minimize any discomfort associated with palatal anesthesia. In addition, the following are important:

1. Topical anesthesia
2. Pressure anesthesia

3. Control of the needle
4. Slow deposition of solution
5. Positive attitude by the administrator

Interestingly, an area of considerable interest among practicing dentists is palatal anesthesia and how to increase patient comfort. Over the years I have received many devices designed by dentists in an attempt to minimize or eliminate pain during palatal injections, and I have also been told of many techniques. These include vibrating wands, "letting the needle trace along the palate for a second or two so they know its coming and its not a 'shock,' " and avoiding the use of palatal injections unless they are absolutely necessary.

The introduction of electronic dental anesthesia (EDA) permits the administration of local anesthetics to proceed virtually painlessly in all areas of the oral cavity. Several of the manufacturers of EDA units provide a device that is applied to the site of needle penetration, producing a very localized area of soft tissue anesthesia and permitting painless needle penetration to follow.

Question: Why do I miss inferior alveolar nerve blocks more often than any other injection?

Of all nerve blocks in dentistry and, with few exceptions, in medicine too, the inferior alveolar is the most elusive of consistent success. A success rate, bilaterally, of 85% or greater indicates that one's basic technique is correct. However, many factors can affect this rate of success:

1. *Anatomical variation.* It is well known that if there is any one aspect of human anatomy that is consistent it is its inconsistency. Strict adherence to injection technique will not always produce adequate inferior alveolar anesthesia.
2. *Technical errors.* The most common technical error I observe with the inferior alveolar nerve block is insertion of the needle too low on the medial side of the ramus (below the mandibular foramen). A second common technical error is insertion of the needle too far anteriorly (laterally) on the medial side of the ramus (thus contacting bone quite soon after penetration).
3. *Accessory innervation.* When isolated regions of mandibular teeth remain sensitive when all other areas are insensitive, the possibility of accessory innervation should be considered. The technique used in eliminating this problem (which is usually produced by the mylohyoid nerve) is described in Chapter 14.

Question: Why do I have a much higher failure rate with inferior alveolar nerve blocks on one side than on the other?

Because of significantly different operator positions during the administration of the inferior alveolar nerve block on contralateral sides of the mouth, it is not uncommon for some doctors to encounter great variation in their success rate. This is the only intraoral nerve block for which significant differences in success rates are noted on opposite sides of the mouth. Although basic protocols are the same on the right and on the left side, the view of the target area by the administrator, the angle of needle entry, and other factors may be responsible for an increased failure rate on one side. The solution to this problem is to evaluate critically one's technique on the less successful side and seek to correct it without interfering in the success on the opposite side. Patience is often required.

Question: How can I achieve adequate pain control when gaining access in pulpally involved teeth?

The recommended sequence of injection techniques for pulpally involved teeth follows:

1. Local infiltration, if possible and not contraindicated
2. Regional nerve block
3. Intrapulpal injection
4. Intraosseous injection
5. Periodontal ligament (PDL) injection, if not contraindicated by the presence of infection
6. Intraseptal injection
7. Psychosedation, if pain control techniques have proved unsuccessful in completely blocking pain impulses from reaching brain
8. Electronic dental anesthesia (Chapter 19)
9. Prayer . . . when nothing else works!

For all teeth in the mouth, with the probable exception of mandibular molars, clinically adequate pain control for pulpal extirpation will be obtained with either local infiltration or nerve block injection. Difficulties arise most often in the mandibular molars. A working knowledge of alternative mandibular anesthesia techniques, such as the Gow-Gates mandibular block or the Vazirani-Akinosi mandibular block, will increase the likelihood of obtaining anesthesia. In addition, the use of intraosseous anesthesia—periodontal ligament injection (in the *absence* of infection) or intraseptal injection, or traditional intraosseous anesthesia—will greatly increase success rates in mandibular molars.

Mandibular premolars and anteriors can be anesthetized adequately for pulpal extirpation with the incisive nerve block.

Question: What special concerns are involved with local anesthesia in pediatric dentistry?

Pain control is generally easier to achieve in pediatric dentistry. There are, however, two concerns that should always be considered:

1. *Increased overdose potential* exists because (most) children are smaller and weigh less than adults. Use milligram-per-weight formulas to minimize doses in children.

2. *Prolonged anesthesia* can lead to traumatization of the lips and tongue, unless shorter-duration drugs are used and both patient and parent are warned of this possible complication.

A third concern relates to injection technique and the appropriate needle to be used in specific techniques. In those injections described in this book for which a considerable thickness of soft tissue was to be penetrated, a long dental needle was recommended. The rationale for this is the rule of thumb that "a needle should not be inserted into tissue all the way to its hub, unless it is absolutely necessary for the success of that injection." If it is possible for an injection technique to be administered in a child with a short (20 mm length) needle within the parameters of this rule, then use of this needle is warranted. Psychologically, sight of a long needle is more traumatic than is the sight of a short needle (in point of fact, needles and syringes should always be kept out of a patient's line of sight, if possible).

Question: What is the recommended method of achieving hemostasis in surgical areas?

The recommended technique is *local infiltration* of a vasopressor-containing anesthetic into the region of the surgery. Only small volumes are required for this purpose. Epinephrine in a concentration of 1:100,000 is recommended (although 1:50,000 may also be used).

REFERENCES

1. American Dental Association Council on Dental Therapeutics: *Accepted dental therapeutics*, Chicago, 1984, The American Dental Association.
2. Gill CJ, Orr DL: A double blind crossover comparison of topical anesthetics, *J Am Dent Assoc* 98:213, 1979.
3. Perusse R, Goulet J-P, Turcotte J-Y: Contraindications to vasoconstrictors in dentistry, *Oral Surg* 74:679-697, 1992.
4. Bennett CR: *Monheim's local anesthesia and pain control in dental practice*, ed 7, St Louis, 1984, Mosby–Year Book.
5. American Dental Association Council on Dental Therapeutics, and American Heart Association: Joint report: management of dental problems in patients with cardiovascular disease, *J Am Dent Assoc* 68:333-342, 1964.

INDEX

TABLE 4-2 Approximate Duration of Action of Local Anesthetics

Short duration (pulpal about 30 min)
Chloroprocaine 2%†
Lidocaine 2%
Prilocaine 4% (infiltration)
Mepivacaine 3%

Intermediate (pulpal 60 min)
Articaine 4% + epinephrine 1:100,000*
Articaine 4% + epinephrine 1:200,000*
Lidocaine 2% + epinephrine 1:50,000
Lidocaine 2% + epinephrine 1:100,000
Mepivacaine 2% + levonordefrin 1:20,000
Mepivacaine 2% + epinephrine 1:200,000*
Prilocaine 4% (nerve block)
Prilocaine 4% + epinephrine 1:200,000
Procaine 2%/propoxycaine 0.4% + levonordefrin
   1:20,000*

Long (pulpal 90+ min)
Bupivacaine 0.5% + epinephrine 1:200,000
Etidocaine 1.5% + epinephrine 1:200,000 (nerve block)

*Not available in the United States (April 1996).
†Not available in glass cartridges for use in a dental aspirating
   syringe (April 1996).

TABLE 4-6 Contraindications for Local Anesthetics

Medical problem	Drugs to avoid	Type of contraindication	Alternative drug
Local anesthetic allergy, documented	All local anesthetics in same chemical class (e.g., esters)	Absolute	Local anesthetics in different chemical class (e.g., amides)
Sulfa allergy	Articaine	Absolute	Non–sulfur containing local anesthetic
Bisulfite allergy	Vasoconstrictor-containing local anesthetics	Absolute	Any local anesthetic without vasoconstrictor
Atypical plasma cholinesterase	Esters	Relative	Amides
Methemoglobinemia, idiopathic or congenital	Articaine, prilocaine	Relative	Other amides or esters
Significant liver dysfunction (ASA III-IV)	Amides	Relative	Amides or esters, but judiciously
Significant renal dysfunction (ASA III-IV)	Amides or esters	Relative	Amides or esters, but judiciously
Significant cardiovascular disease (ASA III-IV)	High concentrations of vasoconstrictors (as in racemic epinephrine gingival retraction cords)	Relative	Local anesthetics with epinephrine concentrations of 1:200,000 or 1:100,000 or mepivacaine 3% or prilocaine 4% (nerve blocks)
Clinical hyperthyroidism (ASA III-IV)	High concentrations of vasoconstrictors (as in racemic epinephrine gingival retraction cords)	Relative	Local anesthetics with epinephrine concentrations of 1:200,000 or 1:100,000 or mepivacaine 3% or prilocaine 4% (nerve blocks)